Integrated Pharmacy Case Studies

Integrated Pharmacy Case Studies

SALLY-ANNE FRANCIS

FELICITY SMITH

JOHN MALKINSON

ANDREW CONSTANTI

KEVIN TAYLOR

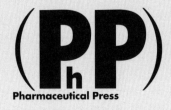

Pharmaceutical Press

Published by Pharmaceutical Press

66-68 East Smithfield, London E1W 1AW, UK

Copyright © The Royal Pharmaceutical Society 2015

(**P₁P**) is a trade mark of Pharmaceutical Press

Pharmaceutical Press is the publishing division of the Royal Pharmaceutical Society

Typeset by Data Standard Limited, UK

Printed, 2015, in Great Britain by Ashford Colour Press Ltd,

Gosport, Hampshire.

Reprinted 2018.

Print ISBN 978-0-85369-884-5
PDF ISBN 978-0-85711-045-9
ePub ISBN 978-0-85711-219-4
mobi ISBN 978-0-85711-220-0

Contents

Foreword

For many years there has been a debate across the profession of pharmacy about the 'divide' between science and practice. The argument has often centred on the apparent dilution of the science in pharmacy, alongside a strengthening clinical role whereas, in fact, the opposite is true. Clinical practitioners use their science at every stage of every drug intervention and patient encounter, and are able to demonstrate their unique contribution as a direct result. These contributions form the basis for the interactions that pharmacists have with patients every day: from the drug and formulation choice, to managing drug stability issues; from assessing the patient's ability to swallow, to recommending the best route of administration; the assessment of the impact of prescribed and non-prescribed drugs on the pharmacokinetics of a newly prescribed drug; all this together with doing the best for the confused patient, no matter what the age or stage of life, understanding the challenges behind medicine preparation and taking.

Across the profession, we want to ensure that clinical practice is strengthened by the integration of pharmaceutical science. *Integrated Pharmacy Case Studies* is a hugely valuable and unique text, covering major disease systems, rare and common, providing a text for all: for those learning the concepts from scratch, as well as for those at experienced stages of career development. Each case study presented is usefully set out with clear learning outcomes and questions that target the needs of the patient through the underlying science. The focus is on the patient, whereas the text provides details and information on the disease/condition, the drugs involved in its management, their pharmacological mechanism of action (according to current understanding), their chemical structures and active groups, formulations, stability and interactions, relevant to the case in hand. The cases navigate the issues behind the science, pharmacokinetics, interactions and side effects and are followed by some pertinent questions, references and further reading for the reader to consult. The work is a true collaboration between academic pharmacists and practitioners so that the clinical cases are used to illustrate clearly that the best patient care results from clinical practice being truly integrated with the pharmaceutical sciences.

DR CATHERINE DUGGAN
PhD, FRPharmS, Director of Professional Development and Support
Royal Pharmaceutical Society

Acknowledgements

The editors would like to take this opportunity to acknowledge those who have assisted in the preparation of this book. We are very indebted to the following:

The authors: for the time and effort that they have put into their respective case discussions. Professional life provides few spare moments, so the time that these individuals have made available to make such knowledgeable contributions is greatly valued. The nature of this book has meant that the cases returned to the original authors for approval were often very different from those originally submitted, as they had been edited and added to, to ensure that they met the objectives of this project. The authors' flexibility and positive responses at all stages have been greatly appreciated.

Catherine Baumber (Pharmaceutics Department, UCL School of Pharmacy): for her considerable secretarial, administrative and organisational support throughout this book's preparation from inception to submission to the publisher.

Our respective partners and families: for their help, support, patience and tolerance as this book was written, edited and prepared in what euphemistically might be called our 'spare time'.

About the editors

SALLY-ANNE FRANCIS, BPharm, PhD, MRPharmS, FHEA is an Honorary Senior Lecturer in the Department of Practice and Policy at UCL School of Pharmacy, having previously held academic appointments at the school for 10 years. During this time, she was responsible for the curriculum design and delivery of postgraduate MSc programmes in Clinical Pharmacy; she has also taught and examined on the MPharm and PhD programmes of study. She is co-author of *International Research in Healthcare*, a textbook for students and researchers undertaking multicentre research projects in health services, medicines use and professional practice.

FELICITY SMITH, BPharm, MA, PhD, FRPharmS is currently Professor of Pharmacy Practice at UCL School of Pharmacy. After a few years in hospital and then community pharmacy, she completed an MA in African Studies at SOAS and a PhD at St Bartholomew's Medical College. She then joined the academic staff of the School of Pharmacy, University of London, now UCL School of Pharmacy. Professor Smith has 25 years' experience in teaching and research in pharmacy practice. During this time she has been actively involved in curriculum design and teaching in pharmacy practice across all 4 years of the MPharm degree, as well as MSc and PhD programmes. She is author of other texts including *Conducting Your Pharmacy Practice Research Project* which is intended for students or other first-time researchers in pharmacy.

JOHN MALKINSON, BPharm, PhD, MRPharmS, MRSC, CChem, FHEA is Senior Lecturer in Pharmaceutical Science Applied to Practice at UCL School of Pharmacy. Dr Malkinson registered as a pharmacist in 1997, before completing a PhD in pharmaceutical chemistry and then post-doctoral research at the University of London. Dr Malkinson has nearly 15 years of teaching experience across all 4 years the MPharm programme and on several MSc programmes. His teaching focuses primarily on organic and medicinal chemistry and on applied science in a clinical context. He has an active interest in the application of technology for the enhancement of teaching and learning and is a Fellow of the Higher Education Academy.

ANDREW CONSTANTI, BSc(Pharm), PhD, FBPhS is a Reader in Pharmacology in the Department of Pharmacology at the UCL School of Pharmacy. He studied for his PhD while employed as a Research Assistant at St Bartholomew's Medical College and received his PhD in Pharmacology from the University of London in 1975. He then joined the academic staff of the School of Pharmacy, University of London (now UCL School of Pharmacy) as a teaching fellow, later being promoted to lecturer, senior lecturer and reader. Dr Constanti has 40 years of experience in teaching and administration in all 4 years of the MPharm degree course as well as contributing to MSc courses and the training of PhD students. He is also a Visiting Professor of Neuroscience at the University of Trieste, Italy, where he currently teaches in the international neuroscience MSc course. His research in neuropharmacology/neuronal electrophysiology has led to the publication of over 100 original articles in refereed journals and he was the main author of the textbook *Basic Endocrinology: for students of pharmacy and allied health sciences*, intended primarily for pharmacy undergraduates. He is a member of the Physiological Society and an elected Fellow of the British Pharmacological Society.

KEVIN TAYLOR, BPharm, PhD, FRPharmS is Professor of Clinical Pharmaceutics at UCL School of Pharmacy. Professor Taylor has more than 25 years' experience in teaching and research in the areas of formulation science, medicines manufacture and drug delivery. During this time he has been actively involved in curriculum design and teaching in pharmaceutics across all 4 years of the MPharm degree as well as MSc and PhD programmes. He has been external examiner for a number of MPharm programmes in the UK. He is co-author or co-editor of several other texts, including *Aulton's Pharmaceutics* and *Pharmacy Practice*, which are intended for use by undergraduate pharmacy students.

List of contributors

BOTHAINA B JERAGH ALHADDAD, BSc, MSc, PhD | Assistant Professor and Lecturer in Clinical Pharmacy, Department of Pharmaceutical Sciences, Public Authority for Applied Education and Training, Shwaikh, Kuwait

FATEMAH MOHAMMAD ALSALEH, BPharm, MSc, PhD | Assistant Professor, Department of Pharmacy Practice, Faculty of Pharmacy, Kuwait University, Kuwait

SOTIRIS ANTONIOU, MRPharmS, MSc, DipMgt | Independent prescriber; Consultant Pharmacist, Cardiovascular Medicine, Bart's Health NHS Trust, London, UK

ANA ARMSTRONG, BPharm, PgDipClinPharm | Lead Pharmacist, Medical Division, Surrey and Sussex Healthcare NHS Trust, UK

NELA RONČEVIĆ ASHTON, BSc, PgDip | Clinical Tutor, School of Pharmacy and Biomedical Sciences, University of Central Lancashire; Advanced Primary Care Pharmacist, Cumbria and Lancashire Clinical Support Unit, UK

ZOE ASLANPOUR, BPharm, PhD | Member of UKPHR, FRSPH, Head of Pharmacy and Public Health Practice, University of Hertfordshire; Consultant in Public Health, NHS Bedfordshire, UK

PAUL BAINS, DipClinPharm, MRPharmS | Independent prescriber; Senior Lead Pharmacist for Medicine, Imperial College Healthcare NHS Trust, Pharmacy Department, Hammersmith Hospital, London, UK

JOANNE BARTLETT, BPharm, ClinDipPharm | Specialist Clinical Pharmacist, End of Life Care, John Taylor Hospice, Birmingham, UK

GORDON BECKET, BPharm, PhD, MRPharmS, MRSC, FNZCP | Professor of Pharmacy Practice, School of Pharmacy and Biomedical Sciences, University of Central Lancashire, Preston, Lancashire, UK

SIÂN BENTLEY, BPharm, MRPharmS, DipClinPharm | Specialist Pharmacist, Paediatrics, Royal Brompton and Harefield NHS Foundation Trust, London, UK

RANIA BETMOUNI, BPharm, DipClinPharm | Independent prescriber; MSc Quality and Safety in Healthcare, Clinical Pharmacist – BUPA Cromwell Hospital, London, UK

ANNETT BLOCHBERGER, DipClinPharm | Independent prescriber; Lead Pharmacist, Neurosciences, St George's NHS Healthcare Trust, London, UK

LISA BOATENG, BSc, MSc, MRPharmS, Certificate in Clinical Pharmacy | Independent prescriber; Highly Specialised Pharmacist, Antimicrobials and Infection Control, London, UK

MARK BORTHWICK, MPharmS, MSc | Consultant Pharmacist, Critical Care, John Radcliffe Hospital, Oxford University Hospitals NHS Trust, Oxford, UK

SIMONE BRACKENBOROUGH, BSc, DipClinPharm | Independent prescriber; Senior Lead Pharmacist for Medicine at Imperial College Hospitals NHS Trust (St Mary's Hospital Site), London, UK

NADIA BUKHARI, BPharm, MRPharmS, PgDipFHEA | Clinical Lecturer, MPharm Student Support Manager & Pre Registration Coordinator, UCL School of Pharmacy, London, UK

MEE-ONN CHAI, MSc, DipClinPharm, BPharm | Clinical Pharmacist, Team Leader – Renal Services, King's College Hospital NHS Foundation, London, UK

BARBARA CLARK, MPharm(Hons), GPhC, ClinDip | Lead Clinical Pharmacist, London Bridge Hospital; Chair UKCPA Haemostasis, Anticoagulation and Thrombosis (HAT) Group, London, UK

JESSICA CLEMENTS, MPharm, CertPharm Pract, DipPharmPract, Cert Independent prescribing practice | Highly Specialised Pharmacist HIV at Medway Maritime Hospital, Gillingham, Kent, UK

LOUISE COGAN, BSc, MRPharmS, PgDipFHEA | Teacher Practitioner, University of Central Lancashire, Preston, Lancashire, UK

ANDREW CONSTANTI, BSc, PhD, FBPharmacolS | Reader in Pharmacology, UCL School of Pharmacy, London, UK

SHANI CORB, MRPharmS, MSc | Independent prescriber; Lead Pharmacist, Paediatric Oncology, Royal Alexandra Children's Hospital, BSUH NHS Trust, Brighton, Sussex, UK

JOYETA DAS, MPharm, DipClinPharm | Independent prescriber; Lead Pharmacist, Hepatology, Imperial College London NHS Trust, London, UK

HALA M FADDA, MPharm, PhD | Assistant Professor, College of Pharmacy and Health Sciences, Butler University, Indianapolis, IN, USA

JOSEPHINE FOLASADE FALADE, BPharm, MSc, FHEA | Highly Specialist Pharmacist, Bart's Health NHS Trust; Clinical Lecturer, UCL School of Pharmacy, London, UK

SALLY-ANNE FRANCIS, BPharm, PhD, MRPharmS, FHEA | Honorary Senior Lecturer, UCL School of Pharmacy, London, UK

CLAIRE GOLIGHTLY, MPharm ClinDipHosp, PGCertEd | Lecturer in Professional Practice, Bradford School of Pharmacy, University of Bradford, Bradford, UK

LARRY GOODYER, PhD, MRPharmS, FFTMRCPS(Glas), FRGS | Professor, Head of the Leicester School of Pharmacy, Faculty of Health and Life Sciences, De Montfort University, Leicester, UK

NICOLA J GRAY, BSc, PhD, MRPharmS, FHEA, FSAHM(US) | Independent pharmacist researcher; Director, Green Line Consulting Limited, Manchester, UK

KATIE GREENWOOD, MRPharmS, PGCertTLHE, FHEA | Lecturer in Pharmacy Practice, Placement Co-ordinator and Pre-Registration Facilitator, School of Pharmacy and Biomedical Sciences, University of Central Lancashire, Preston, Lancashire, UK

ELIZABETH HACKETT, BSc, MSc | Independent prescriber; Principal Pharmacist for Diabetes, University Hospitals Leicester, Leicester, UK

DELYTH HIGMAN JAMES, PhD, MSc, BPharm, MRPharmS, AMBPsS, FHEA | Senior Lecturer, Programme Director, MSc in Pharmacy Clinical Practice (Community and Primary Care), Cardiff, South Wales, UK

TIM HILLS, MRPharmS, DipClin | Independent prescriber; Lead Pharmacist Antimicrobials and Infection Control, Nottingham University Hospitals NHS Trust, Nottingham, UK

STEPHEN HUGHES, MPharm | Specialist Renal Pharmacist, Central Manchester Foundation Trust, Manchester, UK

LYNN HUMPHREY, BPharm, DipPharmPrac, IPP | Senior Lead Pharmacist – Cardiovascular, Imperial College Healthcare NHS Trust, London, UK

ANDY HUSBAND, DProf, MSc, BPharm, MRPharmS | Dean of Pharmacy, Durham University, Durham, UK

MATTHEW D JONES, MPharm, PhD, MRPharmS | Senior Pharmacist – Medicines Information, Royal United Hospital Bath NHS Trust, Bath, UK

SARAH C JONES, MPharm, MSc, MRPharmS | Locality Lead Pharmacist, Avon and Wiltshire Mental Health Partnership NHS Trust, Bath, UK

NAVEED IQBAL, MPharm, PGClinDip, MSc | Teaching Fellow, Aston University; Prescribing Support Pharmacist for NHS, Birmingham Cross City CCG; community pharmacist

KUMUD KANTILAL, BSc(Pharm), DipPharmPract, Postgraduate award in clinical oncology | Macmillan Principal Pharmacist, Lead for Cancer Education and Training, Guy's and St Thomas' NHS Foundation Trust, London, UK

NAZANIN KHORSHIDI, MPharm, PGDip | Highly Specialist Pharmacist; Orthopaedics and Plastics at Guy's and St Thomas' NHS Foundation Trust, London, UK

STEPHANIE KIRSCHKE, PhD | Senior Lead Pharmacist Haematology, Imperial College Healthcare NHS Trust, London, UK

ROGER DAVID KNAGGS, BSc, BMedSci, PhD, MRPharmS | Associate Professor in Clinical Pharmacy Practice, University of Nottingham; Advanced Pharmacy Practitioner – Pain Management, Nottingham University Hospitals NHS Trust, Nottingham, UK

SARAH KNIGHTON, MPharm, MPharmS | Independent prescriber; Clinical Pharmacy Team Leader, Liver and Private Patient Services, King's College Hospital NHS Foundation Trust, London, UK

ROMAN LANDOWSKI, BSc(Pharm), DipClinPharm | Ward Pharmacist, Maternity Care Unit, University College Hospital, London, UK

JEREMY LEVY, MBBChir, PhD, FHEA, FRCP | Consultant Nephrologist, Imperial College Healthcare NHS Trust, London, UK

NATALIE LEWIS, MPharm, ClinDipPharm, PGCertEd | Senior Pharmacist – Teacher Practitioner, Aston University and University Hospitals Birmingham NHS Foundation Trust, Birmingham, UK

TRACY LYONS, BSc(Pharm), MSc | Lead Pharmacist, Infection, Imperial College Healthcare NHS Trust, London, UK

FIONA MACLEAN, MSc, MRPharmS | Independent prescriber; Lead Clinical Pharmacist, Cancer and Neurosciences, NHS Greater Glasgow and Clyde, Glasgow, UK

JANET E MCDONAGH, MB BS, MD, FRCP | Clinical Senior Lecturer in Paediatric and Adolescent Rheumatology, University of Birmingham and Birmingham Children's Hospital NHS Foundation Trust, Birmingham, UK

DUNCAN MCROBBIE, MSc, FRPharmS | Associate Chief Pharmacist, Guy's and St Thomas' NHS Hospital Trust; Clinical Reader, Kings College London, London, UK; Visiting Professor, UCL, UK

CARL MARTIN, PhD, GPhC registrant, MRPharmS, PGCHE | Senior Clinical Teacher, Department of Practice and Policy, UCL School of Pharmacy, London, UK

JAYMI MISTRY, MPharm, DipGPP | Highly Specialist Pharmacist – Acute Medicine (general medicine) and Medicines Safety, London, UK

SANDEEP SINGH NIJJER, MPharm, MBA, GPhC | Pharmacist, UK

LELLY OBOH, BPharm, DipClinPharm | Independent prescriber; Consultant Pharmacist, Care of Older People, Guy's and St Thomas' Community Health Services, London, UK

JIGNESH PATEL, PhD, MRPharmS | Clinical Senior Lecturer/ Honorary Consultant Pharmacist, Anticoagulation, King's College London/King's College Hospital, London, UK

NEIL POWELL, MPharm, ClinDip, MRPharmS | Antibiotic and HIV Pharmacist, Royal Cornwall Hospital Trust, Truro, UK

ANNA PRYOR, MPharm, MRPharmS | Lead Pharmacist, A&E and Admissions, Imperial College Healthcare NHS Trust (St Mary's site), London, UK

GEMMA QUINN, PGDip, MRPharmS | Course Director MSc Clinical Pharmacy (Hospital) and MPharm Stage Tutor (Stage 4), University of Bradford, Bradford, UK

TIMOTHY RENNIE, MPharm, PhD | Head of School of Pharmacy (Associate Dean), University of Namibia, Namibia, Africa

IAN ROWLANDS, MRPharmS, DipClinPharm | Independent prescriber; Lead Pharmacist Stroke Services, Imperial College Healthcare NHS Trust, London, UK

IMOGEN SAVAGE, BPharm, PhD, MRPharmS | Senior Lecturer (retired), UCL School of Pharmacy, London, UK

JENNY SCOTT, BSc, PhD, MRPharmS | Independent prescriber; Senior Lecturer in Pharmacy Practice, University of Bath, Bath, UK

LOUISE SEAGER, BPharm, ClinDipPharm, MRPharmS | Senior Specialist Clinical Pharmacist End of Life Care, John Taylor Hospice, Birmingham, UK

RITA SHAH, BPharm, MRPharmS, MSc | Senior Clinical Pharmacist, Critical Care, King's College Hospital NHS Foundation Trust, London, UK

KATE SHARDLOW, MBBS, BPharm, MRCGP | GP and speciality doctor in genitourinary medicine, Chelmsford, Essex, UK

NEELAM SHARMA, BA, PGCert Psychiatric Therapeutics | Registered Pharmacy Technician, Chief Pharmacy Technician, Medicines Management and E&T, South London and Maudsley NHS Foundation Trust, London, UK

ROB SHULMAN, BScPharm, MRPharmS, DipClinPharm, DHC (Pharm) | Lead Pharmacist – Critical Care, Pharmacy Department, University College Hospital; Honorary Associate Professor in Clinical Pharmacy Practice, UCL School of Pharmacy; Honorary Lecturer, Department of Medicine, University College London, London, UK

MERVYN SINGER, MBBS MD MRCP | Professor of Intensive Care Medicine; Head, Research Department of Clinical Physiology, Division of Medicine, University College London, UK

TIMOTHY J SNAPE, PhD MSci MRSC, CChemCSci | Lecturer in Medicinal Chemistry, University of Central Lancashire, Preston, Lancashire, UK

NUTTAN KANTILAL TANNA, MRPharmS, DComP, PhD | Pharmacist Consultant, Women's Health and Older People, Women's Services and affiliated with the Arthritis Centre, NW London Hospitals NHS Trust, London, UK

NEIL TICKNER, MPharm, MRPharmS, PGDipClinPharm | Lead Pharmacist Paediatrics, St Mary's Hospital, Imperial College Healthcare NHS Trust, London, UK

ADAM TODD, MPharm, PhD, MPharmS, MRSC | Lecturer in Pharmacy Practice, Division of Pharmacy, Durham University, Durham, UK

MARK TOMLIN, PhD, FRPharmS | Independent prescriber; Consultant Pharmacist Critical Care, Southampton General Hospital, Southampton, UK

STEPHEN TOMLIN, BPharm, FRPharmS | Consultant Pharmacist – Children's Services, London, UK

CHARLES TUGWELL, BPharm, MSc, MRPharmS, MCLIP | Specialist Clinical Pharmacist, Neurology/Neurosurgery, Royal London Hospital, Bart's Health NHS Trust, London, UK

SINEAD TYNAN, MPharm, IP, ClinDip, MSc, MRPharmS | Senior Clinical Pharmacist – Liver Services, King's College Hospital, London, UK

SAMIR VOHRA, BPharm | Lecturer in Clinical Pharmacy Practice, School of Pharmacy and Biomedical Science, University of Central Lancashire, Preston, Lancashire, UK

PETER S WHITTON, BSc, MSc, PhD | Senior Lecturer in Pharmacology, UCL School of Pharmacy, London, UK

HELEN WILLIAMS, BPharm, PGDip(Cardiol), MRPharmS | Independent prescriber; Consultant Pharmacist for Cardiovascular Disease, South London, hosted by Southwark CCG, London, UK

ELIZABETH M WILLIAMSON, BSc, PhD, MRPharmS, PhD, FLS | Professor of Pharmacy and Director of Practice, University of Reading School of Pharmacy, Reading, UK

KEITH A WILSON, BSc, PhD | Professor, Aston University, Birmingham, UK

STEWART WILSON, BPharm, ClinDipPharm | Lead Pharmacist Cardiology, Imperial College NHS Healthcare Trust, London, UK

KAY WOOD, BSc, DipClinPharm, PhD, MRPharmS, PGPCTL | Senior Lecturer in Clinical Pharmacy, Birmingham, UK

KIRSTY WORRALL, BSc, MRPharmS | Teacher Practitioner working with Boots and UCL School of Pharmacy, London, UK

PAUL WRIGHT, MRPharmS, MSc | Specialist Cardiac Pharmacist, Bart's Health NHS Trust, London, UK

Abbreviations

^{18}F-FDG	[^{18}F]fluorodeoxyglucose
5ARI	5α-reductase inhibitor
5-FdUMP	5-fluorodeoxyuridine monophosphate
5FU	5-fluorouracil
5-HT	5-hydroxytryptamine/serotonin
A&E	accident and emergency
Ab	amyloid-b
AAD	autoimmune Addison's disease
ABG	arterial blood gas
ABMS	Abbreviated Mental Test Score
ABPA	allergic bronchopulmonary aspergillosis
ABPM	ambulatory blood pressure monitoring
ABW	actual body weight
ACE	angiotensin-converting enzyme
acetyl-CoA	acetyl-coenzyme A
AChEIs	acetylcholinesterase inhibitors
ACS	acute chest syndrome/acute coronary syndromes
ACTH	adrenocorticotrophic hormone
AD	Alzheimer's disease
ADH	antidiuretic hormone
ADP	adenosine diphosphate
AED	antiepileptic drug
AF	atrial fibrillation
AIDS	acquired immune deficiency syndrome
ALL	acute lymphoblastic anaemia
ALP	alkaline phosphatase
ALT	alanine aminotransferase/alanine transaminase
AMI	acute myocardial infarction
AMPK	adenosine monophosphate-activated protein kinase
AMR	antimicrobial resistance
AMD	age-related macular degeneration
anti-dsDNA	antibody to double-stranded DNA
anti-Sm	anti-Smith antibody
API	active pharmaceutical ingredient
APP	amyloid precursor protein
APTT	activated partial thromboplastin time
ARB	angiotensin II receptor blocker
ARR	(absolute risk reduction)
ART	antiretroviral treatment
ASD	autistic spectrum disorder
AST	aspartate aminotransferase/aspartate transaminase
AT-II	angiotensin II
ATP	adenosine triphosphate
ATRA	all-*trans*-retinoic acid
AUC	area under the curve
b.d.	*bis die* (twice daily)
BBB	blood–brain barrier
BCG	bacillus Calmette–Guérin
BDNF	brain-derived neurotrophic factor
BE	base excess
BHIVA	British HIV Association
BMD	bone mineral density
BMI	body mass index
BMR	basal metabolic rate

BNF	*British National Formulary*
BNP	B-type natriuretic protein
BOPA	British Oncology Pharmacy Association
BP	blood pressure
BPH	benign prostatic hyperplasia
BRB	blood retinal barrier
BS	British Standard
BSAC	British Society of Antimicrobial Chemotherapy
BTS	British Thoracic Society
BuChE	butyrylcholinestersae
CABG	coronary artery bypass graft
cAMP	adenosine cyclic monophosphate
CBT	cognitive–behavioural therapy
CCB	calcium channel blocker
CD56	cluster of differentiation antigen 56
CDH	chronic daily headache
CF	cystic fibrosis
CFC	chlorofluorocarbon
CFTR	cystic fibrosis transmembrane conductance regulator
CgA	chromogranin A
cGMP	cyclic guanosine monophosphate
CHF	chronic heart failure
CHM	Commission on Human Medicines
CHMP	Committee for Medicinal Products for Human Use
CIN	cervical intraepithelial neoplasia
CINV	chemotherapy-induced nausea and vomiting
CKD	chronic kidney disease
CMHT	community mental health team
CNS	coagulase-negative staphylococci
CNS	central nervous system
CNV	choroidal neovascularisation
CO	cardiac output
CO_2	carbon dioxide
COMT	catechol-O-methyltransferase
COPD	chronic obstructive pulmonary disease
COX	cyclooxygenase enzyme
COX-1	cyclooxygenase-1
COX-2	cyclooxygenase-2
CPB	cardiopulmonary bypass
CrCl	creatinine clearance
CRF	chronic renal failure
CRH	corticotrophin-releasing hormone
CRP	C-reactive protein
CSCI	continuous subcutaneous infusion
CSF	cerebrospinal fluid
CSII	continuous subcutaneous insulin injection
CT	computed tomography
CTZ	chemoreceptor trigger zone
CVD	cardiovascular disease
CVP	central venous pressure
CVVHD	continuous venovenous haemodialysis
CVVHF	continuous venovenous haemofiltration
CYP	cytochrome P450 enzymes
DAFNE	dose adjustment for normal eating

DALY	disability-adjusted life-year
DAS	disease activity score
DC	direct current
DDW	dose-defining weight
DEHP	di-2-ethylhexylphthalate
DES	drug-eluting stent
DESMOND	Diabetes Education and Self Management in Ongoing and Newly Diagnosed
DXA	dual-energy X-ray absorptiometry
DHFR	dihydrofolate reductase
DHP	1,4-dihydropyridine
DHT	dihydrotestosterone
DKA	diabetic ketoacidosis
DLB	dementia with Lewy bodies
DMARDs	disease-modifying anti-rheumatic drugs
DNA	deoxyribonucleic acid
DNase	dornase alpha
dNTP	deoxynucleoside triphosphate
DOT	directly observed therapy
DPI	dry powder inhaler
DPP-4	dipeptidyl peptidase 4
DQLI	dermatology quality-of-life index
DSM-IV	*Diagnostic and Statistical Manual of Mental Disorders*, 4th edn
DTPA	diethylenetriamine pentaacetic acid
DVT	deep vein thrombosis
DXA	dual-energy x-ray absorptiometry
EBW	excess body weight
ECG	electrocardiogram
ECoG	echocardiogram
ECG-SR	electrocardiogram–sinus rhythm
EDSS	expanded disability status scale
EDTA	ethylenediaminetetraacetic acid
EEG	electroencephalography
eGFR	estimated glomerular filtration rate
EGFR-TK	epidermal growth factor receptor tyrosine kinase
EMA	European Medicines Agency
EPO	erythropoietin
EPSEs	extrapyramidal side effects
ER	endoplasmic reticulum
ESA	erythropoietic-stimulating agent
ESR	erythrocyte sedimentation rate
ETC	electron transport chain
ETT	exercise tolerance test
EU	European Union
FBC	full blood count
FDA	Food and Drug Administration
FDG	fluorodeoxyglucose
FEV_1	forced expiratory volume in 1 second
FT_4	free thyroxine
FTD	frontotemporal dementia
FTU	fingertip unit
FVC	forced vital capacity
GABA	γ-aminobutyric acid
GAD	general anxiety disorder
GALC	galactosylceramidase gene
GARFT	glycinamide ribonucleotide formyltransferase
GAS	Group A Streptococci
GC	guanylyl cyclase
GCS	Glasgow Coma Scale
GBL	γ-butyrolactone
GC	gas chromatography
GFR	glomerular filtration rate
GGT	γ-glutamyl transferase/γ-glutamyl transpeptidase
GI	gastrointestinal
GIRK	G-protein inwardly rectifying K^+
GISN	Global Influenza Surveillance Network
GLP-1	glucagon-like peptide-1
GMP	good manufacturing practice
GORD	gastro-oesophageal reflux disease
Gs	stimulatory G-protein
GP	general (medical) practitioner
GSK-3	glycogen synthase kinase-3
GSL	general sales list
GTN	glyceryl trinitrate
GTP	guanosine-5'-triphosphate
HAART	highly active antiretroviral therapy
HAI	hospital-acquired infection
Hb	haemoglobin
HbS	sickle haemoglobin
HbSS	haemoglobin sickle cell disease
HbA1c	glycated haemoglobin
HbF	fetal haemoglobin
HCAI	healthcare-associated infection
HCC	hepatocellular carcinoma
HCV	hepatitis C virus
HD	haemodialysis
HDF	haemodiafiltration
HDL	high-density lipoprotein
HF	haemofiltration
HF	heart failure
HFA	hydrofluoroalkane
HIV	human immunodeficiency virus
HMG-CoA	3-hydroxy-3-methylglutaryl-coenzyme A
HPA	Health Protection Agency, now part of Public Health England
HPA	hypothalamic–pituitary–adrenal
HPC	history of presenting complaint
HPLC	high-performance liquid chromatography
HPMC	hydroxypropyl methylcellulose
HPTLC	high-performance thin layer chromatography
HPV	human papillomavirus
HR	heart rate
HRT	hormone replacement therapy
HSV	herpes simplex virus
HTN	hypertension
i.m.	intramuscular
i.v.	intravenous/intravenously
IBD	inflammatory bowel disease
IBW	ideal body weight
ICH	intracerebral haemorrhage
ICU	intensive care unit
IDSA	Infectious Diseases Society of America
IgE	immunoglobulin E
IGRA	interferon-γ release assay
IMiD	immunomodulatory drug
INR	international normalised ratio
IPSS	international prostate symptom score
iPTH	intact parathyroid hormone
IU	international unit
JIA	juvenile idiopathic arthritis
JVP	jugular venous pressure
K_{ATP}	ATP-sensitive K^+ channels

K_m	plasma concentration at which the rate is one half the maximum
LAD	left anterior descending (coronary artery)
LANSS	Leeds assessment of neuropathic pain symptoms and signs
LDL	low-density lipoprotein
LFT	liver function test
LMWH	low-molecular-weight heparin
LPL	lipoprotein lipase
LTBI	latent tuberculosis infection
LUTS	lower urinary tract symptoms
LV	left ventricular
LVF	left ventricular function
LVH	left ventricular hypertrophy
MALA	metformin-associated lactic acidosis
MAOI	monoamine oxidase inhibitor
MAP	mean arterial pressure
MAPT	microtubule-associated protein tau
MCP	metacarpophalangeal (joints)
MDRD	modification of diet in renal disease (equation)
MELD	model for end-stage liver disease
MEP	medicine, ethics and practice
MHRA	Medicines and Healthcare products Regulatory Agency
MI	myocardial infarction
MIC	minimum inhibitory concentration
MMR	measles, mumps and rubella
MMSE	Mini-Mental State Examination
MOH	medication-overuse headache
MR	modified release
MRCF	medication-related consultation framework
MRI	magnetic resonance imaging
MRSA	meticillin-resistant *Staphylococcus aureus*
MS	multiple sclerosis
MSH	melanocyte-stimulating hormone
MSSA	meticillin-sensitive *Staphylococcus aureus*
MTX	methotrexate
MU	million units/mega unit
MUPS	multiple unit pellet system
MUR	medicines use review
NAAT	nucleic acid amplification test
NAPQI	*N*-acetyl-*p*-benzoquinoneimine
NaTHNaC	National Travel Health Network and Centre
NF-κB	nuclear factor κB
NG	nasogastric
NHS	National Health Service (in Britain)
NICE	National Institute for Health and Care Excellence (formerly National Institute for Health and Clinical Excellence)
NK	neurokinin
NKDA	no known drug allergy
NMDAR	*N*-methyl-D-aspartate receptor
NMS	new medicines service
NNRTI	non-nucleoside reverse transcription inhibitor
NNT	number needed to treat
NO	nitrous oxide
NPSA	National Patient Safety Agency
NRT	nicotine replacement therapy
NRTI	nucleoside reverse transcription inhibitor
NSAID	non-steroidal anti-inflammatory drug
NSCLC	non-small cell lung cancer
NSTEMI	non-ST-segment elevation myocardial infarction
NTS	nucleus tractus solitarius
NVQ	national vocational qualification
o.d.	*omni die* (every day)
ODU	oncology day unit
OM	obtuse marginal (coronary artery)
o.m.	*omni mane* (every morning)
o.n.	*omni nocte* (every night)
OGTT	oral glucose tolerance test
OTC	over the counter
p.o.	per oral
p.r.n.	*pro re nata* (as required)
$PaCO_2$	partial pressure of carbon dioxide in blood
PaO_2	partial pressure of oxygen dissolved in blood
PASI	psoriasis area and severity index
PBR	payment by results
PCA	patient-controlled analgesia
PCI	percutaneous coronary intervention
PCR	protein (or albumin) : creatinine ratio
PCR	polymerase chain reaction
PDD	Parkinson's disease dementia
PE	pulmonary embolism
PEARL	pupils equal and reactive to light
PEF	peak expiratory flow
PEFR	peak expiratory flow rate
PEG	polyethylene glycol
PET	positron emission tomography
P-gp	P-glycoprotein
PGD	patient group direction
PHI	primary HIV infection
PI	protease inhibitor
PID	pelvic inflammatory disease
PIL	patient information leaflet
PIP	proximal interphalangeal (joints)
PKG	cGMP-dependent protein kinase G
pMDI	pressurised metered-dose inhaler
PML	progressive multifocal leukoencephalopathy
PMR	patient medication record
PN	parenteral nutrition
POBA	plain old balloon angioplasty
PPAR-γ	peroxisome proliferator-activated receptor γ
PPD	*p*-phenylenediamine
PPD	purified protein derivative
PPI	(proton pump inhibitor)
PSS	portosystemic shunting
PT	prothrombin time
PTB	pulmonary tuberculosis
PTH	parathyroid hormone
PTHrP	PTH-related peptide
PTS	post-thrombotic syndrome
PUD	peptic ulcer disease
PXR	pregnane X receptor
q.d.s.	*quater die sumendum* (four times daily)
RA	rheumatoid arthritis
RAAS	renin–angiotensin–aldosterone system
RAS	renal artery stenosis
RAST	radioallergosorbent test
RBC	red blood cell
RCA	right coronary artery
RCT	randomised controlled trial
RDS	respiratory distress syndrome
REMS	rapidly evolving multiple sclerosis
RPS	Royal Pharmaceutical Society

RNA	ribonucleic acid
RR	respiratory rate
RRMS	relapsing–remitting multiple sclerosis
RTA	road traffic accident
rTPA	recombinant tissue plasminogen activator
s.c.	subcutaneously
SA	surface area
SACT	systemic anti-cancer therapy
SaO_2	oxygen saturation of arterial blood
SBP	systolic blood pressure
SCD	sickle cell disease
SCLC	small cell lung cancer
SDS	sodium dodecylsulphate
SERM	selective estrogen (oestrogen) receptor modulator
SGLT2	sodium–glucose co-transporter 2
SIGN	Scottish Intercollegiate Guidelines Network
SLE	systemic lupus erythematosus
SLS	sodium lauryl sulphate
SMART	single inhaler maintenance and reliever therapy
SmPC	Summary of Product Characteristics
SNRI	serotonin–noradrenaline reuptake inhibitor
SOB	shortness of breath
SOBOE	shortness of breath on exertion
SOP	standard operating procedure
SPC	Summary of Product Characteristics
SPECT	single photon emission computed tomography
SpO_2	blood oxygen saturation
SSI	surgical site infection
SSRI	selective serotonin reuptake inhibitor
SST2	somatostatin type 2
STEMI	ST-segment elevation myocardial infarction
STI	sexually transmitted infection
SV	stroke volume
SVR	sustained virological response
t.d.s.	*ter die sumendum* (three times daily)
T_3	triiodothyronine
T_4	tetraiodothyronine (thyroxine)
TB	tuberculosis

TBA	total bilateral adrenalectomy
TCA	tricyclic antidepressant
TDM	therapeutic drug monitoring
TENS	transcutaneous electrical nerve stimulation
THMPD	Traditional Herbal Medicinal Product Directive
THR	Traditional Herbal Registration
TIA	transient ischaemic attack
TLC	thin-layer chromatography
TNF-α	tumour necrosis factor alpha
TOE	transoesophageal echocardiography
TPMT	thiopurine methyltransferase
TPN	total parenteral nutrition
TRD	treatment-resistant depression
TS	thymidylate synthase
TSH	thyroid-stimulating hormone
TST	tuberculin skin test
TxA_2	thromboxane A_2
U&Es	urea and electrolytes
UA	unstable angina
UKONS	United Kingdom Oncology Nursing Society
UKPDS	United Kingdom Prospective Diabetes Study
ULN	upper limit of normal
UPCR	urine protein: creatinine ratio
UTI	urinary tract infection
UV	ultraviolet
VaD	vascular dementia
VCI	vascular cognitive impairment
V_d	volume of distribution
VEGF	vascular endothelial growth factor
VGSC	voltage-gated sodium channel
V_m	maximum rate of metabolism
VOC	vaso-occlusive crisis
VR	venous return
VRE	vancomycin-resistant enterococcus
VTE	venous thromboembolism
WBC	white blood cells
WCC	white cell count
WHO	World Health Organization

Introduction

An integrated approach to learning

Within the healthcare team, pharmacists are the recognised medicines experts. They have a breadth and depth of understanding about all aspects of medicines that set them apart from other health professionals. As a result of their extensive, specialist education and training, pharmacists can conceptualise a drug molecule, together with its formulation and delivery, as a medicine, and can ensure its safe and effective use by patients. Pharmacists also have a deep understanding of pharmacology and therapeutics, the physicochemical properties of drugs and excipients, biopharmacy and pharmacokinetics, side effects, contraindications and drug interactions. This is combined with knowledge of the legal and ethical framework in which medicines are supplied, as well as biological causes of disease, and the social and behavioural factors that determine whether a patient will obtain optimal benefit from their medication. This hugely varied, complex, integrated, expert knowledge allows pharmacists to make professional judgements relating to medicines, giving them an unchallengeable sphere of expertise, which, when utilised for patient benefit, legitimises pharmacists' professional status.

To be effective, pharmacists' education must prepare them to be scholars, scientists, practitioners and professionals – no mean feat. A modern undergraduate Masters pharmacy curriculum recognises the importance of both pharmaceutical science and pharmacy practice, which, when seamlessly integrated, prepares graduates for the many professional roles and activities that they will be called upon to undertake now and in the future. Nowadays, pharmacy programmes aim to achieve this integration during a student's studies, increasingly incorporating opportunities for workplace learning to provide a context in which they learn and apply their scientific knowledge.

In the UK, the General Pharmaceutical Council (GPhC) regulates the education and training of pharmacists. The GPhC is responsible for accrediting pharmacy degrees and ensuring that they are fit for purpose. It has published a document containing a comprehensive set of standards and outcomes against which programmes are accredited and reaccredited (GPhC, 2011). This document highlights: 'Curricula must be integrated ... the component parts of education and training must be linked in a coherent way' and 'Learning opportunities must be structured to provide an integrated experience of relevant science and pharmacy practice'.

The conception and design of this book

Integration of science with practice, together with its practical application, is at the core of modern pharmacy programmes. The need for pharmacy students to integrate their learning has been a guiding principle in the design and production of this book. True integration of all the elements that contribute to pharmacists' knowledge is difficult. This text aims to present the fundamental aspects of pharmaceutical chemistry, pharmacology, pharmaceutics and therapeutics within a patient-care context. Traditional attempts at integration commonly begin with sections of 'underpinning' science, and then build clinical and professional elements onto it. This approach can be superficial and undermines the credibility of any resultant learning exercise. By contrast, in this text, with the help of many experienced practitioner colleagues, each case study is grounded in a real-life clinical setting, which has then been used as a starting point to illustrate how pharmacists' practice and decision-making are informed by pharmaceutical science.

Thus, the case studies in this book were initially written by pharmacist practitioners, based on their own practice and experience, with additional science content being incorporated later through collaboration with the editorial team. In this way, the science concepts included have a direct relevance to contemporary practice. In particular the science is included in the case because it helps inform understanding and decision-making in real-life practice settings: it has earned the right to be there!

The cases have been organised into sections, broadly based on the *British National Formulary*, the most widely used reference source in pharmacy, where the chapters relate to particular systems of the body (e.g. the cardiovascular system) or to aspects of medical care (e.g. infections). Although this has allowed us to impose some structure, our cases are very diverse and reflect the fact that real patients experience multiple pathologies. They include material relevant to the wider clinical picture.

We have striven to include cases covering the broadest range of clinical conditions, from both community and hospital practice. All the case studies have a similar structure. Within each case we have integrated a significant science component from one or more of pharmaceutical chemistry, pharmacology or pharmaceutics, and in many cases all three. We have included what we believe are the key science concepts. However, it would be impossible to cover in a single set of case studies all the pharmaceutical, clinical and behavioural science that appears in an undergraduate pharmacy programme. The goal here is to demonstrate the potential diversity of clinical scenarios and the relevance of science across all.

Most cases describe the use of many drugs in a particular clinical setting. Again it has not been possible to detail the chemistry, pharmacology, indications, posology, contraindications, side effects and formulations for every drug. However, these case studies can be used as a starting point to expand learning and application of knowledge across the science and practice disciplines. Each case ends with references/further reading and extended learning points, designed to take the reader's learning beyond the specific case; highlighting other relevant, tangential areas of science and practice.

How to use this book

This book has been designed primarily for use by undergraduate pharmacy students and pre-registration trainees. However, it may also be useful for qualified pharmacists, pharmacy technicians and other health professionals. It will also provide a resource for tutors and lecturers to plan and use in learning activities.

We intend this book to be free standing: a learning and teaching aid to promote integration and contextualisation of material learned during undergraduate studies. It is not a textbook. There are plenty of excellent textbooks that will provide a detailed understanding of the subjects that are introduced here. The case studies provided are of varying complexity, independent of each other and not intended to be read sequentially.

Each case begins with a set of **Learning outcomes** which provides an overview of what is contained in the case study and highlights what the reader should be able to do having studied the case.

Each, detailed **Case study** begins with contextual information about a patient, including the medical and drug histories. This equates to the level of information likely to be available to a pharmacist on consulting medical notes, or talking with other members of the healthcare team or to the patient and/or their carer. The cases are interspersed with, and followed by, a series of questions. These are the sort of questions that pharmacists will ask themselves when encountering such a case in practice, or questions that might be asked of pharmacists by patients or other health professionals. We recommend that readers consider each question based initially on their current knowledge, before accessing additional sources such as the current *British National Formulary*, lecture notes, NICE guidance, websites and textbooks. At times, supplementary information may be revealed as the case progresses, which may take readers in a different direction or cause them to reflect and re-evaluate their previous responses and recommendations.

The cases and questions are followed by a section entitled **Case discussion**. We have chosen not to supply discrete answers for each question. Such an approach gives the impression that a definite answer is possible; that all questions have right and wrong answers. Professional practice demonstrates that real-life issues cannot be considered in such a black-and-white manner, and what demarcates the professional is their appreciation and acceptance of uncertainty and their ability to make judgements based on the available evidence. 'Answers' to the questions can be found in this section, but there is much more besides, because the case is considered in its clinical, practice and science context. Having read this section, refer back to the questions posed in the case, consider how you might answer them in light of this information, and think of what additional questions you might now ask and what further information you would like. This is the spur to **References and further reading**. We have also provided some **Extended learning** questions, representing our own thoughts for how this case might encourage useful further study. Hopefully, you will also have formulated your own questions. Finally, although all the cases are 'practice' focused, in some instances we have included **Additional practice points**, highlighting supplementary practice issues that may be tangentially linked to the substance of the case study, or alluding to pertinent debates and concerns within pharmacy.

The cases have been written by practitioners with academic input, representing current clinical and scientific knowledge, and are informed by the experience, expertise and opinions of the authors. They should not be taken as a template for professional practice. Readers are reminded that knowledge, pharmacotherapy and treatment guidelines are continually changing and that pharmacists are called on to make judgements based on their own knowledge and experience. Be prepared, at times, to disagree with what you read!

Conventions used in the text

With the widely different backgrounds of the contributing authors, there were inevitably differences in terminologies, units of measurement, etc., between cases. Also clinical and science conventions often diverge. Thus, in this text we express drug doses as mg, micrograms (written in full), etc., as is accepted in clinical practice (to minimise the risk of prescribing errors), but follow scientific conventions for clinical data and other measurements, e.g. we have used μg throughout (rather than microgram or mcg) to express 10^{-6} grams.

Most cases include medicines that are currently being used or are to be used by a patient. Note that all doses are for the oral route (p.o.), unless otherwise stated; dosing instructions are indicated as standard Latin abbreviations, e.g. t.d.s. We have ensured that the names of the medicines referred to in the case studies are as found in the most current version of the *British National Formulary* (*BNF* 68, September 2014) at the time of writing. Occasionally, the proprietary name of a product

has also been included, where this is appropriate to the context of the case.

The editorial team and the case study authors

The authors of the cases were chosen because of their experience as practising pharmacists, their unique knowledge of a particular area of practice or therapeutics, and their ability to communicate to early years pharmacists. The large majority of the authors currently practise as pharmacists in the community and hospitals, and the cases reflect that contemporary practice. Their enormous, learned contributions to this text are testament to the vast expertise that UK clinical pharmacists now possess and use daily for patient benefit.

The editorial team, all with pharmacy degrees, has extensive experience in teaching undergraduate and postgraduate pharmacists, as well as pharmacy technicians. Between them, they conduct research and teach in the core disciplines of pharmacy, namely pharmacy practice, pharmaceutics, chemistry and pharmacology. They have worked together building up the case studies supplied by the authors to ensure that each case integrates current science and practice, is coherent, and provides a tool for effective learning.

The authors and editors have worked together with the shared belief that this is a valuable and worthwhile project. The collaboration has led to an innovative learning resource, which has drawn on the collective knowledge and experience of a very diverse group.

This collection of case studies has been a great pleasure to produce. In the process, we have realised the enormous range of subjects of which pharmacists require a deep knowledge and understanding, in order to make their unique contribution to healthcare. We hope that readers will derive the same enjoyment, and that this book clearly illustrates how the various disciplines that comprise pharmacy can complement, support and inform each other, such that pharmacists truly are medicines experts.

Reference

General Pharmaceutical Council. *Future Pharmacists: Standards for the initial education and training of pharmacists.* London: GPhC, 2011.

1

Gastrointestinal, liver and renal cases

INTRODUCTION

This section comprises 10 cases centred on patients with gastrointestinal (GI), liver and renal diseases. The GI cases include uninvestigated dyspepsia, inflammatory bowel disease and threadworm infestation. Liver disease is the topic of four cases: liver disease in an elderly patient, alcoholic cirrhosis, liver disease with ascites and a case of paracetamol poisoning. Three renal cases focus on chronic kidney disease and haemofiltration/renal replacement therapy.

Case 1
Uninvestigated dyspepsia ▶ 3

This case concerns a middle-aged man who presents in a community pharmacy with epigastric discomfort after eating. The case considers approaches to questioning patients to gather information to enable a judgement to be made about the appropriate course of action. The case then enables an examination of the advantages and disadvantages of non-invasive tests for *H. pylori*, interpretation of test results and the treatment of *H. pylori* infection.

Case 2
Inflammatory bowel disease ▶ 7

This case concerns a patient with long-standing Crohn's disease. The case distinguishes Crohn's disease from ulcerative colitis in terms of its definition, symptoms, signs and course of the disease. Mesalazine is often central to treatment of inflammatory bowel disease. Its mechanism of action is discussed as well as its formulation as modified-release oral preparations, necessitating prescribing by proprietary name. Other pharmacological agents are also considered, including the place of anti-TNF-α antibody treatment.

Case 3
Treatment of threadworm ▶ 10

Treatment of threadworm takes place in a community pharmacy. This case focuses on the signs and symptoms of infestation, recommended treatments and additional advice for patients (in this case the mother of young children). Mebendazole is the drug of choice and its mode of action is discussed. Mebendazole is available in liquid form (often preferable for younger children). Using mebendazole as an example, this case distinguishes different liquid oral dosage formulations: solutions, suspensions and emulsions. A further complication of the case is that one family member has epilepsy, so potential drug–drug interactions must be considered.

Case 4
Liver disease in an elderly patient ▶ 13

This is the first of four liver cases and describes an elderly patient with liver disease. This case introduces the basic structure and functions of the liver, first-pass metabolism, the main enzymes that are used to monitor liver function and how liver enzymes are interpreted to indicate liver failure.

Case 5
Alcoholic liver cirrhosis ▶ 15

This case describes a female patient with alcoholic liver cirrhosis admitted to an accident and emergency department (A&E). It focuses on the interpretation of liver function tests to assess disease severity. It includes the operation and application of the Child–Pugh classification of liver insufficiency. The case examines some implications of liver disease in drug handling and prescribing. The case also discusses the signs, symptoms and management of acute alcoholic hepatitis.

Case 6
Liver disease with ascites ► 19

This case involves a male patient diagnosed with alcohol-induced liver cirrhosis, who is admitted to hospital because of decompensated liver disease. This case considers the impact of liver disease on drug handling: pharmacodynamic and pharmacokinetic effects. In particular, the bioavailability of the drug, drug metabolism and volume of distribution are discussed. The case also addresses the management of hepatic encephalopathy and the management of ascites.

Case 7
Management of paracetamol overdose with acetylcysteine ► 22

Paracetamol is a widely used mild analgesic and antipyretic, which when taken at recommended therapeutic doses is safe and often effective. However, higher doses are dangerous and paracetamol overdose is one of the most frequently presented drug poisonings. This case describes the metabolic pathways and mechanisms of liver damage that are a consequence of paracetamol poisoning. It outlines the signs, symptoms and presentation of paracetamol overdose and the importance of establishing the number of tablets and timing of ingestion to aid the development of a treatment plan. The case discusses the use and administration of acetylcysteine as an antidote.

Case 8
Chronic kidney disease ► 26

This case concerns a patient with chronic kidney disease and co-morbidities: type 2 diabetes and hypertension. After the definition, causes, signs and symptoms of chronic kidney disease and how kidney function is assessed are considered; the case then addresses the rationale for prescribing drugs for a patient with chronic kidney disease. This involves a review of the patient's current medication. There is also a particular focus on furosemide, including its chemistry and mechanism of action.

Cases 9 and 10

Cases 9 and 10 discuss haemofiltration (renal replacement therapy) with regard to two patients who experience an acute decline in renal function.

Case 9
Haemofiltration ► 31

In this case, the patient undergoes cardiac surgery which leads to a decline in cardiac output and renal function. The relationship between cardiac and renal output is discussed, and the impact of medicines used to improve cardiac function. Haemofiltration is started to address the decline in renal function. The case concludes with a comment on how the chemical properties of a drug can influence renal clearance and dosing regimens.

Case 10
Renal replacement therapy ► 35

This case distinguishes the processes of haemofiltration and haemodialysis, with particular regard to implications for the clearance of medications. This patient has a viral infection that is resistant to first- and second-line antivirals. A new unlicensed medication (that has reached phase 2 clinical trials) is considered. This case also outlines the classification of clinical trials into phases 1–4.

Case 1
Uninvestigated dyspepsia
NAVEED IQBAL AND KAY WOOD

LEARNING OUTCOMES

At the end of this case, you will be able to:

- Outline questions you may ask a patient about upper gastrointestinal (GI) symptoms to decide whether to treat over-the-counter (OTC) or refer
- Discuss the advantages and disadvantages of the available non-invasive tests for *H. pylori*
- Discuss the terms *specificity* and *sensitivity* in relation to tests for *H. pylori*
- Recommend appropriate management for *H. pylori*.

Case study

You are working as a community pharmacist. A middle-aged man, Mr AS, presents asking for something for epigastric discomfort after eating.

❷ What questions would you ask Mr AS initially?

Mr AS says that he is the patient and that he has been suffering from discomfort after eating, on and off, for the last 2 weeks. He has not tried anything for this condition and he is not taking any other medicines. He has no 'ALARM' symptoms.

❷ What are ALARM symptoms?
❷ When should you refer?
❷ What lifestyle advice would you offer Mr AS?

After discussion with the pharmacist, the patient took ranitidine 75 mg tablets.

▶ **Four months later …** *you have a phone call about Mr AS from your local GP. The GP outlines the following:*

Mr AS is a 40-year-old private tutor with dyspepsia. He has no 'ALARM' symptoms and is being managed according to the 'uninvestigated dyspepsia' pathway in the NICE guidance (NICE, 2004). The GP has judged that it is appropriate to test Mr AS for *H. pylori* infection. NICE guidance states that *H. pylori* can be initially detected using either a ^{13}C-urea breath test or a stool antigen test, or laboratory-based serology where its performance has been locally validated.

CASE NOTES

History of presenting complaint
- A 4-month history of intermittent non-specific epigastric discomfort after eating

Past medical history
- Knee arthroscopy (keyhole surgery used to investigate knee joint pain) and partial meniscectomy (knee cartilage removal) in 2002

Medical history
- Dyspepsia

Social history
- Married
- Four children
- Runs a private tuition centre
- No history of alcohol consumption
- Non-smoker
- Came to the UK from Pakistan 20 years ago

Drug history
- Lansoprazole 30 mg capsules
- Multivitamins (purchased without a prescription)
- Reports rash with penicillin

The GP asks for your advice on non-invasive tests available for H. pylori

❷ Review the advantages and disadvantages of key non-invasive testing methods for *H. pylori*.

The GP has decided that Mr AS should undertake a ^{13}C-labelled urea breath test. He has chosen Helicobacter Test INFAI – a simple proprietary breath test for H. pylori *and advises Mr AS to discontinue taking the PPI before taking the test and not to eat or drink anything (including water) for 4 hours beforehand.*

Mr AS read in the patient information leaflet that the ^{13}C-labelled urea breath test has a sensitivity of 97.9% and a specificity of 98.5%. He asks you what this means.

3

> On examination
> - Weight: 89 kg
> - Height: 1.80 m
> - BMI: 27.4
> - BP: 138/85 mmHg

❷ How would you respond to Mr AS's question?

The practice nurse conducts a ^{13}C-labelled urea breath test on Mr AS, and the result is negative. The prevalence of H. pylori *infection in men of Mr AS's age is around 25% (Logan and Walker, 2001). The GP asks your opinion on this result as Mr AS had a high pre-test probability of* H. pylori.

❷ How does the test work?
❷ What could have led to the negative test result for Mr AS?

Mr AS admitted that he continued with the PPI, in spite of instructions to the contrary, as he was concerned that his symptoms would have had an effect on his work commitments. Mr AS still continues to complain of symptoms. The GP reassures him of the reasoning behind discontinuing PPI therapy before undertaking the Helicobacter test again. The retest is issued as the previous results were invalid. The results are now positive for H. pylori. *The GP asks for your advice on the most suitable regimen as combination packs are no longer available.*

❷ What advice would you give to the GP?
❷ Why was it necessary to discontinue taking the PPI before the *H. pylori* test?

Case discussion

— Questioning patients with upper gastrointestinal symptoms

On first meeting a patient, it is advisable to have a systematic approach to understanding a patient's problems and determining when it may be appropriate to refer to another health professional. The WWHAM questions can be used as a guide to appropriate questioning (Rutter, 2013). This mnemonic should be used as an aide-memoire; do not fire questions at patients in a manner that may affect the flow of the consultation:

Who is the patient?
What is the problem?
How long has it been a problem?
What Action has been taken?

What other Medicines are being taken (prescribed or non-prescription)?

❶ Remember, medication includes non-oral medicines such as inhalers, and herbals, homeopathic medicines and 'GSLs' (general sales list medicines). Patients' perceptions of what they consider to be medication can be different from those of healthcare professionals.

— ALARM symptoms
In addition to this, you should be aware of 'ALARM' symptoms. This mnemonic is used to help in the assessment of symptoms of dyspepsia, and to identify cases that may signify a more serious condition and warrant further investigation.

Anaemia (iron deficiency)
Loss of weight
Anorexia
Recent onset of progressive symptoms
Melaena/haematemesis (passage of black tarry stools/vomiting of blood)
Swallowing difficulty

— Referral of patients
Immediate (same day) specialist referral is indicated for patients presenting with dyspepsia and significant GI bleeding (e.g. vomiting large amounts of blood).

Urgent (within 2 weeks) specialist referral or endoscopy is indicated for patients of any age if they present with dyspepsia and any of the following (NICE, 2004):

- Chronic gastrointestinal (GI) bleeding (e.g. vomiting small amounts of blood, blood in stools)
- Progressive dysphagia (difficulty swallowing)
- Progressive unintentional weight loss
- Persistent vomiting
- Iron deficiency anaemia
- Epigastric mass
- Suspicious barium meal result.

— Lifestyle advice
Lifestyle modification may help with GI symptoms. Advice could be given on weight reduction and avoiding provoking factors, such as eating fatty or spicy foods or heavy meals at night, drinking coffee or alcohol, and smoking (NICE, 2004). If it is to be effective, questioning should elicit the patient's perspectives and the advice should be responsive to their needs and situation.

Tests for *H. pylori*

— Non-invasive testing methods for *Helicobacter pylori*

There are several different methods to test for *H. pylori* infection (De Korwin, 2003):

- *Urea breath test* (also called the carbon isotope-urea breath test): the patient takes a urea product that contains ^{13}C-labelled urea as in Helicobacter Test INFAI. If *H. pylori* is present, the bacteria convert the ^{13}C-labelled urea to ^{13}C-labelled carbon dioxide which is detected on the patient's breath. This is an effective and reliable test for the presence of *H. pylori* infection. Patients should normally be advised to avoid taking PPIs (at least 2 weeks prior) or antibiotics (at least 4 weeks prior) to undergoing a urea breath test.

- *Antibody serology:* blood tests can measure antibodies to *H. pylori*. Thus, these tests will detect an infection if present, but antibodies may remain long after an infection has cleared.

- *Stool antigen test:* this test detects genetic traces of *H. pylori* in the faeces. It is reliable in diagnosing infection and to confirm eradication.

— Sensitivity and specificity of tests

A test with high *sensitivity* is good at correctly identifying patients *who do have H. pylori* infection.

A test with high *specificity* is good at correctly identifying patients *who do not have H. pylori* infection.

In this case, Mr AS needs to be aware that a *sensitivity* of 97.9% indicates that the ^{13}C-labelled urea breath test will correctly identify, from a cohort of 100 patients, 98% patients with *H. pylori*. This means that around 2% patients who have *H. pylori* infection will not be identified by the test as having it. These patients will be labelled incorrectly as not having the infection – a so-called 'false-negative' result (National Prescribing Centre, 2005).

In turn, a *specificity* of 98.5% for the ^{13}C-labelled urea breath test will correctly identify most people who do not have *H. pylori* infection in a cohort of 100 patients, 98.5% patients will not have *H. pylori* infection. That means that 1.5% of patients who do not have *H. pylori* infection will be identified by the test as having it. These patients will be labelled incorrectly as having the

infection – a so-called 'false-positive' result (National Prescribing Centre, 2005).

These results should not be the only factors to be considered when deciding if the results could be a false negative or positive. We need to take into account the prevalence of this disease in the population to which the patient belongs (National Prescribing Centre, 2005). You need to consider the patient's pre-test probability of having *H. pylori* infection. In this case, be aware that Mr AS grew up in Pakistan; rates of *H. pylori* infection are higher in less-developed countries (Logan and Walker, 2001).

— Helicobacter test INFAI: how it works

After oral ingestion, ^{13}C-urea labelled urea tablets will rapidly disintegrate on reaching the stomach. In the case of infection with *H. pylori*, ^{13}C-labelled urea is metabolised by the urease enzyme present in *H. pylori*.

$$(NH_2)_2{}^{13}CO \;+\; H_2O \;\xrightarrow{\;\text{urease from}\; H.\ pylori\;}\; 2\,NH_3 \;+\; {}^{13}CO_2$$

The ^{13}C-labelled CO_2 liberated diffuses into the blood vessels and is transported as bicarbonate to the lungs where it is liberated as $^{13}CO_2$ in exhaled air, mixed with $^{12}CO_2$; this is the product of normal respiration. Infection with *H. pylori* will significantly change the ratio $^{13}C:{}^{12}C$ in the exhaled CO_2 (Klein et al., 1996). The relative abundance of naturally occurring ^{13}C (six protons and seven neutrons) is around 1% of all carbon isotopes; essentially all of the remaining 99% is made up of ^{12}C (six protons and six neutrons). ^{12}C and ^{13}C are the only non-radioactive isotopes of carbon. Comparison of the $^{13}C:{}^{12}C$ ratio in exhaled CO_2 before and after the ingestion of ^{13}C-labelled urea can therefore indicate the presence or absence of *H. pylori* urease in the gastrointestinal tract.

The proportion of $^{13}CO_2$ in the breath samples is determined by isotope-ratio mass spectrometry (IRMS). In this analytical technique, the breath sample is ionised using a powerful electrical current in the form of a beam of electrons. As these electrons collide with CO_2 molecules in the breath sample, they cause the removal of electrons from the CO_2 molecules, resulting in positively charged ions. The CO_2 ions are accelerated and then deflected around a curved path. Heavier ions ($^{13}CO_2$ has a relative molecular mass of 45, whereas $^{12}CO_2$ has a relative molecular mass of 44) with the same charge are deflected less than lighter ions, allowing separation and counting of the relative amounts of $^{13}CO_2$ and $^{12}CO_2$. In a positive test, the ratio $^{13}CO_2 : {}^{12}CO_2$ will be higher *after* ingestion of ^{13}C-labelled urea than before. The rate-limiting step is the *H. pylori* urease activity. The activity of this enzyme and its implications on screening can have a huge impact on the validity of test results.

— **False-negative results**

In this case, Mr AS is taking lansoprazole, a proton pump inhibitor (PPI) that has a direct antibacterial effect on *H. pylori* and has been shown to inhibit *H. pylori* urease activity (Stoschus et al., 1996). PPI contribution to false-negative test results has been reported to occur in as many as 40% of individuals taking a PPI (Laine et al., 1998). The mechanism of this effect still remains unclear.

The THREE most common hypotheses that have been investigated to explain this occurrence are:

1 PPIs have an effect on intragastric pH, which could make the intragastric environment unfavourable for *H. pylori*; this could lead indirectly to a lower bacterial load (Scott et al. 1998).

2 The high pH from PPI consumption could close the proton-gated urea channel (HpUreI) that facilitates bacterial cell entry of urea and therefore reduce urea's access to cytoplasmic *H. pylori* urease, which produces NH_3 and CO_2 (Scott et al., 1998).

3 Direct antibacterial activity of *H. pylori* could result in a reduction in bacterial load (Stoschus et al., 1996).

— **Advising on the treatment of *H. pylori* infection**

In this case, Mr AS's claim to have an allergy to penicillin should be questioned to determine the likelihood of true allergy, and assess whether the symptoms described are consistent with a type 1 allergic reaction. This questioning will also ensure a correct recording of his allergy status and reduce the risk of withholding effective drug treatment. A safety first approach would exclude the use of a penicillin for Mr AS.

NICE recommends a 1-week triple therapy regimen as first-line *H. pylori* eradication therapy (NICE, 2004). The optimum regimen consists of a full-dose PPI, with either amoxicillin 1 g and clarithromycin 500 mg, or metronidazole 400 mg and clarithromycin 250 mg, all given twice daily. Eradication is effective in 80–85% of patients on triple therapy using either combination (NICE, 2004).

We need to take into account Mr AS's antibiotic history. This is pertinent to Mr AS's case because each course of clarithromycin or metronidazole increases the risk of resistance (McNulty et al. 2012), which could ultimately lead to treatment failure. The importance of compliance should be stressed to Mr AS for increasing eradication rates.

As Mr AS claims to have an allergy to penicillin the regimen that would be favoured will consist of full dose PPI, with metronidazole 400 mg and clarithromycin 250 mg, all given twice daily for 1 week. This information is available in Chapter 1 of the *British National Formulary* (BNF): *Gastro-intestinal system*.

EXTENDED LEARNING

- Describe different types of allergy/hypersensitivity reactions
- How are antibiotics classified? Give examples of each group
- What medicines can cause symptoms of dyspepsia as an adverse effect? How would you question and advise patients about concurrent use of these drugs?

References and further reading

De Korwin JD (2003). Advantages and limitations of diagnostic methods for *H. pylori* infection. *Gastroenterology Clin Biol* 27:380–90.

INFAI (2012). ^{13}C-urea breath tests for *Helicobacter pylori* infection. Available at: www.infai.com/products/helicobacter.php (accessed 20 September 2012).

Klein PD, Malaty HM, Martin RF, Graham KS, Genta RM, Graham DY (1996). Noninvasive detection of *Helicobacter pylori* infection in clinical practice: the 13C urea breath test. *Am J Gastroenterol* 9:690–4.

Kusters JG, van Vliet AH, Kuipers EJ (2006). Pathogenesis of *Helicobacter pylori* infection. *Clin Microbiol Rev* 19:449–90.

Laine L, Estrada R, Trujillo M, Knigge K, Fennerty MB (1998). Effect of proton-pump inhibitor therapy on diagnostic testing for *Helicobacter pylori*. *Ann Intern Med* 29:547–50.

Logan RPH, Walker MM (2001). ABC of the upper gastrointestinal tract: Epidemiology and diagnosis of *Helicobacter pylori* infection. *BMJ* 323:920–2.

McNulty C, Lasseter G, D'Arcy S, Lawson A, Shaw I, Glocker E (2012). Is *Helicobacter pylori* antibiotic resistance surveillance needed and how can it be delivered? *Aliment Pharmacol Ther* **35**:1221–30.

National Institute for Health and Clinical Excellence (2004). *Management of Dyspepsia in Adults in Primary Care*. Clinical Guideline 17. London: NICE. Available at: http://guidance.nice.org.uk/CG17 (accessed 2 October 2013).

National Prescribing Centre (2005). Using evidence to guide practice-supplement. *MeRec Briefing* **30**(Suppl).

Rutter P (2013). Introduction. In: *Community Pharmacy: Symptoms, diagnosis and treatment*. Edinburgh: Churchill Livingstone.

Scott DR, Weeks D, Hong C, Postius S, Melchers K, Sachs G (1998). The role of internal urease in acid resistance of *Helicobacter pylori*. *Gastroenterology* **114**:58–70.

Stoschus B, Dominguez-Munoz JE, Kalhori N, Sauerbruch T, Malfertheiner P (1996). Effect of omeprazole on *Helicobacter pylori* urease activity in vivo. *Eur J Gastroenterol Hepatol* **8**:811–13.

Case 2
Inflammatory bowel disease

PAUL BAINS

LEARNING OUTCOMES

At the end of this case, you will be able to:

- Discuss the definition, signs and symptoms of Crohn's disease and ulcerative colitis
- Describe the treatment options for relapses of Crohn's disease and ulcerative colitis
- Outline the place in therapy for anti-TNF-α antibody treatment in Crohn's disease
- Outline the concept of modified release for oral dosage forms
- Describe the chemistry and mechanism of action of aminosalicylates

Case study

Mr PB is a 45-year-old white man. He was diagnosed with Crohn's disease 10 years ago and has since been controlled on maintenance mesalazine MR 400 mg three times daily.

- Name the two main forms of inflammatory bowel disease (IBD)
- What are the symptoms of these two forms?
- What are the common side effects of mesalazine/aminosalicylates? What are the important counselling points for patients taking mesalazine?
- Draw the structure of mesalazine. What structural features are important to its pharmacological and clinical use?
- Mesalazine has been prescribed as a modified-release product. Why is such a product appropriate for mesalazine?

- What are the formulation approaches that can be adopted to produce modified-release solid dosage forms?

Mr PB has been admitted to hospital. He has been opening his bowels six to seven times a day and has confirmed that his diarrhoea is bloody. He has a fever and feels generally unwell. It is clear to his medical team that Mr PB's Crohn's disease has relapsed.

- Discuss the role of corticosteroids and aminosalicylates as treatments for relapse of IBD.

Mr PB is improving on prednisolone 40 mg each morning. His dose is slowly reduced, but he complains of feeling very unwell when his dose is reduced to below 10 mg each morning.

- What is the treatment option to avoid the need for long-term prednisolone?
- What may be measured before starting this treatment?
- What parameters should be monitored before and during therapy?

▶ Twelve months later … *Mr PB has been readmitted to hospital with another relapse. His Crohn's disease is now severe, as he is opening his bowels on a frequent basis and his quality of life is very poor. Mesalazine had been stopped some time ago, because it had no effect. His initial response to azathioprine was good, but he is now losing response. He has been started on prednisolone 40 mg each morning, but his dose cannot be reduced as his Crohn's disease relapses.*

- What is the best treatment option for Mr PB?

Case discussion

— The main forms of inflammatory bowel disease and their symptoms

IBD encompasses ulcerative colitis and Crohn's disease. Ulcerative colitis is limited to the colon, whereas Crohn's disease may affect any part of the gastrointestinal (GI) tract. Both conditions are characterised by chronic relapsing inflammation.

Ulcerative colitis can be divided into distal or more extensive disease. Distal disease includes inflammation of the rectum alone (proctitis) or of the rectum and sigmoid colon (proctosigmoiditis). Extensive disease includes pancolitis: inflammation of the whole colon. Ulcerative colitis always involves inflammation of the rectum. Although Crohn's disease can affect any part of the GI tract, it is usually limited to the ileum and colon.

The causes of ulcerative colitis and Crohn's disease are unknown. It is believed that a combination of environmental triggers (e.g. infection) and genetic predisposition leads to inflammation of the GI tract.

In ulcerative colitis, the symptoms are linked to the area inflamed. Proctitis is associated with the passage of mucus and blood, but less often diarrhoea. Ulcerative colitis affecting more of the colon beyond the rectum is accompanied by bloody diarrhoea. Crohn's disease is associated with abdominal pain, which is often the first symptom of the disease. The pain is usually (but not always) right sided and can mimic appendicitis. Diarrhoea and weight loss are also present. The diarrhoea is not always bloody. The abdominal pain of Crohn's disease is related to the site of inflammation.

— Structure, chemistry and mechanism of action of mesalazine

mesalazine

Mesalazine (also known as 5-aminosalicylic acid or mesalamine) is an aminosalicylate non-steroidal anti-inflammatory drug (NSAID) used to treat inflammatory bowel diseases, such as ulcerative colitis and Crohn's disease. Mesalazine acts locally in the GI tract, with minimal systemic side effects. Sulfasalazine (another NSAID) is metabolised to sulfapyridine and the active mesalazine.

The mechanism of action of mesalazine's anti-inflammatory activity is related to the mechanism of action of other NSAIDs such as ibuprofen (although there is evidence that mesalazine acts through a variety of mechanisms). Mesalazine binds reversibly to the active site of the cyclooxygenase enzymes (COX-1 and COX-2), inhibiting the production of prostaglandins involved in the inflammatory response. Similar to most NSAIDs, the presence of a carboxyl group (which is deprotonated and negatively charged at physiological pH) attached to a hydrophobic group (the aromatic ring in mesalazine) is important for interaction with the COX active site. These features mimic the structure of arachidonic acid, the normal substrate for the COX enzymes.

— Side effects and counselling points

Common side effects include headache, diarrhoea, nausea, vomiting, abdominal pain and rash. Mesalazine is tolerated better then sulfasalazine. Patients receiving aminosalicylates should be advised to report any unexplained bleeding, bruising, sore throat, fever or malaise while on treatment, due to the risk of blood disorders. Treatment should be stopped if blood dyscrasia (abnormal cellular elements) occurs.

— Formulation approaches for modified-release, solid dosage forms and their application to mesalazine

Modified-release oral formulations aim to deliver drugs at specific rates, times or specific physiological sites within the GI tract. Production of a modified-release formulation may result in extended release (allowing a reduction in the frequency of dosing), delayed release (drug is not released immediately after administration) or release of drug at a specific site in the GI tract (e.g. in the small intestine or colon). Gastroresistant coatings, also known as enteric (pH-controlled) coatings, protect a drug as it passes through the stomach and can be used for drug delivery to the small intestine or colon. This may be employed to reduce the adverse effects of drugs (such as NSAIDs) in the stomach, as is the case here. Modified-release can be achieved by using matrix polymer tablets, polymer-coated pellets or osmotic-based systems.

The drug release characteristics of oral mesalazine preparations are different and thus the products should not be considered as interchangeable. Prescribers must specify the proprietary name of mesalazine to be dispensed (e.g. Asacol, Pentasa, Salofalk). Patients should be counselled to identify which form of oral mesalazine they take; this is done best by the patient remembering the brand name.

— Corticosteroids and aminosalicylates for treating relapse of IBD

Corticosteroids are indicated for moderate-to-severe relapses of Crohn's disease or IBD. They act through the inhibition of several inflammatory pathways. Oral glucocorticoid steroids such as prednisolone or budesonide, or intravenous hydrocortisone (for severe relapse) are all options. Topical preparations (in the form of enemas, foams or suppositories) are useful for relapses of ulcerative colitis to control inflammation of the rectum. Topical and oral preparations can be used together. Budesonide is poorly absorbed and undergoes extensive first-pass metabolism. Prednisolone is started at a dose of 40 mg each morning, with higher doses being no more effective, while increasing the risk of adverse effects. Once the patient is in remission, prednisolone should be withdrawn slowly and not be stopped abruptly. Too rapid a withdrawal can lead to a further relapse. A typical withdrawal regimen would involve prednisolone being reduced by 5–10 mg every 7–14 days.

— Treatment options avoiding the need for long-term prednisolone and associated patient monitoring

For a mild relapse of ulcerative colitis or Crohn's disease, mesalazine at a dose of ≥4 g/day may induce remission. Topical rectal preparations of aminosalicylates are effective for proctitis or distal ulcerative colitis and these can be combined with oral forms for greater effect, particularly in moderate or severe relapses of ulcerative colitis.

The thiopurines, azathioprine and 6-mercaptopurine, would be indicated at this stage. The main role for thiopurines in IBD is steroid sparing. Thiopurines should be considered for any patient who requires two or more courses of corticosteroids within a calendar year, or those whose disease relapses when prednisolone is reduced to <15 mg each morning or within 6 weeks of stopping prednisolone. Both azathioprine and 6-mercaptopurine are started at low doses and titrated upwards, aiming for doses of azathioprine 2–2.5 mg/kg per day or 6-mercaptopurine 1–1.5 mg/kg per day. The maximum dose will differ from person to person and is largely dependent on the dose at which leukopenia (a decrease in the number of white blood cells) develops.

Thiopurine methyltransferase (TPMT) is an enzyme required to metabolise thiopurine drugs. Patients with low or absent levels of TPMT are at much greater risk of thiopurine-induced leukopenia resulting from accumulation of the unmetabolised drug. TPMT activity should be assessed before starting thiopurine treatment. If activity is very low or absent, alternative treatment should be considered. If TPMT activity is below normal but not absent, both azathioprine and mercaptopurine should be prescribed at lower doses.

Patients should have a full blood count (FBC) pre-treatment, and then weekly for the first 6–8 weeks, followed by 3-monthly if no problems arise. Patients should be advised to report any unexplained bleeding, bruising, sore throat, fever or malaise while on treatment because of the risk of blood disorders. Liver function tests should also be performed at the same time as the FBC due to the low risk of hepatotoxicity with these drugs. Liver function tests (LFTs) provide information about the diagnosis and treatment of liver disease, and monitoring of liver activity. The liver-associated enzymes that are measured are alanine aminotransferase (ALT), aspartate aminotransferase (AST), alkaline phosphatase (ALP) and γ-glutamyltransferase (GGT). In addition, bilirubin and serum albumin may be measured. The values of these parameters will provide a clinical picture of liver function, and the ability of the liver to metabolise drugs.

— Further treatment options

The National Institute for Health and Care Excellence (NICE) reviewed the monoclonal antibodies against tumour necrosis factor α (TNF-α) – infliximab and adalimumab – for the treatment of severe Crohn's disease. Both drugs are approved for severe active Crohn's disease where disease has not responded to corticosteroids and/or immunosuppressants, or in patients who are intolerant of, or have contraindications to, them. Infliximab is given as an intravenous infusion at a dose of 5 mg/kg at weeks 0, 2 and 6, and then every 8 weeks thereafter. Adalimumab is given by subcutaneous injection at a dose of

160 mg at week 0, 80 mg at week 2 and then 40 mg every 2 weeks thereafter.

- What are the therapeutic uses of NSAIDs?
- What is the role of methotrexate in the treatment of IBD?
- What is the role of ciclosporin in treating ulcerative colitis?
- What is the role of infliximab for severe ulcerative colitis, including guidance from NICE?
- What are the processes involved in the formulation and manufacture of modified-release oral dosage forms and rectal dosage forms?

- Other than the risk of relapse, why, in general, should oral glucocorticoid steroid therapy never be stopped abruptly?

References and further reading

McConnell EL, Basit AW (2013). Modified-release oral drug delivery. In: Aulton ME, Taylor KMG (eds), *Aulton's Pharmaceutics: The design and manufacture of medicines*, 4th edn. London: Elsevier, 550–65.

Mowat C, Cole A, Windsor A, et al. (2011). Guidelines for the management of inflammatory bowel disease in adults. *Gut* **60**:571–607.

National Institute for Health and Clinical Excellence (2010). *Infliximab and Adalimumab for the Treatment of Crohn's Disease.* Technology Appraisal 187. London: NICE. Available at: http://publications.nice.org.uk/infliximab-review-and-adalimumab-for-the-treatment-of-crohns-disease-ta187 (accessed 2 July 2013).

Case 3
Treatment of threadworm

CLAIRE GOLIGHTLY

LEARNING OUTCOMES

At the end of this case you will be able to:

- Describe the signs and symptoms of a threadworm infestation
- Identify the correct course of treatment
- Explain the implications for treatment of a patient with epilepsy
- Describe the pharmacology of the recommended treatment
- Outline the differences between common liquid dosage forms
- Differentiate between flocculated and deflocculated suspensions and their associated properties
- Give the correct additional advice to a family presenting with a case of threadworm

Case study

A mother with 4-year-old twin boys (Tom and Daniel) approaches your pharmacy counter and asks for a quiet word with the pharmacist. You take them into the consultation room. On questioning she describes the following:

Tom started to complain his back passage was itchy and has been pulling at his shorts and in particular his pyjama bottoms in the night. I just assumed he was getting too hot in this recent warm weather, but now Daniel is doing the same. I have heard that itching may mean there is a threadworm infection, but I don't know if that is what it is.

❓ What further questions would you ask?

After discussing the symptoms with the mother, it is clear that this is a threadworm infestation.

❓ What is the drug of choice for treating threadworm infestation?
❓ What is its mode of action?
❓ What dosage forms might be considered for treatment?

When you inform the mother that it is a threadworm infestation she is taken aback and is very eager to assure you that her house is very clean and that the boys are bathed regularly.

❓ How would you address her concerns?
❓ What additional hygiene advice should you give her?

When you discuss how to treat the infestation, she informs you that her husband has epilepsy. He hasn't had a seizure for 3 years but takes tablets (carbamazepine).

❓ What advice would you give about appropriate treatment for her husband?

Case discussion

— Appropriate questions to ask

- How long have the boys been uncomfortable with these symptoms?
- Have you noticed any soreness or broken skin around the anus?
- Have they complained of being unwell in any other way? For example, upset stomach, sickness, raised temperature?
- Have you noticed any little white threads in their stools?
- Have you looked for, or seen, any thread-like worms around the anus?
- Has any other member of the family displayed the same symptoms?
- Has the family travelled abroad recently?
- Does any member of the family take medication prescribed by the GP?
- Is the mother pregnant or breastfeeding?

Threadworm (*Enterobius vermicularis*) is a common and yet easily treated infestation. It is common for the public to consider that it results from poor hygiene, but studies have shown that there is no relationship with hygiene, and it occurs across all sectors of society.

Children transfer the threadworm infestation easily between each other. This would be particularly so in this family because twins are likely to play together regularly.

The signs of the infestation are a child scratching his or her bottom, particularly at night, and worms appearing as small white threads in the stools and around the anus. These are more visible at night. The infestation does not have any GI symptoms or fever.

Alternative diagnoses may be eczema, dermatitis or another type of worm: roundworm or tapeworm. These infestations are more likely if the family has travelled abroad recently.

Symptoms requiring referral to the GP would include:

- Foreign travel: possible exposure to other infections

- Broken skin, discharge around the anus, possibly indicating secondary infection
- Treatment failure.

— Mebendazole in the treatment of threadworm infestation

Drugs that are used to immobilise and expel parasitic worms from the body are termed anthelmintics. Each member of the family should be treated, whether or not showing signs of infestation.

The drug of choice for treating threadworm infestation is mebendazole (e.g. Ovex, Vermox). It is available as a chewable orange-flavoured tablet (100 mg), which is taken as a single dose and then repeated after 14 days, or as a banana-flavoured suspension (100 mg/5 mL) given as a single 5 mL dose. Mebendazole kills the worms, which are then expelled in the faeces. The second dose is to ensure that any eggs that may have subsequently hatched during the 2 weeks are also removed. It is considered to have in the region of 60–82% effective cure rate.

mebendazole

— Mode of action

Mebendazole is believed to work by selectively interfering with the synthesis of microtubules by binding to tubulin in the parasitic worms. As threadworm is common in young children, age-appropriate dosage forms are required. Proprietary products are formulated as chewable tablets, which may also be swallowed. But the liquid may be more appropriate for younger children (aged ≥ 2 years).

— Liquid dosage forms

Liquid oral dosage forms are solutions, suspensions or emulsions, which differ in their properties (Table 1.1).

As a highly lipophilic drug (log P = 3.10), mebendazole (methyl 5-[benzoyl]benzimidazole-2-carbamate) has only limited aqueous solubility (71.3 mg/L), which means that a conventional solution will not be possible, so it is formulated as a fruit-flavoured suspension. Suspensions are often less preferred (than solutions) than oral liquid

▼ TABLE 1.1
Liquid oral dosage forms

	Solution	Suspension	Emulsion
Description	Drug dispersed at the molecular level with solvent molecules	Solid particles dispersed in a liquid	Liquid droplets (usually oil) dispersed in another liquid (usually aqueous)
Physical appearance	Clear	Opaque	Opaque
Physical stability	Stable	Unstable: caking, sedimentation, flocculation	Unstable: creaming, flocculation, coalescence, cracking

formulations because accurate dosing is dependent on the suspended particles being evenly dispersed throughout the liquid. Sedimentation occurs in suspensions as a result of gravity (described by Stokes' law). A number of factors affect the sedimentation of particles, including: suspended particle size and density, and the density and viscosity of the suspending medium. Small, dense particles (deflocculated) tend to settle slowly. However, once settled a 'cake' may be formed, which is hard to re-disperse, leading to unacceptable, varied dosing. Sedimentation behaviour may be controlled by formulating a flocculated system, whereby the attractive and repulsive forces between the suspended particles are controlled, leading to the formation of low-density loose aggregates of particles (floccules), which are readily re-dispersed on shaking, allowing reproducible dosing. Note that drug absorption is faster from a solution than other oral dosage forms, but in this case absorption is not an issue because the drug has a local effect in the gastrointestinal tract. Here, the very low aqueous solubility of mebendazole is beneficial because systemic absorption is undesirable; very little drug dissolves in the contents of the GI tract, so very little is available for absorption. Any small amount of mebendazole that is absorbed undergoes very extensive first-pass metabolism in the liver (a common feature of low-polarity drugs). Most of an oral dose of mebendazole is excreted unchanged in the faeces, after having exerted its local anthelmintic effect.

— General advice on management and hygiene

To avoid causing the skin to break around the anus, pyjama bottoms should be worn, and if necessary mittens. Hot baths should be avoided before going to bed to reduce irritation. Showering or bathing each morning is recommended.

If the anal area is sore, Sudocrem or Vaseline can be applied for symptomatic relief.

The children's nursery/school should be informed and the children kept away until the first treatment has been taken and threadworms cannot be seen. Advise the mother to follow the advice of the nursery or school as policies on the length of time required for children to be away from school differ between areas.

A pharmacist should reassure the mother that threadworm infestation is not necessarily caused by poor hygiene; however, hygiene is a key factor in successful eradication. The infestation is easily cleared and should pose no further harm to the children.

Fingernails should be cut short, because worms and their eggs are often harboured here after scratching. Hand washing should be scrupulous after using the toilet and before eating. In addition, recently used clothing, towels and bedding should be washed as a precaution.

— Interactions with carbamazepine and other antiepileptic drugs

In this case, the recommended treatment for the twins and their mother would be mebendazole tablets. For their father, there is a significant interaction listed in *Stockley's Drug Interactions* (Baxter and Preston, 2013) between mebendazole and carbamazepine. Carbamazepine lowers the plasma levels of mebendazole. It is well known that several commonly used antiepileptic drugs, such as carbamazepine, phenytoin and phenobarbital, are able to induce the synthesis of a broad range of drug-metabolising liver enzymes (e.g. the cytochrome P450 [CYP450] system). This will affect the metabolism of other drugs that are taken in combination and share similar clearance pathways, resulting in a reduction in their duration, action and therapeutic effectiveness.

Thus, an increased dose of mebendazole may be required for treatment. However, this interaction is significant only for the treatment of systemic intestinal infections and is of no importance where its action has a local effect on the worms in the gut.

EXTENDED LEARNING

- How are solutions, suspensions and emulsions formulated and manufactured?
- Describe the factors influencing the physical stability of suspensions and emulsions. How is this instability controlled and measured?

References and further reading

Baxter K, Preston CL, eds (2013). *Stockley's Drug Interactions*, 10th edn. London: Pharmaceutical Press.

Brayfield A, ed. (2014). *Martindale: The Complete Drug Reference*, 38th edn. London: Pharmaceutical Press.

Robertson AP, Martin RJ (2007). Ion-channels on parasite muscle: pharmacology and physiology. *Invert Neurosci* 7:209–217.

Rutter R (2009). *Symptoms, Diagnosis and Treatment. A guide for pharmacists and nurses.* Philadelphia, PA: Elsevier.

Case 4
Liver disease in an elderly patient

NADIA BUKHARI

LEARNING OUTCOMES

At the end of this case, you will be able to:

- Outline the basic structure of the liver
- Outline the basic functions of the liver
- Outline first-pass (pre-systemic) metabolism and its implications for the fate of orally administered drugs
- State the main enzymes used to monitor liver function
- Describe how liver enzymes are interpreted to indicate liver failure

Case study

Mr GV is a 65-year-old man. He is a non-smoker and admits to drinking a glass of wine a day, sometimes two, since his wife's death 5 years ago. He was diagnosed with liver disease 3 years ago. Apart from his liver disease, he is otherwise healthy and has been prescribed aspirin 75 mg for prevention of coronary events.

- Describe the basic structure of the liver
- What are the main functions of the liver?

When Mr GV was diagnosed with liver disease 3 years ago, a series of investigations was conducted to confirm his diagnosis.

- List the tests commonly used to diagnose liver disease
- Describe each test and how it is used to diagnose liver disease

Case discussion

— Structure of the liver

The liver is the largest internal organ in the body. It is a dark reddish-brown organ weighing roughly 1.5 kg, located right, below the diaphragm. It is divided into four lobes. The main lobes are the right and left lobe, each lobe being made up of many hexagonal lobules. Most livers have between 50 000 and 100 000 lobules, each lobule consisting of a central vein surrounded by hepatocytes grouped in sheets or bundles. These cells perform the work of the liver. Cavities known as sinusoids separate the groups of cells within a lobule; the sinusoids give the liver a spongy texture.

The liver has its own blood supply, which constitutes approximately 25% of the resting cardiac output, and receives oxygenated blood from the heart. This blood enters the liver through the hepatic artery. The liver also receives blood, filled with nutrients from the small intestine, which enters the liver through the portal vein. The hepatic artery and the portal vein branch into a network of tiny blood vessels that empty into the sinusoids. The hepatocytes absorb nutrients and oxygen from the blood as it flows through the sinusoids; they also filter out waste and toxins, and secrete sugar, vitamins, minerals and other substances into the blood. The sinusoids drain into the central veins, which join to form the hepatic vein. Blood leaves the liver through the hepatic vein.

Each lobule also contains bile capillaries, tiny tubes that carry the bile secreted by the liver cells. The bile capillaries join to form bile ducts, which carry bile out of the liver.

Functions of the liver

The main functions of the liver are:

- Synthesis of bile: emulsifies fats in the small intestine during digestion
- Synthesis of cholesterol
- Synthesis of certain proteins, e.g. albumin
- Metabolism of drugs and hormones, e.g. aldosterone
- Conversion of excess glucose into glycogen for storage
- Regulation of blood levels of amino acids, which form the building blocks of proteins
- Storage of iron and fat-soluble vitamins (A, D, E, K)
- Conversion of toxic ammonia to urea
- Detoxification of drugs and toxins
- Regulation of blood clotting
- Synthesis of immune factors.

— Hepatic drug metabolism

Drugs absorbed from the stomach, small intestine and the upper region of the colon enter the hepatic portal system and pass through the liver before passing to the systemic circulation. The liver is the primary site for drug metabolism, and hence a drug must be resistant, at least in part, to metabolism by the enzymes of the liver if it is to become available in the systemic circulation. In general, the most lipophilic (low-polarity) drugs undergo the most extensive metabolism in the liver. Such metabolism (often oxidative) introduces or unmasks polar functional groups that can be utilised for further conjugation of even more polar moieties. The wall of the GI tract contains metabolising enzymes and so is also a site of drug metabolism. Such metabolism in the liver and wall of the GI tract, before a drug enters the systemic circulation, is called first-pass or pre-systemic metabolism. A number of routes of drug administration avoid first-pass metabolism, including parenteral, rectal, buccal, sublingual, transdermal, pulmonary and nasal routes.

Liver function tests and their place in disease diagnosis

Liver function tests (LFTs) are a standard group of tests that are conducted to indicate how the liver is functioning. They do not assess genuine liver function but are useful for detecting the presence of liver disease and placing liver disease in a broad category (i.e. is the liver damaged or is there some kind of blockage?). LFTs cannot be used independently to make a diagnosis. Further imaging techniques would have to be used to make a confirmed diagnosis. The tests are also useful to follow the progress of the disease once treatment has commenced.

— Serum albumin

Serum albumin is a globular protein synthesised by the liver and is important for transporting a number of cations, small molecules and hormones in the blood (e.g. Ca^{2+}, bilirubin, steroids, fatty acids, thyroid hormones) including certain drugs (warfarin, phenytoin), as well as maintaining the colloidal osmotic pressure of the plasma. In liver disease, the patient would present with abnormally low blood albumin levels (hypoalbuminaemia <3.5 g/dL: normal range: 3.5–5.0 g/dL). As albumin has a long biological half-life (approximately 20 days), this would feature in advanced liver disease.

— Serum bilirubin

Bilirubin is a yellow ferrous iron-containing breakdown product of haemoglobin catabolism. An adult normally produces about 250–300 mg bilirubin a day. It is insoluble in water and transported in the plasma bound to albumin; it is then taken up by the liver for conjugation. The conjugated bilirubin is more soluble in water than unconjugated bilirubin. The conjugated bilirubin gets excreted in the bile and some gets re-excreted through the enterohepatic circulation. Bile is responsible for the emulsification of dietary fats. Bile salts are surface-active, solubilising the fats (triglycerides and phospholipids) in food, aiding their dispersion prior to digestion by pancreatic lipase. When the biliary tract becomes blocked, bilirubin accumulates in the blood, as it is not excreted; the patient then becomes jaundiced (characteristic yellowish colouration of the skin and whites of the eyes), which is one of the early signs of liver disease.

— Aspartate aminotransferase and alanine aminotransferase

Aspartate aminotransferase (AST) and alanine aminotransferase (ALT) are important aminotransferase or transaminase enzymes found in the liver that are involved in amino acid metabolism. These enzymes are released into the plasma when hepatocellular damage (damage to the liver cells) occurs and are therefore useful clinical markers of liver function. In liver disease, levels of both enzymes in the blood can increase to 5–8 times their normal value (AST: 10–34 IU/L; ALT: 10–40 IU/L).

— Alkaline phosphatase

Alkaline phosphatase (ALP) is a hydrolase enzyme responsible for dephosphorylation of many types of molecules, including proteins and nucleotides. When blood levels of this enzyme are raised, it usually indicates liver blockage (bile duct obstruction). ALP is then released in high amounts in the blocked liver (4–6 times the normal value: 20–140 IU/L).

— γ-Glutamyl transpeptidase

GGT is an enzyme responsible for transferring γ-glutamyl functional groups. This enzyme is more liver specific. If both ALP and GGT levels (normal: 0–51 IU/L) are raised, it confirms there is some type of blockage in the liver.

— Prothrombin time

The liver is responsible for the synthesis of prothrombin and other blood clotting factors. If the liver were damaged, the prothrombin time (PT – a measure of blood clotting tendency: usually around 12–13 s) would increase, as synthesis of prothrombin would be reduced. In addition, there would be a deficiency of vitamin K (important for blood coagulation), because vitamin K is stored in the liver. These would all contribute to an increased risk of bleeding in the patient. This is an early sign of liver disease because prothrombin has a very short half-life (6 hours).

EXTENDED LEARNING

* What are enzymes? What is their function in biological systems?
* Which enzyme groups are important in the metabolism of drugs in the liver?
* What are the features of drugs that are metabolised by the liver?

References and further reading

Kumar P, Clark M (2012). *Clinical Medicine*, 8th edn. London: Saunders.

Lefkowitch JH (2011) Anatomy and function. In: Dooley JS, Lok ASF, Burroughs AK Heathcote EJ (eds), *Sherlock's Diseases of the Liver and Biliary System*, 12th edn. London: Wiley-Blackwell

Walker R, Whittlesea C (2012). *Clinical Pharmacy & Therapeutics*, 5th edn. London: Churchill Livingstone.

Case 5
Alcoholic liver cirrhosis

SINEAD TYNAN

LEARNING OUTCOMES

At the end of this case, you will be able to:

* Understand LFTs and use them to assess the severity of a patient's liver disease
* Understand the effect of liver disease on drug handling
* Describe the diagnosis and management of acute alcoholic hepatitis.

Case study

Ms AB is a 55-year-old, 45-kg woman, with known alcoholic liver cirrhosis admitted through the accident and emergency department having been found collapsed at home. She has a long history of excess alcohol consumption. She has been admitted to hospital in the previous month with haemoptysis (coughing up of blood).

Blood tests on admission were as shown in Table 1.2.

❷ Would you define this patient's liver dysfunction as acute or chronic?
❷ How can the severity of liver disease be assessed?
❷ Explain how a patient's liver function may influence prescribing decisions
❷ How would you decide if a drug was appropriate for this patient and/or if an altered dose was required?
❷ What is the definition of acute alcoholic hepatitis?
❷ What are the treatment options?

▼ TABLE 1.2

Blood tests on admission for Ms AB

Blood test	Level	Normal range
Na$^+$ (mmol/L)	142	135–145
K$^+$ (mmol/L)	4.3	3.5–5.0
Urea (mmol/L)	6.6	2.5–8.0
Creatinine (μmol/L)	56	50–90
Bilirubin (total) (μmol/L)	468	<35
Alkaline phosphatase (ALP) (IU/L)	277	35–100
Aspartate aminotransferase (AST) (IU/L)	333	0–35
γ-Glutamyltransferase (GGT) (IU/L)	594	5–36
Albumin (g/L)	37	35–50
Platelet count ($\times$ 10^9/L)	198	130–400
INR (international normalised ratio)	1.48	0.9–1.2
Haemoglobin (g/dL)	10.1	12.3–15.7
White blood cell (WBC) count ($\times$ 10^9/L)	18.57	4–10

Case discussion

— Acute and chronic liver dysfunction

Liver disease can be classified according to both the damage pattern and the time course over which the damage is seen. The pattern of liver damage can be described as cholestatic or hepatocellular, both of which can lead to fibrosis; this in turn can lead to cirrhosis. Cholestasis, in which bile flow is reduced or impaired, leads to bile accumulation in the liver and injury to the hepatocytes. Cholestasis often results in elevated blood levels of substances excreted via the bile and of liver enzymes associated with the biliary tract, notably conjugated bilirubin, ALP, GGT, bile acids and cholesterol. Injury to hepatocytes will result in hepatocellular damage causing ALT and/or AST to be released from hepatocytes with consequent raised serum levels.

Acute liver disease is defined when the history of disease does not exceed 6 months. Diseases of longer duration are classified as chronic liver disease. An additional term, 'acute on chronic', is used to describe a sudden clinical complication in a previously stable patient with chronic liver disease.

A clotting screen, including PT and INR, is essential in the assessment of the patient's liver function. A raised INR and low serum albumin may indicate a reduction in the synthetic function of the liver. Albumin has a long half-life, approximately 20 days and therefore a low albumin level may indicate chronic liver disease.

It is essential to look at trends in LFTs, in addition to other factors (e.g. diagnosis, signs and symptoms of liver disease), rather than an isolated result, when assessing a patient's liver function.

— Assessing the severity of liver disease

The severity of chronic liver disease is usually assessed by using the Child–Pugh classification, which is based on five parameters: ascites (accumulation of fluid in the abdomen), encephalopathy, total bilirubin, serum albumin and prothrombin INR. These parameters carry equal weighting towards a total score, with 15 being the highest attainable score (Table 1.3). The score is then converted into a designation of either Child–Pugh class A (5–6), Child–Pugh class B (7–9) or Child–Pugh class C (10–15), with C representing the most advanced disease.

The Child–Pugh scoring system is used to predict disease outcome and mortality from liver disease. It has limited use in predicting the effects of liver disease on drug handling.

The model for end-stage liver disease (MELD) is a scoring system that is used as a method of prioritising patients awaiting liver transplantation. The score is based on the results of LFTs. Patients with a higher score are deemed to have a greater

▼ TABLE 1.3

Scoring for Child–Pugh classification of liver insufficiency

Parameter	Score		
	1	2	3
Bilirubin (total) (μmol/L)	<35	35–50	>50
Albumin (g/L)	>35	28–35	<28
International normalised ratio	<1.7	1.8–2.3	>2.3
Grade of hepatic encephalopathy	None	1–2	3–4
Ascites	None	Moderate or easily treated	Severe or intractable

risk of dying and therefore to require a liver transplantation more urgently than those with a lower score.

— Prescribing in liver disease

As abnormal LFTs do not always indicate hepatic dysfunction and may not be drug induced, changes to patients' medications may not always be necessary. However, if enzyme levels are more than twice the upper limit of normal (ULN), this is generally considered to be significant (note that some variation can exist in the 'normal' ranges usually quoted in the literature and online, most likely as a result of differences in the assays used by different laboratories; values may also vary by gender and age). Consideration should be given to whether the liver dysfunction could be drug induced, and also to the pharmacokinetic and pharmacodynamic effects of the drugs prescribed, to decide whether any of the medicines require dose reduction or cessation.

To consider whether any of the medicines could be contributing to the patient's liver impairment the following questions need to be considered:

- When were the patient's medications started?
- Does the patient have a history of hepatotoxic reactions?
- Have any other tests been performed that offer alternative explanations for the abnormal LFTs?

The liver is the main site of drug metabolism. Drug metabolism is normally divided into three phases – phase 1 reactions (e.g. oxidation catalysed by CYP450 enzymes), phase 2 reactions (conjugation) and phase 3 pathways (e.g. active transport systems). The effect of liver disease on drug metabolism depends on various factors including:

- The severity of the liver disease
- The enzyme responsible for drug metabolism – with phase 2 metabolic enzymes being affected to a lesser extent than phase 1 enzymes
- The type of liver disease – a cholestatic pattern is more likely to affect drug-transported proteins (phase 3 pathways), whereas acute hepatic inflammation is more likely to downregulate CYP450 enzyme expression.

Liver disease can affect drug absorption due to reduced gut motility and gut oedema. Once the drug has been absorbed into the systemic circulation, the extent of its distribution to the tissues depends on a number of factors: plasma protein and tissue binding and lipid solubility. Chronic liver disease is characterised by hypoalbuminaemia. This may result in a higher fraction of free drug, particularly when the degree of protein binding is high. The volume of distribution of hydrophilic drugs, such as aminoglycosides, will be increased in patients with oedema and/or ascites; this may require higher loading doses (based on the patient's weight), but maintenance doses may not need to be changed unless renal function is also affected. Changes in liver blood flow may be decreased generally, or may bypass the liver as a result of portosystemic shunting (PSS) (bypassing of the liver via the circulatory system). The effect of this depends on the drug and the degree of the extraction by the liver: the higher the extraction by the liver, the more important the blood flow (in relation to metabolism) in determining pharmacokinetics. High extraction drugs will show a marked increase in bioavailability, and both the loading and maintenance dose will need to be decreased.

As a guide, dose modification in liver disease should be considered in the following situations:

- Drug with a narrow therapeutic index that is principally hepatically cleared
- Drug predominantly metabolised by CYP450-1A2, -2CY19, -2D6 and -3A4
- PT >130% of normal
- Bilirubin (total) >100 μmol/L
- Presence of hepatic encephalopathy
- Presence of ascites.

Misinterpretation of total drug concentration measurements may occur if serum albumin concentration <30 g/L and the drug >80% bound to the albumin.

Pharmacodynamics can be altered, making effects and side effects more pronounced, and the complications of liver disease may increase the risk of adverse effects (Table 1.4).

— Signs and symptoms of acute alcoholic hepatitis

Alcoholic hepatitis is a clinical syndrome of jaundice and liver failure that generally occurs after decades of heavy alcohol intake (mean intake approximately 100 g/day). One unit of alcohol in the UK (10 mL: small glass of wine, half a pint of beer/cider or a single measure of spirits) equates to about 8 g alcohol. The principal sign of alcoholic hepatitis is the rapid onset of jaundice,

▼ TABLE 1.4

Types of drugs to be used with caution or avoided in liver disease

Types of drugs	Relevance in liver disease
Sedating drugs	Encephalopathy
Constipating drugs	Encephalopathy
Antiplatelets/Anticoagulants	Increased risk of bleeding
Nephrotoxic drugs	Hepatorenal disease
High sodium-containing drugs	Ascites

caused by a build-up of bilirubin in the blood. Other common signs and symptoms include fever, ascites and proximal muscle loss. Patients with severe alcoholic hepatitis may also present with encephalopathy. Typically, the liver is enlarged and tender.

Laboratory findings of an elevated AST (>300 IU/L), a total serum bilirubin level >35 μmol/L, an elevated INR and neutrophilia (increased neutrophil white cells in the blood) in a patient with ascites and a history of heavy alcohol intake are indicative of alcoholic hepatitis, until proven otherwise.

— **Treatment options**

Maddrey's discriminant function is a measure of liver dysfunction (based on, for example, PT and serum bilirubin) that is used to indicate which patients may benefit from corticosteroid therapy. Corticosteroids (prednisolone 40 mg/day for 1 month) are indicated in patients with Maddrey's discriminant function ≥32 (MELD >21) in the absence of sepsis, hepatorenal syndrome, chronic hepatitis B infection and GI bleeding. Five patients will need to be treated with corticosteroids to prevent one death: this corresponds to an NNT (number needed to treat – see below) of 5. A fall in bilirubin at 7 days is highly predictive of survival in corticosteroid-treated patients and they should probably be stopped in patients whose bilirubin rises or remains static after 7 days.

Raised serum creatinine and older age are associated with reduced survival. Pentoxifylline (Trental), at a dose of 400 mg three times daily for 28 days, has been shown to be beneficial in reducing short-term mortality in patients with alcoholic hepatitis and Maddrey's discriminant function ≥32. Pentoxifylline is thought to reduce

the development of hepatorenal syndrome in these patients.

pentoxifylline

Pentoxifylline is a derivative of caffeine (a xanthine). It is a competitive, non-selective, phosphodiesterase inhibitor and an inhibitor of TNF-α synthesis (a proinflammatory cytokine), high levels of which are associated with the development of hepatorenal syndrome and poor prognosis.

Immediate and lifetime abstinence from alcohol is essential to prevent the progression to cirrhosis, at which stage damage to the liver is irreversible.

Transplantation is contraindicated in acute alcoholic hepatitis. People will be considered for liver transplantation only if they have not had alcohol for at least 3 months.

The NNT is an epidemiological measure that has been developed as an indicator of the effectiveness of a therapy. It is the number of patients who need to be treated to prevent one poor outcome. Thus, an NNT of 5 indicates that, for every five people who receive a given therapy, one adverse outcome will be prevented (or positive outcome achieved as a consequence). The NNT is the reciprocal of the absolute risk reduction (ARR), i.e. the amount that a therapy reduces the risk of an adverse outcome. Thus, an NNT of 5 corresponds to an ARR of 0.2 (NNT = 1/ARR).

EXTENDED LEARNING

- What are the common causes of liver disease and how is it managed?

- Describe the stages of progression of liver disease through fatty liver disease, hepatitis and cirrhosis. At what stage is damage considered irreversible?

- What screening tools are used in practice to diagnose liver disease?

- How does liver function influence prescribing decisions?

- How will you identify and provide advice to patients who may be at risk of liver disease?

References and further reading

National Institute for Health and Clinical Excellence (2010). *Alcohol-use Disorders – Preventing the development of hazardous and harmful drinking.* Public health guidance, 24. London: NICE. Available at: http://guidance.nice.org.uk/PH24 (accessed 07 October 2013).

North-Lewis P (2008). *Drugs and the Liver.* London: Pharmaceutical Press.

Case 6
Liver disease with ascites

RITA SHAH

LEARNING OUTCOMES

At the end of this case, you will be able to:

- List the signs and symptoms of liver disease
- Describe the drug pharmacokinetic and pharmacodynamic parameters that need to be considered in patients with liver disease
- Describe the management of patients with complications of liver disease

On examination

- Underweight
- Jaundiced
- Some bruises on arms
- ++ Ascites (excessive fluid in abdomen)
- Swollen ankles and feet
- Pruritis (itchy skin)
- No haematemis (vomiting of blood)

Case study

Mr BC is a 56-year-old man. Before admission to hospital, he was hearing voices (he was hearing his brother talking) and felt as though he was 'on another planet.' He did not know that there was anything wrong with him. The care workers in the hostel noticed that he was deteriorating and therefore admitted him to hospital.

CASE NOTES

Drinking history

- Been drinking alcohol for about 40 years
- Drank cheap cider – one bottle (about 2 L) at least once a day, sometimes more
- Stopped drinking now for about a year.

Social history

- Not worked for years
- Lives in a hostel

Past medical history

- Nil

Drug history

- Thiamine 200 mg once daily
- Vitamin B compound, strong, 1 tablet three times a day
- Smoker: used to smoke about 20–30 cigarettes each day until 5 years ago. Currently smokes about 10 cigarettes a day
- NKDA (no known drug allergies)

In view of long history of alcohol abuse Mr BC is diagnosed with alcohol-induced liver cirrhosis. He is now admitted because of decompensated liver disease.

❷ List the signs and symptoms of liver disease
❷ With what signs and symptoms does this patient present?

Mr BC has hepatic encephalopathy.

❷ What is hepatic encephalopathy?
❷ What are the precipitating factors?

▼ TABLE 1.5
Blood test results

Na$^+$	135 mmol/L
K$^+$	3.9 mmol/L
Urea	3.4 mmol/L
Creatinine	94 μmol/L
Albumin	30 g/L
Bilirubin (total)	150 μmol/L
AST	300 IU/L
GGT	800 IU/L
ALP	200 IU/L
Haemoglobin	10 g/dL
INR	1.78

❷ What is the treatment for hepatic encephalopathy? For each treatment option, describe the mechanism of action

❷ What monitoring criteria would you use to check if the treatment is working?

Mr BC has ascites.

❷ Why do liver failure patients develop ascites?

❷ What is the treatment for ascites? For each of the drugs, describe the mechanism of action

❷ What monitoring criteria would you use to check if the treatment is working?

Mr BC had an endoscopy, which showed that he has oesophageal varices (large dilated veins) for which he is prescribed propranolol at a usual dose of 40 mg three times a day.

❷ Why was he prescribed propranolol? Is this an appropriate dose for this patient? Give your reasons (hint: think about the pharmacokinetic profile of propranolol)

❷ What pharmacokinetic and pharmacodynamic parameters would one consider before prescribing a medicine to a patient with liver disease?

Case discussion

— Signs and symptoms of liver cirrhosis

Liver cirrhosis can arise from many causes including (Kennedy and O'Grady, 2002):

- Chronic alcohol abuse
- Viral hepatitis
- Autoimmune conditions, such as primary biliary cirrhosis
- Metabolic conditions, such as Wilson's disease, haemochromatosis.

Most patients with cirrhosis will have minimal symptoms. Patients could have symptoms such as general malaise, fatigue, anorexia and weight loss. However, decompensation of the liver (a precipitating factor that causes the cirrhotic liver to undergo stress and fail) will lead to the complications below. The main reason for decompensation is infection, but could also be GI bleeding, alcoholic hepatitis and prerenal failure due to use of diuretics.

Signs and symptoms include ascites (accumulation of body fluid in the abdomen), portal hypertension, oesophageal varices (swollen veins) and variceal bleeds, spontaneous bacterial peritonitis (SBP), jaundice and pruritus, hepatic encephalopathy, easy bruising and bleeding, deranged liver function tests.

Drug handling in liver disease

— Pharmacodynamic effects

Patients with liver disease are very sensitive to the effects and side effects of medicines, e.g.:

- Drugs that cause sedation: patients with liver disease are very sensitive to these drugs, which can lead to hepatic encephalopathy. Therefore, avoid these drugs.
- Drugs that cause GI ulceration: need to avoid or use such drugs with caution because liver patients are at higher risk of bleeding.
- Drugs that cause constipation: use such drugs cautiously because constipation can precipitate hepatic encephalopathy

— Pharmacokinetic parameters

Bioavailability of the drug: in liver disease, the bioavailability of the drug may reduce or increase depending on the nature of the drug and changes to the anatomy of the blood vessels, e.g. propranolol (a non-selective β-blocker prescribed to help reduce blood pressure in the portal vein, and thus reduce the risk of variceal bleeding), being lipid soluble, has a high first-pass metabolism. In patients with liver disease, the bioavailability of the drug is increased. The reason for this can be due to the liver's reduced metabolising power, or because of the formation of collateral circulation as a result of portal hypertension, which means that the drug bypasses the liver.

propranolol

The reason for propranolol's high lipid solubility is its low polarity. Propranolol is one of the least polar β-adrenergic antagonists. Although the drug contains a few electronegative atoms and highly polar O-H and N-H bonds, most of its structure consists of non-polar C-H and C-C bonds. Similar to many low-polarity drugs, propranolol is well absorbed after oral administration, but is then subject to extensive first-pass metabolism, because eventual elimination of low-polarity drugs depends first on metabolism to more polar metabolites. Hepatic clearance is often a feature of low-polarity drugs.

For other drugs, the bioavailability may reduce, e.g. for drugs that undergo enterohepatic circulation, this will be reduced in patients who have cholestasis (build-up of bile acids in the bloodstream, causing persistent skin itching), and this in turn means that the bioavailability of the drug will reduce. Absorption of lipid-soluble drugs will reduce in patients with cholestasis in whom the bile excretion into the duodenum is reduced. Bile salts solubilise fat which aids absorption from the GI tract.

Drug metabolism: it is extremely difficult to predict how drug metabolism is affected by liver cirrhosis. This is because LFTs do not tell us about the function of the liver. The only parameters that will tell us about the synthetic function of the liver are albumin and INR. Patients like Mr BC with low serum albumin (30 g/L; normal range: 35–50 g/L) and high INR (1.78; normal: 0.9–1.2) mean that the liver's synthetic function is low, so the metabolism of the drug may be affected. However, the degree to which it will be affected is not known. Therefore, it would be advisable to start medicines at low doses and monitor patients closely. Dose reduction is a common feature of low-polarity drugs when used in patients with hepatic impairment. Their ability to clear the drug from the systemic circulation can be reduced, potentially resulting in unwanted accumulation, an exaggerated biological response and increased adverse reactions. A 40-mg starting dose of propranolol is typical in portal hypertension secondary to liver disease.

Volume of distribution: in patients with liver disease the following parameters will affect the volume of distribution of the drug:

- Low albumin: for drugs that are highly protein bound, low serum albumin means higher free drug concentration and therefore increased clinical response. In reality, the clinical consequences may be negligible, but close monitoring of the drug is advisable.

- High bilirubin: high bilirubin (total) (Mr BC 150 μmol/L; normal range: 5–17 μmol/L) can displace the protein bound drug, resulting in higher free drug concentration. However, the clinical significance of this may be negligible although close monitoring of the drug is advisable.

- Ascites and peripheral oedema: this could affect the volume of distribution of some water-

soluble drugs because the drug will distribute in this third space. This could potentially be an issue, especially for drugs with a low narrow therapeutic index, e.g. gentamicin, and hence close monitoring is required.

- Low fat mass: this could affect the volume of distribution of drugs, such as lipid-soluble drugs, resulting in increased levels in the plasma. Therefore, for these drugs it would be advisable to start with low doses and monitor patients closely.

— **Management and treatment options for hepatic encephalopathy**

Hepatic encephalopathy is a neuropsychiatric complication of cirrhosis that could develop into a medical emergency and therefore require urgent hospitalisation (Blei and Cordoba, 2001). Increased ammonia levels in the plasma (due to reduced degradation in the liver) lead to increased brain ammonia levels – this is central in the pathogenesis of hepatic encephalopathy. The earliest manifestation is an altered sleep pattern, which eventually progresses to coma.

There is a grading system for hepatic encephalopathy (Blei and Cordoba, 2001):

- Grade 0: no overt neuropsychological symptoms
- Grade 1: short-term memory loss, difficulty in concentrating, reversal of sleep–wake cycle
- Grade 2: liver 'flap' (asterixis: involuntary jerking movements in the hands), daytime sleepiness, confusion, disorientation, slurred speech
- Grade 3: drowsy/asleep but rousable; airways at risk
- Grade 4: coma.

The goal of therapy is to reduce ammonia levels and is based on reducing its generation and absorption in the colon (Blei and Cordoba, 2001):

- Lactulose, which works by increasing the bowel movement through osmotic action. In the colon, lactulose is broken down into acetic acid and lactic acid, thereby creating an acidic environment. The ammonia produced by the bacteria will be converted to ammonium ions and there will be the incorporation of ammonia into bacterial protein, reducing plasma ammonia concentration.

- Other laxatives, such as sodium docusate, senna, phosphate enemas and glycerine suppositories work by stimulating the bowel movement through an increase in intestinal motility, thereby ensuring at least two bowel movements a day. In the case of docusate sodium, it also softens stools.

Treatment of ascites and the mechanism of action of drug therapy

— Management of ascites

Treatment of ascites includes the following:

- Salt restriction (60–90 mmol/day, equivalent to 1500–2000 mg salt/day) will shift the ascites and delay reaccumulation of fluid (Gines et al., 2004).
- Fluid restriction: fluid intake is restricted only if dilutional hyponatraemia is present (Gines et al., 2004).
- Diuretics: first line is spironolactone and the second-line drug is furosemide together with spironolactone (Kennedy and O'Grady, 2002). Aldosterone is a mineralocorticoid released by the adrenal cortex. Spironolactone works as an aldosterone receptor antagonist in the distal

convoluted tubules, enhancing salt and water excretion. Furosemide works as a loop diuretic at the ascending limb of loop of Henle, also enhancing salt and water excretion. It is important to start with low doses and to increase doses gradually. The aim of therapy is to reduce weight by 500 g to 1 kg/day.

EXTENDED LEARNING

- Distinguish between the terms pharmacodynamics and pharmacokinetics
- What are the modes of action of different classes of laxative?
- What are the recommended 'safe' limits for alcohol consumption?

References and further reading

Blei A, Cordoba J (2001). Hepatic encephalopathy. *Am J Gastroenterol* **96**:1968–76.

Gines P, Cardenas A, Arroyo V, Rodes J (2004). Management of cirrhosis and ascites. *N Engl J Med* **350**:1646–54.

Kennedy P, O'Grady J (2002). Diseases of the liver. Chronic liver disease. *Hospital Pharmacist* **9**:137–44.

Case 7
Management of paracetamol overdose with acetylcysteine

SARAH KNIGHTON

LEARNING OUTCOMES

At the end of the case, you will be able to:

- Describe the metabolism of paracetamol, how it causes liver damage in overdose and the factors that increase susceptibility to liver damage
- Understand the diagnosis of paracetamol overdose, signs and symptoms with which patients may present and key investigations
- Describe the treatment options for paracetamol overdose including the recommendations by the Medicines and Healthcare products Regulatory Agency (MHRA) on usage of intravenous acetylcysteine
- Discuss the calculation of the dosage of acetylcysteine, practical aspects of administration and potential adverse effects

Case study

Miss MP is a 25-year-old woman who is brought into the accident and emergency department by paramedics after an intentional paracetamol overdose at home. On admission she is awake and oriented. She admits feeling depressed after a recent break-up with her boyfriend and states that she has taken 30 paracetamol 500 mg tablets (total dose 15 g).

- What is the recommended therapeutic dose of paracetamol and what factors does it depend on?
- What doses of paracetamol may cause serious liver damage?
- How is paracetamol metabolised?
- What happens to paracetamol's metabolism when a patient takes an overdose?
- What factors may increase the risk of liver damage after an overdose of paracetamol?

On further questioning, Miss MP says that she took the paracetamol tablets about 6 hours ago. She took 30 tablets over approximately 15 minutes. She states that she has taken no other medication, drugs or alcohol. She has no past medical history, is on no regular medication and has no known drug or food allergies.

> **On examination**
>
> - Blood pressure: normal (122/78 mmHg)
> - Pulse rate 98 beats/min
> - Temperature 36.9°C
> - Weight 70 kg
> - She has vomited once at home and feels nauseous and tired

- What signs and symptoms of paracetamol overdose does Miss MP exhibit?
- What would you expect?
- What if she had presented to A&E later (e.g. 36 hours after the overdose)?
- Why is it important to know when and how the paracetamol was taken?
- What investigations (e.g. blood tests) would you expect to be performed at this stage?

Miss MP remains clinically stable. She is given an antiemetic to help with the nausea and intravenous fluids for hydration. It is decided that she is not appropriate for activated charcoal treatment.

- What does activated charcoal do and when may it be useful in management of paracetamol overdose?

Results from blood tests taken on admission become available. A serum paracetamol level, taken at 6 hours post-overdose, is reported as 90 mg/L. Liver and kidney function tests and full blood count are reported as normal. Her clinical observations remain stable.

- How can the paracetamol level be interpreted?
- What guidance is available for the treatment of paracetamol overdose and where can this be accessed?

It is decided to start her on intravenous acetylcysteine treatment. The nurse is unfamiliar with this treatment and wants to ask you some questions.

- What is acetylcysteine and how does it work in the treatment of paracetamol overdose?
- How is the dose calculated and what treatment regimen would you recommend for this patient?
- How is acetylcysteine administered?
- What are the potential adverse effects?
- How will Miss MP be monitored both during and after treatment?

Miss MP tolerates the acetylcysteine treatment well and completes the recommended treatment course. She is discharged from hospital after 4 days.

Case discussion

— Paracetamol: recommended dosage and toxicity

Paracetamol is a low-cost, popular and widely available mild analgesic used alone for minor aches and pains, headaches, and symptomatic treatment of cold and flu symptoms, or in combination with more powerful analgesics such as opiates (codeine, dihydrocodeine) for management of more severe postoperative pain or in palliative cancer care. Unfortunately, in view of its wide availability, it is the drug most commonly taken in overdose suicide attempts. The recommended therapeutic dose of paracetamol is dependent on age and in some circumstances also weight and concurrent clinical conditions (e.g. malnutrition or hepatocellular insufficiency). The most current dosage recommendations can be obtained from the *British National Formulary* (*BNF*) or the summary of product characteristics. It is important to refer to these regularly because recommendations can change. The current recommended oral dose of paracetamol for an adult is 0.5–1 g every 4–6 h (up to a maximum dose of 4 g [8 tablets] in any 24-hour period).

Paracetamol is a safe and effective analgesic and antipyretic when taken at recommended therapeutic doses. However, in overdose it can cause irreversible liver damage and death and this is a leading cause of acute liver failure in the UK. Single or repeated doses of paracetamol totalling as little as 10–15 g (20–30 tablets) or 150 mg/kg taken within 24 hours may cause serious liver damage. For patients considered at higher risk of liver damage (see below), this can be as low as approximately 5 g (10 tablets) or 75 mg/kg.

— **Paracetamol: metabolic pathways, mechanism of liver damage and potential risk factors**

At therapeutic doses, paracetamol is mainly metabolised by conjugation (*O*-glucuronidation and *O*-sulphonation) to form inactive paracetamol conjugates. These conjugation reactions produce highly polar, readily excreted metabolites. A minor route is oxidation by CYP450 enzymes to form the reactive metabolite *N*-acetyl-*p*-benzoquinoneimine (NAPQI). This is subsequently conjugated by glutathione to form a non-toxic, highly polar metabolite.

When excessive doses of paracetamol are taken (overdose) then the major conjugation route of metabolism becomes saturated. Therefore oxidation by CYP450 becomes more significant and is used to metabolise the excessive paracetamol. This leads to the formation of excessive amounts of NAPQI. Although glutathione conjugates some NAPQI, this pathway also becomes saturated. The excess NAPQI therefore starts to bind to sulfhydryl groups in cellular proteins, causing cell damage and inflammation, which then leads to liver damage.

The extent of liver damage is affected by the rate of NAPQI formation and the availability of glutathione. NAPQI formation can be accelerated when enzyme induction occurs. Long-term treatment with enzyme-inducing drugs, such as carbamazepine, phenytoin or rifampicin is thought to increase the risk of paracetamol-induced liver damage. It is therefore important to obtain an accurate medication history for all patients presenting with paracetamol overdose. Regular consumption of excessive alcohol also causes enzyme induction.

Availability of glutathione depends on nutritional status. Those with a high chance of glutathione depletion (and thus increased risk of liver damage) include those who are malnourished due to an underlying medical condition or recent fasting, or who have an eating disorder or chronic alcoholism.

— **Presentation, signs and symptoms of paracetamol overdose**

Patients who have taken an overdose often present for treatment within a few hours. At this early stage they tend to be asymptomatic or exhibit relatively non-specific symptoms such as nausea, vomiting and fatigue. Often LFTs will appear normal. Evidence of hepatotoxicity is often delayed and there is a danger that patients may be discharged without appropriate treatment, which could be potentially fatal.

— **Timing of ingestion and presentation to A&E**

Patients who present after 24 hours may start to show signs of severe liver damage, such as right upper quadrant tenderness, jaundice and impaired consciousness. Serum hepatic aminotransferase levels can increase significantly. Serum bilirubin and INR can also rise. Severe liver necrosis and liver failure can occur 48–96 hours post-overdose.

Key investigations to be performed include a timed serum paracetamol level, assessment of liver function, clotting (including INR) and renal function.

— **Paracetamol levels and their interpretation**

It is important to know how many paracetamol tablets were taken, over what time period and the timing of the overdose. Some patients may take all the paracetamol tablets over a very short time period. Other patients may, either deliberately or inadvertently, take them over a longer period of time (1 hour or more). This is known as a 'staggered overdose'. Knowing the details about the timing of ingestion helps to determine a treatment plan.

Where possible, a timed serum paracetamol level is taken. This is usually taken between 4 and 15 hours post-ingestion and can then be interpreted using a treatment nomogram. Serum levels taken earlier than 4 hours cannot be interpreted, because absorption is not complete. Levels taken after 15 hours are also difficult to interpret due to the potential effect of liver damage.

— Activated charcoal in the management of paracetamol overdose

Activated charcoal is highly porous charcoal that consequently has a very high surface area. This large surface area will adsorb drug in the stomach, preventing absorption lower in the GI tract. The sooner it is given after ingestion of the material to be adsorbed the better. Adsorption is the increase in concentration of a material at an interface (here solid/liquid), compared with the concentration in the bulk. In the case of poisoning or overdose, the drug (adsorbate) is concentrated at the surface of the charcoal (adsorbent). Binding between the adsorbant and adsorbate may be chemical or physical. In paracetamol poisoning, activated charcoal should be considered only if the drug has been ingested in the previous hour, which is not the case here.

— Acetylcysteine and the treatment nomogram

Acetylcysteine is the antidote used to treat paracetamol overdose. It spares (and indirectly replenishes) glutathione stores, acting as a sulfhydryl (-SH) donor, binding NAPQI and forming a non-toxic NAPQI conjugate (see metabolic scheme above). It is virtually 100% effective at preventing liver damage if given *within 8 hours of overdose*. After this time, efficacy reduces and therefore there is a limited time window in which to administer it to successfully prevent serious liver damage.

The decision to treat with acetylcysteine is based on assessment of risk of serious liver damage. For patients who are able to have a timed serum paracetamol level checked within the appropriate time period, the treatment nomogram should be used to assess this risk. If the reported serum paracetamol level appears on or above the treatment line, then the patient should receive treatment. A treatment nomogram is published by the MHRA and is available in the *BNF*.

For patients in whom there is doubt over the timing of ingestion or timing is not known, or for those who have taken a 'staggered overdose' treatment should be started with intravenous acetylcysteine straight away and the nomogram should not be used.

For patients who present late after paracetamol overdose (>24 hours) it is recommended that the National Poisons Information service be contacted for advice.

— Acetylcysteine administration

Acetylcysteine is given intravenously as three sequential infusions. The dose for each infusion is calculated using the patient's body weight. Current recommendations are as follows:

First infusion: 150 mg/kg in 200 mL 5% glucose over 1 hour
Second infusion: 50 mg/kg in 500 mL 5% glucose over 4 hours
Third infusion: 100 mg/kg in 1000 mL 5% glucose over 16 hours

Adverse effects of acetylcysteine include nausea. Anaphylaxis can also occur, which is mediated by mast cell histamine release and related to serum acetylcysteine concentrations. It is recommended that the first dose be administered over 1 hour to reduce the risk of reaction. If a reaction occurs, this can be treated by temporarily interrupting the acetylcysteine treatment and giving symptomatic relief (e.g. with an antihistamine, nebulised salbutamol or steroids if required). The acetylcysteine can then be recommenced, possibly at a slower rate of infusion.

— Advice to patients on the safe use of paracetamol-containing products

Paracetamol is considered a safe product when used appropriately and dose recommendations are followed, but it is very dangerous in overdose. Many patients may not be aware that a relatively small number of extra tablets can lead to serious problems. Patients who intentionally overdose may be aware that they are inflicting self-harm, but not that this might be life-threatening. Inadvertent overdose also occurs. Paracetamol is the sole active ingredient or an active component of many non-prescription products that people buy in a pharmacy or other retail outlets. Patients need to be alert to the ingredients and aware that they could be taking higher doses of paracetamol than they realise. Care is required to ensure that storage is not accessible to young children.

A warning not to exceed the maximum recommended single and daily dose is a requirement for all paracetamol-containing products. Also, in the UK general sales of paracetamol products are now legally restricted to small pack sizes (16 tablets).

EXTENDED LEARNING

- Describe the basic anatomy and function of the liver
- Outline the classification and types of liver disease
- How is liver function assessed? How are the results of liver function tests interpreted?
- What is the difference between absorption and adsorption?
- Describe the causes and measurement of surface phenomena, such as adsorption at interfaces, wetting and surface tension

ADDITIONAL PRACTICE POINTS

- Be aware of over-the-counter products containing paracetamol. What is the role of pharmacists and pharmacy staff in reducing the potential for paracetamol poisoning?

References and further reading

Drug Safety Update. September 2012, vol 6, issue 2:A1. Available at: www.mhra.gov.uk/home/groups/dsu/documents/publication/con185631.pdf (accessed 22 July 2014).

Ferner R, Dear J, Bateman D (2011). Management of paracetamol poisoning. *BMJ* **342**:d2218.

North-Lewis P, ed. (2008). *Drugs and the Liver – A guide to drug handling in liver dysfunction*. London: Pharmaceutical Press.

Pettie J, Dow M (2013). Assessment and management of paracetamol poisoning in adults. *Nurs Stand* **27**(45):39–47.

Prescott LF (2001) *Paracetamol (Acetaminophen): A critical bibliographic review*, 2nd edn. London: Taylor & Francis.

— Resources

British National Formulary December 2012. Available at: www.medicinescomplete.com/mc/bnf/current (accessed January 2013).

eMC. *Summary of product characteristics*. Parvolex 200 mg/ml solution for infusion. Available at: www.medicines.org.uk/emc/medicine/1127 (accessed 20 September 2013).

MHRA webpage on new guidance for treatment of paracetamol overdose with acetylcysteine. Available at: www.mhra.gov.uk/Safetyinformation/Safetywarningsalertsandrecalls/Safetywarningsandmessagesformedicines/CON178225 (accessed 30 July 2014).

Case 8
Chronic kidney disease

RANIA BETMOUNI AND JEREMY LEVY

LEARNING OUTCOMES

At the end of this case, you will be able to:

- Describe the causes of chronic kidney disease
- Recognise the signs and symptoms of chronic kidney disease
- Identify methods for assessment of renal function and their pitfalls
- Describe the type and rationale for medicines use in chronic kidney diseases
- Describe the chemistry and mechanism of action of furosemide

Case study

Mrs CK is a 65-year-old Asian woman with chronic kidney disease. Her past medical history includes type 2 diabetes and hypertension. Recently, she has been complaining of nausea, tiredness and pruritus, and an increasing shortness of breath.

Over the last few months she has noticed increased ankle swelling.

- What are the most common causes of chronic kidney disease?
- What is the most likely cause in this case?
- What are the classic symptoms of chronic kidney disease?
- Explain the classification/staging of chronic kidney disease and what the advantages of this system are
- How would you assess Mrs CK's kidney function?

A month later Mrs CK is admitted to hospital unwell and grossly oedematous. She was started on high-dose furosemide 250 mg twice a day.

- What sort of drug is furosemide and what is its mode of action?
- Draw the structure of furosemide. Is the drug an acid or a base?

Intravenous administration of furosemide is by slow intravenous infusion. Would dextrose saline (about pH 4) or physiological saline (about pH 5.5) be most suitable for the infusion?

Explain the rationale for using furosemide. How would you monitor Mrs CK while she is taking furosemide?

You see Mrs CK on your ward and she has been prescribed metformin, gliclazide, amlodipine, ferrous sulfate, aspirin and simvastatin. She has a blood pressure of 165/85 mmHg and her blood results are as shown in Table 1.6.

▼ TABLE 1.6
Blood results for Mrs CK

Na^+	137 mmol/L	HCO_3^-	18 mmol/L
K^+	5.2 mmol/L	PO_4^{3-}	2.3 mmol/L
Urea	18.5 mmol/L	Corrected Ca^{2+}	2.1 mmol/L
Creatinine	220 μmol/L	Glucose	10.8 mmol/L
eGFR	21 mL/min per 1.73 m^2	Hb	9.8 g/dL

Urinalysis: protein 3+
Urine protein : creatinine ratio: 220 mg/mmol
eGFR, estimated glomerular filtration rate.

What would you advise when reviewing her medicines? What alternatives, if any, would you recommend and why?

The team are keen to prescribe an erythropoiesis-stimulating agent (ESA) in view of her anaemia.

Explain the rationale for using ESAs. What advice would you give when starting ESA treatment and what would you monitor?

Mrs CK is also prescribed a phosphate binder.

What are the advantages and disadvantages of each of the phosphate binders currently available?

Case discussion

— Incidence, prevalence and classification of chronic kidney disease

Chronic kidney disease (CKD) is usually asymptomatic in the early stages but, when advanced, it carries a high risk of morbidity and mortality. Morbidity of a disease can be expressed as incidence or prevalence. The *incidence* refers to the number of new cases in a defined population in a specified period, often a year. The incidence rate is calculated by dividing the number of new cases in the specified period by the total population. The *prevalence* is the number of cases at any one time in a defined population. The *mortality rate* is the ratio of the total number of deaths from one or any cause, in a year, to the number of people in the population. Latest figures reported a diagnosed prevalence rate of 4.3% of the population aged >18 years in England, who had stages 3–5 CKD. However, total prevalence is considered to be higher due to a substantial number of undiagnosed cases. Obtaining accurate prevalence rates can be difficult due to different sources of data being used to identify the number of new and pre-existing cases (such as hospital data, primary care registers), and these do not account for undiagnosed cases.

CKD is defined as a progressive and irreversible loss of kidney function. A five-stage classification system (stages 1–5) for CKD has been widely adopted. This is based on the four-variable Modification of Diet in Renal Disease (MDRD) equation, which calculates an estimated glomerular filtration rate (eGFR) based on serum creatinine, age, sex and race.

The aim of the classification system is to identify patients in stage 3 (and later) CKD (GFR 30–59 mL/min per 1.73 m^2, or worse), ensure early referral to a nephrologist where appropriate, or better management of CKD and management of vascular risk factors in primary care. Most management of CKD is about preventing cardiovascular events, such as stroke and cardiac disease, but also preventing further decline in renal function.

— Causes of kidney disease

The major causes of CKD are diabetes, hypertension, chronic glomerulonephritis, renal vascular disease and polycystic disease. Acute kidney injury can occur from a wider variety of insults, including prerenal factors (volume depletion, hypotension) causing a reduction in the perfusion of the kidneys, intrinsic renal disease such as damage to tubules (acute tubular necrosis or acute interstitial nephritis) or glomerulus (acute glomerulonephritis), and finally postrenal factors resulting in obstruction of urine flow (e.g. prostate disease, bladder tumours). It is important to remember that medication can also contribute to prerenal, renal and (less commonly) postrenal causes of kidney failure. Distinguishing acute from chronic kidney injury is always important and patients with CKD are also more likely to get acute kidney injury.

— **Signs and symptoms of CKD**

Patients with CKD may present at a time of an acute deterioration of kidney function: acute-on-chronic kidney disease. In stage 3 CKD, most patients are completely asymptomatic but may have hypertension, and are usually diagnosed after abnormal blood tests or urine analysis. In stage 4 CKD (eGFR 15–29 mL/min per 1.73 m^2) patients may present with extrarenal symptoms, such as ankle swelling, shortness of breath, tiredness, fatigue and anaemia. Many patients will still remain asymptomatic even at this stage. In stage 5 CKD (eGFR <15 mL/min per 1.73 m^2) most patients will present with uraemic symptoms, such as nausea and vomiting, weight loss, pruritus and general malaise.

— **Assessment of kidney function**

The GFR is a measure of excretory kidney function (how well the kidneys 'clean' the blood and get rid of waste products). GFR is ideally calculated by measuring the clearance of a substance that is freely filtered, neither secreted nor reabsorbed in the tubules. Inulin or radioisotopes (EDTA) have been used as exogenous markers, but routine use is cumbersome. Equations have therefore been developed to estimate renal function using serum creatinine as an easier measure.

Serum creatinine itself is not an accurate predictor of kidney function. If the baseline is low, it can double (e.g. 60–120 μmol/L) and still be within normal range, and yet the renal function has deteriorated. Kidney function declines with age, but this change is not reflected in serum creatinine. Gender, race, dietary protein intake and muscle mass all affect serum creatinine.

The Cockcroft–Gault formula estimates creatinine clearance (CrCl), which approximates GFR. As creatinine is secreted as well as filtered, CrCl does overestimate GFR:

$$CrCl = \frac{[F \times (140 - age) \times \text{weight in kg}]}{\text{serum creatinine}}$$

where $F = 1.04$ in females and 1.23 in males.

The MDRD equation has been shown to provide a more accurate estimate of GFR than the Cockcroft–Gault formula. It is based on four variables: the patient's age, gender, race and serum creatinine; it is expressed as mL/min per 1.73 m^2, normalised for body surface area. Both equations have their own limitations and it is important to understand which equation is being used to assess renal function. Both are based on serum creatinine, which is affected especially by muscle mass and nutritional status, and can be affected by drugs. For adjustment of drug doses in renal impairment, the Cockcroft–Gault formula, which gives an estimate of GFR, not normalised for body size, is preferred.

— **Prescribing in kidney disease**

In kidney disease, pharmacokinetic and pharmacodynamic changes will alter how drugs are handled in the body. If a drug (or its metabolites) is cleared by the kidney, accumulation will occur, resulting in increased toxicity. The volume of distribution (V_d) of a drug can change in CKD. The patient's fluid status is likely to have an impact on drugs with a small V_d. CKD patients may be uraemic or malnourished, or have high protein loss affecting V_d of protein-bound drugs, resulting in increased free/unbound drug. The mechanism/site of action of drugs is important.

— **Chemistry and pH solubility of furosemide and implications for practice**

Furosemide is an acidic drug. It contains a carboxylic acid functional group that has a pK_a of 3.9. The nitrogen of the sulfonamide is not basic because it does not have a lone pair of electrons available to accept a proton (sulfonamides are in fact often weak acids). The remaining (secondary amino group) nitrogen is an extremely weak base (its lone pair is partly delocalised over the aromatic ring), and will not behave as a base under the conditions of pH found in the body.

furosemide

For an acidic drug, the higher the pH, the greater the proportion of drug that will be deprotonated and therefore negatively charged. We therefore expect acidic drugs to be more soluble at high pH values, because a greater proportion will be in the charged and highly polar form. In dextrose saline at pH 4, approximately 50% of a dose of furosemide will be protonated (-COOH) and 50% deprotonated (-COO$^-$). The 50% (125 mg in this case) that is protonated (uncharged) is unlikely to dissolve fully in the infusion solution, presenting a significant danger if administered intravenously. In physiological saline at pH 5.5, around 98% of a dose of furosemide will be deprotonated (charged) and only 2% will be protonated (uncharged). Solubility will be considerably better at pH 5.5 in physiological saline. The very small uncharged proportion (2% is 5 mg in this case) is very likely to dissolve in the large volume of the infusion. The proportion of furosemide that will be charged at any given pH can be calculated using the Henderson–Hasselbalch equation (see example calculation in the extended learning points at the end of the case). This equation relates the ratio of deprotonated : protonated drug to the difference between pH and pK_a.

Loop diuretics such as furosemide are so called because they exert their principal action on the luminal side of the thick ascending loop of Henle in the kidneys where the Na$^+$/K$^+$/2Cl$^-$ symporter (co-transporter) is located, and, in so doing, they inhibit the absorption of Na$^+$ (and consequently water) from the filtered luminal fluid. Normally about 25% of urine Na$^+$ is reabsorbed at this position, so a drug that inhibits transport here would be expected to show a relatively powerful diuretic effect. The increased delivery of unabsorbed Na$^+$ to the distal convoluted segment of the distal tubule now stimulates the aldosterone-sensitive Na$^+$/K$^+$ ATPase transporter and Na$^+$/H$^+$ exchanger, resulting in excessive loss of K$^+$ and H$^+$ in the urine, which can lead to hypokalaemia and metabolic alkalosis.

Thiazide diuretics, such as bendroflumethiazide, on the other hand, inhibit the Na$^+$/Cl$^-$ co-transporter in the distal convoluted tubule, where only about 5% of filtered Na$^+$ is normally absorbed. Hence, this class of diuretic is less effective than loop diuretics in producing urinary Na$^+$ loss and diuresis.

Furosemide acts on the luminal side of the tubule and reaches the site of action by glomerular filtration. As the GFR decreases, higher doses of furosemide will be required. Loop diuretics are used in preference to thiazides, as thiazides become ineffective once the GFR <25 mL/min.

The furosemide will help manage Mrs CK's oedema, but she will need a high dose given her significantly reduced GFR. While on furosemide, it is important that Mrs CK is monitored closely to avoid her becoming dehydrated and precipitating acute or chronic renal failure. Her weight, urine output, blood pressure, serum creatinine, fluid balance and serum potassium should be monitored closely (daily probably).

— **Reviewing current medication**
As Mrs CK's eGFR is 21 mL/min per 1.73 m^2 her metformin should be stopped. Although metformin use is contraindicated in patients with GFR <60 mL/min, it is used in patients with mild renal impairment (30–50 mL/min) but at a reduced dose of 500 mg twice daily. However, in severe renal impairment it should not be used because there is a risk of lactic acidosis. Mrs CK's diabetic management should be monitored closely and adjusted. Her gliclazide dose could be increased if her blood glucose levels become significantly increased or a second oral hypoglycaemic agent could be added. Blood sugars should be monitored closely to avoid hypoglycaemic episodes.

Management of hypertension in CKD can delay the progression of kidney disease and reduce cardiovascular risk. The threshold for treatment is 140/90 mmHg, aiming for a target of 130/80 mmHg. In the presence of proteinuria, tighter blood pressure control is advocated. Proteinuria is the presence of albumin in urine detected by urine dipstick analysis. This is followed up by laboratory testing of protein (or albumin) : creatinine ratio (PCR) and increased levels make progression of kidney disease more likely

Angiotensin-converting enzyme (ACE) inhibitors and angiotensin receptor blockers (ARBs) have been shown to reduce proteinuria and are first choice agents in treating hypertension in CKD patients, irrespective of their diabetic history. Both have been shown to reduce the progression of kidney failure and lower cardiovascular mortality. The best evidence is in patients with diabetes, but also in others with proteinuria from other causes.

The amlodipine should be switched to ramipril (an ACE inhibitor) only if the patient's serum potassium has come down from its initial high level. However, when initiating an ACE inhibitor, consider the presence of renal artery stenosis and history of renovascular disease in patients. In addition, repeat blood creatinine and electrolyte measurements should be taken and compared with baseline results after 2–3 weeks. It is usual for the creatinine to rise slightly, but treatment with ACE inhibitors and ARBs should be stopped if there is an increase in serum creatinine >20% or reduction in eGFR >15%.

Serum potassium should be closely monitored. Both ACE inhibitors and ARBs can cause hyperkalaemia. Mrs CK is on a high-dose furosemide, which should (by promoting K^+ loss) help to control the hyperkalaemia. Other causes of hyperkalaemia (e.g. metabolic acidosis) should be investigated and corrected: prescribing oral sodium bicarbonate often improves potassium balance and may reduce the progression of CKD.

— **Management of anaemia and ESAs**

Anaemia in CKD is a common complication brought about by low production of the hormone erythropoietin (EPO) by the kidney. EPO is responsible for the production of red blood cells, needed to carry oxygen and haemoglobin. Anaemia of CKD can be corrected using synthetic EPO, such as short-acting erythropoietin-α, -β, -ζ and longer-acting agents such as darbepoietin and methoxypolyethylene glycol-epoetin β.

Before initiating ESA therapy, other factors contributing to anaemia should be investigated and corrected. These include iron deficiency anaemia, and often CKD patients will require a course of intravenous iron alongside (or before starting) ESA therapy. Iron is usually given intravenously because the absorption of orally administered iron is impaired in CKD. ESA therapy is started when Hb concentration <10–11 g/dL and the patient is symptomatic, and the recommended target is 11–12.5 g/dL.

Haemoglobin and serum ferritin are monitored regularly (e.g. *every 1–3* months) during therapy.

— **Renal bone disease**

Serum phosphate, calcium and parathyroid hormone levels are regulated through feedback mechanisms. Tight control of these parameters is essential in the management of renal bone disease, avoiding complications, such as soft-tissue and vascular calcification. Keeping serum phosphate

<1.8 and calcium in the normal range is important (see UK Renal Association Guidelines).

As Mrs CK's GFR <30 mL/min per 1.73 m², phosphate excretion is reduced and accumulation begins. Her phosphate is elevated at 2.3 mmol/L and a phosphate binder is indicated. Mrs CK's calcium is at the lower end of normal at 2.1 mmol/L. This should be monitored closely before replacing with active vitamin D: calcitriol or alfacalcidol.

Aluminium hydroxide is the most potent phosphate binder. Concern about aluminium toxicity has, however, severely limited its use. Calcium-containing binders are the most widely used. They are effective binders, but there is a risk of hypercalcaemia contributing to vascular calcification. Newer agents such as sevelamer (an anion-exchange resin) and lanthanum carbonate (a non-aluminium/non-calcium phosphate binder) are equally effective binders, but are more expensive. The results of studies looking at the effects of sevelamer on vascular calcification and cardiovascular outcomes have been mixed.

— **Lifestyle modification and adherence**

Both lifestyle and adherence are equally important in the management of CKD. Stopping smoking, reducing alcohol intake, reducing weight and increasing exercise will have a positive impact on hypertension, diabetes management, proteinuria and cardiovascular risk. Compliance with the medication regimen is equally important. Mrs CK will have received lots of information about new dietary restrictions (low-potassium, low-phosphate and if needed low-salt diets) and new medicines. It is essential to work with Mrs CK to develop a plan that suits her in managing these new changes and to optimise her compliance. Clear explanation of the value and importance of her medications will be crucial especially because most will not change any symptoms.

EXTENDED LEARNING

- Describe the basic structure and function of the kidney
- What are the major complications of CKD?
- Compare the signs and symptoms of CKD with those of acute kidney injury
- What are the main classes of diuretic drugs, and what is their mechanism of action?

- How are diuretics used therapeutically and what are their major side effects?
- What are haemodialysis and intraperitoneal dialysis? What are their major advantages and disadvantages?
- The Henderson–Hasselbalch equation:

Example calculation from above (at pH 5.5):

$$pH = pK_a + \log \frac{[\text{Deprotonated}]}{[\text{Protonated}]}$$

So $\dfrac{[\text{Deprot}]}{[\text{Prot}]} = 10^{(pH-pK_a)} = 10^{(5.5-3.9)} = 39.8$

Hence [Deprot] = 39.8 [Prot]

For percentages, [Prot] + [Deprot] = 100

So [Prot] + 39.8 [Prot] = 100

and therefore 40.8 [Prot] = 100

Then [Prot] = 2.5% and [Deprot] = 97.5%

References and further reading

Ashley C, Morlidge C, eds (2008). *Introduction to Renal Therapeutics*. London: Pharmaceutical Press.

James M, Hemmelgarn BR, Tonelli M (2010). Early recognition and prevention of chronic kidney disease. *Lancet* 375:1296–309.

Lewis R (2012) *Understanding Chronic Kidney Disease: A guide for the non-specialist*. Keswick: M& K Publishing.

National Institute for Health and Clinical Excellence (2008). *Chronic Kidney Disease*. NICE Clinical Guideline 73. London: NICE. Available at: www.nice.org.uk/cg73 (accessed 2 July 2013).

Steddon S, Sharples E (2010). *UK Renal Association Guidelines. CKD-Mineral and Bone Disorders (CKD-MBD)*. Available at: www.renal.org/guidelines/modules/ckd-mineral-and-bone-disorders#sthash.pt7BSyDF.dpbs (accessed 8 April 2014).

Case 9
Haemofiltration

MARK TOMLIN

LEARNING OUTCOMES

At the end of this case, you will be able to:

- Describe the principles and determinants of urine output, the effect that some drugs have on urine output and how they are affected by it
- Understand the link between cardiac and renal output and the indirect influence of drugs that alter cardiac performance
- Calculate cardiac output and creatinine clearance
- Describe the different processes of haemofiltration and dialysis and give an example of how they will modify drug clearance

Case study

Mr AM is a 65-year-old retired plumber who was admitted for a cardiac angiogram that shows partial occlusion or stenosis of four cardiac arteries. These narrowings are unsuitable for cardiac stenting so he is admitted to hospital for coronary artery bypass grafting (CABG).

Ten years ago, he was diagnosed with hypertension, which is currently controlled by ramipril and bendroflumethiazide. He is obese (height 5 feet 10 inches or 1.78 m) with an actual body weight (ABW) of 110 kg. He is also taking low-dose aspirin and simvastatin.

❓ Why is he taking his current medication?
❓ Describe how his current medication works
❓ What are the renal effects of ramipril?

Renal perfusion represents a quarter of the cardiac output. Cardiac surgery shocks the heart in a similar way to acute myocardial infarction (AMI). Mr AM is about to have an operation in which his coronary artery stenoses will be bypassed using a section of saphenous vein that has been removed from his leg. It is a major operation and the anaesthetist assesses the risks by discussing his medical history and noting some biochemical results such as his preoperative serum creatinine, which was 100 µmol/L (normal: 45–90 µmol/L).

❷ What is his ideal body weight, excess body weight, dose-defining weight and calculated creatinine clearance preoperation?

During theatre, the patient is put on a cardiopulmonary bypass (CPB) machine which takes over the pumping effect of the heart and the oxygenating effect of the lungs. The heart is arrested to allow the vascular surgery to be undertaken. At the end of surgery the heart must be re-stimulated and adrenaline and dobutamine infusions are started to improve the cardiac output sufficient to withdraw CPB and remove the ventilator tube (extubation). The patient develops a cardiac arrhythmia called atrial fibrillation (AF), which can reduce cardiac output.

❷ What is normal cardiac output?
❷ What is the pharmacology of adrenaline and dobutamine?
❷ How would giving an intravenous infusion of fluid help this patient?
❷ What drugs can inhibit renal output and why?

After surgery the patient's urine output has decreased to <30 mL/h and his serum creatinine has risen to 400 μmol/L. His creatinine clearance is now a quarter of its previous value (20.9 mL/min). An artificial renal replacement machine is started to support his kidneys and remove fluid and toxins from carbohydrate metabolism. This is called haemofiltration and is used for acute renal dysfunction or failure. The filter has a pore size that will allow the passage of solutes with a molecular weight <70 000 Da, just like the renal glomerulus. In many ways, haemofiltration more closely resembles normal kidney function than haemodialysis. Haemodialysis is usually used for chronic renal failure.

❷ How does haemofiltration differ from haemodialysis?

On recovery, the patient develops a sternal wound infection and the microbiologist recommends vancomycin and gentamicin. As the clinical pharmacist, you are asked to recommend a dosing regimen.

❷ What principles will be relevant?
❷ What differences, if any, can you predict between the way these drugs are handled by haemodialysis and haemofiltration?

Case discussion

— Current medication

Mr AM, presenting in this case, takes ramipril, bendroflumethiazide, low-dose aspirin and simvastatin.

Ramipril is an ACEI, licensed for hypertension, which also aids cardiac remodelling. Hypertension is a risk factor for AMI. Antihypertensive vasodilators may divert blood away from the kidneys or reduce renal perfusion pressure. This is called renal 'steal'. Ramipril is a vasodilator and may produce renal steal, especially if there is any renal artery stenosis (RAS). ACE is responsible for converting the inactive circulating precursor angiotensin I (formed through the renin–angiotensin hormone system) to angiotensin II (ATII), which then stimulates production of the mineralocorticoid hormone aldosterone from the adrenal cortex (zona glomerulosa) and therefore promotes Na^+/water retention and an increase in blood volume. ATII also has a powerful direct vasoconstrictor effect on blood vessels; ACEIs counteract these effects. If ramipril reduces afterload, it may enhance cardiac output and renal perfusion and therefore indirectly increase urine output. If there is no RAS, this effect predominates.

Bendroflumethiazide is a thiazide diuretic also licensed for hypertension, but no longer recommended as a first-line antihypertensive agent, ACEIs and calcium channel blocking agents being preferred.

Aspirin at subanalgesic doses (low dose: typically 75 mg daily – a quarter of a regular strength aspirin) is an antiplatelet agent given prophylactically for secondary MI prevention. It upsets the balance between thromboxane A_2 and prostacyclin (epoprostenol), thereby reducing platelet adhesion.

Simvastatin is a cholesterol-lowering agent that acts through inhibition of hydroxymethylglutaryl coenzyme-A reductase (HMG-CoAR) – a key enzyme in cholesterol biosynthesis. High cholesterol is another risk factor for AMI.

Calculating creatinine clearance for this patient

To calculate Mr AM's creatinine clearance, the Cockcroft–Gault formula is used, using his actual body weight (ABW) of 110 kg and his height, 5 feet and 10 inches.

Ideal body weight (IBW) for a male is given by:

$$IBW = 50 + (2.5 \times \text{inches over 5 feet})$$

So IBW = $50 + (2.5 \times 10) = 75$ kg

Excess body weight (EBW) = ABW − IBW

So EWB = $110 - 75 = 35$ kg

The dose-defining weight (DDW) is equal to the ideal body weight plus 40% of the excess body weight:

DDW = $75 + (0.4 \times 35) = 89$ kg

Using the Cockcroft and Gault formula to calculate creatinine clearance (CrCl):

$$CrCl = \frac{[(140 - \text{age}) \times \text{weight}]}{\text{serum creatinine}} \times 1.25$$

$$CrCl = \frac{[(140 - 65) \times 89]}{100} \times 1.25$$

Creatinine clearance = 83.4 mL/min

What is normal cardiac output?

A normal stroke volume (SV) might be 70 mL out of a ventricular volume (capacity) of 100 mL. This gives an ejection fraction of 0.7. A normal heart rate (HR) might be 70 beats/min. Cardiac output (CO) is the product of SV and HR = $70 \times 70 = 4900$ mL/min. Thus, normal cardiac output is about 5 L/min. In this case, Mr AM's cardiac output is 2.8 L/min and is therefore low. The CO can be increased by increasing SV or HR. Increasing HR in this patient will predispose to arrhythmias.

Adrenaline (the natural sympathetic hormone released from the adrenal medulla) is an agonist at adrenergic α-, β_1- and β_2-receptors.

- α_1-Agonists produce peripheral vasoconstriction and therefore raise blood pressure
- β_1-Agonists produce positive cardiac inotropy – an increase in the ventricular SV and contractility of heart muscle
- β_2-Agonists produce skeletal muscle arteriolar *vasodilatation* and chronotropy; this *decreases* blood pressure, enhances perfusion and increases HR.

Dobutamine might be preferred as a cardiotonic agent to increase SV and therefore CO. This would be less arrhythmogenic than adrenaline.

Hypovolaemia (significant decrease in blood volume) after surgery is one of the primary causes of AF in the perioperative period. This is because a low blood volume will reduce venous return

(VR) to the heart, and the heart compensates by increasing HR. VR is the maximum CO possible: restoring normovolaemia could resolve the rhythm disturbance. It will also increase CO by restoring preload to normal levels. Many elderly patients with chronic heart failure may rely on renal vasodilatory prostaglandins to maintain renal perfusion. If you inhibit this with any NSAID, the urine output can dramatically fall.

Acute renal failure can also be caused by dehydration, i.e. there is insufficient blood volume to enable the kidney to produce urine. Long-term treatment with diuretics may produce dehydration. Drinking water or giving an intravenous fluid bolus may increase urine output.

Thus, increasing CO will increase renal perfusion and consequently renal output. Increasing blood volume with fluid will increase cardiac and renal output (the kidney must have sufficient blood volume in order to make urine). NSAIDs inhibit renal perfusion: *this* all corrects the prerenal cause of a low urine output.

Giving a diuretic increases the amount of urine from a given renal perfusion.

— Haemofiltration and haemodialysis

Haemofiltration (HF) is a convective mass transfer process. In HF, the water and solutes pass at the same time and direction through a filter that retains cells and macromolecules such as red blood cells and albumin. Similar to normal kidney filtration, for limit of <70 kDa, molecular size is unimportant. However, flow of blood (perfusion) to kidneys or pumping of blood to a HF is the rate-limiting step. HF is usually slow, low pressure, continuous and ideal for a patient such as Mr AM, with a shocked, sensitive heart after surgery.

Haemodialysis (HD) is a diffusive, osmotic process. In HD, the water moves across a semipermeable membrane down a hydrostatic pressure gradient (ultra (small)-filtration). The solutes diffuse across the membrane down an osmotic pressure gradient and therefore are highly dependent on molecular size. Solute moves in the opposite direction to the ultrafiltration of water. The dialysis membrane has a smaller pore size than the filter. HD is usually fast, high blood pressure, high blood flow and requires 6-hour sessions, two or three times a week (intermittent). The size-dependent differential clearance in HD produces problems such as disequilibrium

vancomycin

gentamicin

amiodarone

syndrome which is cardiotoxic and so could not be used in Mr AM's case.

In both types of machine, the pump controls the perfusion of the membrane so giving intravenous fluids, or increasing CO with cardiac inotropes (stimulating force increase) or chronotropes (stimulating rate increase), will have no effect on the output of the artificial kidney. Diuretics will be similarly useless.

— **Drug clearance: vancomycin and gentamicin**
The values in Table 1.7 are based on experience and are variable between hospitals that run HF at different blood speeds – because this changes the perfusion of the artificial kidney relative to the cardiac output. Also important is the porosity of the filter membrane used.

Both vancomycin (a glycopeptide) and gentamicin (an aminoglycoside) are highly water-soluble antibiotics as a consequence of their high polarities. Both have small volumes of distribution (V_d) and are dependent on renal function for clearance. Thus, vancomycin and gentamicin doses will be reduced in the case of Mr AM. This would be in contrast to a drug with lipophilic properties (e.g. amiodarone, an antiarrhythmic drug, also shown in the diagram), which is lipophilic, has a large V_d, undergoes hepatic clearance and therefore would require no dose modification.

▼ TABLE 1.7

Drug clearance for vancomycin and gentamicin

	Vancomycin	Gentamicin
Normal major route of clearance	80–90% renal	90% renal
Hydrophilic	Yes	Yes
Molecular weight (kDa)	1449	477
V_d (L/kg)	0.47	0.25
Usual dose	500 mg four times daily	80 mg three times daily
Dose at GFR 20 mL/min	250 mg daily	80 mg daily
Dose in HF	1000 mg daily	80 mg daily
Dose in HD	500 mg/48 h	80 mg after each session

EXTENDED LEARNING

- What is chronic kidney disease?
- How do peritoneal dialysis and haemodialysis differ?
- What is end-stage renal failure?
- What are the risks associated with receiving a donated kidney?

ADDITIONAL PRACTICE POINTS

- What do you understand by the NHS organ donor register?
- What are the ethical concerns with regard to organ donation?

Further reading

Ashley C, Currie A (2009). *The Renal Drug Handbook*, 3rd edn. Oxford: Radcliffe Publishing.

Case 10
Renal replacement therapy

MARK BORTHWICK

LEARNING OUTCOMES

At the end of this case, you will be able to:

- Explain the differences between haemofiltration and haemodialysis
- Describe factors that affect clearance of medications in continuous renal replacement methods
- Advise on dose adjustments for medications in patients receiving continuous renal replacement therapies
- Outline the phases (1–4) of clinical trials

Case study

Mr RR is a 20-year-old university student with a past medical history of asthma that is well controlled with a corticosteroid inhaler. He weighs 68 kg. He is brought to the hospital A&E by his flatmates because they are alarmed at his level of difficulty in breathing (audible polyphonic wheeze) and a 4-day history of coryzal symptoms (cold like: runny nose, sneezing), fever and aching muscles. The Health Protection Agency has issued advice that the levels of circulating influenza had passed the threshold necessary to trigger flu pathways involving antiviral use 3 weeks before Mr RR's presentation. Mr RR had received a course of prednisolone 2 weeks ago for an exacerbation of his asthma, and questioning has elicited that he has not been immunised against flu.

Arterial blood gases reveal a relative hypoxia. Mr RR is admitted to a general medical ward, and is prescribed oxygen, steroids, bronchodilators, antimicrobial and antiviral agents. He deteriorates on the ward, and within 24 hours is intubated and ventilated on the intensive care unit.

Mr RR's urine output steadily falls to zero. His blood biochemistry is as shown in Table 1.8.

His drug therapy is as follows:

- *Paracetamol 1 g orally, via nasogastric tube four times daily*
- *Co-amoxiclav 1.2 g intravenously three times daily*
- *Oseltamivir 75 mg via nasogastric tube twice a day*
- *Clarithromycin 500 mg intravenously twice a day*
- *Prednisolone 40 mg via nasogastric tube each day*
- *Salbutamol 5 mg nebulised every 2–3 hours*
- *Ipratropium 500 micrograms nebulised four times a day*
- *Dalteparin 5000 units subcutaneously once daily*
- *Ranitidine 50 mg intravenously three times daily*

Renal replacement therapy is commenced (continuous haemofiltration) with an exchange rate of 2500 mL/h.

❓ What adjustments need to be made to Mr RR's drug therapy?

The Health Protection Agency (HPA), now part of Public Health England, reports that a new influenza mutation has been identified and Mr RR's viral infection is resistant to first- and second-line antivirals. A new unlicensed antiviral medication, 'goodovir', is suggested. It has already been given as a 500-mg dose by infusion three times daily in phase 2 clinical trial studies.

❓ What are the different phases of clinical trial studies and what do they involve?
❓ What information is required to make an informed decision about the dose of goodovir in Mr RR?

▼ TABLE 1.8
Blood biochemistry results for Mr RR

	Day 1	Day 2	Day 3
Na+ (mmol/L)	143	146	148
K+ (mmol/L)	5.2	5.6	5.9
Urea (mmol/L)	9	13	16
Creatinine (μmol/L)	152	214	283

Normal ranges: Na+ 135–145 mmol/L; K+ 3.5–5.0 mmol/L; urea 2.5–8.0 mmol/L; creatinine 70–120 μmol/L.

The following pharmacokinetic information is available for goodovir:

- *Volume of distribution, V_d = 0.65 L/kg*
- *Half-life (normal), $t_{\frac{1}{2}}$ = 12 h; expected to be longer in renal failure*
- *Route of excretion: renal*
- *Protein binding: 35%*
- *Oral bioavailability: negligible*
- *Molecular weight: 7850 Da*

② What type of drug do you expect goodovir to be, based upon these parameters?

② What dose of goodovir will you recommend?

Case discussion

Acute renal failure is a common organ failure in patients admitted to critical care. It often results from acute tubular necrosis secondary to poor oxygenation, or the direct toxic effects of drugs, although there are other causes. There are many reasons to start renal replacement therapy in critical care, some more pressing than others. They include control of acidosis, removal of potassium, removal of fluid, and enhanced excretion of drugs and waste substances such as urea and creatinine.

Haemofiltration (HF) is the process whereby blood is passed through tubes comprising a membrane with holes large enough to allow the passage of largish-molecular-weight molecules, often up to about 30 000 Da. The blood is pushed through the tubes under pressure, so fluid leaks out of the holes, carrying dissolved molecules with it, provided that they are smaller than the holes in the membrane. This fluid is removed, and a replacement fluid given back to the patient.

Haemodialysis (HD) is the process whereby blood is passed through tubes comprising a semipermeable membrane, with very small holes, allowing the passage of solutes up to perhaps 2000 Da. The tubes are bathed in dialysis fluid, so dissolved molecules flow from the blood, through the holes into the fluid along a concentration gradient, i.e. by diffusion.

Haemodiafiltration (HDF) is a hybrid process whereby a dialysis fluid surrounds a haemofiltration membrane. This means that, as well as the filtrate produced under pressure in the haemofiltration method, there is an additional diffusion process because the fluid filtered off is diluted by the dialysate, creating a concentration gradient for substances in the blood to follow.

Continuous methods are generally used in practice because it was thought that these cause less haemodynamic compromise than intermittent haemodialysis, although this view is being challenged. Blood is usually taken from a vein using a large-bore catheter and returned to a vein.

These factors are abbreviated and form a system of nomenclature. Continuous venovenous haemofiltration thus becomes CVVHF; such abbreviations are common in the medical literature and standard texts.

Factors that affect substance (including drugs) removal include the molecular weight, water solubility, protein binding, ionic charges, and the likelihood that the substance will adsorb onto the surface of the renal replacement membranes. Generally, small, water-soluble molecules with low protein binding are removed to some degree by renal replacement therapy.

Published texts can aid in determining the dose adjustments required to effectively dose a patient while avoiding toxicity. Care must be taken to ensure that data for the correct mode of renal replacement therapy are utilised, e.g. vancomycin is cleared by haemofiltration (CVVHF) because of the large pore size in the membrane, but is not cleared at all well by haemodialysis (CVVHD), where the pore size is smaller than the molecular size of vancomycin (molecular weight 1.5 kDa).

The data provided about the new unlicensed antiviral *goodovir* suggest that it is a polar macromolecule, most likely a small protein. This is consistent with the very high molecular weight (7850 Da), its administration by infusion and relative lack of oral bioavailability. Renal clearance is characteristic of polar drugs. Protein drugs are not orally bioavailable because they are chemically and enzymatically unstable in the contents of the GI tract, and too large and too polar to diffuse across the GI epithelium.

— Calculating dose adjustments in haemofiltration

It is possible to calculate a measure of drug removal by haemofiltration by using the following equation:

Clearance = Ultrafiltrate flow rate $\times$ S

where S is the sieving coefficient for the drug in question. In the vast majority of cases, the sieving coefficient approximates to the free fraction of drug, so protein binding becomes the greatest determinant of drug removal. Ultrafiltration refers to filtration though a filter that is capable of removing very small (ultramicroscopic) particles.

$$\text{Clearance} = \frac{\text{Ultrafiltrate}}{\text{flow rate}} \times \left(1 - \frac{\text{Protein-bound}}{\text{fraction}}\right)$$

For *goodovir*,

$$\begin{aligned}\text{Clearance} &= 2500\ (\text{mL/h}) \times (1 - 0.35) \\ &= 2500 \times 0.65 \\ &= 1625\ \text{mL/h (or 27 mL/min)}\end{aligned}$$

This is the clearance from HF. We can calculate the normal clearance using the standard pharmacokinetic equation:

$$\begin{aligned}\text{Clearance} &= \frac{[(\ln 2) \times V_d]}{t_{\frac{1}{2}}} \\[2mm] &= \frac{[0.693 \times (0.65\ \text{L/kg} \times 68\ \text{kg})]}{12} \\[2mm] &= \frac{[0.693 \times (650\ \text{mL/kg} \times 68\ \text{kg})]}{12} \\[2mm] &= 2552\ \text{mL/h (or 42 mL/min)}\end{aligned}$$

$$\frac{\text{Concentration}}{\text{at steady state}} = \frac{\text{Dose}}{\text{Clearance} \times \text{Dosing interval}}$$

Assuming that we want the same concentration at steady state while on HF compared with when there is no renal failure, we can construct a balanced equation:

$$\frac{500\ \text{mg}}{42 \times 8} = \frac{\text{Dose on HF}}{27 \times 8}$$

$$1.488 = \frac{\text{Dose on HF}}{216}$$

Dose on HF $= 1.488 \times 216 = 321$ mg

So, in this case, giving a rounded dose of 320 mg every 8 hours while in anuric renal failure on a haemofilter should give the same steady-state plasma concentration as 500 mg every 8 hours to a patient with no renal impairment.

In some patients there is some residual renal function. The total clearance would thus be the clearance from the residual renal function plus the clearance from the renal replacement therapy.

— Phases of clinical trials

Clinical trials of potential new medicines are conducted in the following phases:

- *Phase 1*: first studies in humans, usually healthy volunteers, studying tolerance, pharmacokinetics, metabolism, pharmacodynamics, different formulations, etc.
- *Phase 2*: first studies in patients with the target disease, studying efficacy, safety and dose finding
- *Phase 3*: pivotal studies, investigating efficacy and safety versus 'standard therapy'. Data generated in these studies form the basis of submissions to regulatory authorities (e.g. MHRA, EMA, FDA) for marketing authorisations
- *Phase 4*: post-registration studies to establish long-term safety.

EXTENDED LEARNING

- Describe the design and features of randomised controlled trials
- What is the legislation for medicines with respect to clinical trials of investigational medicinal products?
- Explain the role of medicines regulatory authorities, good clinical practice (GCP) guidelines, and health professionals in clinical trials of investigational medicinal products.

References and further reading

Ashley C, Currie A (2008). The *Renal Drug Handbook*, 3rd edn. Oxford: Radcliffe Press.

Schetz M (2007). Drug dosing in continuous renal replacement therapy: general rules. *Curr Opin Crit Care* **13**:645–51.

2
Cardiovascular cases

INTRODUCTION

This section contains nine cases concerning patients with various cardiovascular disorders, namely atrial fibrillation, angina, heart failure, acute coronary syndrome, hypertension, blood pressure support in severe hypotension, deep vein thrombosis, ischaemic stroke and secondary stroke prevention. The last case study of a patient with internal bleeding raises the important issue of drug–drug interactions, particularly between conventional medicines and certain readily available herbal preparations.

Case 1
Atrial fibrillation ▶ 43

This case is based on an elderly female patient who is taken to a hospital accident and emergency department (A&E) after a collapse. Based on her history of occasional dizziness and palpitations, and an abnormal electrocardiograph recording (ECG), she is diagnosed with chronic atrial fibrillation (AF). The definition and classification of AF are described, along with a discussion of its main symptoms and various treatment options including direct current (DC) or pharmacological cardioversion, and how the most appropriate management can be chosen for this patient who shows haemodynamic instability. As the antiarrhythmic drug amiodarone is administered, some discussion of its chemical structure and physicochemical properties is presented, together with considerations for prescribing, dosing and monitoring the action of this agent. The problem of AF-related strokes, their risk assessment and prevention with anticoagulants are also outlined. The possible use of heart rate-controlling drugs such as β-blockers, calcium channel blockers or digoxin for the long-term control of AF in this patient is discussed.

Case 2
Angina management ▶ 49

This case deals with a male patient who presents to his GP with worsening symptoms of chest pain and shortness of breath (SOB) during exertion, which he puts down to an 'unhealthy' lifestyle. He was previously diagnosed with angina and received medication, but discontinued it because of the unpleasant side effects that he was experiencing. The case considers the causes (atherosclerosis) and symptoms of stable angina and the associated risk factors (modifiable and non-modifiable), along with information and counselling points that would normally be given to the patient about lifestyle changes, and the drug treatment strategies (short and long acting) currently available. Possible alternative revascularisation options are also mentioned. Finally, the chemistry of amlodipine and its mechanism of interaction with its biological target (L-type calcium channels) are considered.

Case 3
Heart failure ▶ 52

This case describes an elderly man presenting to his GP with chronic heart failure as a consequence of ischaemic heart disease, showing the classic symptoms of cardiac insufficiency – tiredness, SOB and ankle oedema. He is also taking medication for asthma. The pathophysiology, signs, symptoms and diagnosis of chronic heart failure are initially discussed, then the appropriateness and likely advantages of using a low-dose angiotensin-converting enzyme (ACE) inhibitor as a first-line treatment for this patient are considered, together with what monitoring procedures would need to be established while using this drug. The feasibility of using a β blocker to improve the outcome for the patient is also considered, particularly in view of his ongoing respiratory airway disease. The chemical structure and pharmacology of the cardioselective β_1-receptor blocker bisoprolol are outlined (aimed at avoiding unwanted bronchial β_2-receptor blocking activity), along with consideration of what issues might arise in chronic heart failure sufferers after initiation of β-blocker therapy, and what the best advice would be to give to this patient to monitor his condition.

Case 4
Acute coronary syndromes ► 56

This case concerns a male patient who presents to his GP with symptoms of sudden-onset chest pain radiating to his back, neck, shoulders and arms, who is referred to the hospital A&E with a suspected acute coronary episode. After taking a patient history, it is established that he was previously a heavy smoker, who consumes alcohol at an 'above-average' level. A battery of diagnostic blood tests is then carried out, including a test for troponin I, along with standard ECG and echocardiogram recordings to monitor cardiac function. The patient was diagnosed with an obtuse marginal coronary artery thrombus and a stenosis of the distal left and right coronary arteries, requiring drug-eluting stent intervention together with clopidogrel antiplatelet drug therapy. The pathophysiology of an acute coronary syndrome (ACS) is initially discussed together with the symptoms, signs and usual diagnostic criteria, including characteristic changes expected on the ECG. The significance of raised blood troponin levels as an indicator of cardiac muscle damage is also mentioned and the general risk factors for developing cardiovascular disease are outlined. The case ends with a discussion of coronary stent function, and the role of different medications that would normally be prescribed for a patient with ACS to reduce the risk of future cardiac events, including antiplatelet, β-blocker and ACE inhibitor (ramipril drugs), statins and glyceryl trinitrate (GTN). The technique of motivational interviewing by pharmacists to improve patient adherence is outlined.

Case 5
Management of hypertension in black patients ► 61

This case describes the treatment of an African–Caribbean man with hypertension and focuses on why ethnicity may be important in the consideration of such cases. The case starts with a discussion of how blood pressure readings should ideally be taken and interpreted according to NICE guidelines, and what laboratory tests should be completed to establish any evidence of pressure-related target organ damage. The fact that hypertension is more prevalent and often difficult to control in black patients is highlighted, and general lifestyle advice that can be given to hypertensive patients is outlined, together with a description of the currently recommended drug therapies including ACE inhibitors, angiotensin receptor blockers, β-blockers, diuretics and dihydropyridine calcium channel antagonists, the last of which are considered first line for African–Caribbean patients. The reasons why black people may not respond so well to some antihypertensives is also mentioned. The chemical structure and properties of dihydropyridine antihypertensives are then discussed in some detail, in relation to their bioavailability. In addition, the various ingredients contained in amlodipine tablets are considered as an example of what is normally involved in pharmaceutical tablet formulation. Finally, the concepts of cardiovascular disease risk assessment calculations, and ethnicity and health are addressed.

Case 6
Cardiovascular (blood pressure) support in an elderly hypotensive patient ► 66

This case is based on an elderly female patient who is admitted to a hospital A&E with severe hypotension, most probably induced by her ongoing antihypertensive drug therapy, comprising a thiazide diuretic and an ACE inhibitor. The case is also complicated by a severe urinary tract infection that requires urgent antibiotic therapy, coupled with critical dehydration. Routine arterial blood gas measurements are made to assess her $O_2 : CO_2$ status and blood pH (she develops a metabolic acidosis), but the patient goes into septic shock and is transferred to an ICU where emergency treatment is initiated. A description of septic shock and its causes is initially given, followed by a discussion of intravenous fluid resuscitation methods and interpretation of the patient's blood gas values. The use of pharmacological vasoconstrictors such as noradrenaline, adrenaline and dopamine, or the cardioselective sympathomimetic agonist dobutamine, to rapidly restore blood pressure in severe cases of hypotension is also outlined.

Case 7
Deep vein thrombosis and warfarin ▶ 70

This case describes an elderly woman who has fractured her hip after a fall, and who, after surgery and discharge from hospital, develops a painful swelling in her leg, diagnosed as deep vein thrombosis (DVT). The case initially considers the pathophysiology and incidence of venous thromboembolism (VTE), and lists the risk factors that can contribute to its occurrence (including recent surgery, as in the case of this patient). The symptoms, signs and diagnosis of DVT (being one manifestation of VTE) are explained, along with current standard treatment options involving short- and long-term anticoagulant therapy. The chemistry of warfarin and the mechanisms of action of heparin and warfarin on the blood coagulation cascade are discussed, and the method of warfarin tablet manufacture is outlined in some detail, explaining the nature of the tablet excipients and their function in the formulation. This case also considers the possibility of significant pharmacodynamic interactions between warfarin and existing antiplatelet drugs, e.g. aspirin or herbal remedies such as ginko biloba. Finally, the type of advice that would be given by a pharmacist to a patient taking warfarin is outlined, with a particular focus on the importance of adherence and the avoidance of other therapies that might potentially interact to increase the risk of bleeding.

Case 8
Treatment of acute ischaemic stroke ▶ 75

This case deals with an elderly woman patient who is admitted to hospital with a suspected stroke. Some background on stroke definition, incidence, and signs and symptoms is initially given, along with an explanation of a transient ischaemic attack (TIA). The case then describes the use of thrombolytic treatment with recombinant tissue

plasminogen activator (rTPA) alteplase and the associated monitoring process for the patient. Some consideration is also given to whether high blood pressure should be actively reduced in cases of acute stroke, and how supportive therapy with antiplatelet (e.g. aspirin) or anticoagulant drugs after thrombolysis might also be beneficial in some cases. Finally, the chemical structure, properties and mechanism of the antiplatelet action of aspirin are outlined.

Case 9
Secondary stroke prevention ▶ 78

This case continues the theme of stroke and stroke prevention with a male patient who experiences symptoms of a stroke and is investigated at a local hospital stroke centre. In this case, a decision was made not to thrombolyse, and the patient was eventually discharged with prescribed medications for secondary prevention. An overview of secondary prevention measures for patients who survive a stroke is initially given, including drug therapy with antiplatelet drugs and anticoagulants, and also consideration of beneficial reductions in high blood pressure and blood glucose levels, and of high cholesterol levels with statins. The chemical structure, properties and mechanism of action of simvastatin are given as an example of a currently used statin. General lifestyle advice that would be given to post-stroke patients is also discussed, e.g. to stop smoking and avoid excessive intake of alcohol. Finally, haemorrhagic (as opposed to ischaemic) stroke is considered, and there is a discussion of the general issue of non-adherence to long-term medication regimens in some post-stroke patients.

Case 10
Drug interactions ▶ 82

This case describes the treatment of an elderly male patient who is on warfarin therapy after a mitral valve replacement and AF, who is admitted to hospital with major symptoms of internal bleeding, severe nausea and disorientation. The patient is also taking other medications for ongoing conditions including digoxin, diltiazem, fluoxetine, magnesium/aluminium hydroxide antacid mixture, and salbutamol/tiotropium inhalers. In addition, he was recently prescribed ciprofloxacin and prednisolone tablets for a respiratory tract infection. The case progresses to an additional complication of endocarditis which requires rifampicin antibiotic treatment. Blood tests reveal an excessive blood clotting time and a dangerously high serum level of digoxin; there is also some renal impairment. The patient is stabilised, but, after discharge from hospital, a community pharmacist is approached about whether the patient can take the herbal medicine St John's wort along with his other medications. There is a general discussion of why it is so important for pharmacists to be aware of the possible, potentially dangerous, drug interactions (pharmacokinetic and pharmacodynamics) that can occur when patients are taking several medications at the same time, both conventional drugs and certain foods and herbal products. The *British National Formulary* (*BNF*) and *Stockley's Drug Interactions* are highlighted as useful sources of information in this area. In this case, the patient's bleeding symptoms are a consequence of warfarin toxicity, most probably caused by a pharmacokinetic interaction with ciprofloxacin; the mechanism of this effect is explained. The properties, actions and possibility of developing toxicity of digoxin in elderly people are also described. Potential interactions between rifampicin and warfarin are explained. Finally, the risk of developing 'serotonin syndrome' with concurrent use of fluoxetine and St John's wort is explained, and also how certain Mg^{2+}- and Al^{3+}-containing antacids can affect the absorption of other orally administered medications.

Case 1
Atrial fibrillation
DUNCAN MCROBBIE

LEARNING OUTCOMES

At the end of this case, you will be able to:

- Outline the signs, symptoms and classification of AF
- Describe the treatment options in AF
- Outline the place of rate control therapy in AF and describe the medication options
- Describe the practical aspects of assessing the risk of stroke in AF and the choices available to reduce stroke risk

Case study

Mrs OC, a 74-year old woman on a trip to London for the weekend, collapses during the interval of the play that she is watching. An ambulance is called and she is transferred to the local A&E.

On arrival, her clerking notes described the following:

CASE NOTES

History of presenting complaint

- She has been feeling a bit 'off' for the last couple of weeks, but the trip had been booked for ages so she was determined to go. On closer questioning she had been feeling fatigued and had a few odd 'spells' which she described as palpitations followed by episodes of dizziness

Past medical history

- Mrs OC is usually well, still playing tennis once a week, but has been complaining of pains in her legs which were diagnosed as intermittent claudication by the GP at a recent check-up. She has long-standing hypertension which is controlled with ramipril 10 mg and bendroflumethiazide 2.5 mg

Drug history

- She has no known allergies. Apart from the antihypertensive listed above, her GP recently started her on simvastatin and clopidogrel which she has been taking for the last 6 weeks

Social history

- Mrs OC is married and her grown-up children live nearby. All are in good health

Review of systems

- She has no signs of jaundice, anaemia, cyanosis, clubbing (ends of fingers and toes enlarged; nails shiny and abnormally curved) or oedema. Her respiratory, abdominal and neurological examinations were all unremarkable
- Her creatinine clearance was within normal limits.
- Her radial pulse was irregularly irregular, but there was no third heart sound. Her ECG showed an absence of P-waves on the rhythm strip and a ventricular rate of 150 beats/min. Her blood pressure was 100/50 mmHg and her respiratory rate 19 breaths/min

Diagnosis

- A diagnosis of atrial fibrillation was made

- What is the definition of AF?
- How is AF classified?
- Should Mrs OC be cardioverted in A&E?

Mrs OC was prescribed amiodarone intravenously. She was admitted to hospital.

- Was amiodarone a suitable choice for Mrs OC?
- What pharmaceutical considerations are required for the prescribing, administration and monitoring of this drug?
- What is the most appropriate choice of agent to reduce the risk of stroke for Mrs OC?

Although this controlled Mrs OC's ventricular rate, her ECG showed that she was still in AF.

- What medications should be prescribed long term for rate control?

Case discussion

— Definition and classification of atrial fibrillation

Atrial fibrillation is a supraventricular tachycardia characterised by disorganised atrial electrical activity. This electrical disorganisation results in the absence of significant atrial depolarisation, characterised by the absence of distinct positive-going P-waves on the ECG. Instead, there are rapid oscillations or fibrillatory waves that vary in size, shape and timing. This results in a lack of coordinated atrial contraction and progressive deterioration of atrial function. The ventricular rate is usually rapid and irregular. A slower ventricular rate may represent atrioventricular conduction disease, or the effect of rate-controlling drugs such as β-blockers. The first detected event may be because of haemodynamic instability, or the patient presenting with symptoms. Patients without overt symptoms may also be identified as being in AF through opportunistic monitoring for other conditions.

Classification of AF is based on the temporal pattern of the arrhythmia. A single episode of AF in patients with a structurally normal heart and normal clinical examination can be classified as 'lone' AF. These events may be self-limiting or amenable to cardioversion (conversion to normal rhythm) if associated with haemodynamic instability. Patients with 'lone' AF are often considered at lower risk for developing thromboembolic complications.

Recurrence of AF, even self-limiting episodes, changes the patient's thromboembolic risk and is designated chronic AF.

Episodes themselves are termed 'paroxysmal' if they terminate spontaneously, usually within 7 days, or persistent if the arrhythmia continues, requiring electrical or pharmacological cardioversion for termination. AF where cardioversion is not indicated, or has not been successful, is termed 'permanent'.

By this definition, Mrs OC has chronic AF, which is persistent. A rate or a rhythm control strategy may be considered.

— **Management of AF and cardioversion**
The acute management of AF patients should concentrate on relief of symptoms and assessment of AF-associated risk.

Restoration and maintenance of sinus rhythm improve exercise tolerance and cardiac output, protect against the development of cardiomyopathy and relieve symptoms.

Cardioversion is the preferred choice for early single presentation of AF in younger (usually aged <65 years) patients, especially those who are haemodynamically unstable with either ventricular

rates >150 beats/min or ongoing chest pain or poor perfusion. Conversion rate with antiarrhythmic drugs is lower than with direct current (DC) cardioversion, but does not require conscious sedation or anaesthesia.

Patients who have been in AF longer than a few days could potentially have already developed clots in their atria. Cardioversion may dislodge these into the systemic circulation and increase the risk of strokes. Traditionally, patients suitable for cardioversion would be treated with warfarin anticoagulant to achieve an international normalised ratio (INR) >2 for a minimum of 4 weeks before cardioversion was attempted. In many centres, the presence of clots can be excluded by transoesophageal echocardiography (TOE), leading to early attempts at DC cardioversion, which is usually done with low-molecular-weight heparin (LMWH) or unfractionated heparin cover.

Pharmacological cardioversion may be attempted with drugs such as flecainide and propafenone (Na^+ channel blockers) or amiodarone (K^+ channel blocker). Flecainide and propafenone should be avoided in patients with structural heart disease (non-coronary cardiovascular abnormalities of the heart).

In this case, Mrs OC presented with a recent collapse and demonstrated some moderate haemodynamic instability in A&E. However, in light of her age and a suspicion from her medical history of long-standing AF, DC cardioversion was not considered and she was deemed to require rate control acutely.

Ventricular rate control can be achieved by oral administration of β-blockers or non-dihydropyridine calcium channel antagonists in stable patients. Mrs OC's rapid ventricular rate and unstable blood pressure require acute treatment.

— **Amiodarone in the treatment of AF**
In UK clinical practice, amiodarone is the agent most commonly used in the management of patients presenting with AF and haemodynamic compromise. Given intravenously, it rapidly reduces ventricular rate and may convert a number of patients back to sinus rhythm. Oral or intravenous flecainide or propafenone can be used in patients without structural heart disease. Vernakalant (a more recently developed blocker of atrial K^+ channels) has been approved by the

European Medicines Agency for rapid cardioversion of recent-onset AF to sinus rhythm in adults.

Ventricular rate control (without cardioversion) may be achieved with β-blockers or rate-controlling calcium channel blockers. If used intravenously, care should be taken to ensure the correct dose of metoprolol or verapamil. As a result of the high first-pass clearance by the liver of the oral formulations of these drugs, the intravenous doses are significantly lower.

In this case, intravenous amiodarone was prescribed for Mrs OC to control her rapid ventricular rate.

— Pharmaceutical considerations for the prescribing, administration and monitoring of amiodarone

The standard recommended dose of amiodarone is 5 mg/kg bodyweight given by intravenous infusion over a period of 20 min to 2 hours, which may be followed by a repeat infusion of up to 1200 mg (approximately 15 mg/kg bodyweight). In practice, this is given as 300 mg over the first hour, followed by 900 mg over the next 23 hours. Intravenous amiodarone is incompatible with physiological (0.9%) saline and should be administered only in 5% dextrose in water for injection. Amiodarone is unstable if diluted to a concentration of <0.6 mg/mL.

The reason for the incompatibility of amiodarone with 0.9% saline is related to the pH of the infusion solution. Examination of the structure of amiodarone (see below) indicates that it is a basic molecule. This basicity arises due to the presence of a tertiary amino group. The pK_a of the tertiary amino group is 6.6. This pK_a refers to the dissociation of the *conjugate acid* (i.e. the protonated version of the group).

amiodarone

The pH of 0.9% saline is approximately 5.5. This is around 1 unit *lower* than the pK_a of amiodarone. If the pH is lower than the pK_a, we expect protonation to occur – the drug will mainly be in the ionised (positively charged) form. As there is 1 unit difference, around 90% of amiodarone will be ionised, leaving 10% unionised. Unionised amiodarone has, however, very low polarity and very poor solubility. It is unlikely that all of the dose will dissolve in the infusion, because 10% remains unionised at this pH. This presents a very significant risk of introducing solid particles of precipitated drug into the bloodstream.

The pH of 5% dextrose in water for injection is lower at approximately pH 4. This is between 2 and 3 units lower than the pK_a of amiodarone, so between 99% and 99.9% will be ionised. Very little of the amiodarone will be in the unionised form. The solubility will be much better at pH 4 (dextrose) than pH 5.5 (0.9% saline).

Amiodarone injection contains benzyl alcohol as a preservative, which may cause allergic reactions and precipitate hypotension, especially if the administration rate is too fast.

The use of administration equipment or devices containing plasticisers, such as DEHP (di-2-ethylhexylphthalate) in the presence of amiodarone may result in leaching out of DEHP. To minimise patient exposure to DEHP, the final amiodarone dilution for infusion should preferably be administered through non-DEHP-containing sets.

Patients receiving amiodarone intravenously should have continuous ECG monitoring, because amiodarone can have *pro*arrhythmic effects (these generally occur in the context of drug interactions and/or electrolytic disorders), and can cause bradycardia and QT interval prolongation on the ECG (QT is the time between electrical depolarisation and repolarisation of the ventricles). Combination of amiodarone with class Ia (e.g. disopyramide) or class III antiarrhythmic drugs (e.g. sotalol) increases the risk of torsades de pointes (a characteristic type of ventricular tachycardia). Combinations of amiodarone with other drugs known to increase the risk of prolonged QTc (corrected QT interval) (e.g. terfenadine [H_1-receptor antihistamine – now withdrawn], fluoroquinolones [antibiotics: ciprofloxacin], lithium [for bipolar disorder] and tricyclic antidepressants [amitrypyline, desipramine]) should be avoided if possible. Drugs that may cause hypokalaemia (e.g. stimulant laxatives and thiazide/loop diuretics) can also increase the risk of torsades de pointes and should therefore be used with caution.

Amiodarone increases plasma digoxin concentrations; patients on digoxin should have their dosage of digoxin halved to prevent toxicity. Combining amiodarone with β-blockers or rate limiting calcium channel blockers may result in bradycardia.

The main active metabolite of amiodarone, desethylamiodarone, is a potent inhibitor of cytochrome P450 (CYP) enzymes, particularly CYP2C9, CYP3A4, CYP2C19 and CYP2D6, and drugs that are also metabolised by these enzymes (e.g. warfarin and phenytoin, by CYP2D6, and statins, ciclosporin and midazolam by CYP3A4) may have significantly elevated plasma levels and should have their doses titrated accordingly. Drugs with narrow therapeutic indices need particular consideration. Grapefruit juice inhibits CYP3A4 and may increase the plasma concentration of amiodarone, and should be avoided during treatment with oral amiodarone.

In this case, Mrs OC was administered: amiodarone 300 mg in 250 mL 5% dextrose i.v. over an hour, followed by two infusions of 450 mg in 500 mL 5% dextrose.

— **Reducing the risk of stroke**

People with chronic AF are five times more likely to have a stroke than people without it. In addition, AF-related strokes are more severe and associated with more disability than non-AF strokes. Adequately controlled anticoagulation with warfarin reduces the risk of stroke by 68% and can prevent three out of four AF-related strokes.

Risk-scoring systems are needed to balance the benefits of preventing stroke against the risk of bleeding with oral anticoagulants; hence, in patients with fewer risk factors, the bleeding risk outweighs the benefit of treatment, but patients with multiple risk factors, or with prior stroke or TIA (or 'mini-stroke'), the benefits of oral anticoagulation outweigh the risk.

The most commonly used stroke risk assessment system in clinical practice is the $CHADS_2$ score (Table 2.1); patients with a $CHADS_2$ score ≥ 2 should be considered for oral anticoagulation therapy with warfarin, those with a $CHADS_2$ score of 1 should be considered for treatment with warfarin or aspirin depending on

▼ TABLE 2.1
$CHADS_2$ score

Risk factor	Score	Mrs OC's score
History of chronic heart failure	+1	0
History of hypertension	+1	1
Age ≥ 75 years	+1	0
History of diabetes mellitus	+1	0
Stroke previously or TIA	+2	0

bleeding risk, and those with a $CHADS_2$ score of 0 should be offered aspirin as thromboprophylaxis.

Data from clinical trials suggest an annual risk of bleeding of approximately 2% on anticoagulation, so anticoagulation is recommended for all patients with a stroke risk greater than the bleeding risk, with a $CHADS_2 \geq 2$ (Table 2.2).

According to this score, Mrs OC may be considered low risk with an adjusted risk for stroke of 2.8% per year.

The year 2010 saw the introduction of an extended risk factor scoring system to replace $CHADS_2$. The CHA_2DS_2VASc score is recommended by the European Society of Cardiology and identifies a number of other risk factors for stroke not covered by $CHADS_2$ (Table 2.3). Using this scoring system, Mrs OC has a score of 4, which equates to an adjusted stroke risk of 4% per year.

▼ TABLE 2.2
$CHADS_2$ score and stroke risk

$CHADS_2$ score	Stroke risk per 100 patient-years	$CHADS_2$ risk level	Antithrombotic recommended
0	1.9	Low	Aspirin or no treatment
1	2.8	Low	Aspirin or oral anticoagulation (anticoagulation preferred)
2	4.0	Moderate	Anticoagulation
3	5.9	Moderate	Anticoagulation
4	8.5	High	Anticoagulation
5	12.5	High	Anticoagulation
6	18.2	High	Anticoagulation

▼ TABLE 2.3

CHA$_2$DS$_2$VASc score

Risk factor	Score	Mrs OC's score
History of chronic heart failure	+1	0
History of hypertension	+1	1
Age ≥75 years	+2	0
History of diabetes Mellitus	+1	0
Stroke previously or TIA	+2	0
History of vascular disease	+1	1
Age 65–74 years	+1	1
Sex category (female)	+1	1

As Mrs OC's stroke risk (4% per year) is greater than her bleeding risk (2% per year), the option of starting anticoagulation should be discussed with Mrs OC.

Warfarin inhibits vitamin K-dependent clotting factors and therefore delays clotting time. Individual dose adjustment is required with the aim of maintaining the International Normalised Ratio (INR) between 2 and 3. Warfarin can reduce protein C and protein S levels and cause a prothrombotic state. Enoxaparin should be continued until the INR is more than 2, particularly if patients have an already established clot, e.g. a deep vein thrombosis. There is less evidence for concomitant therapy in low risk patients with AF.

New oral anticoagulants are now available. Dabigatran (in higher doses), a direct thrombin inhibitor, and apixaban (a factor Xa inhibitor) have been shown to be superior to warfarin in reducing the risk of stroke with similar bleeding risks. Rivaroxaban (another factor Xa inhibitor) and lower doses of dabigatran have been shown to be at least as effective as warfarin. Due to a reliable dose response none of these drugs requires INR monitoring. While there are fewer dietary restrictions than with warfarin, these agents have a number of drug interactions particularly with other drugs that utilise the cytochrome P-450 or p-glycoprotein systems. A number of other oral anticoagulant agents are currently being developed and undergoing clinical trials.

— Prescribing to achieve long-term rate control
A rate control strategy is recommended for patients with persistent AF who are aged >65 years, have coronary artery disease and contraindications to antiarrhythmic therapies or are unsuitable for cardioversion, or patients with permanent ('long-standing' or 'chronic') AF.

An irregular rhythm and a rapid ventricular rate in AF can cause symptoms including palpitations, dyspnoea, fatigue and dizziness. Guidelines differ in their recommendations and in practice a resting heart rate between 60 and 80 beats/min is considered acceptable.

The choice of rate-controlling agent is based on the autonomic sympathetic and parasympathetic tone, other concomitant diseases that may limit the choice of therapy, the side-effect profile of individual medicines and patient choice. In a number of patients, combinations of drugs may be required to control the rate.

β-Blockers or rate-limiting (non-dihydropyridine) calcium channel blockers have similar effectiveness at controlling ventricular rate. *β*-Blockers should be considered first choice in patients whose symptoms are worse with exercise, or who have myocardial ischaemia. *β*-Blockers are highly effective at controlling both resting heart rate and heart rate during exercise. However, they may cause the unpleasant side effects of cold hands and feet and fatigue, and should be used cautiously in respiratory disease and diabetes.

Rate-limiting calcium channel blockers (verapamil, diltiazem) may be suitable for patients who have contraindications or side effects from *β*-blockers. They should be avoided in patients with heart failure because they have negative ionotropic activity.

Amiodarone is sometimes continued after the initial attempt at rhythm control. However, a number of serious side effects can occur with long-term use, including severe pulmonary and liver complications. Cutaneous side effects (increased photosensitivity and skin discoloration) are unpleasant for patients. Amiodarone's high iodine content also affects thyroid hormone levels. Unless safer agents are unsuitable, amiodarone should be avoided for long-term use. Dronedarone has fewer side effects than amiodarone, but is contraindicated in patients with permanent AF.

Digoxin does not have any effect in patients with a high sympathetic nervous system drive, and its role is now limited to sedentary patients or as an adjunct in patients who have AF with underlying heart failure.

In this case, Mrs OC has a previous history of intermittent claudication that would be worsened by β blockers. Long-term amiodarone side effects would be unacceptable. Mrs OC was therefore started on diltiazem. Her GP was asked to monitor her pulse and blood pressure and adjust the dose of diltiazem accordingly.

Mrs OC's discharge prescription was therefore:

- Warfarin, dose adjusted to maintain INR between 2 and 3 for life
- Simvastatin 20 mg every evening and titrated according to her cholesterol level
- Diltiazem sustained release 90 mg twice a day.

EXTENDED LEARNING

- Outline the role of cytochrome P450 enzymes in drug metabolism
- Describe the classification of antiarrhythmic drugs
- What is the mechanism of action of amiodarone in reducing AF?
- What do we mean by drugs having a 'narrow therapeutic index'? What drugs fall into this category?
- Describe the use of polymers and plasticisers in pharmaceutical packaging and devices
- Outline the process of new medicines regulation, and the roles played by the European Medicines Agency (EMA) and the Medicines and Healthcare products Regulatory Authority (MHRA)
- Use the Henderson–Hasselbalch equation to determine exactly what proportion of amiodarone is ionised in 0.9% saline (pH 4) and 5% dextrose saline (pH 5.5). The actual values are 99.7% and 92.6%. respectively.

References and further reading

Camm AJ, Lip GY, De Caterina, R, et al.; ESC Committee for Practice Guidelines (2012). 2012 focused update of the ESC Guidelines for the management of atrial fibrillation: an update of the 2010 ESC Guidelines for the management of atrial fibrillation. Developed with the special contribution of the European Heart Rhythm Association. *Eur Heart J* 33:2719–47.

European Heart Rhythm Association, European Association for Cardio-Thoracic Surgery; Camm AJ, Kirchhof P, Lip GY et al. (2010). Guidelines for the management of atrial fibrillation: the Task Force for the Management of Atrial Fibrillation of the European Society of Cardiology (ESC). *Eur Heart J* 31:2369–429.

Gage BF, Waterman AD, Shannon W, Boechler M, Rich MW, Radford MJ (2001). Validation of clinical classification schemes for predicting stroke: results from the National Registry of Atrial Fibrillation. *JAMA* 285:2864–70.

Lévy S, Camm AJ, Saksena S et al. (2003). International consensus on nomenclature and classification of atrial fibrillation; a collaborative project of the Working Group on Arrhythmias and the Working Group on Cardiac Pacing of the European Society of Cardiology and the North American Society of Pacing and Electrophysiology. *Europace* 5:119–22.

National Collaborating Centre for Chronic Conditions (2006). *Atrial Fibrillation: National clinical guideline for management in primary and secondary care.* London: Royal College of Physicians.

Stellbrink C, Nixdorff U, Hofmann T et al.; for Anticoagulation in Cardioversion using Enoxaparin Study Group (2004). Safety and efficacy of enoxaparin compared with unfractionated heparin and oral anticoagulants for prevention of thromboembolic complications in cardioversion of nonvalvular atrial fibrillation: the Anticoagulation in Cardioversion using Enoxaparin (ACE) Trial. *Circulation* 109:997–1003.

Case 2
Angina management

SOTIRIS ANTONIOU AND PAUL WRIGHT

LEARNING OUTCOMES

At the end of this case, you will be able to:

- Outline the pathophysiology, signs and symptoms of stable angina
- Describe the treatment options in angina, particularly in relation to symptom control
- Discuss treatment options for secondary prevention of angina
- Outline the formulation options for glyceryl trinitrate, in the context of the drug's first-pass (presystemic) metabolism
- Outline the chemistry of amlodipine
- Outline the place of potential non-drug further interventions

Case study

Mr SW is a 48-year-old man going through a stressful time at work who, for the past 6 months, has been increasingly short of breath while walking to the bus. He has put this down to his 'unhealthy' lifestyle. Although he has cut down from two packets to one packet of cigarettes a week, reduced his alcohol intake from about 40 units to 25 units a week and is trying to lose weight (currently 1.8 m tall, weighing 100 kg), he sometimes finds himself short of breath with mild chest tightness, especially when he is running late. He has a strong family history of cardiovascular disease with his father having a stroke in his early 50s and his older brother having had a coronary artery bypass graft 2 years ago. Both have encouraged Mr SW to see his GP due to his worsening symptoms.

- What is angina?
- What are the classic symptoms of angina?
- How is a diagnosis of angina confirmed?
- What are the modifiable and non-modifiable risk factors?

Mr SW was seen by a GP 2 years ago who prescribed aspirin 75 mg daily, atenolol 50 mg daily and a GTN spray to be used if he experiences chest pain. Since this time, he has stopped taking the aspirin, because he feels that he does not need

it and he has stopped the atenolol for more than a year because he was feeling tired and read that it can cause impotence. He has used the GTN once but, after experiencing a headache and facial flushing, he has not used it since and he does not carry it with him.

After his current GP visit, he goes to the pharmacy to collect a prescription with the following items:

Aspirin 75 mg daily
Simvastatin 40 mg at night
Amlodipine 5 mg daily
GTN spray when required

The GP rings ahead of the prescription and asks you to counsel the patient on all of the prescribed items because they had no time for an explanation during the consultation.

- What information and counselling points would you include?
- How is stable angina managed?
- Draw the structure of amlodipine and describe how the molecular shape is important for its interaction with its biological target
- What options are there if Mr SW experiences further symptoms despite the use of amlodipine?

Despite good adherence to the prescribed treatment regime, Mr SW still experiences chest pain during physical exertion and organises a further appointment with the GP.

- What options would you now suggest for Mr SW?

Case discussion

— Angina and its pathophysiology

Stable angina pectoris is a common and disabling cardiovascular condition. It is a chronic, long-term condition which is managed medically in the first instance, but may require surgical intervention if symptoms worsen despite optimal medical management. Symptoms (typically central chest pain described as 'crushing in sensation') occur during periods of increased physical activity or emotional stress; this causes a mismatch between oxygen supply and demand to the myocardium, causing temporary myocardial ischaemia. Pain may also be typically felt in the shoulders or arms (commonly on the left side, but either or both sides may be involved), the neck, jaw or back. Stable angina symptoms are normally relieved within minutes of rest.

One of the biggest contributing factors to a reduction in coronary artery blood supply is the cross-sectional area of vessels, which can be markedly reduced with build-up of atherosclerotic plaques. Atherosclerosis is common to most ischaemic cardiovascular disease and treatment is often similar. The process begins with infiltration of low-density lipoproteins (LDLs) into the artery wall which brings about an inflammatory response. Further build-up and calcification occurs to such an extent that the diameter of the artery is significantly reduced. Due to the large reserve capacity of the heart, it often requires a significant reduction in lumen diameter before symptoms occur.

Managing stable angina

— Treatment: secondary prevention
Treatments can be divided into those that reduce the risk of future cardiovascular events, thereby reducing mortality (this is secondary prevention – see below) and those that prevent symptoms (which can be further subdivided into short- and long-term relief). Once a patient experiences symptoms, there is already a significant coronary atherosclerotic build-up, which in addition to reducing blood supply is more likely to rupture and cause an acute event such as a myocardial infarction (MI). For this reason, patients with angina are considered to have established cardiovascular disease and treatment with low-dose aspirin and a statin should be considered and discussed with the patient to minimise this risk. Together with initiating medication, modifiable risk factors should be addressed and advice on smoking cessation, exercise, diet and weight loss offered.

Aspirin 75 mg daily is indicated for secondary prevention. In studies, aspirin use has been associated with a reduction in non-fatal MI and vascular events. Accordingly, aspirin should be considered for all patients with angina, but offered only to those for whom expected benefits outweigh the perceived risks.

Statins for secondary prevention have been shown to confer a benefit in reducing the likelihood for all-cause mortality and cardiovascular mortality, although event rates are relatively low in stable angina. The reduction in risk, low price and relative safety of statins make taking them a cost-effective intervention for patients with stable angina. NICE guidelines suggest simvastatin at a starting dose of 40 mg daily; an alternative preparation or lower dose can be used if there are clinical contraindications or drug interactions. If total cholesterol <4 mmol/L or LDL-cholesterol <2 mmol/L is not achieved at the initial dose, titration of simvastatin or alternative (with similar acquisition cost) should be used.

— Treatment: short-acting relief
GTN is used to minimise the discomfort of angina. Used sublingually, it has a rapid onset of action within 1–5 min and can be used before situations that patients know will cause angina symptoms. Short-acting GTN is available as sublingual tablet or spray formulations. The choice should be discussed with the patient and the most appropriate formulation chosen. Tablets lose potency on exposure to air and should be discarded 8 weeks after the bottle is opened; an advantage is that they can be removed from the mouth once angina symptoms have resolved or side effects (such as headache, flushing or dizziness) become problematic. The spray has a longer shelf-life (usually 2–3 years) so may be easier to use and more appropriate for patients who do not require GTN often. However, it can cause difficulties for those with significant arthritis or reduced hand dexterity.

GTN may be given via the sublingual or buccal route in the form of tablets or a metered-dose aerosol spray for the treatment of an angina attack. Sublingual, meaning 'under the tongue', offers advantages over the oral route, with rapid drug absorption, and is a useful route for drugs that undergo first-pass (presystemic) metabolism, which results in reduced systemic drug levels. First-pass metabolism occurs primarily due to enzymes in the liver and GI tract. After absorption of drug in the GI tract, drug in the blood enters the hepatic portal system, passing through the liver and exposing it to metabolising enzymes, before passage to the rest of the body. Some routes of administration, such as sublingual, buccal, pulmonary, rectal and intravenous routes, result in the drug being distributed in the systemic circulation, without first passing through the liver, thus avoiding the first-pass effect. GTN tablets may be given via the buccal route; the drug is also available as an intravenous injection, ointment and transdermal patches.

— **Treatment: longer-acting symptom control**
Generally, treatment for initial management of stable angina consists of one or two anti-angina drugs. Doses should be titrated to the maximum tolerated dose, based on control of symptoms versus side effects. Response to treatment should be reviewed 2–4 weeks after starting or changing drug treatment.

NICE CG126 recommends that first-line treatment should be with either a β-blocker or calcium channel blocker (CCB). In contrast to other guidance, this option allows treatments to be discussed and tailored to individual patients. For patients taking either a β-blocker or a CCB alone, whose symptoms are not controlled, the next step is to swap or add the other (usually avoiding the combination of β-blocker and verapamil). Where there are contraindications or the other agent is not tolerated, adding one of the following medicines should be considered:

- A long-acting nitrate (e.g. isosorbide dinitrate or mononitrate)
- Nicorandil (an ATP-sensitive potassium channel opener)
- Ivabradine (a blocker of the I_f [f = 'funny'] mixed Na^+/K^+ inward pacemaker current activated by hyperpolarisation in the sinoatrial node)
- Ranolazine (a blocker of the cardiac, late inward sodium channel current [I_{NaL}]).

— **Structure and activity of amlodipine**

amlodipine

Amlodipine is a member of the 1,4-dihydro-pyridine (DHP) class of CCBs. The drug interacts

in a specific manner with a binding site within the α_1 subunit of L-type calcium channels, impeding the flow of Ca^{2+} ions. The shape of the drug is essential to this interaction. The presence of a chlorine atom in the *ortho* position (with respect to the DHP ring) greatly restricts rotation about the bond joining the two rings, effectively 'locking' them in a conformation in which they are perpendicular to each other. This conformation, common to all DHP CCBs, appears to be a requirement for biological activity. The low overall polarity of amlodipine also results in good absorption of the drug after oral administration.

Addition of a third anti-anginal medicine should be considered only if a patient's symptoms are not adequately controlled with two drugs, and they are waiting for revascularisation, or revascularisation is not considered appropriate. There are limited trial data looking at combinations of two versus more than two antianginal medicines for symptomatic relief and prevention of cardiovascular events. Furthermore, none is licensed for use as part of triple antianginal therapy. Based on the lack of data supporting triple antianginal therapy, drug combinations should be based on co-morbidities, contraindications, patient preference and drug costs.

Further treatment options in the management of angina

— **Revascularisation options**
Where a patient's angina symptoms are not adequately controlled with medication, the relative merits and risks of coronary artery bypass grafts versus percutaneous coronary intervention to alleviate symptoms should be discussed. A multidisciplinary discussion should take place when the coronary artery disease is more complex.

— **Counselling: lifestyle and risk factors**
Mr SW has already been taking steps to address his unhealthy lifestyle and reduce his cardiovascular risk. Risk factors for cardiovascular disease are commonly distinguished as modifiable and non-modifiable. Modifiable risk factors are those that can be controlled, treated or modified. These include smoking, diet (especially cholesterol and lipids), weight and obesity, physical exercise, blood sugar levels and hypertension. Non-modifiable risk factors are those that cannot be changed, such as age, gender, ethnicity and family history.

Assessment of risk factors and action to reduce these, wherever possible, are part of both primary and secondary prevention strategies of cardiovascular disease. Primary prevention is the delaying or preventing of the onset of cardiovascular disease, and thus should be engaged in by everyone. Secondary prevention follows the early detection of disease process and is the application of interventions (e.g. lifestyle and medication) to prevent progression of disease.

References and further reading

European Society of Cardiology (2006). Guidelines on the management of stable angina pectoris: full text. *Eur Heart J* doi:10.1093/eurheartj/ehl002. Available at: www.escardio.org/guidelines-surveys/esc-guidelines/Documents/ANGINA/guidelines-angina-FT.pdf (accessed 22 July 2014).

Kones R (2010). Recent advances in the management of chronic stable angina I: approach to the patient, diagnosis, pathophysiology, risk stratification, and gender disparities. *Vasc Health Risk Manage* 6:635–56.

National Institute for Health and Clinical Excellence (2011). *Management of Stable Angina*. Clinical Guideline 126. London: NICE. www.nice.org.uk/cg126 (accessed 30 June 2013).

Case 3
Heart failure

HELEN WILLIAMS

Case study

Mr PJ is a 68-year old man who was diagnosed with heart failure secondary to ischaemic heart disease earlier this year, after presenting to his GP with increasing lethargy, SOB and ankle swelling.

- What are the primary signs and symptoms of heart failure?
- How is a heart failure diagnosis confirmed?

Mr PJ is currently taking furosemide 40 mg daily, ramipril 1.25 mg twice daily, aspirin 75 mg daily, simvastatin 40 mg daily and isosorbide mononitrate MR 60 mg once daily, salbutamol inhaler when required and beclometasone 200 microgram inhaler twice daily.

- How do ACE inhibitors improve outcome for patients with heart failure?
- Is the low dose of ACE inhibitor prescribed here appropriate?
- What monitoring is required for patients on ACE inhibitors?

Mr PJ attends the cardiac outpatient department where you provide pharmacy input. He is relatively stable, able to walk for approximately half a mile unlimited by breathlessness, although hills can be more of a struggle. He is sleeping well and denies palpitations.

> **On examination**
> - BP: 105/68 mmHg
> - HR: 92 beats/min
> - Minor ankle swelling without pitting

Mr PJ is initiated on bisoprolol 1.25 mg daily.

❷ How do β-blockers improve outcome for patients with heart failure?

❷ Is a β-blocker appropriate in view of his airway disease?

❷ What issues might arise after initiation of β-blocker therapy?

❷ What advice would you give this man?

Case discussion

— Heart failure pathophysiology

Heart failure may be defined as a condition in which the heart is no longer able to provide an adequate pumping function to maintain the blood flow and oxygen requirements of the body. When the heart begins to fail and cardiac output falls, the body responds through a number of compensatory mechanisms: increased activity of the sympathetic nervous system leads to an increase in blood pressure and heart rate in an attempt to maintain cardiac output. In the longer term, this sympathetic activation can cause a further decline in left ventricular systolic function, cardiac 'energy depletion' and increased risk of arrhythmias. Sympathetic activity is closely correlated to prognosis in chronic heart failure (CHF).

The fall in cardiac output results in stimulation of the renin–angiotensin–aldosterone system (RAAS) which in turn causes peripheral vasoconstriction, sodium and water retention, and stimulation of the sympathetic nervous system in an attempt to improve blood pressure and renal perfusion. Although this may be of benefit in the short term, in CHF it exacerbates the situation as a result of increased myocardial workload, leading to further progression.

— Signs and symptoms of heart failure

Heart failure is a clinical diagnosis. It is a syndrome characterised by breathlessness and reduced exercise tolerance. The main signs are those of fluid retention, in the lungs as pulmonary oedema and as peripheral oedema (Table 2.4).

— Confirming a diagnosis of heart failure

The symptoms of heart failure on presentation are often non-specific (lethargy, breathlessness, ankle swelling, poor exercise tolerance) and it can be difficult to identify heart failure from other medical conditions. Measuring a BNP (B-type natriuretic protein) level can help to exclude heart failure as a diagnosis, because, if the BNP is normal, the patient is very unlikely to have this condition. A raised BNP indicates that heart

▼ TABLE 2.4

Signs and symptoms of heart failure

Symptoms	Signs
Dyspnoea (shortness of breath)	Tachycardia (increased heart rate)
Paroxysmal nocturnal dyspnoea	Tachypnoea (increased respiratory rate)
Orthopnoea (breathlessness on lying flat)	Third or fourth heart sound
Lethargy, fatigue	'Crackles' at lung bases
Pulmonary oedema	Cardiomegaly (enlarged heart)
Peripheral oedema	Pitting oedema
Fatigue	Raised JVP (jugular venous pressure)
Anorexia	Hepatomegaly (enlarged liver)
Nausea	Ascites (abdominal fluid accumulation)
Weight loss or gain	Abdominal discomfort
	Pleural transudates
	Displaced cardiac apex beat

failure may be present, but this must be confirmed objectively, usually by echocardiography, which provides information on cardiac size and function. Complementary investigations include chest X-ray, ECG and coronary angiography.

— ACE inhibitors in the treatment of heart failure

The reduction in renal perfusion as cardiac output falls activates the RAAS as a compensatory mechanism, increasing blood concentrations of angiotensin II (AT-II) and aldosterone. AT-II leads to vasoconstriction and the release of aldosterone from the adrenal cortex, which in turn increases renal perfusion and maintains arterial blood pressure, primarily through Na^+ and water retention. Chronic exposure to increased levels of AT-II, however, results in cardiac hypertrophy (abnormal heart enlargement), vascular smooth muscle growth and sympathetic nervous system activation, and hence contributes to the progression of CHF.

The central role that ACE inhibitors play in the management of all classes of heart failure is now well established. ACE inhibitors block the conversion of circulating AT-I to AT-II, the latter being responsible for mediating many of the effects of RAAS stimulation, including vasoconstriction, stimulating aldosterone release and cross-activating the sympathetic nervous system. Blockade of the RAAS in this way is known to significantly improve long-term prognosis and day-to-day quality of life in CHF patients. Meta-analysis concludes that ACE inhibitors reduce mortality and cardiovascular hospitalisations to the order of 35% in patients with heart failure caused by left ventricular (LV) systolic dysfunction.

ACE inhibitors should be initiated at low doses to avoid precipitating hypotension and allow monitoring of the effect on renal function. Low doses of ACE inhibitors are beneficial in HF and do confer a mortality benefit. However, studies have shown that increasing the dose is associated with improved outcomes for patients, including significantly fewer hospital admissions with higher doses. The aim should be to increase the ramipril dose to 10 mg daily if tolerated, but clinicians should pay careful attention to blood pressure and renal function.

— Monitoring patients on ACE inhibitors

Renal function should be monitored before, within a month of starting therapy or a change in dose and at least 6 monthly thereafter. A rise in plasma creatinine concentration of up to 20% is expected when ACE inhibitors are initiated; if a greater increase is seen, then dose titration should be approached cautiously. ACE inhibitors should be withdrawn if creatinine increases on initiation by 50% or more, and further advice on management sought.

Blood pressure should be checked before and after dose changes, but hypotension is common in heart failure patients and this should not inhibit dose increases, unless the patient is symptomatic. Most clinicians would increase the dose of ACE inhibitor with systolic BP as low as 85 mmHg, provided the renal function is stable.

How do β blockers improve outcome for patients with heart failure?

In addition to stimulating RAAS activity, a fall in cardiac output leads to chronic activation of the sympathetic nervous system. This compensatory effect increases the rate and force of myocardial contraction and hence increases cardiac output. As with activation of the RAAS, this response is helpful in the short term, but, in the long term, it increases the pressure on an already failing heart, as well as increasing the risk of arrhythmias and episodes of ischaemia. Despite these deleterious effects, patients with chronic heart failure become dependent on this sympathetic overdrive in order to maintain their cardiac output, and therefore

blockade of this system must be undertaken slowly and cautiously to avoid precipitating an acute deterioration in HF status.

β-Adrenoceptor blockers are currently the only drug class used to suppress sympathetic activity in the management of CHF. Blocking the β-adrenoceptors reduces the heart rate and force of contraction, hence reducing overall cardiac workload. This results in a number of beneficial effects, including reduced risk of arrhythmias and ischaemia, improved diastolic filling time, which improves systolic efficiency, and reduced blood pressure. Overall, β-blockers reduce mortality from heart failure by approximately 30–35%, which includes a significant reduction in the risk of sudden cardiac death. In addition, patients on β-blockers have a reduced risk of hospital admission and report improved symptom control and quality of life.

— Appropriateness of β-blockers in airway disease

β-Blockers are clearly contraindicated in patients with severe bronchial asthma or severe COPD (chronic obstructive pulmonary disease) due to risk of bronchoconstriction. Therefore, lung function tests may be appropriate to establish if there is a significant element of airway reversibility before making a decision about the initiation of a β-blocker. Studies have concluded that β-blockers can be safely used in patients with mild-to-moderate, reversible airway disease with cautious initiation and careful monitoring. In view of the compelling evidence that β-blockers improve prognosis and quality of life in patients with heart failure, a trial of a β-blocker is appropriate. Clinicians should choose a cardioselective agent with reduced β_2-receptor-blocking activity to minimise any effects on the lung. Bisoprolol is a cardioselective β_1-receptor blocker suitable for use in these patients.

— Selectivity properties of bisoprolol

Bisoprolol has very good selectivity for β_1-adrenergic receptors over β_2-receptors (around 75:1), resulting in good cardioselectivity because β_1-receptors are found primarily on cardiac muscle. Although both β_1- and β_2-receptors have similar structures (due to similar amino acid sequences), small differences in the structures of ligands can result in different selectivities for the two subtypes. A drug's structure and shape are the key determinants of its ability to interact with other molecules (such as receptors and enzymes) because the correct parts of the drug must be in the correct relative positions for binding. Bisoprolol is also manufactured and administered as a racemic mixture (1:1 mixture of two enantiomers). Only the enantiomer with the S configuration is active because it has the correct three-dimensional shape to bind to the β_1-receptor in a complementary manner.

bisoprolol

What issues might arise after initiation of β-blocker therapy?

Initiation of β-blockers in heart failure does present some challenges. The reduction in sympathetic activity resulting in a slower heart rate and reduced force of contraction can precipitate an initial worsening of heart failure symptoms. This may manifest as minor ankle swelling or reduced exercise tolerance, which resolves within a few days of initiation or dose titration. Occasionally, the symptoms can be more significant, with pitting oedema of the legs (skin holds imprint of finger when pressed) or increasing breathlessness, and may require additional diuretic therapy for control. Patients with significant symptoms after initiation or dose titration may need to be maintained on the same β-blocker dose for a number of weeks to stabilise before the next dose increase, or occasionally the dose may need to be stepped down.

Heart rate and blood pressure should be monitored during treatment. Bradycardia (heart rate at rest <50 beats/min) can occur and may limit the dose in some patients. As with ACE inhibitors, the aim should be to increase the dose to ensure the benefits seen in clinical trials are attained.

In this patient, monitoring of the peak expiratory flow rate (PEFR) would be valuable to determine if the β-blocker has any deleterious effect on lung function. Adverse effects should be dealt with promptly to encourage ongoing compliance. Poor adherence by people taking medicines for long-term conditions is common

and early experiences of side effects, doubts about benefits or other problems can lead to non-adherence within a short period of starting a new therapy. Indeed, this is the basis for the New Medicines Service: an advanced service offered by community pharmacists in England, although heart failure is not one of the initial conditions for which the New Medicines Service is offered.

Patient advice in this case

Mr PJ should be advised of the benefits of initiation a β-blocker. He should be made aware that, in the short term, he may experience a deterioration in symptoms, but that these usually resolve within a few days. If he experiences significant deterioration, he should seek advice from his GP or heart failure team. He should be advised to monitor his peak flow and report any decline in lung function, particularly should he experience breathlessness. The importance of taking his regular 'preventer' inhaler should be emphasised. He should be asked to seek advice should he experience any other side effects that become troublesome.

EXTENDED LEARNING

- What is the role of aldosterone antagonists in the management of heart failure?
- What non-pharmacological strategies are available for heart failure management, including lifestyle changes?
- What is the role of the multidisciplinary team in heart failure care?
- Why would the plasma creatinine concentration be expected to rise in CHF patients initiated on ACE inhibitor treatment?
- What is the New Medicine Service (NMS) offered by community pharmacists in England?
- What other services do community pharmacists offer to support patients in the use of their medicines?

References and further reading

National Institute for Health and Clinical Excellence (2010). *Chronic Heart Failure: Management of chronic heart failure in adults in primary and secondary care*. NICE Clinical Guideline, CG108. London: NICE.

Sani M (2009). Heart failure: clinical features and diagnosis. *Clin Pharmacist* 1:113–19.

Williams H (2009). Heart failure management. *Clin Pharmacist* 1:120–5.

Case 4
Acute coronary syndromes
LYNN HUMPHREY AND STEWART WILSON

LEARNING OUTCOMES

At the end of this case, you will be able to:

- Outline the signs, symptoms and diagnosis of acute coronary syndromes

- Describe the intervention and drug treatment options for patients with coronary heart disease

- Describe the mode of action of nitrates and ACE inhibitors

- Describe how drugs used for the secondary prevention of cardiac events should be monitored, reviewed and optimised

- Acknowledge the importance of adherence to secondary preventive medicines and the possible value of motivational interviewing in achieving this

Case study

Mr TR, a 54-year-old man, presented to his GP with sudden-onset epigastric pain that started the previous night and 'felt like trapped wind'. This radiated through his back, up to his neck and into both shoulders/arms. He was extremely flatulent. He walked to his GP's surgery without recurrence of the pain. His GP referred him to A&E for further investigation.

The following significant history was obtained.

CASE NOTES

Past medical history
- GORD (gastro-oesophageal reflux disease)/ PUD (peptic ulcer disease) 20 years ago, but no surgery or gastrointestinal (GI) bleed

Social history
- He denies recreational drug/sildenafil use
- Alcohol: drank ½ bottle of vodka last night
- Gave up smoking recently, previously smoked 25 cigarettes a day for 40 years
- Last cholesterol test 8 months ago – total cholesterol 4.9 mmol/L, LDL (low-density lipoprotein) 2.9 mmol/L, HDL (high-density lipoprotein) 1.07 mmol/L

Family history
- Father MI (myocardial infarction) in his 60s

Drug history
- Nil regular

Allergy
- Pistachios, 'some types of penicillin'

On examination

- Weight: 98 kg
- Height: 1.72 m
- Abdomen soft, no guarding (tensing of the abdominal muscles to guard inflamed organs)
- Blood pressure (BP) and heart rate (HR) normal
- On questioning: pain free at present

❓ What are the common differential diagnoses?
❓ What further diagnostic tests should be arranged?
❓ What risk factors does this patient have for cardiovascular disease?

Results of diagnostic tests carried out

- FBC (full blood count) and U&Es (urea and electrolytes): nil of note
- ECG–SR (electrocardiogram – sinus rhythm): subtle changes in T waves 'slightly elevated'
- Echocardiogram: good LV function

A blood sample for a troponin I test was taken and the results are awaited. The patient discharged himself before the results were known.

❓ What are troponins?
❓ What is their diagnostic use?

Blood result
Troponin I raised.

The patient was recalled to hospital.

> ## On examination
>
> - BP 132/86 mmHg
> - HR 86 beats/min
> - SpO_2 (oxygen saturation) 96%
> - RR (respiratory rate) 12/min
> - JVP not raised
> - ECG as before

❷ What is the likely diagnosis now?

The patient was referred for coronary angiogram/ percutaneous coronary intervention (PCI), which was carried out on site the same day.

It showed the presence of a thrombus in the OM (obtuse marginal coronary artery). The distal LAD (distal left anterior descending coronary artery) and the RCA (right coronary artery) were 80% and 60–70% stenosed, respectively. Two drug-eluting stents were inserted into the OM.

The following drugs were prescribed post-PCI:

- *Aspirin 75 mg daily*
- *Clopidogrel 75 mg daily*
- *Bisoprolol 2.5 mg daily*
- *Ramipril 1.25 mg at night*
- *Atorvastatin 40 mg at night*
- *Lansoprazole 30 mg daily.*

❷ What is a coronary stent and how is it normally inserted?

❷ Why is clopidogrel required post-PCI and stent insertion?

❷ What is the difference between drug-eluting stents and bare metal stents?

❷ How does this affect the duration of clopidogrel treatment?

❷ What type of drug is clopidogrel?

❷ To what class of drugs does ramipril belong? Draw its structure and explain which structural features of the drug are important in its pharmacological and clinical use

Mr TR was discharged after 3 days, after an uneventful inpatient stay, with the drugs listed above and a GTN spray to be used sublingually. Arrangements were made for an exercise tolerance test (ETT) in 6 weeks to determine whether further

PCI was indicated, and for Mr TR to enter the local cardiac rehabilitation programme.

❷ How would you counsel the patient about his medication?

❷ How should the patient's drugs be monitored and optimised as an ongoing process?

❷ What is sublingual administration?

❷ Why was it necessary to prescribe GTN in this case, and what alternative routes of administration are there for this drug?

Case discussion

— Acute coronary syndromes and their pathophysiology

ACS is an umbrella term used to describe the following diagnoses: ST-segment elevation myocardial infarction (STEMI), non-ST-elevation myocardial infarction (NSTEMI) and unstable angina (UA). ACSs usually occur in association with rupture of an atherosclerotic plaque, initiating platelet aggregation and thrombus formation in a coronary artery. The reduced blood and oxygen flow to the myocardial muscle will lead to ischaemia, and can ultimately result in cell damage or necrosis.

A STEMI occurs when the coronary artery is fully occluded; the resulting ischaemia leads to an elevation in the ST segment above the baseline when a 12-lead ECG is carried out. NSTEMI and UA usually occur when there is an incomplete or transient occlusion of the artery. The aims of treatment in ACS are to improve blood flow and reduce the ischaemic burden and myocardial damage. In STEMI, complete occlusion of the artery requires urgent treatment to restore blood flow, either mechanically using PCI or with thrombolytic agents. In NSTEMI/UA, treatment is tailored to prevent complete occlusion of the artery, followed in most cases by referral for angiography.

— Symptoms, signs and diagnosis of ACS

Patients may present with 'classic' symptoms such as chest pain or tightness, radiating to the left arm, neck, shoulders and jaw (referred pain), breathlessness, and nausea and vomiting. However, many will experience atypical symptoms such as epigastric (upper central region of abdomen) discomfort. Non-specific symptoms can make diagnosis difficult, and require further investigations to be performed to exclude other conditions with similar presenting symptoms, e.g. gastric and respiratory conditions.

When an ACS is suspected, patients should have a 12-lead ECG performed. The presence, or absence, of a raised ST segment will guide the treatment choice. It may also identify the presence of myocardial ischaemia, e.g. ST-segment depression, T-wave inversion or rhythm abnormalities.

Troponins I, T and C are proteins found in cardiac and skeletal muscle (I and T are specific to the heart). A raised level of troponin I and T in the blood indicates necrosis of the myocardial muscle, with levels peaking 12–24 hours after the event. Testing for troponin I or T levels before 12 hours may result in a false result, and require a repeat sample at a later time to confirm the troponin status. A positive troponin test helps to differentiate UA (where levels will be normal) from an NSTEMI or STEMI (where levels will be raised, due to some damage to the heart). There can be some variation between hospital troponin tests and reference ranges. The reader should familiarise him- or herself with recommended reference ranges for troponin in his or her hospital.

In this case, Mr TR had a 'normal' ECG with a raised troponin I level and pain suggestive of a cardiac origin. Therefore, the most likely diagnosis was NSTEMI, confirmed by angiogram, which identified thrombosis and stenosis in the coronary arteries (obtuse marginal [OM], left anterior descending [LAD] and right coronary artery [RCA]), requiring the deployment of drug-eluting stents (DESs).

The patient also had an echocardiogram (cardiac ultrasonography) performed to identify whether the ischaemia had caused sufficient cell damage to impair the heart muscle function. The LV function was normal in this case.

— **Cardiovascular risk factors**

Risk factors for developing cardiovascular disease can be broadly characterised as modifiable and non-modifiable.

- **Modifiable**:
- Cigarette smoking
- Hypertension
- Elevated total and LDL-cholesterol
- Low HDL-cholesterol
- Diabetes mellitus
- Obesity
- Sedentary lifestyle
- Stress
- Cocaine or amphetamine use
- **Non-modifiable**:
- Advancing age
- Male gender
- Ethnicity (south Asian heritage a greater risk)
- Family history of premature cardiac event.

— **Coronary stents and PCI**

PCI is a procedure to open an occluded or partially stenosed coronary artery, restoring blood flow. It involves the insertion of a thin guide wire (normally via the femoral or radial artery), along which a balloon catheter is manoeuvred. Real-time X-ray imaging with contrast media is used to locate the occlusion. Inflation, and subsequent deflation, of the balloon increases the artery lumen size, leading to increased blood flow.

Most PCI procedures utilise a stent to maintain the patency of an 'opened' coronary artery. This prevents rebound elastic recoil and reduction in lumen size once the angioplasty balloon has been removed. If a stent is not deployed, the term plain old balloon angioplasty (POBA) may be used.

A coronary stent is a short piece of tubular alloy mesh. In its basic form it is referred to as a bare metal stent. DESs are similar to the bare metal stents, but are coated with cytotoxic/immunosuppressant drugs (e.g. paclitaxel or sirolimus). These are slowly eluted locally over time in order to prevent tissue growth at the stent site, and therefore possible reocclusion of the artery (restenosis). However, the reduced endothelial cell growth over the stent increases the risk of thrombus formation on the exposed metallic surface. If a DES is inserted, a longer period of dual antiplatelet therapy is required until re-endothelisation occurs.

— **Antiplatelet use in patients with stents**

Antiplatelet agents such as aspirin, clopidogrel, prasugrel and ticagrelor are used to reduce platelet aggregation and thrombus formation in cardiovascular diseases. Aspirin irreversibly inhibits thromboxane A_2 production within the platelet. Clopidogrel, prasugrel and ticagrelor inhibit $P2Y_{12}$-type adenosine diphosphate (ADP) receptors. These receptors are present on platelet cell membranes, and are responsible for mediating platelet activation and cross-linking with fibrin to form a blood clot at a wound site. Clopidogrel and prasugrel are irreversible inhibitors, whereas ticagrelor is a reversible inhibitor.

In this case, Mr TR was prescribed a combination of low-dose aspirin and clopidogrel. Aspirin (75 mg) would normally be for lifelong use to prevent secondary cardiovascular events, and clopidogrel for a defined period of time. When patients have a STEMI/NSTEMI and/or a DES inserted, the second antiplatelet agent should normally be continued for 1 year. For a patient having a bare metal stent inserted as part of an elective PCI for the treatment of stable angina, clopidogrel treatment would normally be continued for 1–3 months only (this may vary according to local practice).

NICE currently recommends dual antiplatelet therapy with aspirin and clopidogrel, prasugrel or ticagrelor as the second antiplatelet agent post-ACS. Drug choice may vary, and readers should ensure that they are aware of local guidelines.

— Monitoring of drug therapy in primary care or by cardiac rehabilitation service

After an ACS, it would be expected that patients would be prescribed a drug from each of the groups listed below to reduce the risk of future cardiac events. The patient should be encouraged to report any adverse effects from the drugs to their GP.

— Antiplatelet agents

Dual antiplatelet therapy is recommended after an ACS. As this is associated with an increased risk of GI bleeds, treatment courses of the second antiplatelet agent should be kept to a minimum as discussed previously. Patients identified as having a high risk of bleeding, e.g. previous gastric ulcers, or corticosteroid use, should be considered for H_2-receptor antagonist or proton pump inhibitor therapy, in accordance with local policy. The duration and indication for treatment with antiplatelet agents should be recorded in the discharge letter to the GP. The patient should also receive a copy of this information, and receive counselling and an antiplatelet card (if used locally). Response to antiplatelet agents is not routinely monitored.

— β-Blocker

Start the drug, e.g. bisoprolol, at a low dose and increase gradually (at 24- to 48-hour intervals in hospital or at 1- to 2-weekly intervals in primary care) to the maximum tolerated dose. Systolic BP should normally be maintained >100 mmHg, and heart rate >60 beats/min. Heart rate and blood pressure should be monitored after each dose increase.

— ACE inhibitor

Start at a low dose and increase gradually to the maximum tolerated dose. Systolic BP should normally be maintained >100 mmHg. Titration steps should occur at 12- to 24-hour intervals in hospital or at 1- to 2-weekly intervals in primary care. Blood pressure, serum creatinine and potassium levels should be monitored at baseline and after each dose titration. If the patient remains stable, yearly monitoring should be sufficient.

In this case, Mr TR was initiated on ramipril, which is an ACE inhibitor. The structure of the drug is shown in the diagram.

ramipril

ACE is a peptidase that catalyses the conversion of AT-I to AT-II, a potent vasoconstrictor and stimulator of aldosterone (mineralocorticoid) release from the adrenal cortex. ACE inhibitors, such as ramipril, inhibit this conversion and thus the production of AT-II and aldosterone.

— Chemistry and mode of action of ramipril

Ramipril is an ester prodrug. It is well absorbed after oral administration and undergoes ester hydrolysis in the liver to generate the active carboxylic acid metabolite ramiprilat. Ramiprilat itself is not orally bioavailable due to the additional carboxylic acid group. It has three ionised groups (two carboxyl groups and one amino group) at the pH of the small intestine and is consequently too polar to diffuse across the cell membranes of the intestinal epithelium.

Ramiprilat mimics the transition state produced during the ACE-catalysed hydrolysis of the two C-terminal amino acids of the AT-I peptide. In particular the two carboxylic acid groups (which are both negatively charged at physiological pH) are important for making non-covalent interactions with a positively charged region and a Zn^{2+} ion at the active site of ACE.

As ramipril is a prodrug that is activated in the liver, a dose reduction may be required in hepatic impairment. In addition, the highly polar active metabolite ramiprilat primarily undergoes renal clearance from the systemic circulation, so a dose reduction of ramipril may also be required in renal impairment. In general, ACE inhibitors should be used with caution in renal impairment, but they are still routinely prescribed.

A persistent dry cough may develop in up to 15% of patients taking ACE inhibitors. ACE also catalyses the degradation of bradykinin. Thus, ACE inhibitors can lead to unwanted accumulation of bradykinin in the bronchial mucosa, which may (directly and indirectly via prostaglandin biosynthesis) be responsible for causing the dry cough resulting from sensitisation of sensory nerve endings in the lungs. If necessary, a switch to an AT-II receptor blocker (ARB) such as losartan or valsartan may be considered.

— **Statins**
High-intensity statins are recommended after an ACS, with the aim of reducing total cholesterol to <4 mmol/L, with LDL-cholesterol <2 mmol/L. Cholesterol and LFTs (liver function tests) should be measured at baseline, and 8 weeks after starting therapy, or increasing the dose. If stable, annual checks should be sufficient. Creatine kinase should be monitored at baseline, and repeated if the patient experiences muscle ache, pain or weakness (common and sometimes serious side effects of statin therapy).

— **Glyceryl trinitrate**
GTN is used for the treatment of angina, acute MI and severe hypertension. It may be given sublingually (under the tongue) as an aerosol spray or tablet, or intravenously.

GTN and isosorbide mono-/dinitrate are generally believed to produce their beneficial vasodilatory effects by generating nitric oxide (NO) within the body, although the exact mechanism by which they do this is still under debate. The intrinsic generation of NO activates cytosolic soluble guanylyl cyclase (GC) to produce the intracellular cyclic nucleotide messenger cyclic guanosine monophosphate (cGMP) from guanosine-5′-triphosphate (GTP), which then activates cGMP-dependent protein kinase G (PKG), leading to a reduction in intracellular calcium concentration ($[Ca^{2+}]_i$), and vascular smooth muscle relaxation. This results in venodilatation and arterial dilatation, and reduction of cardiac ischaemia, which relieves anginal symptoms.

— **Medicines optimisation: supporting adherence through motivational interviewing**
It is estimated that 50% or more of cardiovascular patients do not take their medicines as intended. This is despite the fact that poor adherence to secondary preventive therapy after MI can lead to an increase in recurrence, hospitalisation and mortality. There are many possible reasons for poor adherence: patients' beliefs about the potential benefits of medicines and/or concerns about adverse effects can be important factors in determining whether a patient continues to take them.

Motivational interviewing is increasingly promoted by health professionals as a potential way to support patients in engaging in positive health adherence behaviours. It has been defined as a form of collaborative conversation for strengthening a person's own motivation and commitment to change. A motivational interview employs techniques such as asking open questions so that patients voice their own perspectives, listening to the patient, and promoting reflection on relevant goals and concerns, so that they build their own priorities and motivation to achieve them. For example, an interview may start with a question asking the patient to rate (e.g. on a 1–10 scale) their motivation and confidence in using their medication. Discussing why a lower rating was not specified encourages patients to recognise positive motivations to take their medicines. Conversely, discussing why the rating was not higher may enable the identification of barriers to medicine use. In the interview, patients may also consider wider values and goals, and explore any connections between these and health behaviours. This may highlight a patient's potential motivations and ability to achieve goals. Techniques, such as motivational interviewing, may provide pharmacists with more effective ways of supporting patients in achieving optimal outcomes from their medicines.

EXTENDED LEARNING

- What are the treatment options for a patient with a STEMI?
- Review the drug therapy used during the PCI procedure, and consider how this may vary depending on the diagnosis, e.g. STEMI, NSTEMI, UA or stable angina
- Review the evidence and recommended use for current antiplatelet agents in your locality
- What is a prodrug? Why might we employ a prodrug rather than a drug as a therapeutic agent?
- Give examples of prodrugs used in practice.

References and further reading

De Luca G, Dirksen MT, Spaulding C et al.; Drug-Eluting Stent in Primary Angioplasty (DESERT) Cooperation (2012). Drug-eluting vs bare-metal stents in primary angioplasty: a pooled patient-level meta-analysis of randomized trials. *Arch Intern Med* **172**:611–21.

Hamm CW, Bassand JP, Agewall S et al. (2011). ESC Committee for Practice Guidelines. ESC Guidelines for the management of acute coronary syndromes in patients presenting without persistent ST-segment elevation: The Task Force for the management of acute coronary syndromes (ACS) in patients presenting without persistent ST-segment elevation of the European Society of Cardiology (ESC). *Eur Heart J* **32**:2999–3054.

National Institute for Health and Clinical Excellence (2009). *Prasugrel for the Treatment of Acute Coronary Syndromes with Percutaneous Coronary Intervention.* Technology Appraisal Guideline 182. London: NICE. Available at: http://publications.nice.org.uk/prasugrel-for-the-treatment-of-acute-coronary-syndromes-with-percutaneous-coronary-intervention-ta182 (accessed 15 August 2013).

National Institute for Health and Clinical Excellence (2010). *Unstable Angina and NSTEMI: The early management of unstable angina and non-ST-segment-elevation myocardial infarction.* Clinical Guideline 94. London: NICE. Available at: www.nice.org.uk/cg94 (accessed 9 July 2013).

National Institute for Health and Clinical Excellence (2011). *Ticagrelor for the Treatment of Acute Coronary Syndromes.* Technology Appraisal Guideline 236. London: NICE. Available at: http://publications.nice.org.uk/ticagrelor-for-the-treatment-of-acute-coronary-syndromes-ta236 (accessed 15 August 2013).

National Institute for Health and Care Excellence (2013). *Secondary Prevention in Primary and Secondary Care for Patients Following a Myocardial Infarction.* Clinical Guideline 172. London: NICE. Available at: http://guidance.nice.org.uk/CG172 (accessed 8 April 2014).

Case 5
Management of hypertension in black patients

KAY WOOD, NAVEED IQBAL AND KEITH WILSON

LEARNING OUTCOMES

At the end of this case, you will be able to:

- Outline the investigations required before starting antihypertensive drug treatment
- Discuss why it is so important to treat hypertension in black patients promptly and aggressively
- List the factors that may be included in a cardiovascular risk assessment, and explain how the result is interpreted
- Recommend appropriate lifestyle advice to reduce blood pressure and cardiovascular risk
- Recommend appropriate antihypertensive drug treatment taking into account a patient's ethnicity
- Identify how ethnicity may be an important determinant of appropriate use of medicines by a patient
- Use the Summary of Product Characteristics (SPC) to ascertain the excipients included in a proprietary pharmaceutical product

Case study

Mr JB is a 45-year-old, 90-kg, African–Caribbean man. During a routine health check, he was found to have a blood pressure (BP) reading of 175/95 mmHg.

- ❓ Why is Mr JB's ethnicity so important?
- ❓ What lifestyle advice should be offered to Mr JB that will help reduce his BP?

After ambulatory blood pressure monitoring (ABPM), Mr JB's readings are usually around 155/95 mmHg. This is known as stage 2 hypertension, and drug treatment should be started.

❓ What would you recommend and why?

Mr JB's BP improves, but is not at the clinic target of 140/90 mmHg despite taking amlodipine 10 mg daily. He claims to be fully compliant with his medication and lifestyle advice.

❓ What are the ingredients of amlodipine tablets and why are they included in the formulation?

❓ What drug treatment would you add and why?

Case discussion

— Interpreting blood pressure readings
On receiving a blood pressure reading, you need to confirm the circumstances in which the reading was taken, e.g. is this is a one-off reading? Was the patient rushed or anxious when the reading was taken? Had the patient been sitting quietly for at least 5 min before taking the reading? The reading should be checked again at the same appointment. If there is a substantial difference between the two readings, check a third time. BP should be measured in both arms, and, if there is a difference of >20 mmHg, repeated.

In Mr JB's case, the BP is high, but not extreme, so if the second (and third) readings are still high, then Mr JB should be offered ABPM. (See National Institute for Health and Clinical Excellence, 2011, for further information on ABPM.)

Mr JB should also be investigated for evidence of target organ damage:

- Urine should be tested for the presence of protein by sending a urine sample for estimation of the albumin:creatinine ratio. Haematuria should be tested for, using a reagent strip.
- Plasma glucose, electrolytes, creatinine, estimated glomerular filtration rate (eGFR), serum total cholesterol and HDL-cholesterol should be measured in a blood sample.
- The fundi should be examined for the presence of hypertensive retinopathy.
- A 12-lead ECG should be performed.

— Importance of ethnicity in hypertension
The prevalence of hypertension (HTN) is high in black patients, with increased prevalence of severe hypertension ($\geq$180/110 mmHg). Compared with white people, there is a higher frequency of co-morbid conditions such as diabetes mellitus, albuminuria, chronic kidney disease (CKD) and pressure-related target-organ injury such as strokes, LV hypertrophy (LVH), heart failure (HF) and CKD/end-stage renal disease. An early study in the UK noted that black patients had a higher incidence of HTN than whites or Asians, but they had fewer heart attacks and more strokes. Subsequent UK studies confirmed the increased incidence and mortality associated with strokes in black people; black people are twice as likely to have a stroke as white people, and the first stroke occurs at an earlier age. It has been estimated that as many as 30% of all deaths in hypertensive black men and 20% in hypertensive black women may be due to high BP.

Black patients often struggle with control of BP. This may be due to inappropriate choice of drug therapy (see later), but it may also be due to non-pharmacological factors, such as health beliefs about the risks of hypertension and/or perceptions of the need for medication that may impact on adherence.

— Hypertension and lifestyle advice
Lifestyle modifications for people with hypertension include the following:

- Lose weight if above target BMI (20–25 kg/m^2). Healthy, low-calorie diets have a modest effect on blood pressure in overweight individuals with raised blood pressure. A meta-analysis published in 2003 contained a simple message: 1 kg in weight lost = 1 mm lowering of diastolic and systolic pressure
  In this case, Mr JB weighs 90 kg. No height is given here, so it is not possible to calculate his BMI, but he is likely to be overweight. Obesity is more common in black people than white people, especially among women. This increases the risk not only of hypertension but also of diabetes mellitus and heart failure. Obesity leads to over-secretion of cortisol and aldosterone from the adrenal cortex. High circulating levels of aldosterone are linked to renal vascular resistance. There is also a link to salt sensitivity.
- Alcohol consumption should be no more than recommended levels (no more than 3–4 units a day for men, with 2 alcohol-free days; maximum of 21 units a week).

- Reduce salt intake (at least to <100 mmol/day sodium intake – approximately 6 g NaCl or <2.4 g sodium), or substitute sodium salt (be careful if using KCl as a substitute if patient has renal failure and/or is taking potassium-sparing drugs).

Black people may consume less potassium in their diet than white people, but a similar amount of sodium. Night-time BP levels are usually 10–20% lower than daytime BP levels. People whose night-time BP falls <10% from daytime levels are termed 'non-dippers'. During ABPM, both normotensive and hypertensive black people exhibit more non-dipping than white people. Nocturnal non-dipping has been linked to high dietary salt intake, salt sensitivity and a lower dietary intake of potassium.

The 2011 NICE guidelines do not recommend potassium supplements as a means of reducing BP, but they do recommend maintaining salt intake to <6 g/day and/or substituting sodium salt. Salt substitutes that contain potassium may be appropriate (depending on the patient's drug therapy and renal function). However, in those patients with low potassium diets, it would be prudent to recommend a review of the diet to see if the potassium content can be increased.

- Partake in regular aerobic exercise, tailored to the individual (e.g. brisk walking at least 30 minutes a day for most days a week).
- Increase intake of fruit and vegetables to at least five portions a day.
- Discourage excessive consumption (five or more cups per day) of coffee and other caffeine-rich products. Studies suggest that excessive consumption of coffee (in participants with or without raised BP) is associated with a small increase in blood pressure.
- Relaxation therapies can reduce BP, and individual patients may wish to self-fund these, because they are currently unavailable from within NHS resources.

Patients should also be encouraged to reduce their risk of cardiovascular disease through:

- Smoking cessation: there is no strong direct link between smoking and BP. However, there is overwhelming evidence of the relationship between smoking and cardiovascular and pulmonary diseases.
- Reducing saturated fat and cholesterol intake.

- Increasing oily fish intake (mackerel, sardines, herrings – high in omega-3 fatty acids).

Whether this is the only form of intervention or part of a strategy for the treatment of a hypertensive patient, adherence to these principles is very important.

— Drug treatment of hypertension

The 2011 NICE hypertension guidelines include an algorithm for treatment, which lays out a clear approach to drug management (see below). At step 1, for patients aged <55 years, an ACE inhibitor or low-cost ARB is recommended. For patients aged >55 years, and black people of African or Caribbean family origin of any age, a calcium channel blocker (CCB) is first line, unless contraindicated.

In this case, Mr JB should be prescribed a CCB. An intrinsically long-acting dihydropyridine CCB such as amlodipine maleate (initially at a dose of 5 mg once daily) is a good choice.

— Chemical properties of dihdropyridine antihypertensives

The structure of amlodipine, along with two other dihydropyridine (DHP)-type CCBs (nifedipine and felodipine), is shown in the diagram on page 64. Note the presence of a phenyl ring with an electron-withdrawing substituent in the adjacent *ortho* position, bonded to C4 of the DHP ring in each drug; this substituent forces the two rings to lie essentially perpendicular to each other, which is essential for interaction with the L-type calcium channel, for which they are high-affinity ligands. In amlodipine (and felodipine, but not nifedipine), the two ester groups are asymmetrical – one ethyl ester and one methyl ester. This lack of symmetry makes C4 a chiral centre. Despite being manufactured and administered as a racemic mixture, the *S*-enantiomer is responsible for its calcium channel-blocking activity. Increasing the length(s) of the carbon chain(s) of the esters increases lipophilicity. Although increased lipophilicity can lead to improved drug absorption from the small intestine, first-pass metabolism can also be increased, resulting in lower overall bioavailability.

The nitrogen atom at position 1 of the DHP ring is effectively non-basic due to resonance delocalisation. Most DHP CCBs are unionised at physiological pH. Amlodipine, however, has an additional basic primary amino group. This group is predominantly ionised (positively charged) at

amlodipine   nifedipine   felodipine   1,4-dihydropyridine

physiological pH, which may contribute to the increased half-life of amlodipine compared with other DHPs. The basicity of the amino group also allows formulation of the drug as a maleate or similar salt. Salt formation is often employed as a strategy to improve the properties of a drug candidate, such as its aqueous solubility and dissolution rate, to enhance the performance of resultant formulations. In this case, the ionic salt is formed by reacting an acid, such as maleic acid, with the weak basic drug.

— Ethnicity and response to medicines

It is well known that black people respond less well to ACE inhibitors, ARBs and β- adrenoreceptor blockers when these are used as monotherapy. The reason for this has been widely reported to result from the low circulating renin of black people. However, most black hypertensive patients do not have fully suppressed circulating renin levels and dietary salt-induced suppression of renin production. Circulating renin and AT-II levels are not a particularly good measure of the activity of the renin–angiotensin system (RAS), because most angiotensin is generated locally in the vasculature. The key to response to drug treatment can be explained by increased salt sensitivity, with expanded plasma volume and increased renal vascular resistance. Thus, black patients respond better to diuretics and CCBs. In fact, a systematic review reported that CCBs were effective antihypertensives across different subgroups of black patients in the study, so a CCB is a logical first-line choice.

Use of agents that block the RAS have been shown to be important in slowing the progression of kidney disease, so ACE inhibitors or ARBs should be considered for black patients. Step 2 of the 2011 NICE hypertension guidelines recommends the addition of 'A' to a CCB (Table 2.5). For a black patient, 'A' would be a low-cost ARB rather than an ACE inhibitor. Black patients are more prone to ACE inhibitor-induced dry cough and angio-oedema, so an ARB is preferred, e.g. losartan (start at a low dose, increasing gradually, checking renal function before commencing and 7–10 days after each dose increase).

— Amlodipine tablets

Amlodipine is available as 5 mg and 10 mg tablets. The most readily available reference source to find the ingredients of a proprietary medicine is the Summary of Product Characteristics (SPC/SmPC).

▼ TABLE 2.5

Summary algorithm of NICE guidance for antihypertensive drug treatment

	<55 years		Patient 55+ years or black person of African or Caribbean origin of any age
Step 1	A		C
	↓		↓
Step 2		A + C	
		↓	
Step 3		A + C + D	
		↓	
		Add further diuretic or α-blocker or β-blocker Consider expert advice	

A, ACE inhibitor or angiotensin II receptor blocker; C, calcium channel blocker; D, thiazide-like diuretic.

These are can be accessed online and provide a wealth of information in a standardised format, including: pharmaceutical form; clinical particulars such as dosage, indications, contraindications and adverse drug reactions; and pharmacology and pharmaceutical particulars, such as excipients, storage conditions and shelf-life. Amlodipine tablets contain the drug (also called the active pharmaceutical ingredient [API] as the maleate, besilate or mesilate salt). The tablet will also contain excipients to ensure optimal properties of the tablet (e.g. dissolution behaviour) and favourable processing conditions for tablet manufacture. The SPC of one commercially available amlodipine tablet product lists the excipients as: microcrystalline cellulose, anhydrous calcium hydrogen phosphate, sodium starch glycollate type A and magnesium stearate. Some excipients have multiple functions.

Microcrystalline cellulose and anhydrous calcium hydrogen phosphate are both used as fillers (diluents) to bulk up the size of a low-dose tablet (as is the case here), so that the tablet is of an acceptable size and as binders, which ensure that the tablets and the granules used in the preparation of tablets are of the required mechanical strength.

Sodium starch glycollate type A is a disintegrant, included in a tablet formulation, so that when the tablet is in contact with a liquid (e.g. the contents of the gastrointestinal tract) it breaks into small fragments, aiding dissolution.

Magnesium stearate is a lubricant, which aids in the tablet manufacturing process, by reducing the friction between the tablet and the walls of the die in which the tablet is formed, by compression between two punches.

— CVD risk assessment

As well as looking for secondary causes of hypertension, Mr JB's cardiovascular risk should be assessed. A risk factor calculator is commonly used to assess the risk of an individual developing a cardiovascular disease (CVD) such as: heart attack, angina, stroke and peripheral vascular disease. These calculations may take into account a range of factors from: blood pressure, blood cholesterol (especially total cholesterol : HDL ratio or TC : HDL), blood sugars, or presence of diabetes, smoking, obesity, diet, physical activity, alcohol consumption, age and sex. Adjustment is also made for strong family history and ethnic origin.

Treatment with lipid-lowering drugs, usually statins, is recommended if an individual has a high risk. The Framingham measure has been used for a long time, but there are a number of other tools, e.g. the QRISK*2 takes into account other factors such as the presence of atrial fibrillation or kidney disease.

The test result is expressed as a percentage, which indicates the chance of experiencing a cardiovascular or cerebrovascular event within the next 10 years. Scores are generally interpreted as follows:

- High risk: ≥20%, i.e. ≥2 in 10 chance of developing a cardiovascular disease within the next 10 years.
- Moderate risk: 10–20% chance of developing a CVD within the next 10 years. This should be re-assessed every year.
- Low risk: <10%. This should be re-assessed every 5 years.

— Ethnicity and health

Ethnicity is complex. Some differences between population groups have a genetic or biological origin that can influence susceptibility to disease and also be a determinant of drug handling. Thus, the recommended therapy for hypertension, as this case illustrates, differs between ethnic groups.

However, ethnicity is also viewed as a 'socially constructed identity'. How people see themselves and interact with society can be important for health beliefs, perceptions of illness, and use of health services and medicines. Membership of an ethnic group can confer an identity that may be linked to certain health risks and needs, although it is also important to recognise that individuals within a group can be diverse.

Inequalities between ethnic groups in health are well recognised. People from ethnic minority communities in the UK are more likely to be from more deprived backgrounds. In general, people from lower socioeconomic groups experience poorer health outcomes; because of this confounding, the picture is complex. Also, there is a huge diversity between ethnic minority groups in their background and identity so it is often not appropriate to make generalisations.

Sometimes experiences such as travel and migration, racism or language barriers can have an impact on health status and uptake of services. Ethnicity can be an important consideration in the prescribing of medicines as well as a determinant of health beliefs, understanding and adherence to therapy.

different ethnic and cultural groups are met?

EXTENDED LEARNING

- What are the common tools that are used for cardiovascular health risk assessment in primary care?
- What is the proposed mechanism underlying the ACE inhibitor-induced cough side effect seen in some hypertensive patients?
- What actions can health providers take to help ensure that the health needs of

References and further reading

Brewster LM, van Montfrans GA, Kleijnen J (2004). Systematic review: antihypertensive drug therapy in black patients. *Ann Intern Med* **141**:614–27.

Flack JM, Sica DA, Bakris G et al. (2010). Management of high blood pressure in Blacks: An Update of the International Society on Hypertension in Blacks Consensus Statement. *Hypertension* **56**:780–800.

National Institute for Health and Clinical Excellence (2011). *Hypertension: Clinical management of primary hypertension in adults*. Clinical Guideline 127. London: NICE. Available at: http://guidance.nice.org.uk/CG127 (accessed 3 October 2013).

Case 6
Cardiovascular (blood pressure) support in an elderly hypotensive patient

MARK BORTHWICK

LEARNING OUTCOMES

At the end of this case, you will be able to:

- Outline the methods and parameters used for monitoring blood pressure and fluid status
- Explain how blood gases may be used to monitor the effectiveness of therapy for hypotension
- Describe the chemistry and mechanism of action of adrenergic agonists and dopamine in the treatment of hypotension
- Describe medicines that can be used to address hypotension

Case study

Mrs CV, a 69-year-old woman, has been brought to A&E by paramedics who found her at home, the alarm having been raised by concerned neighbours. She has had a 3-day history of increasing fever, pain on micturition and deteriorating cognitive function. Her past medical history includes hypertension and ischaemic heart disease. Her drug history is as follows:

- *Bendroflumethiazide 2.5 mg once daily*
- *Lisinopril 10 mg once daily*
- *Aspirin 75 mg once daily*
- *Simvastatin 40 mg once daily*

Her heart rate is 115 beats/min and her non-invasive blood pressure is recorded as 90/45 mmHg, with a mean arterial pressure of 55 mmHg. She is not producing much urine, but it is cloudy and positive for nitrites and leukocytes on a dipped test strip.

She is diagnosed with a severe urinary tract infection (UTI) and antibiotics are started.

- What do the cardiovascular parameters described above tell you?
- How should Mrs CV's low blood pressure be managed?
- What other signs can you look for that will help direct initial management?

Mrs CV becomes increasingly confused in A&E, and a set of arterial blood gas results is obtained. Her respiratory rate approaches 40 breaths/min. The decision is made to intubate and ventilate.

Arterial blood gases (on 30% O_2) are:

pH	7.19	BE (mmol/L)	−12.5
$PaCO_2$ (kPa)	2.7	HCO_3^- (mmol/L)	15.0
PaO_2 (kPa)	18.3	Lactate (mmol/L)	11.5
SaO_2	98%		

BE, base excess; $PaCO_2$, partial pressure of carbon dioxide in the blood; PaO_2, partial pressure of oxygen in the blood; SaO_2, oxygen saturation of arterial blood.

Emergency treatment is initiated.

❷ Interpret the blood gas results. What are the potential causes of the clinical state reflected by the arterial blood gases?

Mrs CV is transferred to the intensive care unit. She is still hypotensive.

❷ What pharmacological agents can be used to restore her cardiovascular function?

❷ How could these agents affect her blood gas results?

Case discussion

— Interpretation of cardiovascular parameters
In this case, Mrs CV has presented in septic shock (i.e. sepsis with hypotension). Her blood pressure is low overall, with a low mean arterial pressure. The production of inflammatory mediators in sepsis (e.g. cytokines) has increased her heart rate, caused her vascular system to vasodilate and made her capillaries very leaky. The circulating blood volume has thus reduced, because plasma has leaked out of capillaries into the interstitial spaces, and the remaining blood is filling a larger space due to vasodilatation. This has resulted in a fall in blood pressure. She has compensated for low blood pressure by further increasing her heart rate, which would increase cardiac output, so increasing blood flow to meet the oxygen/metabolic demands of tissues.

A blood pressure target should be established and therapies started to meet those targets. Target setting can be complicated by other factors, such as pre-existing hypertension and the clinical state of the patient. Normally, the target is set to reach a mean arterial pressure (MAP) of >60 mmHg. At this level, renal perfusion is usually re-established and an anuric patient (not passing urine) may begin to produce urine. In patients with long-standing uncontrolled hypertension, the required MAP to make this occur may well be higher. In this case, prior diuretic use could have further exacerbated the hypovolaemia (low blood volume).

The first step in resuscitation is to replenish the circulating fluid with the administration of intravenous fluid. A fluid challenge should be given, whereby a volume of fluid is rapidly administered to the patient and the response noted, usually in terms of heart rate, blood pressure and urine output. Additional monitoring can be achieved by measuring the central venous pressure (CVP), an invasive method that directly measures pressure in a large vein via a catheter, usually placed in the vena cava. The CVP should respond to the fluid bolus by increasing; however, a large sustained increase would suggest too much fluid has been given, and this risks putting the patient into fluid overload with subsequent pulmonary oedema. This may be a particular problem in this patient given her cardiac history, which puts her at risk of pre-existing inefficient cardiac function.

There are numerous signs that can be used to assess for lack of circulating fluid volume. These include thirst, skin turgor and reduced capillary refill times. The choice of fluid for resuscitation in sepsis has been controversial for many years. However, a picture is emerging that crystalloid (aqueous solution of mineral salts or other small soluble molecules) should be the mainstay of therapy.

Patients who do not meet the oxygen requirements of tissues switch energy production in those tissues towards anaerobic respiration. A consequence of this is the production of lactic acid, which can be measured in arterial blood and which also affects pH. There are confounders, however: lactic acid is broken down by hepatic processes to bicarbonate, so liver failure will also result in a hyperlactataemia. Clearly, ventilatory parameters also affect blood gases. Critical care staff will adjust ventilation and cardiovascular support in an effort to get blood gases into the right range.

The interpretation of blood gases is important, because adjustments in therapy affect the values of the arterial blood gases and give an indication as to whether the therapy is having the desired effect. Arterial blood gases may be measured very frequently and can be examined alongside physical values such as blood pressure, heart rate, ventilator settings, etc., to determine whether to alter therapy and, if so, in which manner.

Normal physiological arterial blood gas values at sea level are:

pH	7.35–7.45	BE (mmol/L)	+2 to −2
$PaCO_2$ (kPa)	4.7–6.0	HCO_3^- (mmol/L)	22–28
PaO_2 (kPa)	>10.5	Lactate (mmol/L)	0.4–1.5
SaO_2 (%)	95–100		

BE, base excess; $PaCO_2$, partial pressure of carbon dioxide in the blood; PaO_2, partial pressure of oxygen in the blood; SaO_2, oxygen saturation of arterial blood.

A simple step process can be taken to interpret the arterial blood gas values.

1. Acidosis, alkalosis or normal? Look at the pH. Abnormally low = acidosis, abnormally high = alkalosis; otherwise, it is normal.
2. Respiratory component? Look at the $PaCO_2$. Abnormally high with an acidosis = respiratory acidosis. Abnormally low with an alkalosis = respiratory alkalosis.
3. Metabolic component? Look at HCO_3^-. Abnormally low with an acidosis = metabolic acidosis. Abnormally high with an alkalosis = metabolic alkalosis.
4. Compensation? Look at the remaining variable(s) and decide if it is/they are adjusted to compensate for the state you think the patient is in.

Base excess (BE), in which a positive value indicates an excess of base and a negative value indicates a deficit, provides a measure of the metabolic component of acid–base balance, whereas $PaCO_2$ is an indicator of respiratory acid–base balance. HCO_3^- is the principal base that contributes to BE.

In this case, Mrs CV has a low pH, so she has an acidosis. The HCO_3^- is low, so it is a metabolic acidosis. The remaining variable, the $PaCO_2$, is low, so she is trying to compensate by breathing off CO_2. She has a partially compensated metabolic acidosis (if it were fully compensated, the pH would be normal).

It is worth noting that respiratory compensation can occur very quickly (minutes), but metabolic compensation takes a while to achieve (hours to days).

If fluid resuscitation is not sufficient to adequately restore blood pressure, the addition of inotropes and vasopressors can be used to manipulate the cardiovascular system in order to restore tissue perfusion.

Inotropes increase the force of contraction of the heart, and thereby increase cardiac output and delivery of blood (and oxygen) to tissues. Commonly, *vasopressors* are used to increase blood pressure, again in an attempt to restore blood supply to tissues. There is a range of such agents used, each with its own receptor profile, which itself is usually dependent on the dose of the drug being infused.

— Noradrenaline

(Receptor profile: adrenergic – α_1^{+++}, β_1^+, β_2^0; dopaminergic – D_1^0, D_2^0)

Noradrenaline is the naturally released neurotransmitter of the sympathetic nervous system. At doses of <0.03 micrograms/kg per min there is predominant cardiac β_1-receptor stimulation that causes an increase in heart rate, stroke volume and cardiac output, whereas at higher doses (>0.05 micrograms/kg per min) α_1-receptor stimulation becomes dominant, leading to peripheral vasoconstriction and a rise in blood pressure. Reflex baroreceptor-mediated bradycardia is possible if the blood pressure rise is sufficiently large.

noradrenaline   adrenaline

— Adrenaline

(Receptor profile: adrenergic – α_1^{+++}, β_1^{+++}, β_2^{++}; dopaminergic – D_1^0, D_2^0)

Adrenaline is a natural hormone synthesised from dopamine in chromaffin cells of the adrenal medulla and released into the circulation as part of the sympathetic nervous system 'fight-or-flight' response. At low doses (<0.01 micrograms/kg per min), there is mainly β_2-receptor stimulation that can cause dilatation of the skeletal muscle vasculature and a paradoxical *fall* in blood pressure. At medium doses (0.04–0.1 micrograms/kg per min) there is increasing cardiac β_1-receptor stimulation that increases heart rate and stroke volume, leading to increased cardiac output. At larger doses (0.1–0.3 micrograms/kg per min), α_1-receptor stimulation dominates, leading to vasoconstriction and so increased blood pressure. At very high doses (>0.3 micrograms/kg per min) the increased α_1-receptor stimulation and vasoconstriction can reduce renal and splanchnic vascular bed perfusion.

Examination of the structures of both noradrenaline and adrenaline shown above reveals their very close similarity. Both are catecholamines and contain a hydroxylated aromatic ring, and the carbon atom in the side chain that is bonded to a secondary aliphatic hydroxyl group has the

dopamine

dobutamine

R-absolute configuration. In addition, both contain an amino group that will be protonated and positively charged at physiological pH. These structural features are common for all agonists at adrenergic receptors. The S-enantiomers of noradrenaline and adrenaline are about an order of magnitude less potent as agonists than the naturally occurring R-isomers.

— Dopamine
(Receptor profile: adrenergic – α_1^{++}, β_1^{++}, β_2^{++}; dopaminergic – D_1^{+++}, D_2^{+++})

Dopamine is an important inhibitory neurotransmitter in the brain, but it can also exert peripheral effects on cardiovascular and kidney function. Dopamine is still commonly used as a first-line vasopressor agent in hypotensive patients and also for blood pressure support in pre-term neonates, due to its effects on adrenergic β- and α-receptors. At low doses (<2 micrograms/kg per min) there is a predominant dopamine D_1-receptor stimulation that leads to a diuretic effect through natriuresis and renal *vasodilatation* with an increased renal, mesenteric and coronary perfusion. The use of low-dose dopamine to preserve renal function has been investigated but shown to be ineffective. At medium doses (2–5 micrograms/kg per min), there is dominant cardiac β_1-receptor stimulation leading to an increase in heart rate, stroke volume and cardiac output. At large doses (>6 micrograms/kg per min), an adrenergic α_1-receptor stimulation predominates, leading to vasoconstriction, which increases blood pressure.

— Dobutamine
(Receptor profile: adrenergic – α_1^+, β_1^{++}, β_2^+; dopaminergic – D_1^0, D_2^0)

Dobutamine is a relatively cardioselective sympathomimetic agonist. At the usual dose (2.5–10 micrograms/kg per min) there is predominant cardiac β_1-receptor stimulation which leads to increased cardiac output. Dobutamine contains a single chiral centre (indicated by an asterisk on the structure above) and is manufactured and administered as a racemic mixture. Interestingly, the two enantiomers have different activities at the different subtypes of adrenergic receptors. The R-enantiomer is the more potent β_1-agonist, but also exerts α_1-*antagonist* activity. The S-enantiomer exhibits weak β_1-agonist activity in addition to be being a potent α_1-agonist, which causes arterial vasoconstriction. The net effect of β_1-receptor agonism (for the racemic mixture) leads to the increase in cardiac output. In addition, (R)-dobutamine has some slight β_2-receptor activity, causing vascular vasodilatation, which can slightly oppose the effects of the α_1-mediated vasoconstriction. However, in fluid-depleted states, dobutamine can cause an unexpected hypotension.

It is possible to consider the properties of each individual agent and choose the one most suited to the clinical condition being treated, carefully titrating the dose to achieve the expected result. In reality, clinicians often use a first-line agent and then tweak the dose while continually monitoring parameters such as heart rate, blood pressure, CVP, urine output, pH, lactate and other measures of adequate cardiovascular function. Combinations of these agents are used to target and affect different receptor types (e.g. noradrenaline may be used for its α_1-effects in combination with dobutamine for its β_1-effects). More advanced monitoring options exist, such as cardiac output monitoring through a variety of techniques, but these are beyond the scope of this case study.

EXTENDED LEARNING

- What is levosimendan and how does it act?
- How does its use compare with that of dobutamine in critically ill patients requiring inotropic support?

References and further reading

Angus DC, van der Poll T (2013). Severe sepsis and septic shock. *N Engl J Med* **369**:840–51.

Cowley JN, Owen A, Bion JF (2013). Interpreting arterial blood gas results. *BMJ* **346**:f16.

Dellinger RP, Levy MM, Rhodes A et al.; Surviving Sepsis Campaign Guidelines Committee including the Pediatric Subgroup (2013). Surviving sepsis campaign: international guidelines for management of severe sepsis and septic shock. *Crit Care Med* **41**:580–637.

Hollenberg SM (2009). Inotrope and vasopressor therapy of septic shock. *Crit Care Clinics* **25**:781–802.

Schulte W, Bernhagen J, Bucala R (2013). Cytokines in sepsis: potent immunoregulators and potential therapeutic targets-an updated view. *Mediators Inflammation* **165**:974.

Seri I, Rudas G, Bors Z, Kanyicska B, Tulassay T (1993). Effects of low-dose dopamine infusion on cardiovascular and renal functions, cerebral blood flow, and plasma catecholamine levels in sick preterm neonates. *Pediatr Res* **34**:742–9.

Case 7
Deep vein thrombosis and warfarin
DELYTH HIGMAN JAMES AND JIGNESH PATEL

LEARNING OUTCOMES

At the end of this case, you will be able to:

- Describe the pathophysiology, signs and symptoms of a DVT
- Explain the treatment options for a DVT
- State the mechanisms of action of heparin and warfarin
- Describe the stereochemistry of warfarin
- Outline the significant drug interactions with warfarin
- Outline the role of the pharmacist in the pharmaceutical care of patients prescribed warfarin therapy
- Understand the role of effective consultation skills when optimising patient medication
- Outline the manufacture of tablets and excipients commonly used in their manufacture

Case study

Mrs MJ is an 81-year-old woman who fractured her hip after a fall at home. She suffers with mild cognitive impairment and has no other relevant medical history, other than significant hearing loss. She lives at home with her husband, who is a retired headmaster. He is the main carer and is able to help administer his wife's medicines. Three weeks after an operation to repair her fractured left hip, she was discharged from hospital with the following prescription:

Calcium and vitamin D₃ (Calcichew D3) tablets – two tablets once daily

Alendronic acid 70 mg – once weekly
Paracetamol 500 mg tablets – two tablets four times a day as required for the pain
Senna tablets – two tablets at night when required for constipation

She was also given compression stockings to wear at home. Six weeks later she developed swelling, pain and redness in her left leg, which was diagnosed as a deep vein thrombosis (DVT).

- What is a DVT?
- How might this be linked to Mrs MJ's recent surgery?
- How is a DVT managed on an outpatient basis?
- How are tablets formulated and manufactured?
- How do chewable tablets differ from conventional tablets?

Mrs MJ's DVT was initially treated with daily subcutaneous injections of a low-molecular-weight heparin (LMWH) which was administered by a district nurse at home. She was also prescribed a loading dose of warfarin and the LMWH was stopped when the INR had reached the target range.

- What are low-molecular-weight heparins?
- How do these differ from unfractionated heparin injections?
- What is an INR?
- What is the target INR for the treatment of a DVT?
- What length of warfarin therapy should the patient receive?

Mrs MJ was also buying ginkgo biloba from a health food shop to help with her memory loss. She also self-medicates with aspirin 75 mg bought from the supermarket because she has heard that this can also help with 'blood flow to the brain'.

❷ Are there any potential clinically significant drug interactions for this patient?

You are the local village community pharmacist and you know the family well. Mrs MJ's husband brings in a prescription for warfarin 4 mg once daily.

❷ What would you do to ensure a thorough pharmaceutical assessment of this patient?

One month later, Mrs MJ's husband returns with a repeat prescription for the other medicines. He tells you that his wife does not like taking this many medicines and she is sometimes reluctant to take them all. He is not sure which day of the week to give the alendronic acid tablet and she is not able to chew the Calcichew tablets because her dentures have broken.

Following a consultation you identify the problems in the box.

PROBLEM LIST

- Possible non-adherence to warfarin (and other medication) because Mrs MJ sometimes refuses to take them
- Potential pharmacodynamic drug interaction between warfarin and aspirin/ ginkgo biloba
- Patient unable to chew Calcichew tablets
- Husband unsure what day of the week to administer alendronic acid tablets
- Patient and carer would like to reduce the number of medicines taken if possible

---

❷ What advice would you give Mrs MJ's husband?

Case discussion

— **Pathophysiology of venous thromboembolism**
Pulmonary embolism (PE) and DVT represent the spectrum of one disease – venous thromboembolism (VTE). The annual incidence of VTE in developed countries is around 1 in 1000 people. VTE commonly manifests as DVT of the leg and the consequences of DVT range from complete resolution of the clot to death due to PE. The main morbidity associated with DVT is post-thrombotic syndrome (PTS), which occurs in

▼ TABLE 2.6
Risk factors for venous thromboembolism (VTE)

Reduced or altered blood flow	Prothrombotic changes	Damage to vessel wall
Immobility Previous VTE Surgery Trauma	Increasing age Pregnancy and the puerperium Cancer Genetic thrombophilia Anti-phospholipid syndrome Myeloproliferative disease Obesity Surgery Trauma Drugs, e.g. combined oral contraceptive pill	Surgery Trauma

between 20% and 50% of patients after an acute DVT.

There are three major factors that contribute to VTE: changes in blood flow, changes in the vessel wall or an increase in blood coagulability. Usually a combination of these factors is present. Specific risk factors for the development of VTE are listed in Table 2.6.

— **Symptoms, signs and diagnosis of DVT**
Pain and/or swelling of the calf or thigh, along with redness of the overlying skin and increased warmth of the affected leg, are classic signs and symptoms of DVT. It is important to note that, in up to half of all cases, no signs or symptoms may be present and the onset of a PE may be the first sign of the presence of VTE in the patient.

Diagnosis of DVT usually involves the use of a diagnostic algorithm. Along with an accurate clinical history, a screening test is completed (D-dimer test or plethysmography). Although these tests are relatively inexpensive, they have a high negative predictive value. However, the results are useful in deciding which patients need to be investigated further for a DVT, using imaging techniques. A number of imaging tests can be done, including contrast venography, ultrasonography, computed tomography (CT) or magnetic resonance imaging (MRI). The aim of these tests is to visualise the thrombus in the leg and obtain a definitive diagnosis of DVT.

— **Treatment options for DVT**
The current standard treatment for an objectively confirmed DVT is short-term subcutaneous

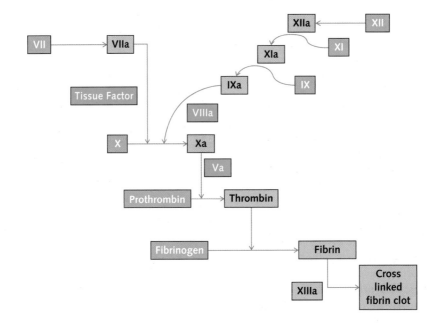

▲ FIGURE 2.1

Illustration of the coagulation cascade and clotting factors.

LMWH therapy (preferably as an outpatient), along with an oral vitamin K antagonist (typically warfarin in the UK), with both usually started at the same time. The LMWH should be continued for at least 5 days and until the INR is >2.0 for 24 hours. The patient then stays on warfarin, aiming for an INR of between 2 and 3. The exact duration of warfarin depends on whether the DVT was provoked, the past medical history of the patient and whether the DVT is a recurrence. Depending on these factors, the duration of warfarin therapy can vary from 3 months to life-long treatment.

In Mrs MJ's case, the DVT was secondary to a transient (reversible) risk factor, so she would typically be given 3 months' warfarin treatment. It is important to note that, with the advent of newer oral anticoagulants, such as dabigatran, rivaroxaban and apixaban, the treatment algorithm described above is already changing. At the time of writing, rivaroxaban is licensed in the UK for the acute treatment of DVT/PE and secondary long-term prevention of VTE, with many NHS organisations now starting to prescribe rivaroxaban monotherapy as first-line treatment for patients with acute DVT.

To minimise the risk of developing PTS, patients should be advised to wear an elastic compression stocking on the affected leg for a minimum of 2 years (assuming no contraindications).

— **Mechanism of action of heparin (unfractionated and low molecular weight) and warfarin**

The heparins belong to a family of sulfated glycosaminoglycans. They are extracted from porcine intestine or beef lung and, as different preparations differ in potency, they are assayed against an international standard. Smaller fragments of heparin are known as LMW heparins. Unfractionated heparin works by activating antithrombin (a natural anticoagulant). Antithrombin inhibits thrombin and other serine proteases in the clotting cascade (Figure 2.1).

By binding to antithrombin, heparin causes a conformational change in antithrombin and accelerates its rate of action. Thrombin is more sensitive to the inhibitory effect of the heparin–antithrombin complex than factor Xa.

LMWHs, due to their smaller size, increase the action of antithrombin on factor Xa, but not on thrombin. Due to their specificity for factor Xa, LMWHs have a predictable pharmacokinetic profile and require little or no monitoring; they have replaced unfractionated heparin as the anticoagulant of choice in many clinical situations.

Warfarin interferes with the post-translational γ-carboxylation of glutamic acid residues in clotting factors II (i.e. thrombin), VII, IX and X. This is done, by inhibiting enzymatic reduction of vitamin K to its active hydroquinone form.

Its effects usually take several days to develop, because of the time that it takes for the degradation of carboxylated factors. Its onset of action is driven by the half-life of the clotting factors that it inhibits. Factor VII has a half-life of 6 hours and is affected first, followed by factors IX, X and II, which have half-lives of 24, 40 and 60 hours, respectively.

Due to their mechanisms of actions, the heparins have an immediate anticoagulant effect, whereas warfarin takes at least a few days to start working – which is why both treatments are used in the initial treatment of a DVT.

— Tablet formulation and manufacture

Warfarin is the most commonly prescribed oral anticoagulant and is available in 500 micrograms (white), 1 mg (brown), 3 mg (blue) and 5 mg (pink) tablets in the UK. Tablets are made by powder compression, i.e. particles are brought into very close proximity by the application of mechanical force. In addition to the active pharmaceutical ingredient (API or drug), tablets contain a series of excipients. During manufacture, a number of processes are employed, including mixing and granulation (a process of particle enlargement to improve the tableting properties of a powder) of active ingredient and excipients. Granules/powder are filled into a powder die (usually by gravity) and the powder is compacted between two punches to form the tablet, which is then ejected from the die. Tableting machines may be of a single punch press or a rotary press design for larger-scale production.

Tablet excipients include:

- Filler (diluent), to ensure the tablet is of a size that can be handled, e.g. lactose, mannitol, calcium phosphate, microcrystalline cellulose
- Disintegrant, to ensure that the tablet/granules break apart when in contact with liquid, e.g. starch
- Binder, to ensure that granules/tablets have sufficient mechanical strength, e.g. starch, polyvinylpyrrolidone, hydroxypropyl methylcellulose, microcrystalline cellulose
- Glidant, to improve the flow properties of powder mixes, e.g. talc, colloidal silica
- Lubricant, to ensure reduced friction between die and punches to permit tablet production and ejection from the die, e.g. magnesium stearate

- Anti-adherent, to reduce adhesion between the powder and the faces of the punches, e.g. magnesium stearate, talc

Formed tablets may also contain a colorant and be film, compression or sugar coated.

— Chewable tablets

Chewable tablets (e.g. Calcichew D3) are designed to disintegrate quickly, producing a more rapid effect than a swallowed conventional immediate-release tablet. Chewable tablets also help in drug administration, particularly where the tablet is large or where patients have difficulty swallowing conventional tablets. Their composition is similar to conventional tablets, although the disintegrant is normally omitted. Sorbitol and mannitol are commonly used as fillers and flavouring and colouring agents are also frequently included.

— Clinically significant drug interactions with warfarin

Warfarin is a racemic mixture of two enantiomers: (*R*)-warfarin and (*S*)-warfarin. A racemic mixture is the name given to any 1:1 mixture of mirror-image stereoisomers (enantiomers). The *S*-enantiomer is up to five times more potent than the *R*-enantiomer and, at steady state, approximately two-thirds of the anticoagulant response is due to the *S*-enantiomer. The *S*-enantiomer is primarily metabolised by cytochrome P450 (CYP) 2C9 enzymes.

Drugs that inhibit the CYP enzyme system (e.g. clarithromycin) or induce it (e.g. rifampicin or St. John's wort) will affect anticoagulation control, and close monitoring along with warfarin dose adjustments will be required.

There is also the potential for pharmacodynamic interactions with warfarin; all antiplatelet therapies (e.g. aspirin, clopidogrel, ginkgo biloba, prasugrel and dipyridamole) interact with warfarin by virtue of the fact that they will increase a patient's risk of bleeding if used together with warfarin therapy.

(*R*)-warfarin   (*S*)-warfarin

— Pharmaceutical assessment of patients prescribed warfarin

Mrs MJ is a good example of a patient who would benefit from a medicines use review (MUR) or full clinical medicine review because she has a number of potential pharmaceutical problems. Before a pharmaceutical care plan can be developed, there is a need to gather further background information from the patient and her husband. To achieve this, it is important that the pharmacist possesses good consultation skills.

The different stages of the pharmaceutical consultation are described in the medication-related consultation framework (MRCF). The first is to build a therapeutic relationship with the patient (and/or carer) in order to set the scene and make sure that the aims and benefits of the consultation are clearly understood. Next is the data collection and problem identification stage, which includes taking a comprehensive medication history, plus a thorough assessment of the patient's adherence to the prescribed treatment regimen. This is followed by the actions and solutions stage in which the pharmacist establishes an acceptable management plan with the patient. The last stage is closure of the consultation in which safety-netting strategies are discussed with the patient. Competent consultation behaviours are needed throughout the interaction, in particular the need to adopt a structured and logical approach. Effective communication skills are also essential and it is important that these are tailored to the individual.

For Mrs MJ, it is important to involve her husband in the consultation due to her hearing loss and forgetfulness. It is particularly important to ascertain exactly how much warfarin has been taken because this will influence the interpretation of the INR test result.

— Additional considerations and advice in this case

- Advise that warfarin is the most important medicine to take and to prioritise this when giving medicines. Give these tablets first and check that the tablet has been swallowed.
- Advise to stop taking the aspirin and ginkgo biloba while she is taking warfarin due to the potential risk of bleeding. She may be able to reintroduce these after stopping the warfarin following discussions with the GP. This

information should be communicated to the GP.
- Advise Mrs MJ's husband that he can first crush the Calcichew tablet with a spoon.
- Suggest using a calendar to mark when the alendronic acid tablet is given once weekly to ensure that it is given on the same day each week.
- Remind the husband that the senna and paracetamol should be taken only when necessary.

EXTENDED LEARNING

- What treatment strategies are employed to prevent DVT (VTE) in hospitalised inpatients?
- How do the symptoms and management of a PE differ from those for a DVT?
- How do the newer oral anticoagulants dabigatran and rivaroxaban work, and what advantages do they offer over warfarin therapy?
- Why are certain drugs administered subcutaneously?
- What properties should formulations for subcutaneous injection possess?
- Describe in detail the processes involved in manufacturing tablets, including: particle size control, mixing, drying, granulation (wet, dry and extrusion spheronisation), compaction and coating.
- What quality control tests are carried on tablets following manufacture?
- Outline the role of CYP (cytochrome P450) enzymes in drug metabolism.
- What is alendronic acid? Why would it have been prescribed for this patient?

References and further reading

Abdel-Tawab R, James DH, Fichtinger A, Clatworthy J, Horne R, Davies G (2011). Development and validation of the Medication-Related Consultation Framework (MRCF). *Patient Educ Counsel* 83:451–7.

Abdel Tawab R, James DH, Horne R, Davies JG (2005). Medication Related Consultation Framework (MRCFr). Available at: www.codeg.org/fileadmin/codeg/pdf/MRCFr_Full_Tool.pdf (accessed 9 July 2013).

Alderborn G (2013). Tablets and compaction. In: Aulton ME, Taylor KMG (eds), *Aulton's Pharmaceutics: The design and* manufacture of medicines, 4th edn. London: Elsevier, 504–49.

Kearon C, Akl EA, Comerota AJ et al. (2012). Antithrombotic therapy for venous thromboembolic disease. American College of Chest Physicians evidence-based clinical practice guidelines (9th edition). Chest 141:e419s–94s.

Phillips KW, Dobesh PP, Haines ST (2008). Considerations in using anticoagulant therapy in special patient populations. Am J Health-System Pharmacy 65:s13–21.

Rang HP, Dale MM, Ritter JM, Moore PK, eds (2003). Haemostasis and thrombosis. In: Pharmacology, 5th edn. Philadelphia, PA: Churchill Livingstone, Chapter 20.

Silverman JD, Kurtz SM, Draper J (1998). Skills for Communicating with Patients. Oxford: Radcliffe Medical Press.

Case 8
Treatment of acute ischaemic stroke

IAN ROWLANDS

LEARNING OUTCOMES

At the end of this case, you will be able to:

- Define stroke and transient ischaemic attack (TIA)
- Outline the signs and symptoms of stroke
- Outline the inclusion and exclusion criteria for thrombolysis in acute ischaemic stroke
- Describe the main side effects and monitoring parameters after thrombolysis
- Describe the chemical structure, properties and mode of action of aspirin

Case study

Mrs PP is a 72-year-old woman of Indian origin with a history of type 2 diabetes, hypertension and hyperlipidaemia. While watching television one evening with her family, her daughter noticed that she was slumped over on the sofa and unable to speak. 999 was dialled immediately; the ambulance took her to the nearest hospital which had an associated stoke unit. They were met on arrival at the hospital by the stroke team, who quickly established that the patient had been mobile and communicating normally 1 hour earlier. All examinations were consistent with stroke, so she was sent for urgent brain imaging.

❷ What is a stroke? What symptoms did Mrs PP have that were indicative of stroke?

Based on the scan results, the stroke consultant decided that the patient was suitable for thrombolysis. Mrs PP was unable to consent to treatment, so the risks and benefits were discussed with her family who agreed with the plan to thrombolyse.

❷ What are the main inclusion and exclusion criteria for thrombolysis in acute ischaemic stroke? What other tests are needed before thrombolysis?

Thrombolysis was administered with no adverse effect. Mrs PP's speech has improved but she has failed a safe swallow test. The following day, the junior doctor asks you for advice about antiplatelet prescribing and how to administer her regular medications given her dysphagia (difficulty in swallowing).

❷ What would you advise the doctor to do about antiplatelet therapy? What options may be available for administering medicines to a patient with swallowing difficulties?

Case discussion
— Stroke background

In the UK, approximately 150 000 people a year will have a stroke; it is the third largest cause of death in the UK, and is responsible for 10% of all deaths worldwide. The World Health Organization (WHO) defines stroke as: 'rapidly developing clinical signs of focal (at times global) disturbance of cerebral function, lasting more than 24 hours or leading to death with no apparent cause other than that of vascular origin.' In other words, a stroke is an interruption of the blood supply to the brain, which leads to the disruption of neurological function – the 'focal' aspect means that the symptoms that the patient experiences are directly linked to the specific area of the brain where the stroke occurs. Strokes can be broadly classified as ischaemic or haemorrhagic.

Ischaemic stroke is more prevalent, accounting for around 70% of strokes, and occurs when a thrombus or embolism occludes a cerebral artery, which deprives the surrounding neurons of essential nutrients.

A *haemorrhagic stroke* is responsible for approximately 20% of strokes, and occurs when a blood vessel in or around the brain bursts, affecting not only the local blood supply but also causing localised pressure and damage to brain tissue.

There is a saying in stroke medicine that 'time is brain'; the longer neurones are starved of blood, the worse the damage will be. Early identification and treatment of stroke are therefore crucial. Approximately 10% of strokes are of unknown origin. A TIA, although not classified as a stroke, is very closely linked. The difference between a TIA and a stroke is the duration of symptoms: if the symptoms resolve fully within 24 hours, then it is classed as a TIA. Although the symptoms of a TIA resolve, these patients are at major risk of developing stroke and should be investigated and treated as soon as possible.

— **Signs and symptoms of stroke**
A good way to illustrate stroke symptoms is to use the FAST test, a tool that was designed to allow ambulance crews, and more recently members of the public, to identify potential strokes so that patients could get access to emergency treatment as soon as possible:

Facial weakness: can the person smile? Has his or her mouth or eye drooped?
Arm weakness: can the person raise both arms?
Speech problems: can the person speak clearly and understand what you say?
Time to call 999

Although the FAST test is not 100% specific, most patients will exhibit at least one of motor weakness, facial weakness or communication difficulties, and it also highlights the urgency of the situation. Any of these symptoms should be treated with a high degree of suspicion, so patients who fit the FAST criteria will be admitted to hospital (ideally a specialist stroke unit) for full physical and neurological examination. It is impossible to tell without the assistance of brain imaging (CT scan) whether a patient has had an ischaemic or haemorrhagic event, so obtaining

urgent scanning is essential because the treatments differ greatly.

— **Thrombolysis in acute ischaemic stroke**
Once haemorrhage has been ruled out, ischaemic stroke patients may be considered for thrombolysis to break down the blood clot. The recombinant tissue plasminogen activator (rTPA) alteplase has been shown to improve outcomes in ischaemic stroke and reduce the risk of permanent disability. Timing is crucial, because studies have shown that thrombolysis is most effective if administered within 3 hours of symptom onset, although there is evidence to support an extended window, of up to 4.5 hours and perhaps longer, although there has yet to be a consensus on this. The longer the time after stroke, the more the risks of thrombolysis can outweigh the benefits, so it is essential that an accurate time of onset can be identified. Major bleeding, particularly intracerebral haemorrhage (ICH) within the infarcted region, is the main consequence of thrombolysis. If the patient is at any risk of haemorrhage (e.g. previous ICH, recent history of head injury, major trauma or surgery, gastrointestinal [GI] ulceration, bleeding disorders or therapeutic anticoagulation), then thrombolysis is contraindicated. Hypertension and hyperglycaemia may also increase the risk of ICH, so these need to be closely monitored and treated if necessary (see below). There is also limited evidence for the use of rTPA in patients aged <18 or >80 years and, as such, these patients may also be excluded from treatment. As a result of the risks involved, thrombolysis can be administered only under the supervision of experienced stroke physicians and in centres that allow it to be used safely.

If the decision is made to thrombolyse and the infusion commenced, the patient needs to be monitored very closely. Any worsening in neurological deficit, worsening headache, nausea or seizures could be indicative of ICH. This would warrant stopping the infusion, sending blood samples for urgent FBC, APTT (activated partial thromboplastin time) and INR, and requesting an emergency CT scan to assess the extent of any potential haemorrhage. Cryoprecipitate, fresh frozen plasma and platelet transfusions can be used if appropriate to reverse the effects of rTPA. Other sources of haemorrhage, such as GI bleeds, would also require the rTPA infusion to be stopped, assessed and treated with blood transfusions if required. Allergic reactions are rare complications of rTPA treatment. Minor skin reactions could possibly be managed with antihistamines and corticosteroids; any severe symptoms of allergy, including angio-oedema and bronchospasm, should be dealt with by stopping rTPA and treating as per local or national guidelines for anaphylaxis. Risk of haemorrhage with rTPA is increased by the usage of antiplatelets and anticoagulants, so these should be avoided in the first 24 hours after thrombolysis. The biological response to rTPA can persist for several hours after administration. Patients should therefore not have nasogastric tubes or urinary catheters inserted within 24 hours, and should have strict bed rest and observation for 24 hours, because the consequence of a fall could be catastrophic.

— **Blood pressure in acute stroke**
Most stroke patients will have raised blood pressure (80% >165/95 mmHg on admission), a combination of pre-existing hypertension and a physiological response to the stroke. Reducing blood pressure in the acute setting is controversial, because there is the concern that reducing blood pressure may also reduce cerebral blood flow and therefore increase ischaemic damage. In most cases, this initial rise in blood pressure will settle in the subsequent 4–10 days, and no treatment is required. However, if SBP (systolic blood pressure) is persistently elevated >220 mmHg (>200 mmHg in haemorrhagic stroke or >185 mmHg if for thrombolysis), treatment should be started. Oral agents such as calcium channel blockers may be used, or intravenous labetalol, but it is worth bearing in mind that blood pressure can be labile post-stroke, so GTN patches can be of great use, because their action is easily reversed by removal.

— **Prescribing antiplatelets and anticoagulants**
Large-scale clinical trials have shown that aspirin, administered within 48 hours of an ischaemic stroke (and haemorrhage excluded), reduces the risk of recurrent stroke, without significantly increasing the risk of haemorrhage. Patients should be administered 300 mg aspirin daily as soon as possible, or after 24 hours if thrombolysed, and continued until a long-term plan has been agreed. Anticoagulants are not used in the acute setting, except in minor cases of cardioembolic stroke or TIA, because of the

bleeding risk. Unless patients have past history of DVT or a significant risk of this, prophylactic anticoagulants are not indicated.

— **Structure and mechanism of action of aspirin**
Aspirin (acetylsalicylic acid) owes its antiplatelet and analgesic activity to its ability to inhibit cyclooxygenase enzymes (COX-1 and COX-2). Platelet COX-1 catalyses the conversion of arachidonic acid to the prostaglandin thromboxane A_2 (TxA_2), a potent platelet aggregation inducer. Aspirin inactivates COX by irreversible covalent transfer of an acetyl group (red) to the side chain of a serine residue close to the active site. New platelets have to be produced to overcome this effect.

aspirin

Aspirin's carboxyl group is ionised at physiological pH and this makes an important electrostatic interaction with the active site of COX-1. The aromatic ring is also important for making hydrophobic interactions with the target enzyme. The ester group in aspirin is rapidly hydrolysed to salicylic acid (which can still bind reversibly to the COX active site) and acetic acid under aqueous conditions, as well as by plasma esterases.

This patient has difficulties with swallowing. A test was undertaken that assesses ability to manage oral medication. It takes into account cognitive ability and physiological function.

Aspirin 75 mg dispersible tablets can be dispersed in water to aid swallowing and to provide a means of administration via a nasogastric tube, but such dispersions should ideally be administered soon after preparation to minimise the amount of aspirin that is hydrolysed to salicylic acid (which is less well absorbed, more irritant and less effective as an antiplatelet).

— **Haemorrhagic stroke**
Treatment of haemorrhagic stroke is supportive only: correction of any clotting, treating hypertension if necessary, stopping any drugs that may have contributed to the haemorrhage and treating any complications that may arise.

EXTENDED LEARNING

- What is a CT scan? What does it show?
- What other types of scan are used for imaging?
- Subarachnoid haemorrhage carries a high risk of mortality. What are the principal causes, presentation and approaches to its management?

References and further reading

National Collaborating Centre for Chronic Conditions (2008). *Stroke: National clinical guideline for diagnosis and initial management of acute stroke and transient ischaemic attack (TIA).* London: Royal College of Physicians.

Summary of Product Characteristics: Actilyse (Alteplase). Available at: http://emc.medicines.org.uk/medicine/308/SPC/Actilyse (accessed 13 August 2013).

Case 9
Secondary stroke prevention

IAN ROWLANDS

LEARNING OUTCOMES

At the end of this case, you will be able to:

- Describe the main risk factors for stroke
- Identify the main treatments for secondary stroke prevention
- Outline the mechanisms of action of antiplatelet drugs, anticoagulants and statins
- Outline the chemistry of simvastatin
- Outline the key lifestyle interventions recommended post-stroke
- Recognise the importance of adherence to medication regimens post-stroke, and possible reasons for, and measures of, non-adherence

Case study

Mr MG is a 56-year-old professional man, previously diagnosed with hypertension and hyperlipidaemia, but not taking any regular medication. He woke this morning to discover he had weakness in his right arm and leg and was struggling to speak. He alerted his wife, who called an ambulance. Within 40 minutes he had arrived at his local acute stroke centre and was investigated as a potential candidate for thrombolysis. His blood pressure on admission was found to be 165/92 mmHg; urgent blood tests did not detect any significant abnormalities. Imaging confirmed a left middle cerebral artery infarct with no evidence of haemorrhagic transformation. The decision was made by the stroke consultant not to thrombolyse. Mr MG was subsequently admitted to the stroke unit for further investigation and treatment.

❓ Why might the consultant have decided not to thrombolyse the patient? What should be prescribed now that thrombolysis and haemorrhage have been ruled out?

Mr MG has smoked, on average, 20 cigarettes a day for the past 25 years, and drinks around 4 bottles of wine per week. He knows that he should reduce his tobacco and alcohol intake, but he exercises regularly, keeps his weight under control, and ultimately feels that his lifestyle helps him to cope with his stressful work life. He was diagnosed 18 months ago with hypertension and hyperlipidaemia by his GP, who prescribed amlodipine and simvastatin, but he discontinued treatment after 4 weeks because they made him feel worse. After the stroke, Mr MG makes a full recovery and is started on several new medications for secondary prevention. The nurse in charge informs you, as the ward pharmacist, that Mr MG is fit for discharge.

❓ What medications should be prescribed for secondary prevention? How would you counsel this patient to help maintain adherence to any prescribed medication? What lifestyle modifications would you recommend, and are there any medicines that may help him make these changes?

Case discussion

— Medication for secondary prevention overview

For patients who survive stroke, the risk of recurrence has been estimated at 30–43% within 5 years. Secondary prevention is therefore the cornerstone in the long-term treatment of stroke patients. The main risk factor for stroke is older age, but there are several modifiable risk factors, and so most of the preventive measures used in stroke medicine are targeted at these.

— Prescribing antiplatelet drugs in patients after a stroke

A large proportion of ischaemic strokes are due to thromboembolism from the large arteries supplying blood to the brain, as a result of atheroma in these vessels. After an ischaemic stroke, most patients will therefore receive treatment to reduce the risk of thromboembolism. As soon as haemorrhage has been ruled out, and the decision has been made not to thrombolyse, patients should receive aspirin 300 mg daily, for up to 2 weeks, until a long-term treatment can be decided upon and initiated (National Collaborating Centre for Chronic Conditions, 2008). Clopidogrel 75 mg daily is an alternative in aspirin-allergic patients.

The first-line long-term antiplatelet therapy for patients with ischaemic stroke or TIA of vascular origin is clopidogrel 75 mg daily. If patients cannot take clopidogrel, they should be prescribed the combination of low-dose aspirin (75 mg daily) and modified-release dipyridamole (200 mg twice daily). There is little between these options in terms of efficacy, but the reduced pill burden and more favourable side-effect profile make clopidogrel the best choice. All antiplatelet medications are associated with GI side effects, including dyspepsia, ulceration and haemorrhage. It is not uncommon to have patients on gastroprotective therapy, especially if there is a history of GI ulceration. Patients will frequently experience headaches due to the vasodilatory effects of dipyridamole, so many stroke centres will initiate patients on a lower dose, before increasing to the full dose after a few days, to improve tolerability and compliance. If patients cannot tolerate either of the first- or second-line antiplatelet regimens, aspirin monotherapy is superior to dipyridamole monotherapy, but each offers much less benefit than the combination of the two agents, or of clopidogrel. Antiplatelet therapies should be continued lifelong after ischaemic stroke or TIA. Some centres will stop dipyridamole after 2 years but there is some evidence that the benefits may persist after this.

— Mechanism of action of antiplatelet drugs

Aspirin (acetylsalicylic acid) at low (non-analgesic) doses of 75 mg daily exerts its now well-known prophylactic antiplatelet (antithrombotic) action by irreversibly inhibiting the function of the constitutive platelet COX-1 enzyme responsible for the production of TxA_2 (from membrane arachidonic acid). TxA_2 normally triggers the cascade leading to platelet activation, aggregation and thrombus formation in blood vessels. Recovery from this effect (and re-synthesis of TxA_2) is dependent on platelet turnover (8–11 days). Higher aspirin doses (300 mg daily) may be used to prevent thrombus formation in cerebral and peripheral blood vessels in patients showing the symptoms of a heart attack or stroke.

Dipyridamole is a platelet phosphodiesterase inhibitor that decreases platelet aggregation by blocking the breakdown of intracellular cyclic adenosine $3',5'$-monophosphate (cAMP), normally responsible for controlling events leading to platelet activation by exogenous ADP (adenosine diphosphate – a platelet 'agonist' released from platelet granules). ADP exerts its effects via purinergic $P2Y_1$, $P2Y_{12}$ and $P2X_1$ receptors. Dipyridamole also inhibits the uptake of adenosine into platelets, which is regarded as an endogenous inhibitor of platelet aggregation (acting though platelet adenosine A_2 receptors).

Clopidogrel (a thienopyridine) is a platelet ADP receptor antagonist, and therefore inhibits the ADP-mediated platelet-aggregation process directly.

— Anticoagulants

Atrial fibrillation (AF) is responsible for approximately 12% of all strokes, and a higher proportion of strokes in elderly people. Anticoagulation is recommended for stroke prevention in all patients with AF, including paroxysmal AF, unless contraindicated. In most cases, anticoagulation should not be initiated until at least 2 weeks after the ischaemic event, due to the risk of haemorrhagic transformation. For decades, the mainstay of anticoagulant therapy has been warfarin, with a target INR of 2–3. If warfarin is to be initiated, aspirin 300 mg daily should be continued until the INR is therapeutic. In minor stroke, or in cases of TIA associated with AF, it may be possible to initiate warfarin early in the days after the event, provided that haemorrhage has been ruled out. In such cases, the patient could be co-prescribed treatment dose LMWH instead of aspirin until the INR is therapeutic. The perceived risk of bleeding, and the complicated nature of administration and monitoring, has limited the usage of warfarin, especially in the elderly population. Newer oral anticoagulants, such as the thrombin inhibitor dabigatran, and the factor Xa inhibitors apixaban and rivaroxaban, are viable alternatives to warfarin for stroke prevention in AF, with equivalent risk reductions and potentially lower bleeding risks. These agents also benefit from standardised dosing regimens and reduced monitoring requirements when compared with warfarin, but with the caveat that there are currently no agents to reverse their anticoagulant effect. Antiplatelet drugs offer significantly less benefit than anticoagulants in AF, and should be used only when anticoagulants are absolutely contraindicated.

— Blood pressure

It is widely recognised that the higher the blood pressure the higher the risk of both ischaemic and haemorrhagic stroke. Combined trial data suggest that, for every 1 mmHg reduction in blood pressure, there is a reduction in stroke risk of 3%. After the acute period, a blood pressure <130/80 mmHg is recommended in stroke patients. Treatment should be based on current British Hypertension Society guidelines, bearing in mind that 130/80 mmHg is a challenging target for most patients, and may involve using multiple agents at optimal doses. Management of hypertension after haemorrhagic stroke and TIA is as for ischaemic stroke.

— Cholesterol and statins

Hypercholesterolaemia is a risk factor for the development of atherosclerosis and ischaemic heart disease and, although the relationship between cholesterol and stroke is less certain, the significant volume of available evidence favours cholesterol reduction after an ischaemic stroke. Unless contraindicated, treatment with a statin, such as simvastatin, should be started if total cholesterol >3.5 mmol/L, or LDL-cholesterol >2.5 mmol/L.

Treatment goals should be:

- Total cholesterol <4.0 mmol/L and LDL <2.0 mmol/L, or
- 25% reduction in total cholesterol and 30% reduction in LDL-cholesterol, whichever achieves the lower absolute value.

There is some evidence that statin therapy, while reducing ischaemic stroke risk, may increase the risk of haemorrhagic stroke. For this reason, it is recommended that patients are not initiated on a statin within 48 hours of ischaemic stroke, and statins should not be routinely used in the initial weeks after haemorrhagic stroke unless there are compelling indications.

— Simvastatin

Simvastatin in an inhibitor of 3-hydroxy-3-methyl-glutaryl CoA (HMG-CoA) reductase – the enzyme that catalyses the rate-limiting step in cholesterol biosynthesis. Simvastatin is produced semi-synthetically from a fungal natural product. It is a prodrug. It undergoes chemical and enzymatic (plasma and hepatic esterases) hydrolysis of the lactone ring (in red in the diagram) to form its active metabolite. This metabolite very closely resembles the intermediate produced from HMG-CoA, and has considerably greater affinity for the HMG-CoA reductase active site. Simvastatin has the same stereochemical configuration of the groups bonded to the lactone ring as the HMG-CoA intermediate; the lipophilic ring system is also essential for high-affinity binding.

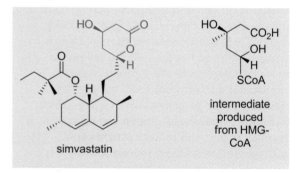

simvastatin

intermediate produced from HMG-CoA

Simvastatin is highly lipophilic. It is well absorbed after oral administration but undergoes significant first-pass metabolism, so only a small fraction of an oral dose is available as the active metabolite. Simvastatin should consequently be used with caution in hepatic impairment. It is metabolised by CYP3A4 and so has the potential to interact with other drugs (e.g. erythromycin) and substances that inhibit this isoform. This is the mechanism of the interaction of simvastatin and grapefruit juice, excessive consumption of which can lead to increased plasma levels of simvastatin and increased risk of ADRs (adverse drug reactions).

— Diabetes
The risk of stroke in people with diabetes is around double that of the average population; however, there are limited data on whether better diabetic control reduces the recurrence of stroke. Despite this, it is common sense to keep blood glucose under tight control to reduce the progression or further development of macrovascular complications.

— Advice on modification to lifestyle
Smokers have twice the risk of ischaemic stroke compared with non-smokers. All patients who smoke should therefore be encouraged to stop smoking at the earliest opportunity. There are a variety of nicotine replacement therapies (NRTs) on the market, the use of which can be based on patient preference. The manufacturers of NRT products advise, in the product literature, avoidance of their use post-stroke due to lack of safety data, but any risk posed by NRT should be weighed against the risk of continuing to smoke. There is no direct evidence to confirm that healthy eating, and weight loss in obese patients, reduces stroke risk, but improvements in blood pressure, cholesterol and blood glucose can be only beneficial. Alcohol intake should also be kept within recommended limits (21 units for men and 14 units for women per week), because high alcohol intake increases the risk of ischaemic and, more significantly, haemorrhagic stroke.

— Haemorrhagic stroke
There are several types of haemorrhagic stroke, the most common being intracerebral haemorrhage (ICH), which is responsible for 10–15% of all strokes. Age and hypertension are the major risk factors for developing ICH, but it can be induced by anticoagulants, antiplatelets, thrombolysis and illegal drugs such as cocaine, and there is the risk of haemorrhagic transformation of an ischaemic stroke. The key to prevention is to reduce any risk factors such as hypertension, and avoid medication that may have precipitated the original bleed. In cases of transformation, drugs such as antiplatelets and statins may be indicated for vascular risk reduction, but should be initiated with caution and only after the bleeding has resolved.

— Promoting adherence to medication regimens
Non-adherence (once commonly called non-compliance) refers to a situation in which a patient does not take a medicine as intended. It is estimated that around 50% of patients prescribed preventive medicines for long-term conditions do not take them as intended. Medication significantly reduces the risk of recurrence of stroke. Thus, non-adherence can have an important impact on clinical outcomes. Non-adherence may be omitting doses, altering doses: taking less or more than intended, not using a product correctly, changing the timing of doses or stopping a medicine altogether.

Reasons for non-adherence are often categorised as follows:

- Patient related, which may include: age, gender, beliefs about the benefits of therapy, concerns about its effect, understanding of how and when to take a medicine, remembering, ability to open containers or manage a device, patient–prescriber relationship, time since diagnosis
- Therapy related, e.g. complexity of regimen and administration device, experience or fear of side effects, route of administration (especially if privacy is required), duration of treatment, whether the treatment is effective
- Healthcare system related, such as obtaining supplies of medicines, costs, availability of advice.

Intentional adherence and non-intentional adherence are also sometimes distinguished. Non-intentional adherence refers to situations in which the patient intends to take a medicine, but is prevented from doing so by factors such as non-availability, poor understanding, memory problems or inability to use a product. Intentionally non-adherent patients opt not to take their medicine as directed. This may be omitting or adjusting doses to fit daily routines, perceiving limited need or benefits, fear of experience of side effects or concern about the appropriateness of a medicine. Clearly, there is overlap in these concepts, e.g. patients who are motivated may be less likely to forget, or take steps to ensure that they understand instructions.

There are a number of methods of measuring adherence, which include checking if patients are obtaining/refilling prescriptions, pharmacy records, pill counts, electronic devices in containers that record opening and closure. These have obvious problems, and may provide only a poor indication of medicine-taking behaviours. A number of self-reported measures have been developed. These take into account the different factors that are known to influence adherence, as discussed above. These measures can also present problems, e.g. some patients may not want to admit to non-adherence, which may be viewed as a lack of cooperation with their health professionals. However, questions are often prefaced with a statement that 'many people, for different reasons, do not always take their medicines as intended'. Although care is required in research into non-adherence, these measures have been widely used and validated.

In addressing problems of non-adherence, an awareness of the wide range of potential influences is essential. Interventions required to support someone with memory problems differ greatly from those required to motivate a sceptical individual.

EXTENDED LEARNING

- What is the evidence for the advantages and disadvantages of established and new anticoagulation therapies?

- Outline the mechanisms of action of anticoagulants: warfarin, LMWH and dabigatran
- Distinguish ischaemic and haemorrhagic stroke in terms of aetiology, pathophysiology and management.

ADDITIONAL PRACTICE POINTS

- How might a pharmacist support smoking cessation and advise on nicotine replacement therapy?

References and further reading

Baigent C, Keech A, Kearney PM et al.; Cholesterol Treatment Trialists' (CTT) Collaborators (2005). Efficacy and safety of cholesterol-lowering treatment: prospective meta-analysis of data from 90,056 participants in 14 randomised trials of statins. *Lancet* **366**:1267–82.

Intercollegiate Stroke Working Party (2012). *National Clinical Guideline for Stroke*, 4th edn. London: Royal College of Physicians.

National Collaborating Centre for Chronic Conditions (2008). *Stroke: National clinical guideline for diagnosis and initial management of acute stroke and transient ischaemic attack (TIA)*. London: Royal College of Physicians.

Case 10
Drug interactions
SANDEEP SINGH NIJJER

LEARNING OUTCOMES

At the end of this case, you will be able to:

- Understand the principles of pharmacokinetic and pharmacodynamic drug interactions
- Apply these principles to some clinically significant interactions
- Outline the mode of action and chemical properties of digoxin
- Describe mechanisms of interaction of some commonly prescribed medicines
- Appreciate interaction potential of herbal products

Case study

Mr QT, a 76-year-old man, has been acutely admitted to hospital due to major symptoms of bleeding. The following information is from his case notes:

CASE NOTES

On presentation
- Blood noted in vomit, urine and faeces. Significant bruising noted on lower leg extremities. Patient feeling disoriented with severe nausea.

Medical history

- Depression (2010), COPD (2006), mitral valve replacement (2001), fast atrial fibrillation with residual permanent atrial fibrillation (1999)

Regular drug history

- Warfarin 1 mg tablets: as directed in anticoagulant book (INR target range: 3.0–4.0)
- Digoxin 125 microgram tablets: one tablet in the morning
- Diltiazem SR 120 mg tablets: one tablet daily
- Fluoxetine 20 mg capsules: one capsule in the morning
- Co-magaldrox suspension (magnesium hydroxide and aluminium hydroxide based antacid): 10 mL after food when required
- Salbutamol 100 microgram inhaler: two puffs when required as directed
- Tiotropium 18 microgram inhaler: one puff once a day as directed

Mr QT's carer has also brought in some medication that was prescribed for Mr QT due to a respiratory tract infection last week:

- Ciprofloxacin 250 mg tablets (20 tablets): one twice a day for 10 days
- Prednisolone 2.5 mg enteric-coated tablets (20 tablets): four daily with breakfast for 5 days

Monitoring: tests conducted on admission

- Warfarin INR: 6.0 (normal range 3.0–4.0). Prothrombin time: 115 s (normal: 19 s)
- Digoxin: 3.0 nmol/L (serum) (reference: 1.2–2.4 nmol/L)
- eGFR (estimated glomerular filtration rate): 80 mL/min per 1.73 m² (classification stage 2: 'mild' chronic renal impairment)

❷ Which medicine is likely to have precipitated an interaction leading to increased bleeding in this case?

❷ What is the most probable underlying mechanism of the interaction?

After Mr QT had been stabilised on the ward, the symptoms of endocarditis (inflammation of the inner tissue of the heart) were noted and the following antibiotic started:

Rifampicin 300 mg capsules. Dosage: one capsule four times a day

❷ What is the likely effect on the INR with the concomitant prescribing of rifampicin and warfarin?

❷ What is the most probable underlying mechanism of this interaction?

❷ Outline the mode of action and pharmacokinetic properties of digoxin

Soon after discharge from hospital, Mr QT's carer comes to the pharmacy and wishes to purchase St John's wort for Mr QT. This is a 'herbal remedy' for depression, which was recommended by her sister, as 'natural and completely safe'.

❷ What is St John's wort and what are the active ingredients?

❷ What is the most probable mechanism of interaction between St John's wort and fluoxetine?

❷ Would you advise the patient to take St John's wort in this case?

❷ What are the potential clinical consequences?

A few months later, the carer is collecting medications for Mr QT from the pharmacy. The pharmacist on duty asks whether Mr QT takes his antacid preparation 'at least 2 hours apart from other medicines'.

❷ Why does the pharmacist ask this question?

Case discussion

— Identifying potential drug–drug interactions as a source of toxicity

This case highlights the importance of the pharmacist being aware of possible drug interactions when patients are taking several medications at the same time. Medicinal products may interact with other medicines taken by patients, potential co-morbidities (*cautions* and *contraindications*) and possibly with certain foods, nutrients and herbal products.

This case illustrates both *pharmacokinetic* and *pharmacodynamic* drug–drug interactions with both conventional medicinal products and herbal therapeutics. *Pharmacokinetic* interactions relate to a change in the measurable plasma concentration of one drug as a consequence of another drug taken concurrently, which affects any of the processes of *absorption, distribution, metabolism* and *excretion*. *Pharmacodynamic* interactions relate to a change in the expected pharmacological action of a drug due to another drug, either directly (at the receptor system) or indirectly (via an effect on an organ system), enhancing (*synergising*) or reducing (*antagonising*) its effects.

digoxin

Reference sources for health professionals to assist in identifying and managing interactions vary on a country-to-country basis, and consequently in interpretation of case reports. Health professionals based within the UK often use the *British National Formulary* (*BNF*) to classify the potential severity of an interaction based on the individual patient's risk factors. Subsequent management is supported via reference sources such as *Stockley's Drug Interactions*.

Effective identification and management of drug interactions require health professionals to understand a patient's medication regimen with respect to the time course of therapy with drug disposition and mechanism of action.

— **Potential interactions in this case**

Mr QT is likely to have warfarin toxicity, given the bleeding symptoms on admission and digoxin toxicity, based on both the clinical symptoms of persistent nausea and disorientation and the recorded serum level at a point above the recommended therapeutic 'window'. Pharmacokinetic changes associated with ageing itself can also have an impact on the metabolism of medications, particularly drugs such as digoxin which have a narrow therapeutic index, thus increasing the risk of toxicity. It should be noted, in older people compared with younger adults, that organs of drug metabolism and elimination (mainly liver and kidneys) can have a dramatic change in function in addition to natural age-related organ atrophy, the loss of muscle mass and gain in fatty tissue. For example, the kidneys can decrease in function and capacity. This can be as much as a 50% reduction compared with 'normal' renal capacity. The symptoms of digoxin toxicity in older patients can include anorexia, cognitive changes, disturbed colour vision (yellow or green halos around objects), arrhythmia and (as in this case) severe nausea/vomiting.

— **Chemistry, mode of action and pharmacokinetic properties of digoxin**

Digoxin is a cardiac glycoside medication derived from the foxglove plant, *Digitalis lanata*. Digoxin can increase intracellular levels of calcium within myocardial cells via an inhibitory effect on the Na^+/K^+ ATPase enzyme. There are numerous actions of digoxin on the heart, including increased contraction force (ionotropic effect) and ejection fraction, and decreased conduction through the atrioventricular node with decreased heart rate. The heart rate-limiting effects have a use within specific arrhythmias such as AF and increases in myocardial contraction and cardiac output are necessary for certain heart failure patients.

Digoxin is a molecule with both hydrophilic and lipophilic substituent groups. It consists of a lipophilic cardenolide steroid core, glycosylated with a hydrophilic trisaccharide (three repeated digitoxose sugars). Although the free drug is poorly water soluble, it is sufficiently polar to be excreted mostly (70–85%) via the renal route, largely mediated by the renal P-glycoprotein efflux pump. Therefore, digoxin would have a small volume of distribution, initially into the plasma compartment, equilibrating into the secondary compartment. As cardiac effects are associated with the larger volume, at least 6 hours post-oral dose would be required before therapeutic drug monitoring should be initiated, with the half-life of digoxin varying between 1.5 and 2 days. Recommendations for therapeutic plasma concentrations of digoxin can vary between countries, although 1–2 micrograms/L is considered to be the limit of the *therapeutic range*, with the range for heart failure being considered between 0.5 and 1 micrograms/L.

Interestingly, the effects of co-morbidities and concurrent medicines can affect the risk of toxicity, e.g. a level of renal impairment could lead to accumulation and the risk of toxicity. Acute illness such as a chest infection in an older person can cause a very rapid decline in renal function. Also, medical conditions requiring medicines that may precipitate electrolyte imbalances can predispose towards digoxin toxicity, e.g. the use of adrenergic β_2-receptor agonists with corticosteroid courses may predispose certain individuals to hypokalaemia (lowered serum potassium levels). which also leads to an increased risk of digoxin toxicity.

— **Potential interactions with rifampicin**
After starting rifampicin, the metabolism and excretion of many medicines can be affected. It has a known potent effect on both the hepatic microsomal enzyme system and the P-glycoprotein efflux transporter. The metabolism of warfarin can be affected, thus leading to a dramatic fluctuation in the INR reading for warfarin, often necessitating a change in warfarin dosage and clinical monitoring. Similarly, the excretion of digoxin can be affected through increasing levels of P-glycoprotein efflux transporters resulting from rifampicin usage.

— **Potential interactions with St John's wort**
Herbal products such as St John's wort derived from the plant *Hypericum perforatum* are well known as an 'alternative' herbal treatment for mild-to-moderate depression and also some forms of anxiety, but can have serious interactions with conventional medicines. Although it contains a large variety of complex components, it is hypericin and hyperforin that are believed to be the most active ingredients, most likely working through inhibition of central serotonin (5-hydroxytryptamine or 5HT) reuptake, akin to the effects of conventional selective serotonin reuptake inhibitor (SSRI) antidepressants (e.g. fluoxetine). St John's wort can have both pharmacokinetic and pharmacodynamic drug interactions. The pharmacokinetic interactions involving St John's wort relate to the induction of hepatic microsomal enzymes (cytochrome P450 isoforms) for hepatic metabolism and P-glycoprotein transporter induction to enhance *renal excretion*.

Pharmacodynamic interactions that involve St John's wort relate to its potential 'serotoninergic' mediated antidepressant activity.

— **Pharmacokinetic enzyme inhibition interaction: warfarin toxicity and the signs of major bleeding**
It should be recognised that acute illness can affect a patient's handling of the dicoumarol anticoagulant warfarin. It is often difficult to separate the effects of illness and disease from the concurrent use of medicines. However, given the relatively rapid increase in INR and signs of major bleeding after prescription and administration of ciprofloxacin in Mr QT, it is most likely that a drug interaction is the cause of the signs of major bleeding.

The *BNF* states:

… anticoagulant effect of coumarins enhanced by ciprofloxacin.

Stockley states:

… altered (usually enhanced) response to anticoagulation with a coumarin has been reported with virtually every class of antibacterial.

Various mechanisms are potentially relevant, including an effect on vitamin K-producing flora and the inhibition of hepatic metabolism of warfarin, decreasing warfarin clearance, and increasing warfarin levels and INR.

Stockley states:

… ciprofloxacin may increase the level or effect of warfarin by affecting hepatic enzyme CYP-P450 1A2 metabolism …

Overall, there would be an enhancement of the anticoagulant effects of warfarin with an increase in prothrombin time and the risk of bleeding (which was seen in this patient's case).

— **Pharmacokinetic enzyme and transporter interaction: the effect of rifampicin on warfarin levels**
The *BNF* states:

… metabolism of coumarins accelerated by rifamycins (reduced anticoagulant effect).

Stockley states:

… the anticoagulant effects of warfarin are markedly reduced by rifampicin, with a two to fivefold increase in dose needed to maintain efficacy in a number of case reports.

Rifampicin is a well-recognised, potent, non-specific and rapid inducer of cytochrome

P450 enzymes and the drug efflux transporter P-glycoprotein. Administration of rifampicin would lead to a genomic effect with increased transcription of drug-metabolising genes via an interaction with the pregnane X intracellular receptor. This would lead to an upregulation of hepatic cytochrome enzymes, increasing warfarin metabolism and clearance, lowering warfarin plasma concentration and decreasing the INR.

This interaction would necessitate an increase in warfarin dosage and monitoring to maintain a therapeutic INR to avoid thrombosis risk. A marked reduction in the anticoagulant effects may be expected within 1 week of starting the rifampicin, and persisting for about 2–5 weeks after the rifampicin has been withdrawn.

— **Pharmacodynamic interaction: the risk of 'serotonin syndrome' with concurrent St John's wort and fluoxetine use**

Concurrent use of fluoxetine and St John's wort would synergistically increase neuronal serotonin levels. The *BNF* confirms this increased serotoninergic effect with all SSRIs and St John's wort use. It is considered a pharmacodynamic interaction, because they can both inhibit the neuronal reuptake of 5HT.

Cases of severe sedation, mania and 'serotonin syndrome' have been reported in patients taking St John's wort with SSRIs. The symptoms of serotonin syndrome can range from tachycardia and shivering in mild toxicity through to death from renal failure, rapid breakdown of skeletal muscle and coagulation of the blood throughout the entire body. Mr QT should therefore be advised to avoid the concurrent use of SSRIs and St John's wort.

— **Pharmacokinetic interactions: antacids and their effects on drug absorption**

Stockley's Drug Interactions provides management advice here. It is believed that certain drug functional groups undergo an electrostatic interaction with the Mg^{2+} and Al^{3+} cations present in antacid preparations forming insoluble chelate complexes. This chelate would not be absorbed. The stability of the chelate formed seems to be an important factor in determining the degree of interaction.

Enteric (gastroresistant) coated preparations (cellulose or polvinyl acetate phthalate) are designed to be non-ionised, and insoluble, at gastric pH (pH 1.3). Therefore, a product that is potentially gastrotoxic (in this case prednisolone) would not undergo dissolution in the stomach.

The enteric coating ionises at the higher pH of the small intestine, hence allowing drug dissolution and absorption. Concomitant temporal administration of an antacid with an enteric-coated preparation would temporarily raise gastric pH, leading to the unintended dissolution of the preparation in the stomach.

Antacids and indigestion remedies containing Mg^{2+} and Al^{3+} salts are commonly purchased over the counter (OTC) as non-prescription medicines. Community pharmacists therefore need to be aware of, and alert patients to, the potential for drug interactions that can lead to treatment failures of regular medication.

EXTENDED LEARNING

- Apart from digoxin, what other commonly used medicines are derived from plants?

- Plants are an important focus in the search for new drugs. Describe some of the current strategies and processes of drug discovery employed in the screening and identification of new therapeutic agents.

- Provide further examples of drugs that are commonly implicated in different types of drug interaction, including non-prescription medicines.

References and further reading

Currie GM, Wheat JM, Kiat H (2011). Pharmacokinetic considerations for digoxin in older people. *Open Cardiovasc Med J* 5:130–5.

Joint Formulary Committee (2013). Appendix 1: Interactions. *British National Formulary*, 65th edn. London: BMJ Group and Pharmaceutical Press.

Mallet L, Spinewine A, Huang A (2007). The challenge of managing drug interactions in elderly people. *Lancet* 370:185–91.

Baxter K, Preston CL, eds (2013). *Stockley's Drug Interactions*, 10th edn. London: Pharmaceutical Press.

3

Respiratory cases

INTRODUCTION

This section contains five cases centred on patients with respiratory diseases, namely: asthma, chronic obstructive pulmonary disease (COPD), cystic fibrosis and cough.

Case 1
Asthma ▶ 89

This case is based on a patient with asthma who is receiving regular treatment with a salbutamol pressurised metered-dose inhaler (pMDI). The pathophysiology, signs and symptoms of asthma are outlined, then the treatment options in asthma are described, particularly in relation to stepping up and stepping down therapy. The mainstays of asthma therapy are inhaled β_2-adrenoreceptor agonists and glucocorticoids, and the chemistry of these agents is briefly outlined. The most frequently prescribed inhalation devices, pMDIs, are described and their formulation considered. To enhance the efficiency of drug delivery in the airways, and ease of use by patients who experience difficulties with pMDIs, they may be used with spacer devices. Alternatively dry powder inhalers may be prescribed as a means of delivering drugs to the lungs. The formulation and use of these devices are outlined. Ultimately, as the case illustrates, the benefit that patients receive from prescribed medicines will depend on their adherence to the prescribed regimen and the ability to use their inhalation device correctly.

Case 2
Treating an acute severe asthma exacerbation ▶ 93

This case continues the theme of asthma, with an acute exacerbation as the focus. It considers the pathophysiology and classifications of acute asthma, and the signs and symptoms of acute asthma exacerbations. Common triggers of an exacerbation, such as medicines, allergens, exercise, non-compliance and infection, are identified. The chemistry and delivery of beclometasone dipropionate are considered, before the various treatment options in asthma exacerbations, such as high-flow oxygen, nebulised β_2-adrenergic receptor agonists, oral steroids and nebulised ipratropium bromide, are outlined. The pharmaceutical monitoring, follow-up and treatment are described. The case also allows for a comparison of the key features of various types of inhalation device (pMDIs, dry powder inhalers, nebulisers) and emphasises the need for patient counselling in the use of these devices.

Case 3
Nebulised therapy for chronic obstructive pulmonary disease ▶ 97

This case describes an elderly ex-smoker, previously diagnosed with, and treated for, COPD, requiring hospitalisation for an exacerbation. The pathophysiology, symptoms, signs and diagnosis of COPD are outlined, followed by the treatment options, particularly in relation to exacerbations. The chemistry and pharmacology of long- and short-acting β_2-adrenergic receptor agonists, particularly salbutamol and salmeterol, are described, and related to their clinical use and adverse effects. The place of nebuliser therapy in COPD is described, together with the operating principles and designs of commercially available nebulisers (air-jet, ultrasonic and mesh). Practical considerations relating to patients' use and maintenance of nebulisers are considered.

Case 4
Paediatric cystic fibrosis ▶ 101

This case describes the treatment of allergic bronchopulmonary aspergillosis (ABPA) in a child with cystic fibrosis (CF). The aetiology of CF and the role of different medications routinely prescribed for a patient with CF are outlined. The chemistry and mode of action of the proton pump inhibitor (PPI), omeprazole, used to treat gastro-oesophageal reflux, frequently presenting in CF patients, are described. Itraconazole is used to treat patients with ABPA. The formulation strategies to enhance this water-insoluble drug's bioavailability are outlined. The clinical use and delivery of nebulised antibiotics and dornase alfa (DNase), an enzyme that cleaves extracellular DNA in the sputum, aiding its removal, are described. The case ends with a discussion of the use of shared-care protocols to ensure consistency of care across the primary care–secondary care interface, and consideration of medicines management in the home, which can be a complex task for this patient group.

Case 5
Cough ▶ 108

This case describes the treatment of cough in a young person, which is, possibly, smoking related. The case starts by considering the pathophysiology, signs, symptoms and diagnosis of different types of cough and the appropriate treatment. The use of mnemonics such as WWHAM is outlined, to ensure effective questioning of a patient when determining a diagnosis. The chemistry and mechanism of action of expectorants and opiate antitussives, widely used to treat coughs, are considered. Symptoms indicating that a patient with a cough should be referred to another healthcare professional are described. The opportunity for a pharmacist to offer lifestyle advice, particularly in relation to smoking cessation, is highlighted.

Case 1
Asthma

GEMMA QUINN

LEARNING OUTCOMES

At the end of this case, you will be able to:

- Outline the pathophysiology, and signs and symptoms of asthma
- Describe the treatment options in asthma, particularly in relation to stepping up and stepping down therapy
- Outline the chemistry of glucocorticoids and β_2-adrenoreceptor agonists used in the treatment of asthma
- Outline the formulation of pressurised metered-dose inhalers
- Describe the use of spacers with pressurised metered-dose inhalers
- Outline the formulation of dry powder inhalers
- Consider the issues that may affect adherence in asthma, and make appropriate treatment recommendations to improve this

Case study

Miss GN is a 19-year-old young woman who is currently studying for a degree in English at the local university. She was diagnosed with asthma when she was 7 years old and her regular prescription is for salbutamol pMDI 200 micrograms when required.

- What is asthma?
- What are the most common signs and symptoms of asthma?
- How is a diagnosis made?
- What non-pharmacological treatment options are available?
- What is the first-line pharmacological treatment in asthma?

Miss GN came to the pharmacy to collect her third prescription for a salbutamol pMDI in 4 weeks. The pharmacist asked to speak to her and discovered that she was currently using her inhaler five to six times a day. Miss GN was referred to her GP and returned a few days later with a prescription for beclometasone (Clenil) 200 micrograms twice daily, via a spacer.

- When is it appropriate to start treatment with inhaled corticosteroids?
- What is a pMDI and what are the benefits of using a spacer?

Miss GN continued to collect her prescriptions for salbutamol and beclometasone, but after a few months she complained that she was still using her salbutamol up to four times a week and was waking at night. She also found it difficult to carry the spacer and two inhalers around with her, meaning that she sometimes missed doses. The pharmacist suggested seeing her GP again for a review. Miss GN subsequently presented with a prescription for budesonide/formoterol (Symbicort 100/6 Turbohaler), two puffs twice daily and one puff when required (SMART regimen: single inhaler maintenance and reliever therapy).

- What sort of inhalation device is a Turbohaler, and how does it differ from a pMDI?
- Draw the structures of budesonide and formoterol. How are they related to other steroids and β_2-adrenergic receptor agonists used in asthma?
- What issues may affect adherence with asthma treatments, particularly in Miss GN's case?
- What is the SMART regimen and when is it recommended?

Miss GN asks you whether she might be able to reduce her inhalers in the future.

- When should inhaler therapy be stepped down?

Case discussion

— Asthma and its pathophysiology

Asthma is one of the most common respiratory diseases in the UK, with about a fifth of children (21%) and 15% of adults affected. It is characterised by 'reversible' obstruction of the airways, caused by a combination of bronchial hyper-responsiveness, inflammatory changes in the airways, and increased numbers of eosinophils and activated T cells. It is usually an allergic condition, with common triggers including pollen, dust, animal dander, respiratory infections, medicines (e.g. β-blockers and non-steroidal anti-inflammatory drugs [NSAIDs]), cold air, strong emotions and exercise.

— Signs and symptoms of asthma
Symptoms characteristic of asthma include wheeze, breathlessness, chest tightness and cough. Symptoms usually occur in response to a trigger and are often worse at night and early in the morning. There is also frequently a family history of asthma or atopic (hyperallergic) disorders.

There is no agreed definition of asthma, so a diagnosis is made based on the pattern of signs and symptoms, where there is no probable alternative diagnosis. Spirometry is the preferred method of demonstrating fluctuating airflow obstruction in asthma, although a normal spirogram does not exclude a diagnosis of asthma.

— Pharmacological and non-pharmacological treatment options for asthma
Many patients can identify triggers for their asthma and, where possible, these should be avoided, particularly where they include dust mites and passive smoking. Where dust mites are felt to be a trigger, patients can try methods such as mattress barrier systems and high temperature washing of bed linen. However, this can be expensive and is not of proven benefit.

Management of asthma is mainly pharmacological, with the aim of achieving 'complete control'. This can be defined as:

- No daytime symptoms
- No night-time awakening due to asthma
- No need for rescue medication (β_2-agonist)
- No exacerbations
- No limitations on activity, including exercise
- Normal lung function (FEV_1 and/or PEF >80% of predicted or best)
- Minimal side effects of medication.

Mild asthma may be managed with a β_2-adrenoreceptor agonist taken only when required. The British Thoracic Society/Scottish Intercollegiate Guidelines Network (BTS/SIGN) guidelines do not recommend one drug over any other, but in practice salbutamol is the usual choice.

— Stepping up treatment: initiating inhaled corticosteroids
Patients should be considered for inhaled corticosteroids if they are symptomatic and/or

need to use their β_2 agonist three times a week or more, if their symptoms wake them at least once a week or if they have had an exacerbation in the last 2 years. The use of two or more canisters of β_2 agonist a month, or 10–12 puffs per day, indicates that patients are poorly controlled and at risk of fatal or near-fatal asthma.

Adults are usually started on the equivalent of 200 micrograms beclometasone twice daily, whereas 100 micrograms twice daily is usually prescribed for children. It is important to note that different formulations of beclometasone are not bioequivalent; some pMDI products are solution formulations in hydrofluoroalkane (HFA) propellants and others are suspension formulations producing different drug deposition profiles within the lung. Consequently, preparations should always be prescribed by brand proprietary name.

— Chemical properties of glucocorticoids and β_2-adrenoreceptor agonists
Budesonide is a glucocorticoid that is closely related to beclometasone dipropionate, and both drugs have essentially the same steroid skeleton. The principal difference is that beclometasone is prepared as the dipropionate ester, whereas budesonide contains an acetal group. Beclometasone dipropionate is a prodrug: the less-hindered ester (at carbon-21) is hydrolysed to give the more active monopropionate metabolite. Budesonide already has a free primary hydroxyl at carbon-21 so is not a prodrug.

Formoterol is structurally similar to other long-acting β_2-adrenoreceptor agonists such as salmeterol. Formoterol has an extended lipophilic substituent on the secondary amine nitrogen. This results in a greater affinity for, and longer residence time, on the β_2-receptor, thereby prolonging its duration of action. Only the (R,R) stereoisomer of formoterol is biologically active.

— Pressurised metered-dose inhalers
The pMDIs comprise an aluminium container/canister containing a liquefied aerosol propellant (HFA 134a or 227). The drug is either dissolved or dispersed as micronised particles (usually 2–5 μm) in the propellant liquid within the canister. Evaporation of propellant within the headspace of the canister provides a pressure (the saturation vapour pressure of the propellant gas), which expels liquid from the canister, via a metering valve; this sits in a plastic actuator. Excipients in

budesonide

beclometasone dipropionate

formoterol

salmeterol

the formulation may include a surfactant, such as sorbitan ester, lecithin or oleic acid, which acts as a suspending agent in suspension formulations, and ethanol as a co-solvent to aid in the dissolution of drug or surfactant.

— Use of spacers

Many patients find using a pMDI very difficult and use it incorrectly. One study found that only 23–43% of patients can use a pMDI correctly; this figure was 55–57% for patients using a pMDI with a spacer.

Spacers are plastic devices used by some patients together with a pMDI. They reduce the velocity of the aerosol emitted from the pMDI, remove large droplets by impaction with the spacer walls, provide time and space for propellant to evaporate from droplets, allowing a fine aerosol to be produced, and remove the need for patients to inhale at the same time as actuating the pMDI.

The use of a β_2-adrenoreceptor agonist with a spacer in mild and moderate exacerbations has been shown to be as effective as treatment with a nebuliser, making a spacer a vital part of an asthma personal management plan. It is important to note that spacers should be cleaned monthly and changed at least every 6–12 months.

The use of a spacer with inhaled corticosteroids may also reduce the risk of oral candidiasis. Rinsing the mouth with water or brushing the teeth after inhaling the dose are also sometimes

tried, but there is little evidence to confirm the effectiveness of any of these interventions.

— Dry powder inhalers

The Symbicort Turbohaler is a dry powder inhaler (DPI) from which drug is inhaled as a cloud of fine particles. DPIs have several advantages over pMDIs. They are propellant free and usually do not contain any excipients, other than a carrier (see below). They are breath actuated, so the problems for patients of coordinating actuation and inhalation are removed.

The drug (with a particle size usually <5 μm) and excipients (if present) is either preloaded in an inhalation device (e.g. Turbohaler, Accuhaler), or put into hard gelatin capsules (e.g. Handihaler), which are loaded into a device before use.

The small drug particles produced by micronisation (milling) have poor flow properties, due to their high surface energy. To improve their flow, and aid device manufacture and delivery of drug from the device, particles are generally mixed with larger 'carrier' particles (30–150 μm) of an excipient, usually lactose. Some formulations also contain fine lactose particles or magnesium stearate to optimise the formulation properties. During inhalation, the turbulent airflow generated within the inhalation device should be sufficient for the deaggregation of the drug/carrier aggregates, with drug particles carried in the inhaled air deep into the airways. Most DPI formulations contain a carrier; some Turbohaler formulations do not. Instead, drug particles are loosely aggregated, and these aggregates are broken up by turbulent airflow created in the device during inhalation by patients.

— Factors affecting adherence with asthma treatments

Patients may find it difficult to adhere to treatments for asthma. This may be intentional or unintentional. As already discussed, achieving correct inhaler technique is very difficult. DPIs may be preferable (53–59% of patients use correct inhaler technique), although alternative devices to a pMDI should be prescribed according to patient preference and local cost. The type of device may be limited by the drug, so it may be appropriate to change the drug, e.g. beclometasone is not available as a Turbohaler, whereas budesonide is. There are also devices available to measure patients' inspiratory flow and match this to the most appropriate device.

The side effects of inhaled corticosteroids may discourage patients from adhering to their prescribed regimen, as may lifestyle issues. As a student Miss GN may have a busy social life and live away from home; this may impact on her ability to have inhalers with her when needed and she may benefit from having more than one of each inhaler available, e.g. one to keep at both her student and her home addresses.

Pharmacists can make a huge impact by teaching patients how to use their inhalers correctly, recommending changes to alternative devices when appropriate and making other practical suggestions that may help with adherence.

— The SMART regimen

Studies have shown that the SMART (single inhaler maintenance and reliever therapy) combination of budesonide/formoterol can safely and effectively be used as an asthma reliever as well as a preventer in primary care asthma management, with formoterol acting as quickly as salbutamol. This can be prescribed if control is not achieved with standard dose inhaled corticosteroids. When this regimen is prescribed, the total daily dose of inhaled steroid should not be decreased, and patients should be advised that the regimen will require review if they need to use the reliever once a day or more on a regular basis.

This may aid adherence because the patient requires only one dry powder inhaler (and therefore no spacer).

— Stepping down treatment

Once a patient's asthma has been controlled, 'stepping down' should be considered. The most appropriate drug to be reduced should be considered in view of current dose, side effects and beneficial effects of the current dose, as well as the severity of asthma and patient preference.

If stepping down inhaled steroids, reductions should be considered every 3 months, with a dose reduction of 25–50% at a time.

EXTENDED LEARNING

- How are inhalation products formulated and manufactured?
- What are the mechanisms whereby inhaled particles are deposited in and cleared from the airways?
- Why is particle size such an important property of inhalation aerosols?
- What methods are used to reduce the size of particles and to measure the size distribution of particles?

ADDITIONAL PRACTICE POINT

- How will you counsel a patient to use a pMDI, pMDI with spacer or DPI?

Further reading

British Thoracic Society/Scottish Intercollegiate Guidelines Network (2012). *British Guidelines on the Management of Asthma*. London: BTS/SIGN, May 2008, updated January 2012.

Murphy A (2010). Asthma: The condition and its diagnosis. *Clin Pharmacist* 2:203–07.

Murphy A (2010). Asthma: Treatment and monitoring. *Clin Pharmacist* 2:209–14.

Taylor KMG (2013). Pulmonary drug delivery. In: Aulton ME, Taylor KMG (eds), *Aulton's Pharmaceutics: The design and manufacture of medicines*, 4th edn, Elsevier: London, 638–56.

Thomas M, Pavord I (2012). Single inhaler maintenance and reliever therapy (SMART) in general practice asthma management: where are we? *Primary Care Respir J* 21:8–10.

Case 2
Treating an acute severe asthma exacerbation
ANNA PRYOR

LEARNING OUTCOMES

At the end of this case, you will be able to:

- Outline the pathophysiology of asthma
- Explain the signs, symptoms and common triggers of acute asthma exacerbations
- Outline the different classifications of acute asthma
- Discuss the treatment options in asthma exacerbations
- Outline the key features of the various inhalation devices (pressurised metered dose inhalers, dry powder inhalers, nebulisers)
- Outline the pharmaceutical monitoring required when looking after asthma patients and be able to make recommendations on therapy

Case study

Miss SA is a 19-year-old white young woman who has had asthma since the age of 5. She has been brought to the A&E by ambulance suffering with an asthma attack after collapsing during a local charity summer fun run.

Her mother tells you that her regular medications are as follows:

Beclometasone pMDI 100 micrograms two puffs b.d. Salbutamol pMDI 100 micrograms two puffs p.r.n.

Past medical history: hay fever

Miss SA has recently been taking ibuprofen 400 mg which she purchased over the counter (OTC) for a knee sprain she sustained while training for the fun run.

She has been admitted to hospital with her asthma before, as a child, but hasn't had any problems for a long time and 'hasn't been using her brown inhaler much lately'.

On admission, she is severely short of breath and unable to speak in full sentences; she is holding on to the sides of the trolley, leaning forward and gasping for breath. Her observations are as shown in the box.

On examination
- Blood pressure (BP) 95/75 mmHg
- Heart rate (HR) 120 beats/min
- Respiratory rate (RR) 30 breaths/min
- Widespread expiratory polyphonic wheeze
- Oxygen saturations PaO_2 = 59 mmHg (7.8 kPa) (normal 80–100 mmHg [10–13 kPa]); SpO_2 = 92% on air (normal >92%)
- arterial blood pH 7.3
- Peak expiratory flow (PEF) = 200 L/min (best = 450 L/min)

❓ What is the underlying pathophysiology of asthma?

❓ What factors could have contributed to Miss SA's asthma exacerbation?

❓ Beclometasone is administered as the dipropionate ester. How is beclometasone metabolised in lung tissue to give its active metabolite?

❓ What is the fate of the beclometasone dipropionate that is NOT deposited in the respiratory tract?

❓ What other investigations should be performed on Miss SA and why?

❓ How would you classify the severity of her asthma attack? What features of her history and presentation give cause for concern?

❓ What treatment should she be given immediately?

She does not respond to initial treatment.

❓ What further therapy could you recommend?

❓ What are the key differences between the various types of inhaler devices available?

Once she has been stabilised, she is taken to the admissions ward.

❓ What recommendations would you make for her further treatment and which specific parameters should you monitor as a pharmacist?

Case discussion

— Pathophysiology of asthma

Asthma is a chronic inflammatory disorder of the airways, characterised by bronchoconstriction, increased vascular permeability, excess mucus production and impaired mucociliary clearance (the process whereby the cilia of the cells lining the airways propel mucus, and deposited materials, upwards towards the throat). Due to airway hyper-responsiveness, both specific and non-specific stimuli can trigger the complex inflammatory response in people with asthma, which is mediated by eosinophils, mast cells lymphocytes and neutrophils.

— Possible trigger factors for an exacerbation in this case

- *Medicines*: NSAIDs, such as ibuprofen, can induce bronchospasm in people with asthma. This is due to the drug's effect on arachidonic acid metabolism: production of prostaglandins is blocked, causing increased production of leukotrienes which cause bronchoconstriction.
- *Allergens*: grass pollen is prevalent in June and July and mould spores (*Cladosporium* and *Alternaria* spp.) are common in late summer. Given that Miss SA is known to have hay fever and was outside participating in the 'fun run', this could have been a contributory factor. No antihistamine medication is mentioned. Of note, in the UK there is a peak of asthma deaths in people aged up to 44 years in July and August.
- *Running*: vigorous exercise causes narrowing of the airways in most people with asthma.
- *Non-compliance with medication*: Miss SA mentioned that she has not been using her steroid inhaler as prescribed.
- *Infection*: respiratory tract infections can provoke a transient increase in airway responsiveness in normal individuals, as well as people with asthma. Upper respiratory tract infections, principally of viral aetiology, are the most common trigger factor for acute asthma.

— Less likely triggers in this case

- Changes in weather, particularly high humidity
- Possible premenstrual component
- Psychological stimuli, such as stress or anxiety.

— Beclometasone dipropionate

Beclometasone is a potent glucocorticoid steroid. In the management of asthma, beclometasone is administered as a diester – the hydroxyl groups at carbon-17 and carbon-21 are both esterified as the propionate (propanoate) esters. After inhalation, the more accessible ester at carbon-21 is rapidly

cleaved by lung esterases to give the highly active beclometasone 17-monopropionate (17-BMP) metabolite. After absorption from the lungs, the 17-BMP is rapidly cleared to inactive metabolites in the liver.

beclometasone dipropionate

Only around 10–30% of an inhaled dose is deposited in the respiratory tract, the remainder being deposited in the oral mucosa and subsequently swallowed. Very little beclometasone dipropionate is absorbed from the gastrointestinal (GI) tract due to its very low polarity and very poor water solubility; most is simply eliminated unchanged in the faeces. Any small fraction that is absorbed undergoes significant first-pass metabolism in the liver, minimising systemic availability.

— Recommended further investigations

- *Chest radiograph*: although not recommended as routine, radiography is useful to rule out other causes for breathlessness, such as pneumothorax or pneumonia.
- *Arterial blood gas (ABG)*: this will help determine the severity of Miss SA's asthma. A low PaO_2 (partial pressure of oxygen dissolved in arterial blood) could be indicative of life-threatening asthma and an SpO_2 (blood oxygen saturation: percentage of Hb molecules bound to oxygen) <92% is associated with a risk of hypercapnia (elevated arterial CO_2; normal $PaCO_2$ = 40 mmHg [5.3 kPa]).
- *Blood tests*: including CRP (C-reactive protein, produced by the liver as a measure of general level of inflammation in the body) and full blood count (FBC) to look for evidence of infection.
- *Temperature*: to diagnose or exclude infection.
- *Echocardiogram (ECoG)*: to exclude a cardiac cause or complication for her symptoms.

— **Signs of acute severe asthma: considerations in this case**

In this case, Miss SA's PEF is <50% of her best, and both her heart rate (HR) and respiratory rate (RR) are elevated. She is unable to complete sentences and is having to use her accessory muscles to breathe (note: 'holding on to the sides of the trolley, leaning forward and gasping for breath').

FEATURES OF ACUTE ASTHMA

- Peak expiratory flow (PEF) 33–50% of best (use percentage predicted if recent best unknown)
- Cannot complete sentences in one breath
- Respirations ≥25 breaths/min
- Pulse ≥110 beats/min

Miss SA is also exhibiting worrying signs that could indicate that she is close to progression to life-threatening asthma, including hypotension and dangerously low oxygen saturation. A blood gas reading would be essential at this stage to determine her risk and plan her treatment.

LIFE-THREATENING FEATURES OF ASTHMA

- PEF <33% of best or predicted
- PaO_2 <8 kPa and/or low pH[a] on ABG
- SpO_2 <92%
- Silent chest, cyanosis or feeble respiratory effort
- Hypotension
- Exhaustion
- Altered conscious level, confusion or coma
- Arrhythmias

---

[a]Normal arterial pH = 7.35–7.45

— **Immediate treatment of an asthma exacerbation**

High-flow oxygen is the most important immediate treatment and should be the first intervention, because hypoxia can put the patient at risk of cell injury and death. Give 15 L O_2 via a re-breathe mask, aiming for an arterial SpO_2 94–98%.

High-dose nebulised β_2-agonist, either salbutamol 5 mg or terbutaline 10 mg: there is no evidence to suggest superior efficacy of either agent. This must be delivered via an oxygen-driven nebuliser with a minimum flow rate of at least 6 L/min because of the risk of desaturation with air-driven devices. Back-to-back nebulisation is recommended, e.g. salbutamol 5–10 mg/h.

Steroids: early administration of steroids is imperative. Their use has been shown to reduce mortality and lower requirements of β_2-agonist therapy. Oral steroids are as effective as parenteral therapy, provided that the patient is able to swallow and retain the tablets. Recommended doses are prednisolone 40–50 mg daily, hydrocortisone 100 mg 6-hourly or methylprednisolone 160 mg intramuscularly.

Nebulised ipratropium bromide (anticholinergic) 500 micrograms 4- to 6-hourly via an oxygen-driven nebuliser: combining an anticholinergic with the nebulised β_2-agonist will produce significantly greater bronchodilatation than the β_2-agonist alone.

— **Possible add-on therapy**

Magnesium sulfate: there is some evidence that, in adults, magnesium sulfate has bronchodilator effects. A single dose has been shown to be safe and effective in acute severe asthma unresponsive to initial therapy. The recommended dosage is 1.2–2 g intravenous infusion administered over 20 minutes.

Intravenous fluid rehydration: patients with acute asthma tend to be dehydrated because they are too breathless to drink adequate amounts of fluid, in addition to experiencing increased fluid loss from the respiratory tract. Dehydration causes the production of more viscous mucus, making clearance more difficult and risking mucus plugging. Consider potassium supplementation to compensate for the hypokalaemic effect of salbutamol and corticosteroids.

Antibiotics: routine prescribing of antibiotics is not indicated in asthma exacerbations. Most infective precipitants are viral in origin. Only if there is objective evidence of bacterial infection, e.g. elevated white cell and neutrophil counts, high temperature and radiological changes, should broad-spectrum antibiotics, such as amoxicillin, be initiated.

Intravenous aminophylline: some patients may derive benefit from the addition of an infusion of intravenous (i.v.) aminophylline; however, it is no longer considered routine therapy. The loading dose is 5 mg/kg over 20 min followed by

Comparison of inhaler devices

Device	A pMDI	DPI	Nebuliser
Principle of operation	Pressurised gas, e.g. HFA	Powder particles dispersed by patient's inhalation	Compressed air/oxygen, or: Ultrasonic Mesh
Drug presentation	Drug dissolved or suspended in liquid propellant	Micrometre-sized drug particles as powder	Drug dissolved or suspended in water
Possible excipients	Propellant, surfactant, co-solvent	Carrier particles, e.g. lactose	Tonicity and pH modifiers
Storage of medication	In inhaler	In inhaler or capsules	As unit-dose 'nebules', independent of device (rarely multidose in vials)
Treatment time	<1 s	One breath	Up to 20 min
Advantages	Small, portable, no preparation	Small, portable, minimal preparation	Ease of use, potential for delivering large doses
Disadvantages	Poor patient compliance	Inspiratory effort required	Relatively large, cost, duration of treatment, non-availability of devices on NHS

DPI, dry powder inhaler; HFA, hydrofluoroalkane; pMDI, pressurised metered-dose inhaler.

continuous infusion of 500 micrograms/kg per hour (maximum concentration 25 mg/mL). Be sure to check the drug history and for interactions. Therapeutic drug monitoring will be required if the infusion is continued for more than 24 hours. *Parenteral β₂-agonist*: intravenous salbutamol may be beneficial in addition to the nebulised route in severe cases, or for patients who are ventilated, although there is limited evidence to support this. Recommend prescribing: 5 mg salbutamol 1 mg/mL diluted in 500 mL 5% glucose or 0.9% sodium chloride and infusing at 0.3–2 mL/min (3–20 micrograms/min) and titrating to response.

— Recommended pharmaceutical monitoring, follow-up and treatment

- PEF: PEF readings should improve, but be careful to watch out for any diurnal variation – asthmatics typically dip first thing in the morning and failure to consider this could lead to inappropriately hasty step-down of treatment and discharge.
- Electrolytes: watch for hypokalaemia in view of the high dose steroid and salbutamol therapy.
- Side effects: monitor for side effects from all drugs, e.g.:
  - Salbutamol: tremor, tachycardia, headaches, palpitations
  - Ipratropium: dry mouth, urinary retention, nausea, headache

- Steroids: hyperglycaemia, hypertension.
- Switch steroids to oral prednisolone 40 mg daily and continue for at least 5 days. At this dose, they can be stopped abruptly on discharge with no need for weaning. Tapering is necessary only if the patient has had repeated courses, doses >40 mg prednisolone or received over 3 weeks of treatment.
- Step-up inhaler therapy: suggest switching to a combination inhaler containing a long-acting β-agonist + corticosteroid, e.g. Symbicort 200/6 or Seretide 125/25 (step 3 of BTS guidelines); this can be stepped down at a later date as control is maintained.

— The key difference between types of inhaler device
See Table 3.1.

— Counselling
It is important to reinforce the need for compliance with treatment, and to ensure that inhalers are used correctly with the optimal devices prescribed. Using these devices to achieve optimum effect is not easy. In particular, pMDIs require coordination of inhaling and actuation, as part of a routine with a number of steps to promote effective drug delivery to the lungs. Patients should be assisted to ensure that they

sustain a good technique in the operation of devices.

A personalised self-management plan should be devised and a written plan issued to the patient on discharge. These, together with self-management education, have been shown to reduce hospitalisation and A&E attendance, particularly in people with asthma who have had recent exacerbations.

The plan should include:

- Structured education, with specific advice about recognising loss of asthma control assessed by symptoms and/or PEF monitoring
- What to do if asthma deteriorates, such as seeking medical attention, increasing inhaled steroids or starting oral steroids, depending on severity.

Consider the need for supplementary treatments such as non-sedating antihistamines, e.g. cetirizine 10 mg daily.

EXTENDED LEARNING

- Outline the British Thoracic Society guidelines for treatment of asthma.
- Describe the pharmacology of long- and short-acting β_2-agonists.
- Describe the anatomy of the lung – how does this impact on the way in which therapeutic aerosols are deposited and cleared from the airways?
- Describe how particles delivered from inhaler devices deposit in the airways, and outline the importance of particle size and density in these mechanisms.

Further reading

Taylor KMG (2013). Pulmonary drug delivery. In: Aulton ME, Taylor, KMG (eds), *Aulton's Pharmaceutics: The design and manufacture of medicines*, 4th edn. London: Elsevier, 638–56.

Case 3
Nebulised therapy for chronic obstructive pulmonary disease
BOTHAINA ALHADDAD

LEARNING OUTCOMES

At the end of this case, you will be able to:

- Outline the pathophysiology, symptoms, signs and diagnosis of COPD
- Describe the treatment options in COPD, particularly in relation to exacerbations
- Outline the place of nebuliser therapy in COPD, and describe the variations in operating principles and designs of available nebulisers
- Describe the practical aspects relating to patients' use and maintenance of nebulisers
- Outline the pharmacological mechanism of action of β_2-adrenergic receptor agonists on bronchial smooth muscle
- Outline the common side effects of β_2-adrenergic receptor agonists
- Appreciate the structural characteristics of long- and short-acting β_2-adrenergic receptor agonists that are important in their pharmacological activity and clinical use

Case study

Mrs MM is a 75-year-old white woman, who has smoked for the previous 40 years. She was diagnosed with COPD 5 years ago, and has since been prescribed bronchodilators, including salmeterol, delivered from a pMDI to relieve her breathlessness. Salmeterol is a long-acting β_2-adrenergic receptor agonist.

- What is COPD?
- What are the classic symptoms of COPD?
- How is a diagnosis of COPD confirmed?
- How is stable COPD managed?

Mrs MM began to feel unwell on Christmas Eve. She was increasingly breathless despite using her inhalers and had just managed to call for an ambulance. The paramedics noted that Mrs MM was out of breath and her PaO_2 was markedly low. She was given oxygen as well as nebulised bronchodilators. During her stay in hospital, Mrs MM was started on an antibiotic and a course of oral steroids. On discharge, she was lent a nebuliser by the hospital for use with prescribed *salbutamol nebules. Salbutamol is a short-acting β₂-adrenergic receptor agonist.*

- ❓ What is an exacerbation of COPD?
- ❓ How is it managed?
- ❓ What is the mechanism of action of salbutamol and salmeterol in the treatment of respiratory disease?
- ❓ What structural characteristics of the salmeterol molecule result in a longer duration of action compared with shorter-acting β₂-agonists, such as salbutamol?
- ❓ What other structural features are important in the clinical use of these agents?
- ❓ What is the rationale for using a nebuliser in the management of COPD?
- ❓ What are the advantages of using a nebuliser rather than a dry powder or pressurised metered-dose inhaler in this case?

Mrs MM's condition improved and she was stabilised after 14 days. She visited her GP who recommended that she continue to use a nebuliser because her COPD had not been adequately controlled with her previous medication; she had increased breathlessness, which limited her daily activities, a productive cough with purulent sputum, and a history of recurrent respiratory infections in the last few years.

Mrs MM is very keen on controlling her symptoms and wanted the GP to help her choose the 'best' nebuliser available.

- ❓ What are the different types of nebuliser systems available?
- ❓ Given the variation between different available nebuliser systems, what factors should influence the choice of the doctor/patient?
- ❓ What factors will determine the proportion of drug in the prescribed salbutamol nebules that will reach the deep lung of a patient using a nebuliser?

Mrs MM comes to the pharmacy and asks you for guidance on the use of her nebuliser.

- ❓ Can you explain when and how the nebuliser should be used, giving clear instructions on cleaning and maintenance?

Case discussion

— COPD and its pathophysiology
Chronic obstructive pulmonary disease, characterised by airflow obstruction that is not fully reversible and does not change over several months, is usually progressive and frequently caused by smoking. COPD is an umbrella term used to describe a range of different overlapping conditions affecting the airways, such as chronic bronchitis, emphysema, long-standing asthma and small airway disease. In COPD, the airways become inflamed as a result of an exogenous factor, often smoking, and produce *elastases* which, over time, result in disruption of the elastin/elastase balance in the lung. This, coupled with inactivation of the protective anti-elastases in the lung (as a result of the oxidants in cigarette smoke), leads to loss of lung elastin, destruction of lung tissue and emphysema. Loss of elastin also causes the lungs to become hyperinflated due to air being trapped in the small airways. In addition, smoking causes inflammation and mucus production, which accelerate the decline in lung function and predispose patients to infections. The consequences of this are breathlessness on exertion, hypoxia, pulmonary hypertension and peripheral oedema.

— Symptoms, signs and diagnosis of COPD
Patients with COPD often experience symptoms of breathlessness on exertion, coughing, sputum production and wheezing. However, clinical signs such as barrel chest, prominent accessory muscle of respiration, recession of lower costal margins, abdominal breathing, weight loss, central cyanosis, peripheral oedema and raised jugular venous pressure (JVP) are seen only when the disease is in the severe stage. Diagnosis of COPD often includes full clinical assessments for symptoms and the presence of any clinical signs, as well as complete history taking. Measurement of lung function by spirometry is essential in making a diagnosis of COPD. However, in uncertain cases, bronchodilator or steroid reversibility testing may be useful.

Spirometry is a standardised measure of a forced expiration (and sometimes inspiration) into a spirometer (a calibrated measuring device). Spirometers usually measure flow and then calculate volume with respect to time. The most common measurements are:

- FEV_1: the forced expiratory volume in 1 s, which is the amount of air blown out in 1 s.
- FVC: the forced vital capacity, which is the total amount of air blown out in one breath.
- A FEV_1:FVC ratio is then calculated.

There are several manufacturers of equipment, and all spirometers need, as a minimum, to meet the standards of measuring and recording as specified in international guidelines. To perform quality-assured spirometry testing and provide valid results for patients, a systematic approach would need to be employed by trained staff according to local standards.

— Treatment options for stable COPD, and during an exacerbation

COPD is mainly managed in primary care with pharmacological and non-pharmacological options. Drug options include inhaled bronchodilators, theophylline, oral or inhaled corticosteroids, and combination therapy of more than one of these. Non-pharmacological options include smoking cessation, pulmonary rehabilitation programmes and oxygen therapy. Exacerbations are common health problems in the natural development of COPD. The National Institute for Health and Care Excellence (NICE) defines an exacerbation as 'a sustained worsening of the patient's symptoms from his or her usual stable state that is beyond normal day-to-day variations, and is acute in onset. Commonly reported symptoms are worsening breathlessness, cough, increased sputum production and change in sputum colour. The change in these symptoms often necessitates a change in medication.' Treatment of an exacerbation includes large doses of inhaled bronchodilators, systemic corticosteroids, antibiotics, intravenous theophylline and oxygen.

— Pharmacology of β_2-adrenergic receptor agonists

The clinical usefulness of drugs such as salbutamol and salmeterol as bronchodilators relies on their ability to 'select' for the β_2-subtype of adrenergic receptor that is present on bronchial smooth muscle cells. Salbutamol was originally introduced into practice for bronchodilatation in 1968 and immediately became successful in asthma and COPD treatment, because it produced fewer serious (particularly cardiac) side effects. (The most common side effects reported for inhaled β_2-adrenergic receptor agonists in the *BNF* are: fine tremor in the hands, nervous anxiety, dizziness, headache, muscle cramps, dry mouth and palpitations/cardiac arrhythmias.)

Up to that time, the less-selective β-adrenergic agonist drugs isoprenaline and orciprenaline were commonly used for such conditions, but their cardiovascular, central nervous system (CNS) and gastrointestinal (GI) side effects were considered too significant and potentially life threatening, and so were withdrawn. The main pharmacologic effects of β_2-adrenergic receptor agonists on bronchial smooth muscle are mediated through a coupling of the β_2-adrenergic receptor with a so-called stimulatory G-protein (G_s), which then activates intracellular adenylyl cyclase, the enzyme responsible for catalysing the conversion of intracellular adenosine triphosphate (ATP) to cyclic adenosine monophosphate (cAMP). The increased intracellular cAMP levels, via activation of protein kinase A, lead to a decrease in intracellular Ca^{2+} concentration and myosin light chain kinase activity, which ultimately causes smooth muscle relaxation (bronchodilatation). In addition, β_2-agonists directly open large (size) conductance Ca^{2+}-activated potassium [BK(Ca)] channels in the cell membrane, leading to hyperpolarisation and relaxation of airway smooth muscle cells. The combination of all these effects is responsible for the beneficial bronchodilator action.

— Chemistry of salbutamol and salmeterol

Salmeterol is considerably more lipophilic than salbutamol due to the extended lipophilic substituent on the nitrogen atom. This extended lipophilic group makes a specific non-covalent hydrophobic interaction with part of the β_2-adrenergic receptor resulting in a higher (10-fold) potency, and localises the drug in the active site for longer.

The secondary amino group nitrogen atom present in both β_2-agonists is basic, with a pK_a value of around 9.0 for the conjugate acid. At physiological pH 7.4, the amino group is protonated and therefore positively charged. This positive charge is essential in making an electrostatic force of attraction with a negatively charged part of the receptor. The basic amino group also means that both agonists can be formulated as salts, which have improved water solubility and dissolution. Hence, salbutamol nebules contain an aqueous solution of salbutamol as the salbutamol sulphate salt.

The carbon atom bonded to the hydroxyl group (-OH) is a chiral centre. Although both salmeterol and salbutamol are manufactured as racemic mixtures (50 : 50 mixtures of *R*- and *S*-enantiomers), only the *R*-enantiomer has the correct shape to bind to the β_2-receptor, because the *R*-enantiomer

salbutamol

salmeterol

has the same relative configuration as the neurotransmitter noradrenaline and the circulating hormone adrenaline.

A bulky substituent on the nitrogen atom and a hydroxymethyl (-CH$_2$OH) substituent on the aromatic ring are important for β_2 selectivity. The hydroxymethyl group also hydrogen bonds with the receptor-binding site and prevents the drug's metabolism by COMT (catechol-O-methyl transferase – the enzyme responsible for metabolising noradrenaline).

— Nebulisers and their modes of operation

A nebuliser is a device that converts a drug solution or, less frequently, a suspension into a fine aerosol for inhalation. The nebuliser system consists of a nebuliser chamber and a driving/energy source. Broadly speaking, there are three types of nebuliser:

1 Air-jet nebulisers, which are most commonly used in practice and comprise a nebuliser chamber and a compressor that generates air at high pressure to atomise the nebuliser liquid
2 Ultrasonic nebulisers, which use high-frequency sound waves to agitate the fluid and cause the drug-containing droplets to be generated from the surface
3 Mesh nebulisers, in which fluid is forced through a mesh with micrometre-sized holes to form droplets.

Each of these devices has advantages and disadvantages. The proportion of available drug that reaches the deep airways depends on the design and mode of operation of the nebuliser, duration of nebulisation, fluid volume (which can be increased by diluting the contents of the nebule) and fluid physicochemical properties, such as viscosity and surface tension. In addition to the device/fluid characteristics, patient technique and breathing pattern are important factors that determine the proportion of drug that reaches the site of action and hence the effectiveness of therapy and clinical outcomes.

— Rationale for using a nebuliser to inhale bronchodilators during an exacerbation

The mode of bronchodilator delivery is changed from regular hand-held inhalers to a nebuliser during an exacerbation. A nebuliser is preferred in this situation as higher doses can be administered to the patient more easily. It is also convenient for healthcare staff to administer, as less patient education and cooperation are required, since the drug is administered during normal tidal breathing, via a mouthpiece or facemask. This is particularly helpful if the patient is distressed. Additionally, the nebulised medication may reduce the viscosity of the mucus and assist in its expectoration from the airways.

— Prescribing nebuliser therapy

Nebulisers are indicated when a patient has severe, distressing breathlessness, despite optimal therapy with pMDIs or DPIs, or is too ill or incapable of using a hand-held inhaler. Domiciliary nebuliser therapy is prescribed after assessment of COPD patients in hospital or general practice. Components of the assessment should include a review of the diagnosis, peak flow rate monitoring at home, and sequential testing of different treatment regimens using peak flow and subjective responses. Only patients who have a clear subjective and peak flow response to domiciliary nebuliser treatment should be advised to continue. If there is a subjective response with <15% improvement over baseline peak flow, a physician should make a clinical judgement, whereas all other outcomes should not result in continued treatment.

— Use and maintenance of nebulisers

When a nebuliser is prescribed, patients (and/or carers) should be provided with the equipment, servicing, advice and support, and should have regular reviews. They are given clear instructions on how and when to use the nebuliser, how to clean it, when to replace parts and when to service the equipment. The nebuliser chamber and the mouthpiece or facemask should be washed in warm soapy water and dried after each use.

Tubing should not be washed because it is difficult to dry. It is advised that air be blown through tubing by running the compressor for a few seconds to dry it out, after the nebulisation session is complete and the chamber is detached from tubing. The chambers should be replaced after 3 months of regular use and the compressor should be serviced regularly according to the manufacturer's recommendations.

EXTENDED LEARNING

- How are COPD and asthma distinguished?
- What are the latest developments in nebuliser design and therapy?
- What conditions other than COPD and asthma may be treated by nebulised therapy?
- What is the place and operation of smoking cessation programmes in the prevention of chronic disease?

ADDITIONAL PRACTICE POINTS

- Familiarise yourself with a nebuliser and its component parts
- Topical use of β-adrenergic receptor *blockers* such as timolol, betaxolol, levobunolol or carteolol in the treatment of glaucoma may lead to sufficient drug being absorbed systemically to pose a threat to

patients with asthma or COPD, due to bronchial β_2-receptor blockade and consequent bronchospastic complications and risk of respiratory failure/death. Practitioners reviewing asthma or COPD therapy should therefore routinely investigate whether there is any ongoing ocular (or systemic) use of β-blockers before formulating a treatment plan

References and further reading

Bellamy D, Booker R (2004). *Chronic Obstructive Pulmonary Disease in Primary Care*. London: Class Publishing Ltd.

Boe, J, Dennis JH, O'Driscoll BR, Bauer TT et al. (2001). European Respiratory Society Guidelines on the use of nebulizers. *Eur Respir J* 18:228–42.

Boe, J, O'Driscoll BR, Dennis JH (2004). *Practical Handbook of Nebulizer Therapy*. London: Martin Dunitz, Taylor & Francis Group plc.

British Thoracic Society (1997). Current best practice for nebuliser treatment. *Thorax* 52(Suppl 2):S1–106.

Levy ML, Quanjer PH, Booker R, Cooper BG, Holmes S, Small IR (2009). Diagnostic spirometry in primary care: proposed standards for general practice compliant with American Thoracic Society and European Respiratory Society. *Primary Care Respir J* 18:130–47.

National Institute for Health and Clinical Excellence (2004). Chronic Obstructive Pulmonary Disease: National guideline for management of COPD in adults in primary and secondary care. *Thorax* 59:(Suppl I).

Primary Care Commissioning (2013). A guide to performing quality assured diagnostic spirometry. Available at: www.pcc-cic.org.uk (accessed 25 May 2013).

Case 4
Paediatric cystic fibrosis

SIÂN BENTLEY

LEARNING OUTCOMES

At the end of this case, you will be able to:

- Outline current knowledge of the aetiology of cystic fibrosis (CF)
- Explain the role of different medications routinely prescribed for a patient with CF
- Describe the presentation and management of allergic bronchopulmonary aspergillosis in a CF patient
- Outline the chemistry and mode of action of omeprazole

- Describe the properties of itraconazole and outline formulation strategies to enhance its bioavailability
- Understand the application of shared-care protocols in prescribing of specialist medication outside the hospital setting

Case study

Charlotte, a 7-year-old girl weighing 21 kg, is admitted to the ward after presenting at her outpatient clinic with increased shortness of breath, increased sputum production (sputum darker than normal), tiredness and generally feeling unwell for the last 3 days.

CASE NOTES

Past medical history
- Cystic fibrosis (CF)
- Pancreatic insufficiency

Allergies
- No known drug allergy (NKDA)

Drug history
- Creon 10 000 with snacks and meals
- Dalivit multivitamin drops 1.2 mL o.d.
- Tocopheryl acetate 100 mg o.d.
- Omeprazole MUPS 20 mg o.d.
- Flucloxacillin 250 mg b.d.
- Colistin (Polymyxin E) 1000 000 units b.d. nebuliser solution
- Salbutamol 100 pMDI two puffs inhaled via a spacer p.r.n. and pre-physiotherapy

On examination
- Temperature 38.5°C

A diagnosis of an infective exacerbation of CF is made. A new sputum sample is taken and sent to microbiology for culture and sensitivity testing. Charlotte is empirically prescribed ceftazidime and gentamicin. The flucloxacillin is increased to a treatment dose:

Ceftazidime: 1000 mg t.d.s. i.v.
Tobramycin: 210 mg o.d. i.v.
Flucloxacillin: 500 mg q.d.s.

- What is CF? Outline the current understanding of its aetiology and symptoms
- Explain what each of Charlotte's medicines on admission are being used for and how they would be administered. Charlotte is unable to take capsules/tablets (Hint: also think about timing with physiotherapy)
- What organisms, common in CF, are the intravenous (i.v.) antibiotics covering?
- Are the doses of the i.v. antibiotics appropriate, and how do they relate to altered pharmacokinetics in CF patients?
- How should the i.v. antibiotics be monitored?

Charlotte receives these antibiotics for a week, but does not improve and becomes progressively more wheezy. Her FEV_1 (% predicted) falls from 65% to 50%. Her blood results show an IgE of 1054 units/mL and Aspergillus fumigatus *RAST (radioallergosorbent test) of 19.8 units/mL, and* Aspergillus *sp. is noted in her recent sputum sample. A diagnosis of ABPA is made and Charlotte is started on prednisolone 30 mg each morning and itraconazole liquid 100 mg twice daily.*

- What does ABPA stand for? What is this? Is the therapy appropriate?
- Comment on the formulation and oral bioavailability of itraconazole in both capsule and liquid form

▼ TABLE 3.2
Blood tests and sputum culture results

Na^+ 136 mmol/L (normal: 134–145 mmol/L)
K^+ 4.5 mmol/L (normal: 3.5–5.2 mmol/L)
Urea 3.3 mmol/L (normal: 2.5–6.5 mmol/L)
Creatinine 35 μmol/L (normal: 32–94 μmol/L)
WBC 17.4 × 10^9/L (normal: 4–13.5 × 10^9/L)
Most recent sputum culture results:
Pseudomonas aeruginosa sensitivity:
Azithromycin R
Ceftazidime S
Chloramphenicol S
Colistin S
Gentamicin S
Tobramicin S
Amikacin S
Temocillin S
Aztreonam R
Timentin S
Meropenem S
Ciprofloxacin R
Staphylococcus aureus sensitivity:
Flucloxacillin S
Penicillin S
Erythromycin R
Gentamicin S

R=resistant; S=sensitive.

● How would you counsel Charlotte and her carer to take itraconazole?

● How would you monitor itraconazole therapy?

Charlotte responds well to the itraconazole and prednisolone. However, her sputum remains difficult to expectorate and she is started on DNase 2.5 mg once daily pre-physiotherapy.

She continues to improve and is ready for discharge after 3 weeks. Her discharge medications are as follows:

Creon 10 000: with snacks and meals
Dalivit: 1.2 mL o.d.
Tocopheryl: 100 mg o.d.
Omeprazole: 20 mg o.d.
Flucloxacillin: 250 mg b.d.
Colistin: 1000 000 units b.d. nebuliser solution
Salbutamol 100 pMDI: two puffs via spacer p.r.n. and pre-physiotherapy
Itraconazole: 100 mg b.d.
Prednisolone: 30 mg mane to be reviewed in clinic in 2 weeks
DNase: 2.5 mg o.d. nebuliser solution

● What is DNase (dornase alfa) and how does it work?

The clinical nurse specialist for CF contacts Charlotte's GP to explain the changes to her regimen, to be told that they are not able to prescribe the DNase under the new commissioning arrangements, and the hospital must provide ongoing supplies. They ask if it can be provided as part of a homecare scheme.

● In the NHS, what is meant by 'homecare'? What are the potential benefits of using such a service?

Case discussion

— Causes and symptoms of cystic fibrosis

Cystic fibrosis is an autosomal recessive, life-limiting disease caused by mutations in the cystic fibrosis transmembrane conductance regulator (*CFTR*) gene (discovered in 1989), which codes for a Cl⁻ ion channel normally present in lung epithelial cells. More than 1900 mutations have so far been found in the gene, but only a relatively small number of these mutations (so-called class I–V, with different biological outcomes) can account for most of the CF patients so far characterised with the condition. The most frequent mutation is a deletion of a phenylalanine amino acid residue at position 508 (ΔF508) which results in misfolding of

the CFTR channel protein in the cell endoplasmic reticulum (ER), thus preventing it from being trafficked to the plasma membrane. The poorly functioning CFTR channel in CF means that there is an imbalance of chloride and subsequently water across the epithelial cell, leading to accumulation of thick mucus secretions at mucosal surfaces in the lungs that are difficult to clear, and therefore particularly prone to bacterial infection and chronic inflammation. The *CFTR* mutations also affect the exocrine functions of the pancreas, intestine, liver, bile duct, salivary and sweat glands.

There has been extensive research in recent years, with limited success, into the use of gene therapy for the treatment of CF, with delivery of the *CFTR* gene directly to the airways. Transfer of genes into the airway cells requires the use of a vector, which may be viral (e.g. adenoviruses, adeno-associated viruses) or non-viral (e.g. liposomes).

Pharmacological treatment in CF: consideration in this case

— Pancreatic insufficiency

Approximately 90% of CF patients in northern Europe are pancreatic insufficient because of the reduction of pancreatic secretions, which leads to poor digestion of fats and malabsorption of proteins and carbohydrates. Patients have steatorrhoea (fatty stools), decreased absorption of fat-soluble vitamins (A, D, E and K), malnutrition and failure to thrive, and therefore require pancreatic enzyme supplementation. Creon 10 000 is usually administered as delayed-release capsules, which contain enteric-coated microspheres of porcine-derived lipases, proteases and amylases. The microspheres are enteric coated to prevent the breakdown of the enzymes in the acidic environment of the stomach. It is taken with all meals and fat-containing snacks. The capsules should be swallowed whole at the start of a meal and the microspheres not chewed to ensure that adequate enzyme levels reach the duodenum. For young children/babies, capsules can be opened and the microspheres mixed with acidic fluid or soft food. This could be apple sauce or yoghurt or any fruit juice with a pH <5.5, e.g. apple, orange or pineapple juice. If the granules are mixed with fluid or food it is important that they are taken immediately and the mixture not stored, otherwise dissolution of the enteric coating may result. They must not be mixed with the food that requires chewing, because this can cause a sore mouth and put children off eating, as well as reducing efficacy as described previously. The number of capsules taken varies from patient to patient, and the dose and strength are adjusted according to the patient's fat intake, stool consistency/frequency and weight. Dieticians usually advise on the enzyme replacement therapy for each patient. High-strength preparations such as Pancrease HL and Nutrizym 22 are not recommended because of their association with colonic strictures in children. However, no association was found with Creon 25 000. It was also recommended that the total daily dose of lipase should not usually exceed 10 000 units/kg.

It follows that all pancreatic-insufficient patients require supplementation with the fat-soluble vitamins A, D and E. Dalivit is a liquid multivitamin preparation (containing mainly vitamins A, B_2, C and D) available in the form of drops, and tocopheryl acetate (vitamin E acetate: the ester form of tocopherol) is a 100 mg/mL liquid formulation. Levels of vitamins A, D and E are usually checked every year at the annual review and supplement doses amended accordingly.

— **Gastro-oesophageal reflux**
Many CF patients also have gastro-oesophageal reflux which is believed to be due to the hyperacidic gastric secretions and relaxed lower oesophageal sphincter tone. Symptom relief is usually obtained with proton pump inhibitors (PPIs) ± prokinetics such as domperidone and low-dose erythromycin. Long-term treatment is usually required.

PPIs (e.g. omeprazole) and histamine H_2-receptor blockers (e.g. ranitidine) may also be prescribed as adjuvant therapy to enhance the effect of pancreatic enzyme replacement therapy, because pancreatic enzymes are inactivated by gastric acid; therefore, by decreasing acidity, the enzyme efficacy is increased.

— **Omeprazole: mode of administration and molecular properties**
Omeprazole may be administered to Charlotte as a MUPS (multiple unit pellet system) tablet formulation. The tablets may be dispersed in 10 mL non-carbonated water and then suspended in a small amount of any fruit juice with a pH <5, e.g. apple, orange or pineapple juice, or in apple sauce or yoghurt after gentle mixing. Milk or carbonated water must not be used. The dispersion

should be taken immediately or within 30 min. The dispersion is stirred just before drinking and rinsed down with half a glass of water. It is important that the tablets should not be crushed or chewed.

omeprazole

The omeprazole MUPS tablets consist of multiple enteric-coated pellets. The polymeric coating is specifically designed to dissolve only in the higher pH environment of the small intestine, hence the need to disperse the tablets in a slightly acidic medium before administration. On reaching the small intestine, the omeprazole (which itself is inactive) is absorbed into the systemic circulation, from where it reaches the highly acidic environment of the parietal cells, undergoing a pH-dependent chemical rearrangement to its active form. This activated intermediate reacts with the thiol (-SH) group of a cysteine residue present on the H^+/K^+ ATPase (the proton pump), covalently modifying and permanently inactivating it. If the omeprazole were not formulated with an enteric coating, this rearrangement would occur in the contents of the stomach, which would prevent the drug from ever being absorbed and reaching the parietal cells.

— *Staphylococcus aureus* **infections**
Long-term prophylaxis against *Staphylococcus aureus* is prescribed in order to reduce the frequency of infective exacerbations caused by this organism. The use of anti-staphylococcal prophylaxis from diagnosis until 3 years of age was shown by a Cochrane review to be effective in reducing the incidence of infection with *S. aureus*, although an improvement in clinical outcomes was not shown. Current guidance is to start it in all CF children identified by newborn screening or diagnosed clinically, unless there is a compelling reason not to, i.e. not tolerated, or allergy. Once aged 3 years, flucloxacillin prophylaxis is reviewed. Although policies vary from institution to institution, an example of such a policy is to continue only if *S. aureus* is repeatedly cultured, i.e. more than two isolates of *S. aureus* in a year. Cephalosporins are generally not used for long-term prophylaxis for *S. aureus* because of worries about increased pseudomonas isolation in a US

cephalexin trial and also evidence from the European database.

In the case of Charlotte, flucloxacillin is administered as the 250 mg/5 mL preparation, taken on an empty stomach to maximise absorption. As prophylaxis it is administered twice daily to facilitate compliance and to fit better with Charlotte's school day.

— Nebulised colistin

Nebulised antibiotics are prescribed for patients who are chronically colonised with *P. aeruginosa* (grown on three or more isolates in a year) or for eradication of first growth. Long-term nebulised therapy has been shown to reduce the frequency of infective exacerbations and the need for intravenous anti-pseudomonal antibiotics, and to improve lung function. The most frequently used nebulised antibiotics are colistin (colistimethate sodium) and tobramycin. It is currently recommended that colistin be used initially in patients chronically colonised with *P. aeruginosa*. Nebulised colistin achieves low systemic and high local concentrations in the lung, which makes it very useful for long-term therapy, because patients do not have the adverse effects associated with the use of these antibiotics administered intravenously.

Patients must have a bronchoconstriction trial before starting therapy to ensure that the nebulised antibiotic does not cause bronchoconstriction. Colistin nebulisers should be administered post-physiotherapy. This enhances their effects because physiotherapy has removed much of the sputum, enabling better penetration to the site of action.

— Salbutamol

Some patients with CF also have asthma (small airway disease) and therefore benefit from the use of bronchodilators, such as salbutamol (β_2-adrenoreceptor agonist). Before starting treatment, patients should undergo a bronchodilator trial in which their lung function is measured before and after treatment. In patients who demonstrate an improvement, bronchodilator treatment is initiated. Nebulised or pMDI bronchodilators are also used by some patients before nebulising antibiotics, in order to prevent bronchoconstriction.

— Intravenous antibiotics in CF: spectrum of activity, dose and monitoring

Ceftazidime is a third-generation cephalosporin and so has greater activity against Gram-negative bacteria, particularly *P. aeruginosa*, compared with second-generation cephalosporins. However, it is less active against Gram-positive bacteria such as *S. aureus* compared with the second-generation cephalosporins.

Tobramycin is an aminoglycoside that is bactericidal and active against some Gram-positive organisms, including *S. aureus* and many Gram-negative organisms, including *P. aeruginosa*. Tobramycin is the aminoglycoside of choice because there is evidence that it is less nephrotoxic than other aminoglycosides in patients with CF.

Larger doses of many antibiotics are used in CF due to altered pharmacokinetics, notably an increased volume of distribution and increased clearance (renal and non-renal). It is not fully understood why this occurs. In addition, due to the severity of the disease, high concentrations of antibiotics are needed at the site of action.

Both ceftazidime and tobramycin have an increased clearance in CF, so the high doses prescribed are appropriate (ceftazidime 50 mg/kg three times daily and tobramycin 10 mg/kg once daily). There is evidence, from a randomised controlled trial of once versus three times daily tobramycin (the TOPIC study), that once-daily treatment is equally efficacious and associated with less nephrotoxicity in children, although the study showed no difference in ototoxicity between the two regimens. In addition, less money is spent on equipment such as needles and syringes and, importantly for the child with CF, fewer blood tests are needed because only trough serum levels need to be monitored. It also saves on nursing time for drug administration.

The antibiotic therapy must be monitored to ensure that it is effective and not causing adverse effects. Temperature and clinical response (general wellbeing, sputum production and lung function) should be monitored to check efficacy.

In this case, Charlotte's trough serum tobramycin level should be measured 23 hours after administration of the second dose (i.e. shortly before the third dose), 48 hours after any adjustment and weekly thereafter, aiming for a trough level <1 mg/L. This will prevent nephrotoxicity or ototoxicity associated with elevated levels of aminoglycosides. Serum urea and creatinine should be measured at the time of first cannula insertion, and with each trough level.

Charlotte's liver function and blood count should also be monitored as ceftazidime can cause disturbances in LFTs (liver function tests) and blood disorders such as leukopenia.

Allergic bronchopulmonary aspergillosis

ABPA is an immune-mediated disease causing bronchiectasis (destruction and widening of the large airways) induced by *Aspergillus fumigatus*, and is not uncommon in CF (occurring in approximately 1–11% of patients). The typical presentation is wheezing, new pulmonary infiltrates on chest radiograph, a rise in serum total IgE and specific IgE to *A. fumigatus*, with a fall in lung function.

The mainstay of treatment is oral corticosteroid therapy to attenuate the inflammatory process, but this may need to be continued for several months and is associated with significant adverse effects. Treatment is with oral prednisolone: an example regimen of 2 mg/kg in the morning (non-enteric coated due to difficulty in absorption of enteric-coated preparations in CF patients as a result of pancreatic insufficiency) for 2 weeks, then 1 mg/kg per day for 2 weeks, and then 1 mg/kg on alternate days for 2 weeks. If an improvement in clinical symptoms, lung function and radiological changes has occurred, and when the IgE levels fall appropriately, prednisolone dose should be tapered to zero over the next 8–12 weeks.

Itraconazole

Itraconazole is used to reduce the antigenic burden of *A. fumigatus* in the respiratory tract. Studies of itraconazole, initially in an uncontrolled setting in CF, and recently in randomised trials in adults with asthma and ABPA, have shown evidence of benefit, including the ability to reduce steroid dosage. It should be given for 3–6 months.

— Formulation, pharmacokinetics and monitoring of oral itraconazole preparations

Itraconazole is a water-insoluble, hydrophobic drug with a log *P* value of 5.66. The poor solubility results in poor bioavailability, particularly from a solid dosage form, because the drug tends to pass through the GI tract without dissolving, ultimately being eliminated in the faeces. As a weakly basic drug, however, dissolution is improved somewhat in acidic conditions. Once in solution, the proportion of drug in the deprotonated (unionised) form can be readily absorbed into

systemic circulation. Dissolution and absorption are enhanced in the case of the capsules by forming a solid dispersion of the drug in the rapidly dissolving polymer, hydroxypropyl methylcellulose (HPMC, hypromellose) coated on to sugar spheres. As dissolution requires an acidic environment for dissolution, acid-reducing therapies should be stopped wherever possible and, if not possible, administered at opposite ends of the day to minimise the effects on absorption. Bioavailability from solid dosage forms is approximately 30%, but, if taken with food, bioavailability is increased to about 55%.

Bioavailability is greater from the liquid preparation, which is formulated in cyclodextrin as a solution. Cyclodextrins are cyclic oligosaccharides comprising six (α-cyclodextrin), seven (β-cyclodextrin) or eight (γ-cyclodextrin) glucopyranose units. They have a 'bucket-like' structure with a hydrophilic outer surface and a hydrophobic cavity that can accept a hydrophobic drug molecule, forming an inclusion complex and bringing the drug into solution.

The liquid preparation is much better absorbed, with a bioavailability >70%. However, it is unpalatable and must be taken on an empty stomach. Liver function tests should be monitored at least after 1–2 months, particularly if there is a history of liver dysfunction. ABPA markers will monitor the progress of the disease, e.g. IgE and *Aspergillus fumigatus* RAST, as well as clinical symptoms, e.g. wheeze, lung function and general wellbeing. Itraconazole levels should also be considered when there is a lack of clinical response, or if there is concern about adequate drug absorption or patient compliance.

DNase (dornase alfa)

Patients with CF have thick tenacious sputum, the retention of which contributes to infective exacerbations and reduced pulmonary function. The thick secretions contain a high concentration of extracellular DNA released by degenerating leukocytes, which accumulate in response to infection and add to the viscosity of the secretions. DNase (recombinant human DNase or rhDNase, Pulmozyme) is a genetically engineered version of the naturally occurring enzyme that cleaves extracellular DNA in the sputum; therefore it reduces its viscosity and aids sputum removal. DNase should be administered 1 hour pre-physiotherapy. DNase should be administered only using a jet nebuliser. Ultrasonic nebulisers are not suitable because they may generate heat within the fluid being nebulised, resulting in the degradation of this biopharmaceutical, and indeed others.

Homecare

Homecare medicine delivery and services can be described as a facility that delivers ongoing medicines supplies and, where necessary, associated care, initiated by the hospital prescriber, direct to the patient's home with their consent. Operating as a registered pharmacy, the homecare provider dispenses against the prescription provided by the hospital (with it effectively being a private prescription) for supply to the name patient. Patients that are typically on homecare are those with chronic diseases, such as cystic fibrosis, and stable regimens that do not require acute care input for each supply.

The benefits of using homecare for a medicine such as DNase is that it minimises the inconvenience of patients having to attend outpatient and day care appointments to receive ongoing supplies, thereby releasing appointment slots for other people and increasing efficiency. There is also an opportunity to improve adherence to treatment through regular contact with, and education of, patients. Homecare providers will often be in direct contact with the pataient, and are ideally placed through checking stocks to identify concerns with stockpiling, which can be brought to the attention of the prescribing team to highlight non-adherence and minimise wastage. Equally, the patient has an addtional point of contact in case of difficulties which can be communicated, via the homecare provider, to the prescribing team.

— Medicines management in the home

In addition to shared care between health professionals in the different healthcare sectors, care in the home will be shared between children/ young people and their parents/carers. Many CF patients are young. Managing the medication for CF on a daily basis can be a complex task. However, as this is a life-long condition many parents become 'experts' in its management, able to judge symptoms and respond appropriately. However, parents and young people will vary greatly in their confidence in making decisions.

Appropriate use of medicines and good adherence are important for daily wellbeing and

longer-term outcomes. Managing medication can be stressful for families. Optimal clinical outcomes depend on optimal use of a wide range of medications: pancreatic enzymes, antibiotics, steroids, vitamins, inhalational therapies. Medicines management activities and ensuring good adherence can be a significant burden for young people and their parents/carers and, when problems and concerns arise, these can be stressful. Shared-care protocols can present additional challenges for parents/carers because formal care is shared between specialists and non-specialists (whose knowledge will be variable and between whom communication can be poor). This can lead to potential inconsistencies in advice and uncertainties for young people and parents with regard to optimal use of medicines.

EXTENDED LEARNING

- Describe recent developments in gene therapy for cystic fibrosis. What are the barriers to successful gene therapy?

- What are biopharmaceuticals? How are they manufactured and formulated into dosage forms? What particular stability problems may they present?

- Liposome delivery of gene therapy is one example of the use of 'nanotechnology' in medicines. What other nano-sized systems have pharmaceutical applications and what benefits do they confer over conventional drug delivery approaches?

- What strategies can formulators employ to enhance the solubility of a drug?

ADDITIONAL PRACTICE POINT

- Consider the particular needs of young people with CF, as they become increasingly responsible for their own medication.

References and further reading

Hanrahan JW, Sampson HM, Thomas DY (2013). Novel pharmacological strategies to treat cystic fibrosis. *Trends Pharmacol Sci* 34:119–25.

Prickett M, Jain M (2013). Gene therapy in cystic fibrosis. *Transl Res* 161:255–64.

Ryan, G, Mukhopadhyay S, Singh M (2003). Nebulised anti-pseudomonal antibiotics for cystic fibrosis. *Cochrane Database System Rev* 3:CD001021.

Smyth A, Tan KH, Hyman-Taylor P et al. (2005). Once versus three-times daily regimens of tobramycin treatment for pulmonary exacerbations of cystic fibrosis – the TOPIC study: a randomised controlled trial. *Lancet* **365**:573–8.

Smyth A, Walters S. (2003). Prophylactic antibiotics for cystic fibrosis. *Cochrane Database System Rev* **3**:CD001912.

Stevens DA, Moss RB, Kurup VP et al. (2003) Allergic bronchopulmonary aspergillosis in cystic fibrosis–state of the art: Cystic Fibrosis Foundation Consensus Conference. *Clin Infect Dis* **37**(Suppl 3):S225–64.

UK Cystic Fibrosis Trust Antibiotic Working Group (2009). *Antibiotic Treatment for Cystic Fibrosis*, 3rd edn. Bromley: Cystic Fibrosis Trust.

Wark PAB, Gibson PG, Wilson AJ (2004) Azoles for allergic bronchopulmonary aspergillosis associated with asthma. *Cochrane Database System Rev* **3**:CD001108.

Case 5
Cough

KATIE GREENWOOD

LEARNING OUTCOMES

At the end of this case you will be able to:

- Outline the pathophysiology, signs, symptoms and diagnosis of different types of cough

- Discuss treatment options for the different types of cough

- Outline the chemistry and mechanism of action of expectorants

- Outline the chemistry and mechanism of action of opiate antitussives

- Know when to refer a patient with a cough to another healthcare professional

- Effectively question a patient to help determine a diagnosis

Case study

John, a 17-year-old student who is one of your regular patient's teenage sons, calls into your pharmacy on the way to college. He has an irritating cough and would like some medicine 'to stop him coughing' so that he can concentrate on his revision and exams. He looks tired and fed up. You notice that John smells of cigarette smoke.

❷ What questions would you ask the patient?

John explains that he has had the cough for about a week, following a cold. He does not take any other medicines and does not have any medical conditions.

❷ What is a cough? Explain the pathophysiology

❷ What are the different types of cough and how would you differentiate between the different types?

You determine that John has a non-productive cough; he has no phlegm and feels that he has an irritation at the back of his throat.

❷ What are the treatments available for the different types of cough?

❷ Would there be any restrictions on the products that you could sell due to the patient's age?

❷ What lifestyle advice, if any, would you provide?

Case discussion

A cough is the most common symptom of upper respiratory tract infection. It may linger after the infection has gone, because the swelling and irritation in the airways can take a while to settle down. The cough can take up to 3 weeks to go completely.

— **Pathophysiology of a cough**
Coughing is a reflex action initiated by stimulation of sensory nerves in the lining of the respiratory passages. The cough reflex is a vital part of the body's defence mechanisms. Normally, the lungs and the lower respiratory passages are sterile. Coughing usually means that there is something in the respiratory passages that should not be there. This can be caused either by breathing in air-borne dust particles or if a piece of food has gone down the 'wrong way'. If dust or dirt gets into the lungs, it could become a breeding ground for bacteria and cause pneumonia or infection in the airways. It could also be a sign that an infection in the lungs is causing the respiratory passages to produce phlegm.

— **Mechanism of cough production**
Mechano- and chemosensitive cough receptors (afferent sensory nerve fibres) in the epithelial

layer of the pharynx and trachea are fired by the stimuli of excessive mucus or perceived foreign body or irritant (tussigenic) chemical stimulus, and impulses are transmitted to the cough centre in the medulla oblongata of the brain stem via vagal afferent nerve fibres. Impulses are sent back, via efferent neurons, to respiratory muscles of the diaphragm, chest wall and abdomen; these contract, producing a deep inspiration followed by a forced expiration of air, forcing open the glottis and producing a cough.

— Classification of coughs: signs, symptoms and causes

There are two classifications of cough:

- Productive: producing sputum
- Non-productive: dry, with no sputum.

Coughs can further be classified as acute or chronic. This is dependent on their duration and frequency. *Acute coughs* last <3 weeks, whereas *chronic* coughs last >8 weeks. Coughs between 3 and 8 weeks' duration are classified as *subacute*.

Productive cough: a productive, chesty cough, is one in which sputum/phlegm is coughed up. The oversecretion of sputum causes the cough. The appearance of the sputum can often help indicate the underlying cause of the cough: clear or white sputum is usually of little significance; pink/frothy sputum may indicate congestive heart failure, because the blood has congested in the lungs and there has been a leakage of plasma into the air pockets. Coloured sputum can indicate a bacterial infection and lower respiratory tract infection, such as bronchitis or pneumonia, where the sputum is yellow, green, rust coloured (particularly in pneumonia) and/or foul smelling, and thicker. However, it may just represent cell debris being cleared from the air passages. Blood might be present: this is not always a serious sign because capillaries can burst due to violent coughing, but it can be an indication for referral because it might also indicate a pulmonary embolism, tuberculosis (TB), bronchitis or lung cancer. The yellow tinge in allergic cough sputum, as can be seen in asthma, is caused by the presence of large quantities of eosinophils from the blood as part of the allergic response.

Non-productive cough: a non-productive cough may be described as dry, tickly or irritating. It produces no sputum and generally is unlikely to be bacterial, although this should be considered along with other symptoms. Non-productive coughs are irritating to the patient and also to those around them, so the treatment is to try to suppress the cough. A non-productive cough is usually the result of a viral infection, smoking or a dry environment. However, it can also indicate asthma (especially if at night) or lung cancer, or may be due to ongoing medication, e.g. ACE inhibitors.

A cough can be caused by:

- Viral cough associated with a cold (tends to be dry and lasts 7–10 days)
- Postnasal drip
- Allergies
- Croup: viral in origin, affects children aged 9–18 months; barking cough. Occurs commonly in the middle of the night, treated with steam inhalation or referral
- Chronic bronchitis (coughing up mucus on most days for more than 3 months for 2 years) associated with smoking and cough worse on waking
- Asthma can present as just a non-productive cough, especially in young children.

A cough can also be provoked by:

- Smoking
- Sucking material into the airways from the mouth
- Gastro-oesophageal reflux
- Medicines, in particular ACE inhibitors used to treat hypertension and heart failure. Cough may develop within days of starting the course of medicine, or after a few weeks or months. ACE inhibitors, in addition to their main therapeutic effects on the angiotensin production system, inhibit the breakdown of bradykinin and other kinins in the lungs and this triggers the characteristic coughing side effect that is dry, non-productive in type and, in some patients, sufficiently irritating and persistent to warrant a switch in therapy to angiotensin receptor antagonists
- Damage to the nerves that supply the vocal folds (known as vocal fold palsy) and chronic cough can occur.

Rarely, coughing can be provoked by:

- Psychological illness
- Heart failure
- TB
- Pneumonia

- Carcinoma of the lung.

— **Differential diagnosis**

A cough with no serious underlying cause will be self-limiting; however, to confirm this, the patient has to be questioned to ensure that all the relevant information is elicited. Various acronyms can be used as an aide memoire for this questioning process, e.g. WWHAM questions:

Who is the patient?
What are the symptoms?
How long have the symptoms been present?
Action that has been taken to date?
Medication already being taken?

Other useful pharmacy mnemonics include ASMETHOD, ENCORE and SIT DOWN SIR: For further details see: www.resourcepharm.com/pre-reg-pharmacist/pharmacy-mnemonics.html

In practice, often a combination or selected questions from these are used depending on the patient's presentation. It is important that you determine the age of the patient, the duration of the cough, whether it is dry or productive and, if productive, the appearance of the sputum. Any associated symptoms such as a cold, or shortness of breath, should be established. The previous history relating to the cough and whether the patient has other medical conditions and medicines should also be established.

— **Treatments available for the different types of cough**

If in doubt about phlegm production, it is best to regard a cough as productive.

Productive coughs: treatment of a productive cough involves encouraging the removal of the sputum and therefore should be treated with an expectorant cough mixture to help loosen the phlegm and make it easier to cough up from the airways. Expectorants contain ingredients such as guaifenesin (a glycerol derivative), ipecacuanha (derived from the dried root of the Brazilian ipecacuanha plant) and ammonium citrate/chloride or sodium citrate. Two mechanisms of action have been suggested: stimulating bronchial mucus secretion making sputum less viscous, or irritation of the GI tract which subsequently affects the respiratory tract, the former being more probable.

Non-productive coughs: these are irritating to the patient and those around them, so the treatment is a cough suppressant to reduce the cough reflex.

Cough suppressants include opiates such as codeine, pholcodine, and dextromethorphan.

guaifenesin

— **Chemical properties and actions of opiate antitussives**

Codeine, pholcodine and dextromethorphan are all examples of opioid receptor agonists and are all structurally related to the principal opium alkaloid morphine. Each contains a polycyclic four- or five-ring system, which includes a six-membered, nitrogen-containing, aliphatic heterocycle. The nitrogen atom in each is therefore part of a basic, tertiary amino group. Codeine is a naturally occurring analogue of morphine, being methylated at the phenolic hydroxyl group to produce a methyl ether. In pholcodine, a synthetic analogue, the methyl group of the ether is replaced by an extended chain with a morpholine ring at the end, which gives the drug an additional basic centre. The configuration of the ring system in dextromethorphan is opposite to that found in codeine and pholcodine; this can clearly be seen when comparing the structures in the diagram because the ring systems are almost mirror images of each other (opposite relative configurations at each chiral centre).

codeine   pholcodine

dextromethorphan

Opiate antitussives exert their effects centrally by acting primarily on μ- and κ-type (G-protein-coupled) opioid receptors present on relay neurons in the brain-stem medullary cough centre (in or around the nucleus tractus solitarius [NTS]) to inhibit neuronal firing and excitability; they do this through inhibition of excitatory (glutamate) neurotransmitter release and by opening postsynaptic neuronal G-protein, inwardly rectifying K^+ (GIRK) channels. The involvement of δ-opioid receptors in the antitussive action is, however, debatable.

Other treatments: demulcents, e.g. simple linctus and glycerin, lemon and honey linctus, coat and soothe the back of the throat. Antihistamines, e.g. diphenhydramine and promethazine, reduce the cough reflex and also dry up nasal secretions, which can be useful for coughs that are caused by a postnasal drip (mucus running down the back of the throat) or associated with a cold. Some cough remedies also contain sympathomimetics, such as pseudoephedrine, for their airway-relaxing and decongestant effects, and can be useful if the patient has a blocked nose as well as a cough. A practical consideration for patients with diabetes is that the cough medicine be sugar free.

It should be noted that there is limited scientific evidence that cough remedies are effective, although some contain ingredients such as paracetamol which reduce pain or fever. Thus, with the exception of antitussives, cough remedies have for many years not been prescribable on the NHS. However, some patients believe that they get some relief and the products are not considered harmful (Schroeder and Fahey, 2002).

There have been questions asked as to whether pharmacists should promote or recommend products with such a doubtful evidence base.

Legal restrictions on the sale of cough medicines
— Codeine
A UK review of scientific evidence has concluded that the risks associated with OTC oral liquid cough medicines containing codeine outweigh the benefits in children and young people aged <18 years. Consequently, OTC oral liquid medicines containing codeine should not be used to treat cough in children and young people aged <18 years (Medicines and Healthcare products Regulatory Agency [MHRA], 2010).

— OTC cough and cold medicines for children
The Commission on Human Medicines (CHM) has advised on a package of measures to improve safe use of cough and cold medicines for children aged <12 years. The advice is that parents and carers should no longer use OTC cough and cold medicines in children aged <6 years: there is no evidence that they work, and they can cause side effects, such as allergic reactions, effects on sleep or hallucinations (MHRA, 2009).

WHEN TO REFER
- Coughing up phlegm that is green, rusty brown, yellow, blood-stained or foul smelling
- Chest pain
- Shortness of breath or wheezing
- Pain and swelling in the calf (deep vein thrombosis)
- Recurrent night-time cough (asthma)
- Whooping cough or croup
- Worsening smoker's cough
- Sudden weight loss
- Fever and sweating
- Hoarseness of the voice with a chronic cough that doesn't clear up spontaneously.

— Lifestyle advice in this case
Pharmacists have a major role to play in the government's public health agenda. The smell of cigarette smoke should lead to a conversation with John about the benefits of smoking cessation and the products available. Smoking will exacerbate the cough and therefore, even if the patient does not want to stop smoking, he or she should be encouraged to limit the number of cigarettes smoked because this will help to resolve the cough.

EXTENDED LEARNING
- What are the respective roles of the MHRA/EMA (European Medicines Agency) and CHM/CHMP (Committee for Medicinal Products for Human Use) in medicines regulation and guidance for health professionals?

References and further reading

Blenkinsopp A, Paxton P, Blenkinsoppp J (2009). *Symptoms in the Pharmacy*, 6th edn. London: Wiley- Blackwell.

Edwards C, Stillman P (2006). *Minor Illness or Major Disease?*, 4th edn. London: Royal Pharmaceutical Press.

Medicines and Healthcare products Regulatory Agency (2009). *Cough and Colds in Children*. London: MHRA. Available at: www.mhra.gov.uk/Safetyinformation/ Safetywarningsalertsandrecalls/ Safetywarningsandmessagesformedicines/CON038908 (accessed 3 August 2012).

Medicines and Healthcare products Regulatory Agency (2010). *Codeine*. London: MHRA. Available at: www.mhra.gov.uk/ SearchHelp/GoogleSearch/index.htm?q=codeine%20over-the-counter%20products (accessed 3 August 2012).

Nathan A (2012). *Managing Symptoms in the Pharmacy*, 2nd edn. London: Pharmaceutical Press.

Rutter P (2009). *Community Pharmacy: Symptoms, Diagnosis and Treatment*, 2nd edn. London: Churchill Livingstone.

Schroeder K, Fahey T (2002). Systematic review of randomised controlled trials of over the counter cough medicines for acute cough in adults. *BMJ* **324**:329–31.

4

Central nervous system cases

INTRODUCTION

This section comprises 14 cases centred on disorders of the central nervous system (CNS) and their treatment. The cases focus on anxiety, schizophrenia, bipolar disorder, depression, the extemporaneous preparation of methadone, neuropathic pain, migraine, epilepsy, Parkinson's disease, smoking cessation and dementia/Alzheimer's disease.

Case 1
Types of anxiety, their treatment and associated issues ▸ 116

This case outlines the pathophysiology of two different presentations of anxiety. The roles of short-term anxiolytic benzodiazepine treatment and adrenergic β_1-receptor antagonists are discussed in relation to the different presentations. Alcohol consumption is briefly explored. Expanding treatment strategies to include cognitive–behavioural therapy is considered.

Case 2
Treatment options in schizophrenia – antipsychotics and side effects ▸ 118

This case focuses on an adult man living in the community with an 8-year history of mental health problems. The case outlines the signs, symptoms, causes, diagnosis and prevalence of schizophrenia. The role of antipsychotic drugs in controlling symptoms and causing side effects are described. Formulation aspects of intramuscular injections of antipsychotic medication, such as the use of aqueous or oily solutions or suspensions to delay or prolong the action of the drug, are discussed. The different treatment options available for people with schizophrenia are reviewed. Wider issues such as the stigma experienced by people with mental health problems and their physical health needs are highlighted at the end of this case.

Case 3
Bipolar disorder and its treatment ▸ 122

This case outlines the diagnosis and pathophysiology of bipolar disorder. Key treatments are explored with a focus on lithium therapy and the need to monitor serum lithium concentrations. The health professionals involved in caring for people with complex mental health problems in the community are described.

Case 4
Treatment-resistant depression in a patient on haemodialysis ▸ 124

This case continues the theme of lithium treatment, and describes a 73-year-old woman who presents with stage 3 chronic kidney disease and a history of treatment-resistant depression (TRD). TRD is defined and the available treatment options are discussed. The chemistry and mechanism of action of lithium are outlined. The ways in which lithium therapy is initiated and monitored are described. The effect of haemodialysis on the pharmacokinetics and dosing of drugs is then summarised. The significance of changes in the oral formulation or drug salt form is highlighted, particularly noting that dose conversion can be a source of error.

Case 5
Self-medication of depression with St John's wort, a herbal remedy ▸ 128

This case focuses on a 27-year-old woman who has occasional episodes of mild-to-moderate depression and is keen to discuss with the community pharmacist the option of self-medicating. Evidence for the efficacy and safety of St John's wort, and the way it is used, are presented. The proposed mechanisms of action of St John's wort and the importance of choosing a standardised product are explained. The mechanisms for drug interactions with St John's wort are detailed, and its roles in inducing cytochrome P450 enzymes and increasing P-glycoprotein expression examined. The rising prevalence of depressive illness internationally and the anticipated impact for population health are outlined. A DALY (disability-adjusted life-year) as a measure of disease burden is explained.

Case 6
Extemporaneous preparation of methadone ► 131

This case identifies the formulation and preparation problems that can occur when a powder is added to a liquid and how these might impact on the plasma level of a drug. The case is set in a drug treatment centre where a pharmacist prescriber notices that one of her long-term patients is experiencing withdrawal symptoms. Best practice when preparing extemporaneous methadone is described, solubility and dissolution rates are distinguished, and the recording and labelling requirements for each batch of extemporaneous methadone mixture that is prepared are highlighted.

Case 7
Neuropathic pain ► 134

This case focuses on an adult female patient with type 2 diabetes mellitus who is a regular customer in her local community pharmacy. The pharmacist notices that she has been buying paracetamol every 3 days for the last 6 weeks. The pathophysiology of inflammatory, neuropathic and functional pain is described. The case continues with a description of the signs, symptoms and aetiology of neuropathic pain, and possible treatment options. The chemistry and mechanism of action of antiepileptic drugs used in the management of neuropathic pain, and the chemistry and mechanism of action of tramadol are detailed.

Case 8
Differential indicators for migraine and medication-overuse headache ► 138

This case concerns a middle-aged man who has been experiencing an increased frequency of headaches. He attends his local pharmacy to explore the possibility that he may be experiencing migraine. Key indicators of headache and migraine are discussed. Treatment approaches to the management of migraine are described. Additional non-drug interventions are outlined. The case concludes with a discussion of medication-overuse headache (MOH).

Case 9
Epilepsy ► 142

This case features a woman with a 6-year history of being diagnosed with generalised tonic–clonic seizures. The definition, signs and symptoms, differential diagnosis and treatment of epilepsy are outlined. The case then focuses on issues that are pertinent to female patients with epilepsy, in particular considering implications for antiepileptic drug (AED) treatment in women of childbearing age. A pharmaceutical care plan and treatment goals for this patient are discussed. The chemistry of valproate, topiramate and lamotrigine is described. The use of the Biopharmaceutics Classification System (BCS) to predict the oral absorption of drugs is summarised.

Case 10
Phenytoin and acute therapeutics ► 146

This case continues the epilepsy theme. A male patient is admitted to an intensive care unit after experiencing tonic–clonic seizures followed by a cardiac arrest, while participating in an alcohol-detoxification rehabilitation programme. Calculation of a phenytoin loading dose is explained. The relevance of chemical structure, pK_a and pH of phenytoin for its formulation and administration in intravenous fluids is discussed. Conversion of an intravenous phenytoin dose to an oral route is demonstrated. A practical approach to phenytoin dose optimisation is considered.

Case 11
Drug therapy of Parkinson's disease ▶ 149

This case considers a woman who was diagnosed with Parkinson's disease 12 months earlier. The signs, symptoms and diagnosis of Parkinson's disease are described. Other causes of parkinsonian symptoms, thereby leading to the misdiagnosis of Parkinson's disease, are outlined. Some of the key drugs used in the pharmacotherapy of Parkinson's disease and their potential adverse effects, and how these can be minimised, are detailed. Disease progression and the use of co-careldopa are discussed. Some clinically significant interactions, which might be caused with drugs used to treat Parkinson's disease, are considered.

Case 12
Smoking cessation in community pharmacy ▶ 153

This case explores the role of a community pharmacist as a trained smoking cessation adviser. Cigarette smoking causes a wide range of diseases and conditions. This case outlines the public health role that a pharmacist can have in helping people to stop smoking. It discusses the behavioural support included in stages of smoking cessation programmes, lists the biomarkers used for smoking cessation and the role of carbon monoxide monitoring, and investigates the pharmacotherapy used in smoking cessation and their mode of action.

Case 13
Dementia/Alzheimer's disease ▶ 159

This case focuses on an elderly man who is referred to the memory clinic at the local hospital and subsequently receives a probable diagnosis of Alzheimer's disease of moderate severity. The definition, signs and symptoms and differential diagnosis of dementia are discussed. The different types of dementia and treatment options are explored. In more detail, the chemical structure and mechanisms of action of donepezil are described. Treatment options for behavioural symptoms are examined, in particular the place of antipsychotic drug therapy. Carers and their role in the management of medicines are acknowledged and the potential contribution that pharmacists can make in supporting carers is highlighted.

Case 14
Dementia and its pharmacotherapy ▶ 163

This case features a woman newly diagnosed with Alzheimer's disease. The Mini-Mental State Examination (MMSE) score is described. The case focuses on a medication review undertaken by the practice pharmacist of a GP's surgery, the choice and effectiveness of treatment options, and when to start drug therapy. In later stages of the disease, swallowing difficulties can occur and alternative formulations may need to be identified. Future considerations for therapeutic approaches are described at the end of the case.

Case 1
Types of anxiety, their treatment and associated issues
PETER WHITTON

LEARNING OUTCOMES

At the end of this case, you will be able to:

- Understand that there are substantially different manifestations of anxiety
- Understand the potential dangers of anxiety
- Be aware of the appropriate treatments for different types of anxiety
- Know the dangers associated with some anxiolytics and how these may be avoided.

Case study

Dr Smith had two patients attend his surgery complaining of conditions that he recognised as anxiety but in quite different forms. Ms JP, a 22-year-old student, complained that she has always been 'highly strung' but with impending examinations she is finding it difficult to sleep and her ability to concentrate has fallen. Mr RJ is a 36-year-old office manager in a business that is struggling due to economic pressures. He has always regarded 'having a drink' as a good way to unwind, but admits that his alcohol consumption has gone up quite a bit. He recently suffered an episode where quite suddenly he felt extremely scared, his heart rate increased for no apparent reason and for a while he thought he was going to die from a 'heart attack'.

- What are the probable descriptive names given to these types of anxiety?
- What would be the appropriate questions Dr Smith might ask to learn more about Ms JP and Mr RJ's problems?

Dr Smith has quite different strategies for the two patients. Ms JP is advised to restrict her caffeine intake and not consume any after 6 o'clock in the evening. She is also put on a low dose of a benzodiazepine for a short duration. Mr RJ is advised to make some drastic lifestyle changes and offered cognitive–behavioural therapy. He is given an open prescription of an adrenergic β_1-receptor antagonist after he shows a blood pressure reading of 170/105 mmHg.

- In the case of Ms JP, why are the advised changes in behaviour relatively modest?
- What are the specific named drug options available to Dr Smith for Ms JP?
- Why is Mr RJ offered behavioural advice?
- Adrenergic β_1-receptor antagonists are of general value in patients with elevated blood pressure. However, what specific effects could β_1-receptor antagonists have in relation to Mr RJ's problem?
- What are the potential problems that might be linked with the treatment strategies for these two patients?

Case discussion

— Types of anxiety and their pathophysiology

Both patients are anxious, but in the case of Ms JP this seems to be an underlying personality trait that has been exacerbated by study and impending examinations. This is not uncommon in individuals who are 'driven' to excellence. Her condition is known as generalised anxiety disorder (GAD), which is a loose descriptor for anxieties where the overall cause is not clear. Mr RJ is also driven, but his anxiety seems more closely linked to his job and attempts to self-medicate. The causes of GAD are unclear but almost certainly involve a dysfunction within the central nervous system (CNS) monoamine pathways. Mr RJ has an increased basal level of anxiety, probably reflecting increased activity of the hypothalamic–pituitary–adrenal (HPA) axis and elevated circulating adrenaline. His sudden severe anxiety attacks are known as panic attacks or panic disorder. The symptoms of these are essentially similar to an injection of an intravenous bolus of adrenaline (increased blood pressure, heart rate and sense of impending doom/death).

— The problems encountered by patients with anxiety

As anxiety can manifest in distinct ways, its treatment is often tailored to the patient. Ms JP is given a benzodiazepine (diazepam 2 mg tablet three times daily) for a short period. She is likely to comply with this treatment strategy but may find discontinuation difficult. These drugs are highly addictive, both psychologically and physically.

Mr RJ has been self-medicating with alcohol. Alcohol offers a challenge because it is socially accepted and graduation from moderate to heavy drinking can be easy to both do and justify. Alcohol is an extremely effective but short-lived anxiolytic. After a few hours the effects wear off and the patient is more prone to the possibility of panic attacks, which can fuel further consumption. β-Blockers are effective because they reduce the frightening physical elements of panic attacks. There are also β-adrenergic receptors in the CNS and blocking them (using a lipophilic β-blocker such as propranolol [80 mg sustained-release tablet daily] that penetrates the blood–brain barrier) is effective in mild-to-moderate anxiety but there is then the risk of developing some rather unpleasant initial side effects, particularly vivid dreams/nightmares and insomnia. Mr RJ should be helped to modify his lifestyle and relationship with alcohol. However, this can be very difficult for many patients.

— Seriousness of chronic anxiety

Chronic anxiety as displayed by both individuals is likely to lead to long-term increases in blood pressure, which can be severe. This can take a toll on peripheral organ systems (such patients are at a higher risk of cardiovascular problems). In addition, long-term anxiety can often evolve into clinical depression, which may be much more difficult to resolve.

— Cognitive–behavioural therapy

Talking therapies are psychological treatments that are used to help people overcome a range of problems such as stress, anxiety and depression. Talking therapies aim to change the ways in which people think about their problems and offer strategies to challenge thinking, help people to behave differently and think about different ways of coping. There are different types of talking therapy including counselling, cognitive–behavioural therapy (CBT) and psychotherapy. The type of talking therapy is matched to the individual and his or her situation.

CBT is one type of talking therapy that focuses on the way that people think and act, with the aim of decreasing negative thoughts and beliefs, and promotes recovery through changed behaviour. CBT is highly structured and tends to offer practical help with regard to current problems. It is often a short-term course of treatment and studies have shown benefit for patients after 2–4 months of treatment.

EXTENDED LEARNING

- How is alcohol dependence treated?
- How are the symptoms of alcohol withdrawal managed?

References and further reading

National Institute for Health and Clinical Excellence (2011). *Generalised Anxiety Disorder and Panic Disorder (with or without Agoraphobia) in Adults: Management in primary, secondary and community care.* Clinical Guideline 113. London: NICE. Available at: http://guidance.nice.org.uk/CG113 (accessed 12 July 2013).

National Institute for Health and Clinical Excellence (2011). *Common Mental Health Disorders.* Clinical Guideline 123. Available at: www.nice.org.uk/guidance/CG123 (accessed 12 July 2013).

Olivier JD, Vinkers CH, Olivier B (2013). The role of the serotonergic and GABA system in translational approaches in drug discovery for anxiety disorders. *Front Pharmacol* 4:74.

Swain J, Hancock K, Hainsworth C, Bowman J (2013). Acceptance and commitment therapy in the treatment of anxiety: A systematic review. *Clin Psychol Rev* 33:965–78.

Case 2

Treatment options in schizophrenia – antipsychotics and side effects

NEELAM SHARMA

LEARNING OUTCOMES

At the end of this case, you will be able to:

- Outline the signs, symptoms, causes, diagnosis and prevalence of schizophrenia
- Describe treatment options for schizophrenia
- Discuss actions and potential side effects of different antipsychotic medications
- Outline the formulation considerations of depot injections
- Acknowledge how and why stigma may be experienced by people with a mental health (or other long-term) condition

Case study

Mr MM, a 36-year-old Turkish man, comes to the pharmacy medication clinic. He has an 8-year history of mental health problems and diagnoses of paranoid schizophrenia and moderate depression. He has had three hospital admissions but has been well in the community for the past 2 years. He is married and has an 18-month-old daughter.

- ❷ What is paranoid schizophrenia?
- ❷ How is it managed?

Mr MM is experiencing blurred vision, erectile dysfunction, tiredness and extrapyramidal side effects (EPSEs) with shaking of his left hand and leg. He has tried switching medication (he was prescribed flupenthixol decanoate 5 months ago) and a dose reduction in his pipotiazine from 100 mg to 80 mg has been made, but there has been no real change to the side effects experienced. The addition of procyclidine has not improved the shaking. Mr MM has also been started on sildenafil recently by his GP but this has not been helpful. Mr MM says that he wears glasses but, whether or not he wears these, he still experiences blurred vision.

Mr MM is satisfied with his antidepressant treatment. He feels that it has helped him and doesn't want to change it.

He is currently prescribed:

Pipotiazine 80 mg injection every 4 weeks for the last 5 months
Venlafaxine 150 mg XL o.n.
Procyclidine 5 mg t.d.s.

- ❷ Why are depot antipsychotics used?
- ❷ What could be causing his blurred vision?
- ❷ What considerations need to be made in selecting an antipsychotic medication for Mr MM?
- ❷ What medication changes would you recommend and why?

After review, Mr MM's prescribed medications were changed to:

Aripiprazole 15 mg o.d.
Venlafaxine 75 mg M/R o.d.

When Mr MM was seen by the team 4 weeks later, he no longer had any perceptible shaking (either subjectively or objectively) and he was no longer experiencing blurred vision. His mental state had remained stable and he was pleased at the improvements seen. The only problem he was still experiencing related to sexual dysfunction.

- ❷ Outline your considerations with regard to Mr MM's sexual dysfunction

Case discussion

— Schizophrenia

Schizophrenia is a serious mental health condition that occurs in about 0.5% of the world's population. It is a psychotic disorder that alters a person's perception, mood and behaviour. Signs and symptoms include hallucinations, delusions, disorganised thought and speech, paranoia, apathy with poor self-care and withdrawal. The suicide risk in people with schizophrenia has been reported to be 10 times that of the general population.

Schizophrenia commonly presents for the first time in males from the age of 18–25 years and slightly later in women, from the age of 25–35 years. There are no specific tests for diagnosis of schizophrenia. Diagnosis is made by observation of symptoms, from accounts of the condition from patients and their family, and also by ruling out organic causes.

Schizophrenia is subclassified into five categories according to the DSM-IV (*Diagnostic and Statistical Manual of Mental Disorders*, 4th edn – American Psychiatric Association, 2000) classification of diseases:

- Paranoid schizophrenia (characterised by delusions and paranoia which may be of a persecutory or religious nature)
- Disorganised schizophrenia (features thought disorder, disorganised speech and behaviour)
- Catatonic schizophrenia (displays immobility with waxy flexibility)
- Undifferentiated schizophrenia (where psychotic symptoms are present but the criteria for the previous three types have not been met)
- Residual schizophrenia (in which psychotic symptoms are no longer of the severity or intensity experienced in a previous episode).

Paranoid schizophrenia is the most common type. A person with paranoid schizophrenia may not experience disorganised thought or speech and may be more highly functioning than people with the other schizophrenia classes.

— Causes

It is not known what causes schizophrenia, but specific risk factors have been identified including genetic factors, substance misuse, environmental factors (urban living, migration), obstetric complications (hypoxia at birth and other complications during delivery) and any permutation of these factors.

— Pharmacological management

Antipsychotic drugs can control the symptoms of schizophrenia, particularly symptoms such as hallucinations, delusions and paranoia, which are known as positive symptoms. They are generally less successful at treating negative symptoms such as apathy, poor self-care and social withdrawal. All antipsychotics have antagonist action at central dopamine receptors, suggesting that schizophrenia, or at least positive symptoms, is linked to dopamine overactivity. First-generation or typical antipsychotic drugs also block dopamine receptors at the basal ganglia; this can result in extrapyramidal side effects (EPSEs) which can sometimes require treatment or a change in antipsychotic, or, in cases of tardive dyskinesia, can be irreversible. Atypical antipsychotics have selective activity for cortical D_2-receptors, which result in a lower propensity to cause EPSEs.

— Depot antipsychotic drugs

Antipsychotic drugs are available in oral and long-acting injection forms (depot injections), which require regular interaction with community psychiatric nurses. These are particularly useful when compliance is an issue and needs monitoring. Although increasingly available as atypical antipsychotics, most depots are first-generation typical drugs. Depot antipsychotics have been shown to reduce the risk of relapse compared with oral treatment.

— Formulation aspects of depot antipsychotics

Intramuscular injection of a drug, formulated into aqueous or oily solutions or suspensions, delays and prolongs the absorption of the medicine from the injection site into the circulation and, thus, the action of the drug can be delayed and prolonged. Some antipsychotic medicines, such as pipotiazine (a typical antipsychotic of the phenothiazine class), are formulated as oily intramuscular injections, permitting dosing every 2–4 weeks, promoting improved compliance compared with daily oral dosing. An oil-soluble derivative of the drug may be synthesised to aid solubility, so the ester, pipotiazine palmitate, is used in the oily injection. This long-chain fatty acid ester prodrug has an extremely low polarity, which facilitates dissolution in the oily vehicle. Non-toxic fixed oils, capable of being metabolised, are used as vehicles, in this case sesame oil. Oily injections are more viscous than aqueous injections; they form a depot within the muscle, from which the drug must partition before being absorbed and entering the systemic circulation. The very poor water solubility of pipotiazine palmitate means that it partitions only gradually into the aqueous extracellular environment before being absorbed. Once in the systemic circulation, the accessible palmitate ester group is rapidly hydrolysed by plasma esterases to generate the active pipotiazine. Relatively stable plasma concentrations of antipsychotic drugs can be achieved using this approach.

— Extrapyramidal side effects

Typical antipsychotics can cause EPSEs, such as shaking, rigidity and muscle spasm. These may require treatment with short-term or regular anticholinergic drugs such as procyclidine or orphenadrine. Anticholinergic medications may in

pipotiazine palmitate

turn cause confusion, dry mouth and blurred vision (paralysis of lens accommodation). For the patient in this case, procyclidine may be causing or making his blurred vision worse due to its antagonistic action at muscarinic M_1-, M_2- and M_4-receptors. As this is not helping the shaking in his arm and leg, it would be best to withdraw the procyclidine and see if any improvement is seen.

Although MM's symptoms are controlled with pipotiazine, he is experiencing intolerable side effects. The blockade of dopamine D_2-receptors in the nigrostriatal pathway causes unwanted EPSEs. Dopamine receptor blockage in tuberoinfundibular pathways causes hyperprolactinaemia (excess pituitary prolactin hormone in the blood), which results in sexual dysfunction due to interference with gonadotrophin function and galactorrhoea (inappropriate breast milk production). All typical depot antipsychotic drugs cause significant blockade of both these pathways. The atypical depots, risperidone and paliperidone, both cause dopamine blockade at the tuberoinfundibular pathway, resulting in prolactin increase, so a suitable alternative atypical antipsychotic is likely to mean a switch to oral medication.

— **Prescribing antipsychotic medication: considerations for this case**

At this stage it would be necessary to consider whether this patient needs a depot medication because of prior poor compliance or whether an oral antipsychotic can be implemented. In this case Mr MM was willing to take oral medication and his care coordinator felt that he was able to switch at this time.

As EPSEs and sexual dysfunction are causing Mr MM the most problems, we would be looking for an atypical antipsychotic with low propensity to cause EPSEs and sexual dysfunction. Olanzapine, quetiapine or aripiprazole may be

options. Aripiprazole is a dopamine receptor partial agonist that rarely causes movement disorders, very rarely causes sexual dysfunction and has low propensity to cause sedation. As Mr MM has mentioned that he has been experiencing tiredness, and both olanzapine and quetiapine are known to cause drowsiness, aripiprazole may be the drug to try first.

First, procyclidine tablets should be stopped because they are not helping with the shaking and may be causing his blurred vision. Then change the antipsychotic medication to aripiprazole starting at a dose of 15 mg once a day. The pipotiazine depot should be stopped once Mr MM has been taking aripiprazole for 3–4 weeks. The patient's mental state, EPSEs, sedation and blurred vision should all be monitored.

As Mr MM had been on a depot antipsychotic, it may take 8 weeks for his prolactin levels to return to normal, but several months for sexual dysfunction to resolve. If this has not improved after a period of 6 months, further investigations such as measurement of blood prolactin levels may be needed. Sexual dysfunction may not always be caused by psychotropic medication and further investigation at a sexual dysfunction clinic may be useful.

— **Medication, stigma and schizophrenia**

People with schizophrenia can feel that others treat them differently because of their illness, i.e. experience 'stigma'. Also mental health legislation, which permits compulsory treatment for the benefit of patients, can amplify their feelings of stigma. The side effects of antipsychotic medication, such as those experienced by Mr MM in this case, can all contribute to the feeling of being different from the rest of society. It is vital that individuals are seen as people in their own right and are not defined by their diagnosis.

Healthcare professionals can help by ensuring that the efficacy of medication for managing symptoms is balanced with the experience of unwanted effects. Careful and considerate language should be used so as not to label individuals with a diagnosis. Families of people with mental health problems can have an essential role in supporting their relative in treatment and care. However, the stigma of mental illness can also be an enormous burden for the family. The separate needs of carers should be acknowledged and addressed.

It has also been reported that people with mental health problems do not feel that their physical health is monitored as closely as their mental health issues. Healthcare professionals need to ensure that physical health problems have equal priority to mental health issues because people with schizophrenia are at an increased risk of developing cardiovascular disease compared with the general population.

EXTENDED LEARNING

- Identify past and current hypotheses regarding the causes of schizophrenia
- Describe the different classes, pharmacology and side effects of antipsychotic drugs
- Provide examples to demonstrate the relevance and application of lipid solubility, partitioning and the partition coefficient in development of pharmaceutical products
- What are the principal considerations for the formulation and administration of parenteral dosage forms?

- How are non-aqueous injections sterilised?
- What are the sources of stigma? How might they impact on the uptake of care and use of medicines?

ADDITIONAL PRACTICE POINTS

- What is meant by 'compulsory treatment'? Understand the role of mental health legislation in the treatment of people with mental health problems
- Why are people with schizophrenia at increased risk of cardiovascular disease compared with the general population?

References and further reading

American Psychiatric Association (2000). *Diagnostic and Statistical Manual of Mental Disorders*, 4th edn, text revision (DSM-IV-TR). Washington DC: American Psychiatric Association.

Leucht S, Tardy M, Komossa K, Heres S, Kissling W, Davis JM (2012). Maintenance treatment with antipsychotic drugs for schizophrenia. *Cochrane Database Syst Rev* 5:CD008016.

Lowe R (2013). Parenteral drug delivery. In: Aulton ME, Taylor KMG (eds), *Aulton's Pharmaceutics: The design and manufacture of medicines*, 4th edn. London: Elsevier, 623–37.

National Collaborating Centre for Mental Health (2010). *Schizophrenia: Core interventions in the treatment and management of schizophrenia in adults in primary and secondary care.* National Clinical Guideline Number 82. London: British Psychological Society and Royal College of Psychiatrists.

Stahl S (2008). *Illustrated Antipsychotics*. Cambridge: Cambridge University Press,

Taylor D (2006). *Schizophrenia in Focus*. London: Pharmaceutical Press.

Case 3
Bipolar disorder and its treatment

PETER WHITTON

LEARNING OUTCOMES

At the end of this case, you will be able to:

- Describe the pathophysiology and symptoms of bipolar disorder
- Outline some of the therapies that are used in the treatment of bipolar disorder
- Describe the side effects of treatments for bipolar disorder
- Demonstrate an understanding of the health professionals involved in caring for people with complex mental health problems in the community

Case study

Mr IN is a 23-year-old student living at home with his parents. They notice that recently he has shown strange changes in his mood. At times, he is withdrawn and will not leave his room unless essential. Mr IN seems very unhappy about his college work although his grades are actually good. Recently, however, he seemed elated and very confident. During this period, he went shopping and spent a large amount of money on expensive clothes using a credit card. In a relatively lucid period, Mr IN reluctantly agrees to a medical assessment.

- Assuming that you are responsible for making the assessment, what is your diagnosis?
- Is Mr IN's behaviour characteristic of this disorder?
- What are believed to be the main causes of this condition?

After a consultation, it is decided that Mr IN should be prescribed either lithium or sodium valproate.

- What are the relative merits of these two treatments, considering their efficacy and side-effect profile?

When given lithium (as lithium carbonate), patients should routinely have their plasma level of the drug checked.

- Why are plasma levels checked specifically for lithium?

- What is a 'safe' therapeutic concentration range for lithium in the plasma?
- What methods are likely to be used to estimate serum/plasma lithium levels?

Case discussion

— Bipolar disorder and its pathophysiology

Bipolar disorder is characterised by the apparent coexistence of two disorders: depression, in which the patient is typically withdrawn, has feelings of low self-worth and usually anhedonia (inability to gain pleasure from experiences that should be enjoyable); these periods may be interspersed with periods of 'mania'. During these, the patient may be outrageously over self-confident and talk of plans that are grandiose and often quite unrealistic. An objective view of practical issues often disappears, which may manifest as spending sprees for items that are either not needed or beyond the person's means. Families are frequently highly stressed by these phases and find themselves having, if possible, to return unwanted purchased items, etc. The pathophysiology of bipolar illness is still unclear, but almost certainly involves an imbalance in function of the dopaminergic and serotoninergic systems in the CNS. There is strong evidence that there is frequently a genetic cause to bipolar disorder.

— Treatment options for bipolar disorder

Medications used to treat bipolar disorder are known as mood stabilisers; these work by reversing manic or depressive episodes and preventing relapses. The 'gold standard' mood stabiliser is lithium, which is effective in treating acute manic episodes, and preventing relapses, more so for manic than for depressive episodes.

The anticonvulsant sodium valproate has become a commonly prescribed treatment, and is particularly effective in treating manic episodes. Other anticonvulsants that may be used to treat bipolar disorder include: carbamazepine and lamotrigine. Carbamazepine was widely used in the late 1980s and early 1990s, but was displaced by sodium valproate in the 1990s. Lamotrigine has been shown to have some efficacy in treating

sodium valproate

lamotrigine

carbamazepine

olanzapine

bipolar depression, and this benefit is greatest in more severe depression. It has also been shown to have some benefit in preventing further episodes.

Atypical antipsychotics have been found to be effective in managing mania associated with bipolar disorder. Olanzapine is effective in preventing relapses, although the evidence is not as good as for lithium. Antidepressants have not been found to be of any greater benefit than mood stabilisers.

— Lithium toxicity and measurement of plasma levels

Although an effective treatment of bipolar disorder, lithium can be quite toxic and its serum levels should be monitored, especially at the start of treatment or in particularly vulnerable patient groups. Lithium toxicity can be acute or chronic but can be the result of an apparently small increase in lithium dose. Symptoms are extensive, depending on the degree of toxicity, but range from stomach discomfort through to coma and death. In the case of lithium toxicity, the protocol is to stop lithium therapy and refer the person urgently to secondary care. There is no specific antidote to lithium poisoning. Referral to secondary care is recommended because the person will require supportive treatment. This may include measuring their lithium levels every 6–12 hours, and administering large amounts of sodium salts and fluids; depending on the severity, dialysis may be required.

— Community mental health teams

In the UK, specialist mental health services exist where mental health professionals work in teams of people with different expert professional knowledge and skills. They provide day-to-day support to people with complex mental health problems to help them to live in the community. They may support those people who have problems maintaining regular support with services, those who experience frequent relapses or have poor symptom control, or those with additional problems such as self-neglect or chronic alcohol and/or drug misuse. The professionals represented in each team may include a consultant psychiatrist, community psychiatric nurse, social worker, occupational therapist and clinical psychologist, as well as many other additional support workers. Composition of teams and the way in which they work may vary widely in different areas. Community mental health teams (CMHTs) work closely with GPs in managing the care of patients in the community. Pharmacists also have a key role in linking with CMHTs to provide expert advice to team members, and being available to patients with mental health problems, and their carers, to discuss their drug treatment.

EXTENDED LEARNING

- What are the most recent ideas concerning the possible mechanisms of action of lithium in bipolar disorder?
- What is the role of neuroinflammation in the pathophysiology of the disease?
- What risks are associated with long-term treatment using lithium?
- What is the role of benzodiazepines in the treatment of bipolar disorder?
- How is mania treated in women of childbearing age?

ADDITIONAL PRACTICE POINT

- What does a lithium treatment pack contain?

References and further reading

Dawda Y (2009). Bipolar affective disorder: long-term management. *Clin Pharmacist* 1:73–9.

Malhi GS, Tanious M, Das P, Coulston CM, Berk M (2013). Potential mechanisms of action of lithium in bipolar disorder. Current understanding. *CNS Drugs* **27**:135–53.

Malone D, Marriott S, Newton-Howes G, Simmonds S, Tyrer P (2007) Community mental health teams (CMHTs) for people with severe mental illnesses and disordered personality. *Cochrane Database Syst Rev* **3**: CD000270.

National Institute for Health and Clinical Excellence (2006). *Bipolar Disorder.* Clinical Guideline 38. London: NICE. Available at: www.nice.org.uk/CG38 (accessed 12 July 2013).

Parker C (2009). Bipolar affective disorder: treatment of acute relapses. *Clin Pharmacist* **1**:80–2.

Sie M (2009). Bipolar affective disorder: symptoms and diagnosis. *Clin Pharmacist* **1**:67–72.

Case 4

Treatment-resistant depression in a patient on haemodialysis

MATTHEW JONES AND SARAH JONES

LEARNING OUTCOMES

At the end of this case, you will be able to:

- Define treatment-resistant depression and outline the available treatment options
- Outline the chemistry and mechanism of action of lithium
- Outline how lithium therapy can be initiated and monitored for this indication
- Describe how haemodialysis affects the pharmacokinetics and dosing of drugs
- Outline how the different salts of a drug can have different pharmacokinetics and dosing requirements

Case study

Mrs VW is 73 years old with polycystic kidney disease, resulting in a gradual decline of her renal function to stage 3 chronic kidney disease. She has a long history of treatment-resistant depression, which initially failed to respond to fluoxetine and then mirtazapine, but has responded well to lithium for many years.

❓ How is treatment-resistant depression defined?

❓ What baseline and ongoing monitoring is recommended for a patient starting lithium who does not have any underlying physical health problems?

❓ Why does lithium require intensive monitoring?

Mrs VW develops urosepsis (spread of urinary tract infection to the bloodstream), resulting in a permanent decline in her renal function. She is diagnosed with end-stage renal failure and requires

haemodialysis. On the advice of her renal physician, her lithium is stopped.

❓ What other treatment options are available for treatment-resistant depression?

Six months later, Mrs VW has failed to respond to alternative treatments for her depression and has been admitted to the psychiatric ward with low mood, anhedonia (inability to experience pleasure from normal activities) and pathological guilt. She is stabilised on three times weekly haemodialysis with very low residual renal function. Her psychiatrist would like to prescribe lithium again and asks for advice on how this drug should be prescribed for Mrs VW.

❓ How does haemodialysis remove accumulated toxins, electrolytes and fluid?

❓ What characteristics of a drug affect its removal during haemodialysis?

❓ Why do the doses of some drugs need to be modified in patients on haemodialysis, whereas standard doses of other drugs can be used?

During your research, you find the following pharmacokinetic characteristics of lithium:

- *Excreted unchanged in urine: >95%*
- *Plasma protein binding: none*
- *Volume of distribution: small (0.5–0.9 L/kg)*
- *Molecular weight: 7 Da (of active ion)*
- *Removed by haemodialysis.*

❓ Based on these characteristics, what would you suggest Mrs VW's initial lithium dose and frequency should be?

❓ When should plasma lithium levels be checked?

Three months later, Mrs VW has responded well to modified-release lithium carbonate tablets. These tablets must be swallowed whole, which she finds difficult, so her psychiatrist changes her prescription to lithium citrate 520 mg/5 mL liquid.

❓ Why must modified-release lithium carbonate tablets be swallowed whole?

❓ What volume of lithium citrate liquid is equivalent to 400 mg lithium carbonate?

❓ How and why do you expect the pharmacokinetics of lithium to differ when formulated as a modified-release tablet or a liquid?

❓ Why can different salts of the same drug affect dosing and pharmacokinetics?

Case discussion

Lithium metal is the third element in the periodic table. The most common isotope of lithium (atomic mass number, $A = 7$) contains three protons (atomic number, $Z = 3$) and four neutrons, giving a relative atomic mass of approximately 7 (g/mol or Da). Neutral lithium atoms have three electrons, but lithium readily donates a single electron to gain a stable, closed-shell configuration in the lithium ion, Li^+, which is the biologically active drug used mainly in the management of bipolar disorder (manic–depressive illness) and other mood disorders, administered orally in the form of the carbonate or citrate salts in controlled-release tablets, capsules or liquids. All salts of lithium are ionic compounds, which dissociate in water to give the Li^+ cation and the appropriate anion, which is dependent on the type of salt used. The Li^+ cation is surrounded (solvated) by water molecules in aqueous solution, and most lithium salts are freely soluble in water.

— Lithium initiation and monitoring in patients starting lithium with normal renal function

The main indications for lithium are acute mania, recurrent depressive disorders (where treatment with other antidepressants has been unsuccessful) and prophylaxis in bipolar affective disorder.

Lithium has a narrow therapeutic window, significant drug interactions, multiple serious side effects and the risk of a severe rebound illness if stopped suddenly. It therefore necessitates careful monitoring.

Before initiating lithium, a baseline physical health screen must be completed. In particular, the prescriber must check renal function, thyroid function and weight. Lithium is most commonly prescribed as a modified-release preparation of the carbonate salt. In a healthy adult, the initiation dose would usually be 400 mg at night.

Drug levels need intensive monitoring while the correct dose is established. The target plasma level depends to some extent on the indication but would usually be between 0.4 and 0.8 mmol/L (12 hours post-dose). Blood tests should be undertaken 1 week after initiation and then 5–7 days after each dose adjustment until a stable and appropriate level has been reached. Once stabilised, patients should have a routine blood level checked every 3 months. Urea and electrolytes (U&Es) blood test and thyroid function tests should be done every 6 months and an overall health check annually.

— Treatment-resistant depression

Despite being a term in wide use, there are no absolute diagnostic criteria for 'treatment-resistant depression' (TRD). However, a widely used definition in the literature is the failure of at least two antidepressants at adequate dose and duration from two distinct pharmacological classes. Estimates of the prevalence of TRD vary widely. STAR*D (a large trial investigating sequential treatments for depression) concluded that up to a third of patients fail to achieve full remission even with repeated pharmacological treatments.

— Treatment options available for treatment-resistant depression

The evidence base to guide the choice of medication after the failure of initial antidepressant therapy is not conclusive and decisions rely extensively on the skill of the prescriber. Despite different treatment comparisons in STAR*D, few significant differences were found.

Antidepressant combinations were once seen as risky due to fear of *serotonin syndrome*, but have become a mainstay in treating TRD. This approach requires agents with complementary pharmacology to be selected. An example is the use of the centrally acting α_2-adrenoreceptor antagonist, mirtazapine, with a serotonin and noradrenaline reuptake inhibitor such as venlafaxine (*enhanced α_2-central adrenoreceptor activity has been suggested as one possible contributing cause of depression*). Some combinations (notably with monoamine oxidase inhibitors) remain higher-risk options and are rarely used. Other strategies with some evidence include: augmentation of an antidepressant with lithium or thyroid hormones, certain atypical antipsychotics (commonly quetiapine, olanzapine or aripiprazole) or mood stabilisers (lamotrigine in particular).

— Mechanism of action of lithium
Despite the fact that lithium salts have been used for more than two decades to treat depressive episodes in bipolar disorders, and to reduce patients' suicidal tendencies, the precise mechanism by which lithium achieves these effects is still controversial and not entirely understood. Extensive experimental evidence showing lithium affecting multiple neurotransmitter systems in the brain (glutamate [NMDAR], dopamine, GABA) has been obtained; however, more recently, it has been suggested that lithium may also exert important central neurotrophic and neuroprotective effects, through induction of brain-derived neurotrophic factor (BDNF) signalling and specific inhibition of glycogen synthase kinase-3 (GSK-3) activity. In addition, it may also reduce cellular inositol metabolism/ signalling (via inhibition of phosphoinositol phosphatases) known to be enhanced in mania and depression.

— Haemodialysis and the dosing of drugs
During haemodialysis, blood is separated from a dialysis fluid (a solution of electrolytes) by a semi-permeable membrane that has sieve-like properties: it allows small molecules (such as water, electrolytes and urea) to pass through, but retains larger structures, such as albumin and erythrocytes. Small molecules can therefore pass through the membrane by diffusion and water by ultrafiltration. Toxins, electrolytes and excess fluid therefore move from the blood into the dialysis fluid, with other electrolytes passing in the opposite direction.

Many drugs are small molecules and can also be removed by haemodialysis. Low molecular weight, low plasma protein binding, a small volume of distribution and high water solubility encourage removal during dialysis. Some drugs are extensively removed, whereas others are not dialysed at all. In addition, if a drug is mainly eliminated by a non-renal mechanism, it will continue to be removed during renal failure. Some drugs therefore require no dosage adjustment in a patient on haemodialysis, whereas others can require significant dose alteration.

— Lithium initiation and monitoring in patients on haemodialysis
Lithium is essentially eliminated only via the kidneys, so, once renal function has been compromised, its excretion is reduced. In someone entirely reliant on haemodialysis, therefore, lithium will be removed only during a dialysis session. The removal of lithium can be predicted from its low molecular weight, limited protein binding and small volume of distribution, all of which suggest a highly dialysable drug. This simple pharmacokinetic picture suggests that, to maintain stable plasma levels, a dose of lithium needs to be given only after each dialysis session.

Plasma level monitoring needs to determine if a therapeutic concentration is being reached and maintained, and to rule out the possibility of a toxic peak level. While establishing a dosing regimen, therefore, plasma levels should be taken pre-dialysis, immediately post-dialysis and at the predicted plasma peak (in the case of modified-release lithium carbonate: 3–4 hours post-dose).

— Lithium dose and frequency: consideration in this case?
In this case, it was decided to start with 200 mg post-dialysis but this gave a subtherapeutic pre-dialysis level (0.2 mmol/L). The dose was increased to 400 mg post-dialysis, which gave appropriate therapeutic levels pre-dialysis, a level within the therapeutic range at peak, and negligible levels immediately post-dialysis (suggesting a low risk of accumulation).

— Clinical significance of changes in oral formulation or drug salt form
There are numerous technologies designed to control the release of a drug from a tablet. Such systems typically involve coating the tablets in a polymer (such as an enteric coating) or embedding the drug in a tablet core made from a polymer with a controlled dissolution rate. Cutting or crushing such tablets can destroy their modified-release characteristics, which may result in adverse effects or loss of efficacy.

The first stages in the absorption of a drug from a tablet are the disintegration of the tablet and dissolution of the drug. These can often be the rate-limiting steps in drug absorption. An aqueous solution of a highly soluble drug (such as lithium) avoids these stages and delivers the drug in an easily absorbable form. In general, therefore, faster absorption with higher peak plasma levels can be expected. However, a modified-release formulation can give more consistent plasma levels, which often has therapeutic advantages.

Drugs can be formulated as different salts for a variety of reasons, e.g. stability, solubility and to circumvent patents. Different salts of a drug may have different solubilities, which can thus affect absorption from tablets or capsules. In practice, this tends not to have clinical significance: licensed formulations must demonstrate bioequivalence, i.e. are equivalent in terms of the rate and extent of absorption.

As different counterions (i.e. the carbonate in lithium carbonate) have different molecular masses (M_r) and can have different stoichiometric relationships with the drug, it is important to bear the salt form in mind when calculating certain doses. In the case of lithium, 200 mg lithium carbonate (Li_2CO_3, $M_r = 73.9$) contains approximately 5.4 mmol lithium:

$$Li_2CO_3 \rightarrow 2Li^+ + CO_3^{2-}$$

No. of moles of $Li_2CO_3 = \dfrac{200}{73.9} = 2.71$ mmol

One mole of Li_2CO_3 dissociates to give 2 moles of Li^+ so:

No. of moles of $Li^+ = 2 \times 2.71 = 5.41$ mmol

To provide the same amount of drug, a much greater amount (509 mg) of lithium citrate (as the tetrahydrate; $Li_3C_6H_5O_7 \cdot 4H_2O$, $M_r = 282.0$) is required:

$$Li_3C_6H_5O_7 \cdot 4H_2O \rightarrow 3Li^+ + C_6H_5O_7^{3-} + 4H_2O$$

One mole of $Li_3C_6H_5O_7 \cdot 4H_2O$ dissociates to give 3 moles of Li^+ so, for 5.41 mmol Li^+:

$\dfrac{5.41}{3} = 1.80$ mmol $Li_3C_6H_5O_7 \cdot 4H_2O$ is required

The mass of $Li_3C_6H_5O_7 \cdot 4H_2O$ required is:

$1.80 \times 282.0 = 509$ mg

This dose conversion is a frequent source of error. Other drugs in which the salt form can affect dosing include phenytoin and iron.

EXTENDED LEARNING

- What are the differences between bipolar and unipolar depression? How is this relevant to a diagnosis of TRD?

- How would lithium dosing be different if the patient was on continuous renal replacement therapy in an intensive care unit, on peritoneal dialysis?

- What are the most significant drug interactions with lithium? How might a patient be managed if he or she was stable on lithium, and then prescribed an interacting drug?

- What are the risks for a patient if lithium plasma levels are outside the normal therapeutic window, and how should this situation be managed?

- Why are frequent thyroid function tests advisable while on lithium therapy?

- What are the differences between absolute bioavailability, relative bioavailability and bioequivalence?

References and further reading

Anderson IM, IN Ferrier, RC Baldwin et al.; on behalf of the Consensus Meeting; endorsed by the British Association for Psychopharmacology (2008). Evidence-based guidelines for treating depressive disorders with antidepressants. *J Psychopharmacol* 22:343–96.

Ashley C, Morlidge M, eds (2008). *Introduction to Renal Therapeutics*. London: Pharmaceutical Press.

Chiu CT, Chuang DM (2011). Neuroprotective action of lithium in disorders of the central nervous system. *Zhong Nan Da Xue Xue Bao Yi Xue Ban* 36:461–76.

McConnell EL, Basit AW (2013). Modified-release oral drug delivery. In: Aulton ME, Taylor KMG (eds), *Aulton's Pharmaceutics: The design and manufacture of medicines*, 4th edn, London: Elsevier, 550–65.

Malhi GS, Tanious M, Das P, Berk M (2012). The science and practice of lithium therapy. *Aust N Z J Psychiatry* 46: 192–211.

Muguruza C, Rodríguez F, Rozas I, Meana JJ, Urigüen L, Callado LF (2013). Antidepressant-like properties of three new α_2-adrenoceptor antagonists. *Neuropharmacology* 65:13–19.

National Institute of Mental Health (2008). *Frequently Asked Questions about the STAR*D Study*. Available at: http://psychcentral.com/lib/2008/frequently-asked-questions-about-the-stard-study (accessed 27 June 2014).

National Patient Safety Agency (2009). *Safer Lithium Therapy Alert*. Available at: www.nrls.npsa.nhs.uk (accessed 27 June 2014).

Case 5

Self-medication of depression with St John's wort, a herbal remedy

ELIZABETH M WILLIAMSON

LEARNING OUTCOMES

At the end of this case, you will be able to:

- Describe the evidence base for the use of St John's wort
- Outline its proposed mechanisms of action and the main components thought to be responsible for its antidepressant activity
- Explain which drugs St John's wort may interact with, and the mechanisms involved
- Comment on the rising prevalence of depressive illness internationally and the anticipated impact for population health.

Case study

Ms DD is a 27-year-old woman who has occasional episodes of mild-to-moderate depression. She has had depression before and was previously prescribed citalopram, but she would prefer to try to manage this herself because she feels that her condition is not too severe and the side effects of the selective serotonin reuptake inhibitor (SSRI) were very uncomfortable. She has read in the press that the herbal remedy St John's wort is suitable for treating mild depression and wishes to discuss with you, a community pharmacist, whether it would be right for her. The BNF *does not currently recommend this medicine but it is extremely popular.*

- ❓ What is St John's wort? Is there any evidence that it is effective against depression?
- ❓ Is it 'safe' for self-medication?
- ❓ What are the main active constituent(s) thought to be responsible for its antidepressant effect and how are they believed to work?

Ms DD mentions in passing that she is prescribed several other medicines that she takes routinely.

- ❓ Is it important to find out what other medicines Ms DD is taking?
- ❓ Why does St John's wort have such a wide drug interaction profile?

Ms DD has a salbutamol and a beclometasone inhaler each month and is on the combined contraceptive pill, Loestrin 20.

- ❓ Can she take St John's wort at the same time as these medicines? What would you advise?

It has been recommended that either St John's wort be avoided in patients taking the contraceptive pill or only preparations with low levels of hyperforin be used.

- ❓ Is the latter suggestion clinically appropriate advice?
- ❓ If not, why not?
- ❓ Why is it important to choose a specific type of St John's wort product?
- ❓ What would you suggest is the best course of action for Ms DD?

Case discussion

— Evidence for efficacy and safety of St John's wort, and the way it is used

St John's wort is a herbal medicine derived from the leaves and flowering tops of the plant *Hypericum perforatum* and is very widely used as an antidepressant, usually by self-medication. There is a substantial body of clinical evidence to show that it can be effective in mild-to-moderate depression (and also some forms of anxiety), although various clinical trials have given conflicting results. This may be partly because there are many different preparations available, of varying composition, and which are thus not equivalent. Extracts of the herb have been shown in animal and *in vitro* studies to inhibit the central neuronal reuptake of serotonin (5HT), noradrenaline and dopamine, and the release of glutamate, which are known characteristics of conventional antidepressant drugs.

One perceived advantage of taking St John's wort, *from the patient's point of view*, is that it can be bought over the counter (OTC) without a prescription, and thus avoids any mention on the patient's medical record. Depression is still perceived as carrying a stigma and many people will avoid going to the doctor if they think that they can treat the condition themselves. However,

hypericin (R = CH₃)
pseudohypericin (R = CH₂OH)

hyperforin (R = CH₃)
adhyperforin (R = CH₂CH₃)

self-diagnosis and self-medication carry their own risks, including the possibility of drug interactions. Patients tend to view 'natural' medicines as safe, which they often are, but this is mainly due to the fact that they have been in use for many years rather than because they are natural! For this reason, they may omit to inform the prescriber and it is important for pharmacists to ask about herbal medicines when counselling patients. St John's wort has a good safety profile, apart from drug interactions, and is suitable for self-medication by those with clinically diagnosed mild-to-moderate depression and who are not on other medication. It may produce GI disturbances, and there is a theoretical risk of photosensitivity (which is rarely reported).

— **Main active constituents of St John's wort**
There are two main classes of active constituents: the naphthodianthrone derivatives, hypericin and pseudohypericin and their derivatives, and the phloroglucinols, hyperforin and adhyperforin and their derivatives, which are thought to contribute to the antidepressant effect. However, hyperforin is now considered to be highly active and it is important that the product chosen is standardised as to its hyperforin as well as its hypericin content. Other components of the extract may have activity themselves, or enhance the bioavailability of the known active components.

— **Drug interactions of St John's wort**
St John's wort is probably the herbal medicine that has the most drug interaction reports of all, and many of these are significant and important, e.g. with immunosuppressants, antiretrovirals, anticonvulsants, cardiovascular drugs and *the contraceptive pill*. So it is most important to check whether the patient is taking any other medication, including OTC remedies. As St John's wort is taken for its antidepressant properties, the conditions mentioned above are particularly likely to be those for which patients choose to take it.

Its wide interaction profile, detailed in the *BNF*, is due to the fact that it can not only induce cytochrome P450 (CYP) enzymes (CYP3A4, -2C19 and -2C9 in particular), thus reducing the blood levels of any drugs metabolised via these pathways, but also increase P-glycoprotein expression, thereby reducing bioavailability.

CYPs comprise a large number of distinct but related haem proteins, which account for about 75% of all drug metabolism in the body. There are important variations in the expression and regulation of these between species as well as genetic variations between human populations and individuals, so animal and *in vitro* studies have given apparently conflicting results and require very careful extrapolation. However, there are enough reliable case reports and mechanistic studies to confirm that St John's wort-CYP interactions are clinically relevant. St John's wort induces the activity of several CYP isoenzymes including CYP3A4, CYP2E1 and CYP2C19. In this particular case, CYP3A4-mediated hydroxylation is the major pathway of oxidative metabolism of ethinylestradiol, a component of the combined oral contraceptive Loestrin 20, and, as such, this mechanism is likely to be the main cause of reduced blood levels. The other constituent of Loestrin 20 is norethisterone (norethindrone) acetate and it is known that its metabolism is also increased when taken together with St John's wort.

Hyperforin has been shown to be an inducer of CYP3A4 via activation of the pregnane X receptor (PXR). St John's wort extracts and isolated hyperforin induce the synthesis of P-glycoprotein

(P-gp) in the epithelial cells of the intestine (involved in the transport of a wide variety of substrate molecules across extra- and intracellular membranes), causing a *reduction* of drug absorption (if P-gp were *inhibited*, this would result in more drug being absorbed and an *increase* in plasma concentration). Hyperforin activation of PXR also leads to an upregulation of P-gp and increased transport activity. However, ethinylestradiol and its first-pass metabolites are not substrates for P-gp, so this mechanism is unlikely to be significant, in contrast to enzyme induction.

Preparations with low hyperforin content have been suggested as suitable for avoiding drug interactions, because hyperforin is such a potent inducer of CYP3A4. A recent study has shown that a preparation devoid of hyperforin did not affect the metabolism of the combined contraceptive pill. However, there is limited evidence for the efficacy of these products compared with that for extracts containing hyperforin. As a significant therapeutic constituent, it is risky to remove it from a herbal product and expect the clinical effect to be the same.

— Clinical issues raised by this case

The patient in this case would normally be an ideal candidate for St John's wort because she has already been diagnosed with mild-to-moderate depression. There is no problem with the fact that she is using the salbutamol and beclometasone inhalers, but she is taking the contraceptive pill so it would first be necessary to find out if she is prepared to use a different method of contraception, or whether she would prefer to go back to the doctor for a different antidepressant on prescription. The side-effect profile of St John's wort is potentially not a problem for her, because it is favourable compared with that of many other antidepressants, with the exception of the potential drug interactions. The possibility of using a product with a low hyperforin content could be considered, but these products are less readily available and their efficacy not widely demonstrated.

— Appropriate course of action in this case

Although the *BNF* currently advises against the use of St John's wort, it remains very widely taken. Patients are entitled to their opinions and in many cases they have had positive personal experience,

so there is an ethical element here. Most pharmacists would try to assess the severity of the condition to decide whether patients should be referred to their GP, and any other issues related to their suitability for self-medication, such as drug interactions. If deemed safe, a THR (Traditional Herbal Registration) product, preferably standardised to both hypericin and hyperforin content, could be recommended for a trial period of 3 months. After that, a decision could be taken as to whether to continue, or perhaps refer to the GP. The dose recommended by the manufacturer for that product should be followed.

— Rising prevalence and impact of depressive illness

Many chronic diseases, including mental health problems, result in significant disability, but as they are not usually a cause of death they do not feature in mortality statistics, which are commonly used to measure and compare health and disease in populations. The WHO projects that, by the year 2030, unipolar depressive disorders will be the leading cause of global disease burden.

To compare the impact (disease burden) of different conditions, the WHO uses a measure called a DALY (disability-adjusted life-year): 1

▼ TABLE 4.1

The *projected* leading causes of burden of disease worldwide, for the year 2030, as measured by disability-adjusted life-years (DALYs) (WHO, 2008)

Disease or injury	Rank	Percentage total DALYs
Unipolar depressive disorders	1	6.2
Ischaemic heart disease	2	5.5
Road traffic accidents	3	4.9
Cerebrovascular disease	4	4.3
COPD	5	3.8
Lower respiratory tract infections	6	3.2
Hearing loss, adult onset	7	2.9
Refractive errors	8	2.7
HIV/AIDS	9	2.5
Diabetes mellitus	10	2.3

COPD, chronic obstructive pulmonary disease.

DALY represents the loss of the equivalent of 1 year of full health; it may also represent 2 years at 50% of full health. This measure provides an indication of the total burden of any disease in a population. Thus, use of DALYs enables comparisons in a population between the impact of diseases that result in early death but little disability, with those that do not cause death but result in disability (Table 4.1).

EXTENDED LEARNING

- How do herbal medicines work? Note that they contain multiple components acting on multiple therapeutic targets, leading to complicated drug interaction mechanisms
- How are herbal medicines formulated and manufactured?
- How are herbal medicines standardised and what is the purpose of standardisation?
- Consider THR as an indicator of quality and safety under the Traditional Herbal Medicinal Product Directive (THMPD). What is the THR certification mark?

- What is the difference between a herbal medicine and a homeopathic medicine?

References and further reading

British National Formulary (current edition). See www.bnf.org for latest edition and recommendations.

Pharmaceutical Press Editorial (2013). *Herbal Medicines*, 4th edn. London: Pharmaceutical Press.

Russo E, Scicchitano F, Whalley BJ et al. (2013). *Hypericum perforatum*: Pharmacokinetic, mechanism of action, tolerability, and clinical drug–drug interactions. *Phytother Res* 28:643–55.

Williamson EM, Driver S, Baxter K, eds (2013). *Stockley's Herbal Medicines Interactions. A guide to the interactions of herbal medicines*. 2nd edn. London: Pharmaceutical Press.

World Health Organization (2008). *World Health Statistics*. Geneva: WHO, 30.

— Useful documents from the MHRA website

The THR scheme: www.mhra.gov.uk/Safetyinformation/ Generalsafetyinformationandadvice/Herbalmedicines/ TheTHRscheme/index.htm

Example THR documents for registration of a St John's wort product: www.mhra.gov.uk/home/groups/par/documents/ websiteresources/con057375.pdf

Case 6
Extemporaneous preparation of methadone

JENNY SCOTT

LEARNING OUTCOMES

At the end of this case, you will be able to:

- Identify formulation and preparation problems that can occur when a powder is added to a liquid and how these might impact on the plasma level of a drug
- Describe best practice when preparing extemporaneous methadone
- Distinguish between solubility and dissolution rate
- Outline the details that need to be recorded for each batch of extemporaneous methadone mixture prepared, and the information with which the pharmacist should label the stock bottle of prepared extemporaneous methadone mixture

Case study

Mrs RT is a pharmacist prescriber. She works in a drug treatment centre. Today she saw one of her long-term patients, Mr FG. He has been stable on methadone at a dose of 90 mg (90 mL of 1 mg/mL liquid), supervised consumption, for a couple of months now, and does not use illicit drugs in addition to this prescription. Mr FG complained that he has been experiencing some withdrawal symptoms over the past week or so. 'It is like somebody has dropped my dose' he said. Mrs RT could see Mr FG was exhibiting some mild withdrawal symptoms. She confirmed that he was not being prescribed any other medicines by his GP, ruling out the possibility of a drug–metabolism interaction. Mrs RT checked her prescribing records to confirm that no error in prescribing had been made, which it had not. She then rang the community pharmacy where Mr FG collects his methadone to confirm that he had been consuming the full measured dose (90 mL) daily, which he had. When Mrs RT spoke with the pharmacist she asked him to confirm which brand of methadone he supplied against her generically written prescriptions. The pharmacist's response was: 'I've started making up my own … I've taken on more patients, so now there is not enough room in my CD safe to store all the methadone I need for a week, so I buy in the diluent and the powder and mix it up in the shop as I need it.' Mrs RT asked when the pharmacist had begun doing so and he confirmed 2 weeks ago.

- Suggest some reasons as to why Mr FG is experiencing withdrawal symptoms.
- How should the pharmacist prepare extemporaneous methadone mixture to avoid these possible problems?
- What should be recorded for each batch of extemporaneous methadone mixture prepared, and how long should this record be kept?
- With which details should the pharmacist label the stock bottle of prepared extemporaneous methadone mixture?
- Extemporaneous methadone mixture is an unlicensed product. Who should the pharmacist inform before supplying extemporaneous methadone mixture?

Case discussion

The case indicates that Mr FG has been receiving extemporaneously prepared methadone for the past 2 weeks. Methadone has a long half-life (24–36 hours typically), so a patient stable on methadone would normally have a lag time of 5–7 days before feeling the full effects of a dose reduction. This concurs with Mr FG's report. His symptoms suggest that he has been receiving inadequate doses of methadone in his 90 mL volume of liquid consumed. The problem may be with the addition of powder to the diluent.

— Practical aspects of extemporaneously preparing methadone mixture

The Royal Pharmaceutical Society (RPS) guidance (MEP 36) states that pharmacists should weigh dry ingredients using class 2 balances and measure liquids in measures that comply with BS 1922, to confirm that the two ingredients will produce a solution of strength 1 mg/mL. If this pharmacist is not doing so and is simply tipping the powder from the container into the diluent then he may not notice if some powder remains in the

container. This could happen, possibly due to adherence of the powder to the side of the container, or clumping if stored inappropriately, e.g. in an environment when moisture can get into the container. Alternatively, the problem may be due to inadequate dissolution and mixing. The pharmacist should stir the liquid thoroughly as the powder is added, to ensure that it all dissolved and no clumping resulted; it should be evenly dissolved in the diluent to provide a consistent solution, with no visible 'lumps'.

The 'methadone powder' for reconstitution in a suitable vehicle (an aqueous syrup) is actually methadone hydrochloride. Methadone, a synthetic opiate receptor agonist now most commonly used for treating opiate addiction, contains a basic tertiary amino group with an available lone pair of electrons. In the presence of hydrochloric acid, the nitrogen atom becomes protonated and positively charged, giving the hydrochloride salt. The formation of this ionic salt greatly increases polarity (compared with the low-polarity methadone free base), allowing greater solubility in water as strong non-covalent interactions are made between the electron-deficient cation and the electron-rich oxygen atoms in the water molecules. The methadone cation becomes surrounded by a 'shell' of water molecules, significantly enhancing water solubility.

methadone hydrochloride

Note that there is a difference between solubility and dissolution rate. In this instance, the methadone (solute) is soluble in the vehicle (solvent), but sufficient attention must be paid to getting the drug into solution. This depends on the dissolution rate. The rate of dissolution of a solid is given by the Noyes–Whitney equation, which is useful for predicting dissolution rates of materials, based on the mass transfer of solute from the surface of particles through a concentrated stationary boundary layer at the solid liquid interface, into the bulk solution:

$$\frac{dm}{dt} = \frac{DA(C_s - C)}{h}$$

where $\frac{dm}{dt}$ is the rate of dissolution, A is the surface area of the drug particles, C_s is the saturated concentration of drug in the dissolution medium and C is the concentration of drug in the dissolution medium at time t, D is the diffusion coefficient and h the thickness of the diffusion layer.

Thus, the rate of dissolution can be increased by considering the parameters of the equation:

- Surface area (A): dissolution rate is increased by milling, ensuring well-dispersed solids (using a wetting agent if appropriate), increasing porosity of particles.
- Solubility of the drug (C_s): dissolution rate is increased by increasing temperature, use of surfactants, alteration of pH and use of a more soluble form of a drug, e.g. the amorphous form or a salt.
- Concentration at time t (C): dissolution rate is increased by increasing the volume of the dissolution medium.
- Diffusion rate constant (D): dissolution rate is increased with decreased solvent viscosity.
- Thickness of the diffusion layer (h): dissolution rate is increased by increased agitation, e.g. stirring or shaking.

Some of these factors are fixed in practice, but some can be modified, e.g. stirring rate and the volume of solvent used for initial dissolution, before making the solution up to its final volume.

— **Making and maintaining records of product preparation**

For each batch of extemporaneous methadone mixture prepared a record must be made of:

- The formula
- The ingredients and quantities used
- The source, batch number and expiry date of the ingredients
- The batch number and expiry date of the extemporaneously prepared mixture
- The people involved in preparing the product, including the identity of the pharmacist assuming overall responsibility.

This should be kept for a minimum of 2 years.

The product must be labelled with:

- The name of the product
- The strength of the product

- The quantity of medicinal product in the container
- Any special handling and storage requirements (e.g. store in safe custody)
- The batch expiry date
- A batch reference number.

The pharmacist should have informed both the prescriber and the patient before he supplied extemporaneous methadone mixture. However, extemporaneous methadone mixture is exempt from the practice requirement to always supply a licensed product where one exists in favour of an unlicensed product. This is because some pharmacies do not have the room to store enough 'made-up' methadone if they dispense a high volume of methadone daily. Therefore, the supply of extemporaneous methadone mixture is permitted if both the prescriber and the patient agree.

EXTENDED LEARNING

- What type of symptoms would you expect to see in a long-term opiate addict undergoing withdrawal? What may be the impact of these symptoms on the health of the individual?
- What are the factors that affect a drug's solubility and dissolution rate?
- What is intrinsic dissolution rate and how is it measured?
- How are solutions formulated and what are their properties?
- What are the physicochemical properties of different polymorphs and solvates of a drug?
- What is the legal provision for non-medical prescribing in the UK?

ADDITIONAL PRACTICE POINTS

- What is the Misuse of Drugs Act? What are the legal requirements for the prescribing of controlled drugs (both handwritten prescriptions and electronic discharge letters)?
- What do you understand by the term 'supervised consumption' of opioid substitution therapy?
- What advice would you give to those travelling abroad with controlled drugs?

References and further reading

Aulton ME (2013). Dissolution and solubility. In: Aulton ME, Taylor KMG (eds), *Aulton's Pharmaceutics: The design and manufacture of medicines*, 4th edn, Elsevier: London, 20–37.

Royal Pharmaceutical Society of Great Britain. (2014). *Dispensing and Preparing Extemporaneous Methadone Quick*

Reference Guide. Available at: www.rpharms.com/support-resources-a-z/dispensing-and-preparing-extemporaneous-methadone-quick-reference-guide.asp (accessed 7 April 2014).

Case 7
Neuropathic pain
ROGER KNAGGS

LEARNING OUTCOMES

At the end of this case, you will be able to:

- Describe the pathophysiology of inflammatory, neuropathic and functional pain
- Describe the presentation and assessment of neuropathic pain
- Outline treatment options for neuropathic pain
- Outline the chemistry and mechanism of action of antiepileptic drugs used in the management of neuropathic pain
- Outline the chemistry and mechanism of action of tramadol
- Discuss the role of opioids in the management of persistent pain

Case study

Mrs AP is a regular customer in your pharmacy. She has type 2 diabetes mellitus. Current medication from her patient medication record includes:

Metformin 1 g b.d.
Gliclazide 160 mg b.d.
Aspirin 75 mg o.d.
Simvastatin 40 mg o.n.

Mrs AP says that she takes her metformin and gliclazide regularly and has no problems with them. She is keen to be fit enough to work because she is supporting her youngest son who is studying to be a doctor. You notice that she has been buying paracetamol every 3 days for the last 6 weeks.

❓ Consider the different types of pain and explain the mechanisms that underlie these

She comes to the pharmacy counter to request a stronger painkiller. When questioned, she explains that, for some time, she has had constant tingling and occasional shooting pain in her legs and feet. Rather than recommending an OTC analgesic, you recommend to Mrs AP that she make an appointment to see her GP to discuss treatment options for her pain.

❓ What pharmacological treatment options are appropriate for the initial management of neuropathic pain?

❓ Outline non-pharmacological treatment options that you can give to Mrs AP

She is prescribed amitriptyline 10 mg at night. A month later Mrs AP returns with a prescription for gabapentin, saying that amitriptyline made her extremely tired and she struggled to arrive at work on time. Over the next few months Mrs AP gradually increases her gabapentin dose. On collecting a repeat prescription several months later she explains that the pain in her feet is worsening. She makes a further appointment to see her GP who prescribes tramadol 100 mg four times a day. He also recommends referral to a specialist pain management clinic.

❓ Describe the role of opioid analgesics in the treatment of persistent non-cancer pain

❓ Draw the structure of tramadol. How is its stereochemistry important in its mechanism(s) of action?

Case discussion

Types of pain and underlying causes

Pain is typically defined as 'an unpleasant sensory and emotional experience associated with actual or potential tissue damage, or described in terms of such damage'. There are three main types of pain:

inflammatory pain, neuropathic pain and functional pain.

— Inflammatory pain

Nociceptive (inflammatory) pain is pain that arises from actual or threatened damage to non-neural tissue and is due to the activation of nociceptors, often by the release of inflammatory mediators, such as prostaglandins, leukotriene B_4 and other cytokines, such as the interleukins and interferons.

— Neuropathic pain

Neuropathic pain may be defined as 'pain arising as a direct consequence of a disease or lesion affecting the somatosensory system' and may occur as a result of pathological damage to nerve fibres in a peripheral nerve or in the CNS. Neuropathic pain may be spontaneous in nature (continuous or paroxysmal) or evoked by sensory stimuli.

Unlike inflammatory pain, which is caused by actual tissue damage, neuropathic pain is the result of changes to the system that normally signals pain. Damage to peripheral nerves can lead to reduced threshold for firing, ectopic discharges and cross-talk with adjacent nerves. Subsequently, this may lead to hyperexcitability and loss of normal inhibitory control within the CNS.

— Functional pain

In functional pain syndromes, no neurological deficit or peripheral abnormality can be detected. Pain is caused by an abnormal responsiveness within the nervous system.

Common causes of nociceptive, neuropathic and functional pain are summarised in Table 4.2.

▼ TABLE 4.2
Common causes of nociceptive, neuropathic and functional pain

Nociceptive (inflammatory) pain	Neuropathic pain	Functional pain
Trauma or injury	Post-herpetic neuralgia	Tension headache
Post-surgical	Diabetic neuropathy	Irritable bowel syndrome
Inflammatory arthritis (such as rheumatoid arthritis)	Phantom limb pain	Fibromyalgia
	Spinal cord injury	

— Neuropathic pain: signs, symptoms and aetiology

In this case, the most likely cause of Mrs AP's pain is diabetic peripheral neuropathy. The underlying aetiology of neuropathic pain is different from inflammatory pain and, typically, patients present with disturbances in sensory function, often describing their pain as 'tingling, shooting or electric shocks'. It is possible for patients to experience pain with sensory loss (i.e. numbness). Unlike inflammatory pain, neuropathic pain serves no biological advantage and can be described as an illness in its own right.

Key components in the diagnosis of neuropathic pain are the identification of painful symptoms, altered sensation and a clinical history that all match a neuroanatomical or dermatomal distribution. There is no standard diagnostic procedure for neuropathic pain, so diagnosis is largely based on clinical judgement and experience. Screening questionnaire tools, such as painDETECT and the Leeds assessment of neuropathic pain symptoms and signs (LANSS) pain scale, are available to support diagnosis.

Pharmacological treatment options for neuropathic pain

Neuropathic pain can be particularly difficult to manage, because it often does not respond to conventional analgesics, such as paracetamol and non-steroidal anti-inflammatory drugs (NSAIDs). Hence other alternatives are required. The underlying cause, such as ensuring optimum diabetic control for Mrs AP, should be treated when possible. A variety of antidepressant and antiepileptic medicines is now considered to be the first-line treatment options for neuropathic pain.

— Antidepressants

Tricyclic antidepressants (TCAs), such as amitriptyline and nortriptyline, have a multimodal action when used in pain management. Their biochemical effects suggest that TCAs inhibit the presynaptic uptake of noradrenaline and serotonin, although they also have blocking effects at some postsynaptic histamine and muscarinic acetylcholine receptors. It can take several weeks for a patient to notice any improvement in their painful symptoms, so it is important to persist with treatment.

The most common side effects of TCAs include sedation, anticholinergic effects (e.g. dry mouth, constipation and urinary retention) and orthostatic hypotension. Secondary amine TCAs, such as nortriptyline, may be preferable because they are better tolerated than tertiary amine TCAs (amitriptyline and imipramine) but have comparable analgesic efficacy.

Initial doses of TCAs should be low (10–25 mg taken 60–90 min before bedtime), and the dosage should be titrated slowly until pain is adequately controlled or side effects limit further dose increases. Although there is a substantial body of evidence about the use of TCAs in neuropathic pain, their use is 'off-label' and this should be explained to the patient.

Duloxetine is a serotonin–noradrenaline reuptake inhibitor (SNRI) licensed for the treatment of diabetic peripheral neuropathic pain. Its improved selectivity for serotonin and noradrenaline (over dopamine) transporters means that it is generally better tolerated than TCAs. The most common adverse events leading to discontinuation are nausea, dizziness, somnolence and fatigue.

Selective SSRIs have been studied in a few trials, some of which have demonstrated a modest analgesic benefit, although the clinical relevance of these compounds is uncertain. Based on these results, citalopram and paroxetine may be considered options for patients who have not responded to an adequate trial of a TCA or an SNRI antidepressant when additional treatment with a medication with analgesic and antidepressant effects is required.

— **Antiepileptic drugs**
Gabapentin and pregabalin are the most commonly used antiepileptic drugs in the management of neuropathic pain. Both drugs are amino acids (more specifically γ-amino acids, as the amino group is separated from the carboxyl group by three carbon atoms), and highly polar. Both the carboxyl and amino groups are ionised at physiological pH, so the drugs exist as doubly charged zwitterions. Both drugs bind to the α_2/δ-subunit of neuronal voltage-gated calcium channels, decreasing the neurotransmitter release of glutamate, noradrenaline and substance P. In some studies of neuropathic pain, treatment was also associated with improvement in sleep, mood and various components of health-related quality of life.

gabapentin   pregabalin

The main dose-limiting side effects of the antiepileptics are somnolence and dizziness, which are reduced by gradual dosage titration and peripheral oedema. Gabapentin and pregabalin are generally safe and have few clinically important drug interactions. It can take several weeks to gradually increase the dose and reach an effective dosage. The onset of activity can be seen as early as the second week of therapy when titration is rapid, but the peak effect usually occurs approximately 2 weeks after a therapeutic dosage has been achieved. As a consequence of their high polarities, both drugs are cleared from the systemic circulation by the kidneys, and dosage reduction is necessary in patients with renal impairment.

In the past, other antiepileptic drugs have been used in the management of neuropathic pain, carbamazepine being used most commonly. However, both limited efficacy and many side effects and drug interactions have prevented widespread use. Nowadays, use of carbamazepine is reserved almost exclusively for trigeminal neuralgia where it is particularly effective. Other antiepileptic drugs, including sodium valproate, phenytoin and lamotrigine, have been used in neuropathic pain conditions with varying degrees of success and tolerability.

— **Topical treatments**
For small areas of localised neuropathic pain, several topical treatments are available. Some randomised controlled trials have demonstrated significantly greater pain relief with a local anaesthetic (lidocaine 5%) medicated plaster (with lidocaine incorporated into the adhesive of the plaster) than with vehicle-controlled patches in patients with post-herpetic neuralgia and other diverse peripheral neuropathic pain conditions, particularly where allodynia (pain resulting from a non-injurious stimulus to the skin) is prominent. However, other more recent studies have produced contradictory results. The only side effects that occur are mild skin reactions (e.g.

erythema and localised rash). Systemic absorption, and hence blood concentrations, are minimal with the approved maximum dose of three plasters a day applied for a 12-hour period.

Topical capsaicin (the active 'hot' ingredient of the chilli pepper) is a $TRPV_1$ (transient receptor potential vanilloid type 1) receptor agonist that has been used in the management of neuropathic pain. Use of older formulations was limited by problems with their application; however, a novel topical formulation has recently been marketed. Capsaicin is available as a large transdermal patch, with an adhesive matrix containing the drug and a protective backing layer. Application of a capsaicin 8% patch is painful and requires prior application of a local anaesthetic, but, where successful, a single application for 1 hour has a long-term effect (sometimes over 12 weeks) with little or only limited systemic exposure and systemic side effects. Health professionals need to wear protective nitrile gloves when handling the patches and when cleaning treatment areas after removal of patches.

Non-pharmacological treatment options

It is essential that all types of chronic pain are managed within a biopsychosocial framework and patients with persistent pain take an active part in the management of their condition. Further information about self-management of chronic pain can be found in the Pain Toolkit (www.paintoolkit.org).

Transcutaneous electrical nerve stimulation (TENS) and acupuncture are non-pharmacological methods of stimulating peripheral nerves and muscles close to the site of pain in order to modulate peripheral nociceptive inputs to the dorsal horn of the spinal cord. Despite limited evidence for efficacy, there are relatively few contraindications and side effects, and these are popular alternatives with patients. For severe persistent neuropathic pain more interventional approaches, such as spinal cord stimulation or intrathecal drug delivery, may be necessary.

Opioid analgesics for treatment of persistent non-cancer pain

The use of opioids is well validated and documented in acute pain, cancer pain and end-of-life care. Over the past 20 years, there have been an increasing number of publications about the use of opioids for persistent non-cancer pain,

including neuropathic pain. Several trials of relatively short duration suggest that certain patients with neuropathic pain may gain adequate analgesia and improvement in function from opioid use. Recently, however, the potential risks of long-term opioid therapy have been highlighted. Very few randomised controlled trials have studied the long-term effects (>3 months) of opioids in persistent non-cancer pain.

Chemistry and mechanism of action of tramadol

Tramadol has a unique pharmacological action, having two different mechanisms of analgesic effect. Tramadol and its only pharmacologically active metabolite, O-desmethyltramadol (denoted as 'M1'), bind to the μ-opioid receptor. In addition, tramadol enhances central noradrenergic and serotoninergic descending inhibition, and hence may offer a theoretical benefit when used in neuropathic pain. Tramadol is associated with less constipation than other opioids, but nausea and vomiting may be a problem. The incidence of respiratory depression is significantly lower than with other opioids at equi-analgesic doses.

tramadol

Tramadol contains two adjacent chiral centres (marked in red as '1' and '2' in the diagram). This results in a total of four possible stereoisomers for the drug: (1R,2R), (1R,2S), (1S,2R) and (1S,2S). The drug is manufactured and administered as a (racemic) mixture of (1R,2R)-tramadol and (1S,2S)-tramadol. As these two isomers have opposite configurations at every chiral centre, they are enantiomers of each other. Interestingly, it is the (1R,2R) isomer (and particularly the more potent O-desmethyl metabolite) that is responsible for μ-opioid agonist activity and the (1S,2S) isomer that is responsible for inhibiting noradrenaline reuptake.

The British Pain Society has published recommendations on the use of opioids for the management of persistent non-cancer pain (see www.britishpainsociety.org for details).

EXTENDED LEARNING

- How is persistent pain self-managed? (see Pain toolkit – available at www.paintoolkit.org)
- What are the treatment guidelines for neuropathic pain?
- Outline the controversies regarding opioid use for non-cancer pain
- Describe combination therapies for neuropathic pain
- Describe the structure of the skin, the 'bricks-and-mortar' model of skin structure, and identify the barriers to dermal drug absorption
- How are transdermal drug delivery patches designed and formulated? How can the penetration of a drug through the skin be enhanced?
- Outline the pharmacology of opioid analgesics
- Describe approaches to the measurement of pain

ADDITIONAL PRACTICE POINT

- When are medicines used off-label? How does this differ from unlicensed medicines and what legal, ethical and safety issues surround the use of unlicensed medicines or medicines used off-label?

References and further reading

Attal N, Cruccu G, Baron R et al.; European Federation of Neurological Societies (2010). EFNS guidelines on the pharmacological treatment of neuropathic pain: 2010 revision. *Eur J Neurol* **17**:1113–23.

Baron R, Binder A, Wasner G (2010). Neuropathic pain: diagnosis, pathophysiological mechanisms, and treatment. *Lancet Neurol* **9**:807–19.

British Pain Society (2010). *Opioids for Persistent Pain: Good practice.* London: British Pain Society.

Dhalla IA, Persaud N, Juurlink DN (2011). Facing up to the prescription opioid crisis. *BMJ* **343**:d5142.

Eisenberg E, McNicol ED, Carr DB (2006). Opioids for neuropathic pain. *Cochrane Database Syst Rev* **3**:CD006146.

Freynhagen R, Baron R, Gockel U, Tölle TR (2006). painDETECT: a new screening questionnaire to identify neuropathic components in patients with back pain. *Curr Med Res Opin* **22**:1911–20.

Freynhagen R, Bennett MI (2009). Diagnosis and treatment of neuropathic pain. *BMJ* **339**:b3002.

National Institute for Health and Clinical Excellence (2010). *Neuropathic Pain: The pharmacological management of neuropathic pain in adults in non-specialist settings.* Clinical Guideline 96. Available at: http://guidance.nice.org.uk/CG96 (accessed 29 September 2013).

Turk DC, Wilson HD, Cahana A (2011). Treatment of chronic non-cancer pain. *Lancet* **377**:2226–35.

Williams AC (2003). *Transdermal and Topical Drug Delivery.* Pharmaceutical Press: London.

Woolf CJ, Mannion RJ (1999). Neuropathic pain: aetiology, symptoms, mechanisms, and management. *Lancet* **353**:1959–64.

Woolf CJ (2004). Pain: moving from symptom control towards mechanism based treatment. *Ann Intern Med* **140**:441–51.

Case 8
Differential indicators for migraine and medication-overuse headache
CARL MARTIN

LEARNING OUTCOMES

At the end of this case, you will be able to:

- Identify key indicators of a migraineur (patient with migraine)
- Demonstrate a raised awareness of the issues around medication-overuse headache
- Demonstrate a raised awareness of the use of headache diaries
- Identify potentially sinister causes of headache

Case study

Mr NH, a 55-year-old white man, presents with a query about use of painkillers; you overhear him telling your assistant that he has read somewhere that shop pharmacists can help with medicines. You are alerted by his manner and indicate to your assistant that Mr NH should be asked to wait next to the consultation room, and that you'll be with him straight away.

Mr NH appears a little reluctant to enter your consultation room and expresses surprise at its availability, muttering something about Mr

Whitecoat never had one of these. You ask him to explain the nature of his initial query about pain relief. He explains that he takes a regular soluble Solpadeine product to help with an old footballing injury (stiff neck/back injury/knee problem) but has noticed recently that he is getting more headaches especially at weekends. He asks whether it could be migraine.

❷ On what basis could you make a differential diagnosis?
❷ What is the recommended first-line treatment for migraine?
❷ What are the components present in the range of soluble Solpadeine products and what is the rationale for the combined use of analgesics?

On further discussion, Mr NH admits that he may be using the soluble analgesics too much but cannot remember how often. He asks if you could recommend something a bit stronger to clear up the pain. He has seen on the internet that Botox is now used.

❷ What are some potentially serious causes of headache?
❷ What are the key elements of his pain profile that Mr NH needs to record, in the form of a diary?

Mr NH agrees to keep a diary of his symptoms and use of analgesics and returns in 14 days. On return, he presents a complex picture: he appears to use the Solpadeine Max Soluble daily and his weekend headaches are associated with nausea and aura/strange flashing lights.

❷ What are the indicators for medication-overuse headache or chronic daily headache?
❷ What are the recognised trigger factors for migraine?

Mr NH thanks you for your help and agrees to visit his GP based on your prepared action plan.

❷ What would be a suitable summary of your findings and an appropriate action plan for Mr NH?
❷ What are the non-drug options available for Mr NH?

Case discussion

— Classification of headaches

The *International Classification of Headache Disorders* (ICHD-II, International Headache Society, 2004) classifies headache disorders under 14 headings and makes a distinction between primary and secondary headaches. Secondary headaches are an indicator of a more serious underlying cause, usually requiring immediate referral (see below).

In the above classification, **primary headaches** are classified based on symptom profiles:

1 Migraine (with or without aura) – episodic and chronic
2 Tension-type headache – episodic and chronic
3 Cluster headache and other trigeminal/ autonomic cephalalgias
4 Neuralgias including trigeminal
5 Other primary headaches, e.g. exertional headache.

A useful aide-memoire can be found in NICE CG150 labelled as 'diagnosis poster' at http:// publications.nice.org.uk/headaches-cg150/ guidance#diagnosis-2

— Migraine diagnostic pointers (IHS 2004)

The duration of headache is from 4 hours to 72 hours in adults. Patients are usually symptom-free between attacks. Headache is at least two of the following:

• Unilateral
• Pulsating
• Moderate to severe
• Aggravated by routine activities.

Accompanying symptoms may include:

• Photophobia (light sensitivity)
• Phonophobia (sound sensitivity)
• Nausea
• Vomiting.

Approximately 25% of migraineurs will experience an aura (early signs heralding the onset of headache). The aura can develop over 5–20 min and last for up to 1 hour. It can either be visual or neurological. Within 60 min of the aura ending, the headache usually occurs.

The pharmacist's role is to facilitate health decision-making in individuals; so rather than the above being used as a guess diagnosis, it is best seen as part of an overall picture. The profile of an average migraineur may be useful. Most migraine sufferers will:

• have approximately one or two attacks a month
• be aged between 25 and 55 years
• rarely experience more than 40 attacks in a year
• have their normal quality of life disrupted.

— Treatment approaches for migraine

It is extremely important that patients are included in all decisions about migraine management. It is the patient who needs to develop the strategy that works specifically for him or her, with minimal disruption of normal day-to-day activities.

The strategy usually includes:

- The avoidance of trigger factors where possible
- Acute intervention for breakthrough attacks
- Use of prophylactic agents where there is a high frequency of attacks

The basis for assessing patients for migraine prophylactic treatment usually involves four elements:

1. Attack frequency: this is usually when number of attacks reaches three to five per month
2. Attack severity: if acute therapy is ineffective and the attacks are particularly severe or prolonged
3. Frequent use of acute medication: generally considered to be more than twice a week
4. Presence of uncommon migraine conditions such as prolonged aura.

paracetamol

codeine

caffeine

Combination analgesic products

Mr NH is taking Solpadeine Max Soluble – one of a number of proprietary combined products containing paracetamol, codeine and caffeine.

Although the analgesic mechanism of action of paracetamol is not fully understood, it is recognised to inhibit the cyclooxygenase (COX) enzymes, which are involved in the biosynthesis of prostaglandins, particularly the COX-3 isoform in the CNS. More recent research suggests that the reactive N-acetyl-p-benzoquinoneimine metabolite of paracetamol may interact with one or more protein targets involved in pain signalling. Codeine (a prodrug) is an opiate analgesic, the metabolites of which, notably morphine, exert their analgesic effect through activation of central μ-opioid receptors. Caffeine is a xanthine alkaloid CNS stimulant that acts as a competitive inhibitor at adenosine receptors. It may offer relief in migraine headache by causing vasoconstriction in cranial blood vessels and/or by increasing the rate at which co-administered analgesics are absorbed.

— Non-drug interventions

The British Association for the Study of Headaches (www.bash.org.uk) lists the following, predominantly as adjuvant therapy:

- Physical therapy: improved physical fitness may have a positive benefit. Physiotherapy by a specialist where there is a specific indication such as neck dysfunction. Dental treatment to correct malocclusion is of unproven benefit but may improve temporomandibular joint dysfunction. Acupuncture has some benefit.
- Psychological therapy: relaxation therapy, stress reduction and coping strategies are first line when they target a specific underlying indication, which limits the success of migraine treatments.
- Alternative remedies: OTC homeopathic medicines are of no proven value. Reflexology also has no scientific basis.

— Headache diaries: recording the pain profile

Headache diaries can be used either as an aid to accurate diagnosis or as support management of the condition. Downloadable diaries can be found at www.migrainetrust.org and both annual and monthly examples at the National Migraine Centre at www.migraineclinic.org.uk.

— Potential secondary causes of headache

Some potentially serious secondary causes of headache include:

- Meningitis
- Subarachnoid haemorrhage
- Giant cell temporal arteritis
- Glaucoma
- Carbon monoxide poisoning
- Conditions causing raised intracranial pressure – intracranial tumours.

Sinusitis is not considered serious unless it fails to respond to usual OTC medication.

— Medication-overuse headache/chronic daily headache

Although the term 'medication-overuse headache' (MOH) was included in the IHS classification, referred to earlier, in 2004, it is also called chronic daily headache (CDH) in the neurology literature. The term MOH usefully highlights the potential role of regular intake of medication (including all medicines used for treating headache) in causing the condition. The current definition is a headache that is present on ≥15 days of the month and has developed or worsened while the patient has been regularly using analgesic or anti-migraine medicines for more than 3 months.

The frequency of analgesic consumption is an indicator of the condition MOH. As a guide, MOH may be an indication for people whose headache has developed or worsened over a 3-month period while using the following medication:

- Triptans ($5HT_{1B}/_{1D}$ receptor agonists: sumitriptan, zolmitriptan), opioids, ergot alkaloids (ergotamine) or combination analgesic medications on ≥10 days/month, or
- Paracetamol, aspirin or a NSAID, either alone or in any combination, on ≥15 days/month.

People with MOH often describe a dull nagging ache that may be present all day, being the first thing that they are aware of on waking, and it never seems to go away. The character of the headache will vary from a dull ache, to a tight pressure, to a dull throb. They will often comment that 'no matter what I take, the headache never goes away' or 'I can't do without my painkillers'.

EXTENDED LEARNING

- Find out about the 'treatment ladder' for migraine

- Explore the available grading scales for measuring the severity of migraine and the impact on the person's quality of life. Together with headache diaries they are also useful in developing care strategies, e.g. the MIDAS (Migraine Disability Assessment Score) used by AJ Dowson at King's College Hospital Headache Service.

ADDITIONAL PRACTICE POINT

- If you are keen to develop your involvement in pain management, possibly running local pain clinics, then become a pharmacist with special interest (PHwSI). You can learn more at the Primary Care Commissioning website at www.pcc-cic.org.uk/article/gps-and-pharmacists-special-interests-gpwsi-and-phwsi

References and further reading

British Association for the Study of Headache (2010). *Guidelines for all healthcare professionals in the diagnosis and management of migraine; tension-type headache; cluster headache; medication-overuse headache.* Available at: www.bash.org.uk (accessed 3 October 2013).

Edvinsson L, Villalón CM, Maassen Van Den Brink A (2012). Basic mechanisms of migraine and its acute treatment. *Pharmacol Ther* **136**:319–33.

International Headache Society, Headache Classification Subcommittee (2004). *International Classification of Headache Disorders*, 2nd edn (ICHD-II). London: International Headache Society.

National Institute for Health and Clinical Excellence (2012). *Headaches: Diagnosis and management of headaches in young people and adults.* Clinical Guideline 150. London: NICE. Available at: http://publications.nice.org.uk/headaches-cg150 (accessed 3 October 2012).

Samsam M (2012). Central nervous system acting drugs in treatment of migraine headache. *Cent Nerv Syst Agents Med Chem* **12**:158–72.

Shahien R, Beiruti K (2012). Preventive agents for migraine: focus on the antiepileptic drugs. *J Cent Nerv Syst Dis* **4**:37–49.

Tepper SJ (2012). Medication-overuse headache. *Continuum* **18**:807–22.

Case 9
Epilepsy
ANNETT BLOCHBERGER

LEARNING OUTCOMES

At the end of this case, you will be able to:

- Understand issues relating to female patients with epilepsy
- Consider implications for antiepileptic drug (AED) treatment in female patients of childbearing age
- Devise a pharmaceutical care plan and treatment goals for patients with epilepsy
- Describe the chemistry of valproate, topiramate and lamotrigine
- Understand the use of the Biopharmaceutics Classification System (BCS) to predict the oral absorption of drugs

Case study

Ms CS is 21 years old and is attending the specialist nurse clinic for an annual review. Ms CS was diagnosed with generalised tonic–clonic seizures at the age of 15. Her seizures are controlled on sodium valproate (as Epilim Chrono) 500 mg twice a day and topiramate 100 mg twice daily. Her last seizure occurred 2 years ago. There is no other significant past medical history.

- How is the diagnosis of epilepsy confirmed?
- What other types of seizure exist? Consider different causes for epilepsy
- Comment on the choice of antiepileptic drugs for this patient

Ms CS explains that she has entered into a long-term relationship and would like to receive advice on suitable contraceptive methods. She is also expressing the wish to discuss cessation of AED therapy versus the risk of having more seizures.

- What advice would you give Ms CS in terms of appropriate contraceptive methods?
- What other advice should she be given at this stage?

Later, on collecting her regular prescriptions, Ms CS mentions to you, as her local community pharmacist, that she is planning to get married

and to have a family. As she is worried about the effect of her medication on an unborn baby, she confides in you that she is considering stopping medication altogether. In fact, she has decided to miss out a tablet occasionally, to see how she gets on without them. You invite her for a medication review to discuss her concerns.

- What are the potential risks of AED therapy to the unborn baby during pregnancy?
- What are the risks of stopping AED medication suddenly?
- How could the risk to Ms CS and a potential baby be minimised?

After the review, Ms CS makes an appointment with the local epilepsy specialist clinic. The consultant reviews her history and the joint decision is being made to withdraw her existing AED therapy with valproate and topiramate, and to initiate lamotrigine.

- Advise on a suitable titration scheme
- Comment on the choice of alternative therapy in view of a potential pregnancy
- What other steps should be taken to support the patient for the future?
- Draw the structures of the three prescribed AEDs in this case and classify them as acidic, basic, both or neither

NICE guidelines for prescribing AEDs include:

Consistent supply to the child, young person or adult with epilepsy of a particular manufacturer's AED preparation is recommended, unless the prescriber, in consultation with the child, young person, adult and their family and/or carers as appropriate, considers that this is not a concern. Different preparations of some AEDs may vary in bioavailability or pharmacokinetic profiles and care needs to be taken to avoid reduced effect or excessive side effects.

- Why is this the case, because, for generic products to be approved by regulatory authorities such as the MHRA, bioequivalence with the innovator (original branded) product must be demonstrated?

Case discussion

— Epilepsy: definition, signs and symptoms, differential diagnosis

Epilepsy is a chronic neurological disorder that is characterised by recurrent unprovoked seizures. The classification of epilepsy is complex and depends on the affected area of the brain, the type and the cause of seizures, and the age of the person. In general, seizures can be divided into partial (focal) seizures and generalised seizures. Partial seizures can be described further as simple partial seizures, where consciousness is not impaired, or complex partial seizures in which there is associated alteration of consciousness. This may, or may not, be associated with secondary generalisation. Generalised seizures can be convulsive or non-convulsive with further subcategorisation into tonic–clonic, tonic, clonic, atonic or absence seizures.

Seizures can be symptomatic of a wide range of neurological conditions, including alcohol withdrawal, chemical intoxication, metabolic disturbances, benzodiazepine withdrawal, encephalitis, head injury, stroke and fever (especially in infants). Correction of the underlying condition may result in resolution of the symptoms.

The diagnosis should always be made by a clinician with expertise in the management of epilepsy, typically a neurologist, to avoid misdiagnosis and to allow for appropriate investigation and initiation of therapy. Due to the transient nature of the symptoms, accurate and extensive history taking is paramount. Collateral history from family, carers or witnesses may need to be sought. Several tests, such as electroencephalography (EEG) and magnetic resonance imaging (MRI), can be useful to support and classify the diagnosis by identifying possible underlying structural or electrical abnormalities (malformations, brain tumours, haemorrhages, etc.). Videotelemetry refers to a form of EEG in which continuous, simultaneous video recording and EEG are performed over a prolonged period, typically days, to provide detailed clinical and electrical description of the seizures.

— Treatment goals

Pharmacological management is usually offered after a second unprovoked seizure, but may be recommended after the first seizure if there is a high risk of reoccurrence as determined on clinical, electrical and radiographic grounds. The aim of treatment for patients with epilepsy is prevention of seizures without experiencing significant toxicity or side effects. Treatment plans differ for individual patients depending on epilepsy classification, personal and social circumstances, and tolerability of medication.

Approximately two-thirds of patients with newly diagnosed epilepsy are well controlled on medication. A good predictor for seizure control is response to the first AED. In cases of treatment failure, the likelihood of achieving seizure freedom is significantly reduced.

— Choice of AED in the general population

There are about 30 licensed AEDs currently available. Factors that need to be taken into account when choosing an AED for an individual patient are epilepsy type, pharmacological profile (including side effects and interactions), gender, age, family planning, co-morbidities and compliance. AEDs can be classified into older drugs, which have been used for decades (sodium valproate, carbamazepine, phenytoin, phenobarbital), and newer AEDs (topiramate, oxcarbazepine, lamotrigine, levetiracetam, lacosamide, zonisamide), although some of the so-called 'newer' agents have been in routine clinical use for over two decades. There are differences in terms of indication; as a rule of thumb, newer AEDs are usually licensed as add-on treatment for partial seizures at the beginning, with an extension to monotherapy once more trial data are available. Such monotherapy licences are now available for a number of the newer agents, such as lamotrigine.

For male patients and women not of childbearing age with generalised tonic–clonic seizures, sodium valproate is considered an effective first-line AED which is usually well tolerated in doses up to 1000 mg. Side effects include weight gain, tremor, sedation, behavioural changes, extrapyramidal symptoms, thrombocytopenia, hepatic toxicity and hair loss. Despite being a GABA (γ-aminobutyric acid) transaminase enzyme inhibitor, valproate is associated with loss of bone mineral density, and may therefore increase the risk of osteoporotic bone fractures. Numerous drug interactions have to be considered alongside a complex pharmacokinetic profile.

— Choice of AED in women of childbearing age

Treatment of epilepsy in women of childbearing age requires comprehensive counselling from early teenage years onwards to avoid unplanned pregnancies and to minimise the risk to a baby. Enzyme-inducing drugs and some others, such as topiramate, can reduce the effectiveness of the oral contraceptive pill. Dose adjustments may be necessary as well as introducing alternative contraceptive methods (intrauterine device). On the other hand, oral contraceptives can reduce the plasma concentrations of lamotrigine. The principal route of clearance of lamotrigine is metabolism to the more water-soluble *N*-glucuronide, followed by urinary excretion. This glucuronidation is induced when co-administered with oral contraceptives.

The advantages of a planned pregnancy are clear. Discussions with the patient should include the additional risk of exposure of potentially teratogenic AEDs to the fetus. The general risk of malformation is about 1–2%. Sodium valproate has been shown to increase the risk up to 6%. Polytherapy can increase the risk of malformations even higher (15%). Most of the data around teratogenicity stem from animal studies and are therefore not fully conclusive: this is particularly true for the newer AEDs. As a result of a higher risk of spina bifida and other neural tube effects, it is recommended that women with epilepsy who are considering pregnancy should take folic acid at a dose of 5 mg daily before conception, and not just after pregnancy has been confirmed.

Ideally, the patient should be seizure free before becoming pregnant. In the case of prolonged seizure freedom (>2 years), the option of withdrawing AEDs can be considered if the risk of reoccurrence is deemed low. Some patients may feel uncomfortable withdrawing their medication. Monotherapy with an AED known to have a low risk of teratogenicity would be the next most favourable option.

Physiological changes that accompany pregnancy include altered renal and hepatic function, decreased albumin-binding capacity, increase in apparent volume of distribution, major hormonal changes and altered metabolism of certain drugs (e.g. lamotrigine). All these factors can have an effect on seizure control, which is more pronounced in patients with poorly controlled epilepsy.

Extensive counselling should include the risk of maternal seizures to the unborn baby (falls, anoxia), birth plan (planned hospital delivery, possible elective caesarean section) and

appropriateness of breastfeeding. Further information about safe childcare must be provided accordingly.

— **Therapeutic considerations in this case**
In the featured case, the decision was made to switch the patient from sodium valproate and topiramate to lamotrigine. In comparison to valproate and topiramate, lamotrigine has a good safety profile in pregnancy (at doses <400 mg/day). This advantage is traded off with a potentially reduced efficacy in generalised seizures. Blood levels drop significantly during pregnancy (increased clearance because of an increase in maternal oestrogen levels, mediated by the mechanism discussed above) and require periodic monitoring. The levels of oestrogen decrease rapidly postpartum which requires further dose adjustments after delivery to avoid lamotrigine toxicity.

— **Chemical properties of valproate, topiramate and lamotrigine**
The structures below demonstrate the diversity that is found among AEDs. Topiramate is neither acidic nor basic. The nitrogen atom present in the sulfonamide ($-SO_2NH_2$) has no available lone pair of electrons due to resonance delocalisation (similar to an amide). In fact, sulfonamides can behave as very weak acids (but rarely at the pH values found in biological systems) because the negative charge formed on deprotonation can also be stabilised by resonance. Valproic acid is clearly acidic due to the presence of the carboxyl group. Valproate, the anion formed by deprotonation, is the conjugate base of valproic acid. Lamotrigine is a weak base; the lone pairs of electrons present on the nitrogen atoms are not as available as the lone pair found on an aliphatic amino group.

— **Principles of switching AEDs**
As a rule of thumb, AEDs should be introduced gradually to avoid side effects. A 'start low–go slow' approach, often different to the recommendations of the *BNF*, is adopted by most clinicians. The first AED should be withdrawn stepwise only once the second drug has been titrated up to an effective dose. Due to the sporadic nature of seizures, this dose may be difficult to establish but can be determined by tolerability.

The patient should be provided with a detailed treatment plan and advice as to what to do when side effects occur or seizure control has not been

topiramate

sodium valproate

lamotrigine

- **Class I**: high permeability, high solubility, e.g. ethosuximide, phenobarbital, lamotrigine, valproic acid, topiramate
- **Class II**: high permeability, low solubility, e.g. carbamazepine, primidone, phenytoin
- **Class III**: low permeability, high solubility, e.g. gabapentin
- **Class IV**: low permeability, low solubility.

Class I is the optimal class; these compounds are well absorbed and there is little risk of absorption variability. Drugs in the other classes are potentially more problematic, especially if this is linked to a narrow therapeutic index, making switching between products potentially problematic.

EXTENDED LEARNING

- How are seizures, and different types of epilepsy, classified according to International League against Epilepsy (ILAE)?
- What is the pharmacology of AEDs?
- Outline the need for, and procedures of, therapeutic drug monitoring for AEDs
- Consider the implications of AEDs on bone health
- What is the role of NICE in prescribing?

achieved. This can result in relatively complex titration schemes, which should ideally be explicitly documented in writing for the patient to avoid misunderstanding.

For generic products to be licensed by regulatory authorities, bioequivalence with the innovator product must be demonstrated. However, in the instance of some narrow therapeutic index drugs, including some AEDs, this may not ensure clinical equivalence, with the result that switching patients between apparently bioequivalent products can have detrimental effects. However, data are often lacking. The key properties of a drug, which may impact on the rate, and extent of drug absorption after oral administration are its solubility and its permeability across absorbing membranes.

The **Biopharmaceutics Classification System** has been established as a means of predicting oral absorption, based on solubility and permeability parameters. Drugs are divided into four classes:

References and further reading

Alcaron G, Nashef L, Cross H, Nightingale J, Richardson S (2009). *Epilepsy – Oxford Specialist Handbooks in Neurology.* Oxford: Oxford University Press.

Brown TR, Holmes GL (2008). *Handbook of Epilepsy*, 4th edn. Philadelphia, PA: Lippincott Williams & Wilkins.

National Institute for Health and Clinical Excellence (2012). *The Epilepsies: The diagnosis and management of the epilepsies in adults and children in primary and secondary care. CG137.* London: NICE. Available at: www.nice.org.uk/CG137 (accessed 30 September 2013).

Case 10
Phenytoin and acute therapeutics
NAZANIN KHORSHIDI, ROMAN LANDOWSKI AND ROB SHULMAN

LEARNING OUTCOMES

At the end of this case, you will be able to:

- Calculate phenytoin loading doses
- Explain the relevance of chemical structure, pK_a and pH of phenytoin for its formulation and administration in intravenous fluids
- Convert an intravenous phenytoin dose to one for an oral route
- Learn about the practical approach to phenytoin dose optimisation

Case study

Mr GY is 33 years old and was admitted to the intensive care unit (ICU) with a cardiac arrest. He was taking part in an alcohol-detoxification rehabilitation programme and had tonic–clonic seizures followed by a cardiac arrest.

Mr GY has a past medical history of alcoholic hepatitis. He was not taking any regular medication before admission.

On admission, the ICU consultant decides to load Mr GY on intravenous phenytoin.

- Why is the intravenous route preferred in an emergency?
- Why is the sodium salt of phenytoin required for intravenous administration? Why is the pH of the injection a concern for phenytoin sodium administration?
- The junior doctor asks you to recommend the loading dose that he should prescribe for Mr GY (patient weighs 85 kg)

On day 1, the patient was prescribed a phenytoin intravenous maintenance dose of 100 mg t.d.s. A phenytoin serum level measured on day 4 was 24 mg/L (96 µmol/L), which is toxic. The next two doses were withheld until the serum levels were within range and then the intravenous maintenance dose was reduced to 100 mg b.d., which he received for 3 days. On day 7 the patient started convulsing and a further phenytoin level was taken. The serum level this time was low at 6 mg/L (24 µmol/L). The consultant asks whether

Mr GY should receive a further loading dose. (Mr GY's albumin level was 30 g/dL; volume of distribution was 0.65 L/kg).

- Recommend an appropriate loading dose and new maintenance dose for Mr GY.

Mr GY's corrected phenytoin level was 8.6 mg/L, so his intravenous maintenance dose was increased by 50 mg daily to the following regimen:

100 mg at 08:00

100 mg at 16:00

50 mg at 22:00.

On day 10, the phenytoin serum level was again at the low end of normal at 11 mg/L; however, the patient had not had further seizures.

- What action would you recommend?

The ICU consultant wants to convert the intravenous route (parenteral) to enteral administration (through a catheter, directly into the gastrointestinal [GI] tract).

- What would the appropriate conversion dose be? What is your advice?

Over the weekend, on day 11 of phenytoin therapy, the patient was discharged from the ICU to a ward and his enteral tube was removed. There was no clear handover of his phenytoin therapy. A few days later, Mr GY complained of blurred vision and was reported as being increasingly drowsy with slurred speech. A serum phenytoin level was 25 mg/L.

- Advise on interpretation and management

Case discussion

The time taken to achieve therapeutic blood concentrations of phenytoin is significantly faster with intravenous phenytoin than oral (average 5.6 h for oral route versus 30 min for the intravenous route). In an emergency situation, it is desirable to ensure patients achieve therapeutic phenytoin levels rapidly.

— Molecular structure and properties of phenytoin
Phenytoin is a weak acid with a pK_a of 8.3. At first glance, it may not be readily apparent as to why it

is acidic, but the drug contains an N-H group situated between two carbonyl (C=O) groups. The hydrogen atom (in red) can be removed under conditions that are sufficiently strongly basic; the resulting negative charge can then be spread out over the molecule (especially the carbonyl oxygen atoms), giving greater stability. Treating phenytoin with sodium hydroxide gives the sodium salt, phenytoin sodium, shown in the diagram. The sodium salt is considerably more polar than phenytoin itself and is sufficiently water soluble for formulation as an aqueous solution for intravenous injection. Phenytoin itself has very low polarity and very poor water solubility.

phenytoin   phenytoin sodium

As the pK_a of phenytoin is 8.3, a pH >11 is required for the drug to remain deprotonated and soluble in water. At this pH, >99% of the drug is in the highly polar, negatively charged form. Mixing a phenytoin injection with physiological (normal) 0.9% saline (pH 5.5) or dextrose saline (pH 4) will reduce the pH significantly, so more of the drug will be in the uncharged, poorly water-soluble form, resulting in precipitation. Aqueous solutions of phenytoin sodium can even gradually absorb atmospheric CO_2 over time, reducing the pH of the solution sufficiently to cause precipitation of free phenytoin, evident from cloudiness (turbidity) of the previously clear solution. Solutions of phenytoin should be administered soon after preparation (within 1 hour) to avoid this, because the consequences of introducing solid particulate into the bloodstream can be severe (so it should be infused via an inline filter).

Mr GY does not usually take phenytoin and therefore a loading dose is necessary to achieve a therapeutic level quickly. The intravenous loading dose of phenytoin in status epilepticus is 20 mg/kg (see *BNF*) at a rate not exceeding 50 mg/min.

20 mg/kg × 85 kg = 1700 mg

The injection is available as 50 mg/mL ampoules, which works out as 34 mL of injection solution.

Phenytoin clearance does not follow first-order kinetics. It has a low therapeutic index and a narrow target range. Small increases in dose can result in greater increases in blood level.

In clinical practice, a trough level (pre-dose) is measured for therapeutic drug monitoring. The recommended therapeutic range for phenytoin plasma concentrations is 10–20 mg/L (40–80 μmol/L). The time required to reach steady state with phenytoin can be very prolonged. In practice, to avoid sustained periods of low or high phenytoin concentrations, plasma levels are measured before reaching the steady state.

When calculating a dose of phenytoin, the serum albumin needs to be considered. Phenytoin is approximately 90% protein bound. Hypoalbuminaemia (reduced serum albumin) increases the proportion of 'free' phenytoin, which is responsible for the pharmacological effect. The actual amount of free phenytoin stays the same although the amount of bound phenytoin will be reduced. Plasma levels represent the total drug concentration, i.e. bound plus 'free' phenytoin, and are therefore open to misinterpretation because an apparently normal level might hide a toxic level of free phenytoin. A formula can be applied to estimate the corrected phenytoin level:

$$\text{Corrected phenytoin level} = \frac{\text{Reported level}}{(0.02 \times \text{Serum albumin}) + 0.1}$$

In Mr GY's case the reported level is 6 mg/L (24 μmol/L):

$$\text{Corrected phenytoin level} = \frac{6 \text{ mg/L}}{(0.02 \times 30 \text{ g/dL}) + 0.1}$$
$$= 8.6 \text{ mg/L}$$

As the patient is convulsing and the corrected plasma level is still low, a repeated loading dose is advised. Administration of the loading dose will result in a more rapid increase of the phenytoin concentration into the desired therapeutic range: To calculate the phenytoin loading dose you need to increase the phenytoin concentration in each litre of the patient's volume of distribution (0.65 × weight in kg), by the change in concentration you desire.

Loading dose (mg) = V_d (0.65 L/kg) × Weight (kg) × Change in plasma concentration required (in mg/L)

If the desired therapeutic concentration is 20 mg/L (80 μmol/L) then:

Loading dose (mg) $= 0.65 \times 85 \times (20 - 8.6)$
$= 629.85$ mg phenytoin.

This mass of phenytoin is present in 629/0.92 mg $= 685$ mg phenytoin sodium, which can be rounded to 650 mg.

The value of 0.92 is the salt fraction for phenytoin, compared with phenytoin sodium. It can be thought of as the mass of phenytoin (in grams) contained in 1 g phenytoin sodium. The relative molecular mass (M_r) of phenytoin ($C_{15}H_{12}N_2O_2$) is 252, and that for phenytoin sodium ($C_{15}H_{11}N_2O_2Na$) is 274. The salt fraction, S, can be determined by dividing these two values of M_r, so $252/274 = 0.92$. In other words, 0.92 g phenytoin contains the same number of moles of the drug (the same number of drug molecules) as 1 g phenytoin sodium.

In practice, a dose of either 650 mg or 700 mg would be appropriate. In Mr GY's case a dose of 650 mg was considered to be sufficient because the patient's weight may have been exaggerated due to the presence of mild oedema (and phenytoin preferentially distributes into fat rather than water).

The patient was administered the loading dose of 650 mg; however, the maintenance dose also needs adjusting. In general, maintenance doses are increased as follows:
<7 mg/L level, increase daily dose by 100 mg
7–12 mg/L level, increase daily dose by 50 mg
12–16 mg/L level, increase daily dose by 25 mg.

Multiple daily intravenous doses are administered before the steady state is achieved in order to help maintain levels throughout the day:

Albumin $= 31$ g/dL

$$\frac{\text{Corrected}}{\text{phenytoin level}} = \frac{11 \text{ mg/L(or } 44 \text{ } \mu\text{mol/L)}}{(0.02 \times 31 \text{ g/dL}) + 0.1}$$
$$= 15.3 \text{ mg/L (or } 61.2 \text{ } \mu\text{mol/L)}$$

Once the level has been corrected for hypoalbuminaemia, it is within the therapeutic target range. There is no need to adjust the phenytoin dose, because the patient is asymptomatic. This highlights the importance of calculating corrected phenytoin levels and the potential for misinterpretation.

The patient has a nasogastric (NG) tube and therefore phenytoin suspension is the most appropriate formulation. The bioavailabilities of the different formulations and the salt fraction ($S = 0.92$) may need to be considered when converting between dosage forms. The injection consists of the sodium salt whereas the suspension contains the acid form and approximately 90 mg suspension is equivalent in phenytoin content to 100 mg injection. However, in practice a 1:1 conversion is acceptable when switching between doses. Enteral phenytoin should be prescribed as a single daily oral dose because enteral feeds significantly reduce the adsorption of phenytoin liquid (phenytoin binds to the feed). You should advise the nurses to stop the feed for 2 hours before and 2 hours after phenytoin administration. If the oral dose was prescribed three times a day, the feeds would be turned off for a total of 12 hours a day, which would severely impair the nutrition, so once-daily dosing is preferable.

You recommend a phenytoin dose of 250 mg once daily via the NG tube. In some cases, where seizures are secondary to another cause (in this case excess alcohol intake), phenytoin therapy should be reviewed once seizures have been controlled, because long-term therapy might not be required. However Mr GY's seizures are not yet adequately controlled.

Albumin $= 31$ g/dL

$$\frac{\text{Corrected}}{\text{phenytoin level}} = \frac{25 \text{ mg/L}}{(0.02 \times 31 \text{ g/dL}) + 0.1}$$
$$= 34.7 \text{ mg/L}$$

This high phenytoin level is likely to be the result of changing from NG to oral administration, and the subsequent increase in bioavailability (NG feeds and tubes reduce phenytoin absorption in practice). You recommend the phenytoin is withheld until the daily levels are within therapeutic range.

To establish the new daily dose it is first necessary to calculate a value for V_m (the maximum rate of metabolism):

$$V_m = \frac{(S)(F)(\text{Dose}/\tau)(K_m + \overline{C}_{ss})}{\overline{C}_{ss}}$$

where S = salt fraction, F = bioavailability, K_m = plasma concentration at which the rate of metabolism is half the maximum, $\overline{C}_{ss}$ = concentration at steady state, τ = dosage interval = 1 (day).

If K_m is assumed to be 4 mg/L (the average K_m reported in the literature), $S = 0.92$ and $F = 1.0$ then:

$$V_\mathrm{m} = \frac{0.92 \times 1 \times (250 \text{ mg/day}) \times (4 + 34.8 \text{ mg/mL})}{34.8 \text{ mg/mL}}$$

$$= 256 \text{ mg/day}.$$

Now we can calculate the dose (D) required to achieve a steady-state concentration of 15 mg/L (this is the average therapeutic range):

$$D = \frac{(V_m)(\bar{C}_{ss})(\tau)}{(K_m + \bar{C}_{ss})(S)(F)}$$

where $\bar{C}_{ss}$ = average steady-state concentration and τ = dosage interval = 1 (day).

$$D = \frac{(256 \text{ mg/day} \times 15 \text{ mg/L} \times 1 \text{ day})}{(4 + 15 \text{ mg/L}) \times 0.92 \times 1}$$

$$= 220 \text{ mg per day}$$

A daily dose of 220 mg would be difficult to administer so this is rounded to 225 mg daily. It is recommended that Mr GY be monitored closely and serum levels checked over the next few days and continue to be monitored until two steady-state phenytoin levels taken 7 days apart are found to be similar.

EXTENDED LEARNING

- Identify the basic parameters of pharmacokinetics and how they determine drug bioavailability and inform dosing regimens
- What are tonic–clonic seizures and how are they treated?
- What is *status epilepticus* and how is it treated?
- Outline the pharmaceutical considerations in the composition and administration of enteral feed solutions
- Why and when is adsorption in pharmaceutical systems important?

References and further reading

Datapharm (2013). Phenytoin electronic Summary of Product Characteristics. Available at: www.medicines.org.uk (accessed 30 September 2013).

Winter M (2004). Phenytoin. In: *Basic Clinical Pharmacokinetics*, 4th edn, Baltimore, Lippincott Williams & Wilkins: pp 321–63.

Case 11
Drug therapy of Parkinson's disease

CHARLES TUGWELL

LEARNING OUTCOMES

At the end of this case, you will be able to:

- Describe the signs and symptoms most commonly associated with Parkinson's disease
- Outline other causes of parkinsonian symptoms that might result in the misdiagnosis of Parkinson's disease
- Identify some of the key drugs used in the pharmacotherapy of Parkinson's disease and their potential adverse effects, and how these can be minimised
- Identify some clinically significant interactions that might be caused with drugs used to treat Parkinson's disease

Case study

Mrs TP is a 68-year-old woman who was diagnosed 12 months ago with Parkinson's disease.

Initially, this caused a tremor just in her left hand, but more recently this has become much worse and is now bilateral. She also finds that she often feels very stiff and she has had to give up her main hobby of embroidery because it is impossible to make the fine movements necessary to do this. She has also noticed that her handwriting has become very small.

- Comment on Mrs TP's presenting symptoms
- What are some of the other signs/symptoms of Parkinson's disease that patients may exhibit and that might develop in Mrs TP as the disease progresses?

Mrs TP is started on ropinirole at a dose of 250 micrograms three times daily. This was increased each week (by a total daily dose of 750 micrograms) until she reached a dose of 4 mg three times daily. She found the drug to be helpful once this dose was reached and was able to resume many of her activities, including her embroidery.

However, she complained of severe constipation, which she felt was caused by the drug, and the doctor noticed some peripheral oedema on examination. Despite these effects, she continues with this treatment, feeling that it is beneficial.

- ❷ Briefly outline how ropinirole works and list other drugs that have a similar pharmacological action
- ❷ Why is the dose increased gradually?
- ❷ Constipation and peripheral oedema are potential adverse effects of ropinirole. What other unwanted effects are associated with this class of drug?

Mrs TP is seen in clinic 6 months later and clearly is not as happy as she was at her previous appointment. She states that the drug is no longer working and finds it increasingly difficult to initiate movements such as getting up out of a chair. The doctor notices that she now walks with a festinating gait (characteristic involuntary movement with short accelerating steps). It is decided that co-careldopa 25/100 tablets should be added to her medication. She is told to increase the dose of this preparation each day (by adding an extra tablet) until she is taking two tablets three times a day. After 3 days, the patient telephones you to say that the new tablets make her feel very sick.

- ❷ Comment on the loss of symptom control that Mrs TP has experienced and the new symptoms she complains of
- ❷ What is co-careldopa? How does each constituent of the preparation work?
- ❷ What could be done to try to reduce the nausea that Mrs TP experiences with co-careldopa?
- ❷ If you were to recommend an antiemetic, which one would you choose and why?

Mrs TP is seen in clinic at 3-monthly intervals and her condition is now reasonably well controlled. Her GP has prescribed fluoxetine for depression and she has been on this for several weeks now, at a dose of 40 mg daily. At her appointment today it comes to light that the effects of her anti-Parkinson's disease medication wear off before the next dose is due. She is prescribed selegiline to help resolve this problem.

- ❷ Briefly comment on the development of depression in this patient
- ❷ In the treatment of Parkinson's disease, what is selegiline particularly useful for?

At the time of adding selegiline, the neurologist is unaware that Mrs TP is now taking fluoxetine. Fortunately, the community pharmacist is fully conversant with Mrs TP's medication and is concerned about the addition of selegiline.

- ❷ Is the pharmacist right to be concerned? If so, why?
- ❷ What other potential interactions might be important?

Case discussion

— Symptoms, signs and diagnosis of Parkinson's disease

Parkinson's disease is a serious central neurodegenerative disorder that results from the progressive death of dopamine-containing cells in the substantia nigra of the midbrain. Mrs TP's presentation is characteristic of Parkinson's disease. About three-quarters of patients present with a tremor. Symptoms are typically initially unilateral. The tremor associated with Parkinson's disease is usually more apparent at rest; if the hand reaches out to pick something up, the tremor reduces or stops. It is important to differentiate the tremor of Parkinson's disease from essential tremor. It is also essential to rule out other causes of tremor such as drug-induced (e.g. cinnarizine, sodium valproate, amiodarone, lithium, metoclopramide, calcium-channel blockers, SSRIs).

Mrs TP experiences stiffness and problems with dexterity; these are common symptoms. She also states that her handwriting has become very small. This is a classic sign of Parkinson's disease, which is known as micrographia.

Other symptoms associated with Parkinson's disease include:

- Hypokinesia and bradykinesia
- Postural instability
- Difficulty swallowing (dysphagia)
- Speech problems
- Depression
- Hallucinations
- Dementia
- Bladder problems
- Constipation
- Sleep problems
- Hyposmia (reduced ability to smell and discriminate odours).

— Drug therapies for Parkinson's disease

The symptoms of Parkinson's disease are due to reduced levels of dopamine in the brain. This is due to progressive degeneration of the dopamine-producing cells in the substantia nigra leading to a deficiency of the neurotransmitter dopamine. The main drug treatments for Parkinson's disease are: dopamine receptor agonists (e.g. ropinirole, see below), levodopa, which increases the amount of dopamine in the brain, and enzyme inhibitors, which block the breakdown of dopamine. These latter include MAO-BI (monoamine oxidase B inhibitors), e.g. selegiline, which inhibit intracellular breakdown in the brain, so that dopamine is effective for a longer period, and COMT (catechol-*O*-methyltransferase) inhibitors (e.g. entacapone), which inhibit breakdown of peripheral levodopa, so increasing bioavailability to the brain. These enzyme inhibitors, used together with levodopa, can help with 'end-of-dose' deterioration in symptoms.

Drug therapy does not halt disease progression, but relieves symptoms and improves quality of life.

— Pharmacology of ropinirole and drugs in the same class

As Parkinson's disease results from degeneration of certain dopaminergic pathways in the brain involved in the control of movement, treatment has always been centred on trying to replace dopaminergic function in those deficient circuits. One way of doing this is to administer directly acting dopamine receptor agonists such as ropinirole. Other drugs that act in a similar way include:

- Apomorphine
- Bromocriptine
- Cabergoline
- Pergolide
- Pramipexole
- Rotigotine.

Mrs TP's dosage of ropinirole was increased gradually to minimise the risk and severity of adverse effects. However, she experienced constipation and peripheral oedema, which are recognised adverse effects of ropinirole. Other unwanted effects that are associated with this class of drug include:

- Nausea/vomiting
- Drowsiness
- Sudden onset of sleep
- Confusion
- Hallucinations
- Hypotension
- Dyskinesias (abnormal movements).

The older, ergot derivatives (bromocriptine, cabergoline, pergolide) also cause serious pulmonary, retroperitoneal and pericardial fibrotic reactions.

— Disease progression and use of co-careldopa

Parkinson's disease is a progressive condition and one for which there is very little evidence that any of the drugs currently available reduce the rate of progression. However, drug therapy can significantly reduce the patient's symptoms, especially in the early stages of the disease. As the disease advances, careful tailoring of dosages and the combinations of drugs becomes necessary, often balancing the beneficial effects against the side effects experienced. Mrs TP's Parkinson's disease has now reached the point where ropinirole alone does not provide adequate control of her symptoms. She is finding it difficult to get out of her chair and she now walks with a significant festinating gait (trunk is flexed forward and legs are flexed at hips and knees, and steps taken when walking are short and become progressively rapid). It is often 5 years or so after initial diagnosis that gait problems become apparent.

Two preparations are available that combine levodopa with a peripheral dopa-decarboxylase inhibitor. Levodopa is a precursor to dopamine, the neurotransmitter that in Parkinson's disease is depleted in certain areas of the brain. Dopamine itself is unsuitable for replacement therapy because it is too polar to penetrate the blood–brain barrier (BBB) for delivery to the brain. Levodopa is an L-amino acid derivative that undergoes active transport across the BBB and into the brain. Levodopa is then converted to dopamine in the striatum, by the enzyme dopa-decarboxylase and thus replenishes levels of the neurotransmitter. As dopa decarboxylase is also expressed in peripheral tissue, this results in the undesirable peripheral production of dopamine and reduced availability of levodopa for CNS delivery. To reduce the amount of levodopa converted outside the brain, a peripheral dopa-decarboxylase inhibitor is included in formulations. Carbidopa (as well as benserazide) is a dopa-decarboxylase inhibitor that does not cross the BBB because it is too polar itself and is not actively transported in the same way as levodopa; this restricts its inhibitory activity to the peripheral tissues alone. Doing this reduces the amount of levodopa that needs to be taken and decreases side effects that result from peripheral utilisation. Two preparations are available: co-careldopa (levodopa + carbidopa) and co-beneldopa (levodopa + benserazide).

— **Domperidone for treatment of nausea in Parkinson's disease?**

Despite starting with a low dose of co-careldopa and increasing this gradually, Mrs TP experienced significant nausea. This is a well-recognised adverse effect. Sometimes these problems can be reduced by increasing the dosage more slowly. In some patients an antiemetic is helpful and reduces the troublesome nausea associated with taking the levodopa preparation. In patients with Parkinson's disease, the antiemetic of choice is domperidone. This drug acts at the chemoreceptor trigger zone (CTZ) in the medulla and, unlike other antiemetics, does not pass across the BBB. This reduces effects on the CNS, such as sedation and dystonia (sustained muscle contractions), the latter being likely to exacerbate the symptoms of Parkinson's disease. A dose of 10–20 mg three or four times daily is often effective.

— **Depression, the use of antidepressants and the potential for interactions with some drugs used to treat Parkinson's disease**

Depression is common in patients with Parkinson's disease. Some studies have shown that up to 50% of these patients have significant depression. In a high proportion of patients, their depression is a more significant factor in reducing their quality of life than the motor symptoms associated with Parkinson's disease. SSRIs are often used, although caution is necessary because antidepressants can worsen some of the symptoms of Parkinson's disease.

— **Selegiline**

Selegiline is a selective MAO-B inhibitor used together with levodopa preparations to reduce

'end-of-dose' deterioration, which is a problem occurring in patients with advanced disease who have been taking levodopa for some time. Selegiline blocks the breakdown of dopamine by the enzyme monoamine oxidase in certain areas of the brain, thus maintaining levels of dopamine available for synaptic transmission. Unlike carbidopa, selegiline is highly lipophilic and is able to penetrate the BBB into the brain, where its action as a MAO-B inhibitor is required. It has been found that this concomitant therapy helps retain control of symptoms until the next dose of levodopa preparation is due.

selegiline

Several reports have been published of a potentially serious interaction occurring when selegiline and fluoxetine (an SSRI) are taken together. It is generally recommended that fluoxetine should be stopped for 5 weeks before starting treatment with selegiline to avoid an adverse effect. The interaction can result in excitation of the CNS and hypertension. In one reported case, the patient's blood pressure rose to 200/120 mmHg. Other effects that have been reported with this combination include: manic behaviour, hyperactivity, confusion, ataxia, palpitations and seizures. Although the mechanism for this interaction is not clear, in many ways it is consistent with the so-called 'serotonin syndrome'.

EXTENDED LEARNING

- Explain the differences between MAO-A and MAO-B inhibitors. How do they differ in terms of potential interactions with food and other drugs?
- Where do other forms of drug therapy, not mentioned in the case study above, fit in to the potential approaches for managing Parkinson's disease?
- What new therapies are in the pipeline for the management of Parkinson's disease?
- Apart from drug therapy, what other forms of therapy can be helpful in managing the symptoms associated with Parkinson's disease?

- What is the blood–brain barrier and what are the implications for drug therapy?
- Outline the pharmacology of SSRIs

ADDITIONAL PRACTICE POINT

- Comment on the need for careful timing of drug administration for patients with Parkinson's disease.

References and further reading

Chan KL, Jagait P, Tugwell C (2004). Parkinson's disease – current and future aspects of drug treatment. *Hosp Pharmacist* 11:18–22.

National Institute for Health and Clinical Excellence (2006). *Parkinson's Disease – Diagnosis and management in primary and secondary care*. Clinical Guideline 35. London: NICE. Available at: http://guidance.nice.org.uk/CG35 (accessed 1 October 2013).

Tugwell C (2008). *Parkinson's Disease in Focus*. London: Pharmaceutical Press.

Case 12
Smoking cessation in community pharmacy
ZOE ASLANPOUR

LEARNING OUTCOMES

At the end of this case, you will be able to:

- Understand the role of pharmacists in promoting public health and smoking cessation
- Outline the behavioural support included in stages of smoking cessation programmes
- List the biomarkers used for smoking cessation and the role of carbon monoxide monitoring
- Describe the pharmacotherapy medications used in smoking cessation and their mode of action

Case study

You manage a pharmacy in a socially and economically deprived neighbourhood. As a trained smoking cessation adviser, you run a weekly smoking cessation clinic from your community pharmacy. Every March you run a 'No smoking campaign' to highlight your services in promoting the health of the community and the hard-to-reach people you serve.

- How does smoking cessation fit into the public health agenda?

Mr RS receives his prescription of antihypertensive and lipid-lowering drugs dispensed at your pharmacy on a regular basis. In March, he comes in for his prescription and asks about the success rate of the 'No smoking campaign' that you are running, because he smokes and hopes to quit.

- How would you use this opportunity to help him stop smoking?
- What information would you provide him with?

Mr RS agrees to attend your smoking cessation clinic. However, he wants to know what it would entail.

- How do you respond to Mr RS?

After attending the first session at your smoking cessation clinic, receiving advice and agreeing on a quit date, Mr RS returns the following day. He has read the leaflets that you provided at the clinic and has some questions. Mr RS would like you to explain what 'biomarkers' are and their use in the clinic, the role of the breath carbon monoxide monitor and what medications are on offer to help him to quit.

- What responses would you provide to Mr RS's questions?

Case discussion
— Smoking cessation and the public health agenda

Smoking is the biggest single cause of inequalities in death rates between the rich and poor in the UK. Babies from deprived backgrounds are more likely to be born to mothers who smoke, and have much greater exposure to environmental (passive) tobacco smoke in childhood. In the past 30 years, there has been a steady decrease in the overall prevalence of smoking in the UK. However, this decline in smoking rates has been much slower among lower-income groups. The evidence suggests that smokers in routine and manual households, and lower socioeconomic groups, are much less successful in their quit attempts and are often more addicted to smoking compared with those in managerial and professional households.

Cigarette smoking causes a wide range of diseases and conditions, including cancers, respiratory diseases, coronary heart and other circulatory diseases, stomach and duodenal ulcers, erectile dysfunction and infertility, osteoporosis, cataracts, age-related macular degeneration (leading to gradual loss of central vision) and periodontitis (severe gum disease). After surgery, smoking contributes to lower survival rates, delayed wound healing and postoperative respiratory complications. There are currently around 8.5 million smokers in England, half of whom will die as a direct result of smoking-related conditions.

The NHS Stop Smoking Services in England are part of a much wider tobacco control strategy that involves the six internationally recognisable strands:

1 Making smoking less attractive to young people
2 Encouraging as many smokers as possible to try to stop
3 Giving as much support as possible to smokers who are trying to stop
4 Protecting non-smokers from exposure to environmental (passive) tobacco smoke
5 Preventing the tobacco industry from promoting its products
6 Stopping the promotion of tobacco.

Smoking cessation interventions have been shown to be one of the most cost-effective of all life-saving treatments provided within the English healthcare system, costing approximately £1000 per life-year gained, compared with >£15 000 for the average life-saving treatment.

Each year, around 75% of all smokers contemplate quitting. However, fewer than half actually go on to make a quit attempt and only a small fraction (<3%) quit successfully. The likelihood of a successful quit is four times higher when smokers use NHS Stop Smoking Services compared with smokers who stop without any form of support. Pharmacists are one of the recognised providers of NHS Stop Smoking

Services, supporting successful implementation of this public health agenda.

— Helping patients stop smoking: behavioural support and the steps in a smoking cessation programme

Smoking cessation clinics use withdrawal-oriented therapy and a behavioural support programme. This treatment model focuses on preventing relapse in the early stages of a quit attempt by providing intensive support when withdrawal symptoms are at their worst, supervising medication use closely and emphasising the importance of complete abstinence.

Typical nicotine withdrawal symptoms include:

● Irritability/aggression
● Depression
● Restlessness
● Poor concentration
● Increased appetite
● Light-headedness
● Night time awakenings
● Craving.

Treatment is delivered by smoking advisers over six or seven sessions at weekly intervals, in groups or one to one. Both formats are shown to increase long-term success compared with minimal interventions. Community pharmacists deliver treatment to individuals on a sessional basis, and provide an alternative to clinic (group) treatment. Evidence suggests that structured smoking cessation interventions provided by trained pharmacists can increase smoking cessation rates.

To provide a smoking cessation clinic, pharmacists should attend an accredited course to enable them to work as a smoking cessation adviser. The following section is adapted from *Helping Smokers to Stop: Advice for pharmacists in England* (McRobbie and McEwen, 2005). There are four main steps in the smoking cessation programme: preparing to quit, the quit date, each week after the quit date and staying stopped.

— 1. Preparing to quit
● Explain the treatment that you offer:
  ● Evidence-based treatment combining support/advice and medication
  ● Five further sessions on a weekly basis.
● Make sure that your client is motivated to quit at this time:

- Ask: 'Are you ready to make a serious attempt to stop smoking?'
- Check that the person can attend all the treatment sessions
- Advise that if the person is not fully committed at this time, he or she can come back and see you at any time in the future.
- Make a quit date
  - Explain the importance of choosing a day to quit smoking
  - Arrange an appropriate date to quit
  - Advise the client to smoke as normal up to the quit date
  - Advise that cutting down does not work
  - Explain that the goal from the quit date onwards is 'not to have a single puff'.
- Explain the withdrawal syndrome:
  - Explain that many smokers experience a range of different symptoms when they stop (see above)
  - Reassure the client that most symptoms last, on average, between 3 and 4 weeks, and will become less severe and less frequent the longer they go without a single puff
  - Explain that medication (nicotine replacement therapy [NRT], varenicline and bupropion) will help reduce the severity of withdrawal symptoms.
- Assess the level of tobacco dependence:
  - Ask: 'How soon after waking do you smoke?' If it is within 30 min, the patient is a highly dependent smoker needing more intensive treatment and higher dose of withdrawal therapy medicine. A more quantitative method is the Fagerstöm test for nicotine dependence, which consists of six questions that assess the urgency of the patient to smoke upon waking or in situations or locations when smoking is not possible, leading to a score out of 10 for low, moderate or high dependence. An average smoker would score 4/10. The number of cigarettes smoked/day is also considered.
- Measure the carbon monoxide (CO) level in expired breath:
  - Explain that CO is one of the many harmful components of cigarette smoke inhalation that would interfere directly with the oxygen-carrying capacity of the blood
  - Explain that the breath CO level gives an indication of cigarette use

- Use the CO reading to provide motivation (the level will drop within a week of the client stopping smoking).
- Discuss available medication and arrange a supply:
  - Explain the three different types of medication currently available to treat nicotine addiction and how they work (there are no magic cures, but medication does reduce the severity of withdrawal symptoms and roughly doubles the chance of quitting success).
  - If either varenicline (Champix) or bupropion (Zyban) is the product of choice, they need to start this a week before quitting. Both are prescription-only therapies.
  - Varenicline acts as a partial agonist at $\alpha_4\beta_2$-nicotinic acetylcholine receptors (nAChRs) in the brain and, in so doing, modulates dopaminergic function in the central pleasure/reward pathway. It competes with circulating nicotine for available receptor-binding sites, but activates them less effectively than nicotine itself, consequently inhibiting nicotine's potent stimulant effect. Bupropion is, however, a non-competitive antagonist at neural $\alpha_4\beta_2$-nAChRs, inhibiting nicotine binding but without any intrinsic activity of its own. Bupropion is also an atypical antidepressant, inhibiting the reuptake of dopamine, noradrenaline and serotonin (5HT) in the CNS. Recent experimental evidence suggests that the central pharmacological activity of bupropion could be mediated by its major metabolite, *hydroxybupropion*. Side effects of both drugs include headache, insomnia and depression.

varenicline   bupropion

- If NRT is the product of choice, discuss the various different types (all available on the general sales list) and offer advice on which product might be most suitable for the patient, e.g. chewing gum (Nicotinell, NiQuitin), transdermal skin patch

(Nicopatch), microtablet (Nicorette), lozenges (Nicopass), nasal spray, mouth spray or inhaler, all designed to assist smokers to break their habit while providing a reduced dose of nicotine to help overcome withdrawal symptoms such as craving and mood changes. NRT allows a measured amount of nicotine into the bloodstream, stopping or reducing the symptoms of nicotine withdrawal without smoking. These dosage forms and routes of delivery allow therapeutic levels of nicotine to be rapidly delivered into the bloodstream on demand, or, in the case of patches, nicotine is delivered at a controlled rate over a prolonged period for up to 24 hours.

- Explain that the client will start NRT on the quit date, and show the patient how to use it.
- Arrange for a supply of medication from the GP.
- Offer advice on preparing to stop:
  - Suggest that, by the quit date, all cigarettes, lighters and ashtrays be cleared out of the house.
  - Ask the client to consider which cigarettes are going to be missed most (e.g. first one in the morning) and how they might be able to deal with this.
  - Offer strategies on how to cope with urges to smoke.
  - Suggest that they tell all their friends, family and colleagues (especially those who smoke) about their quit attempt, and ask for their support.

— 2. **The quit date**

- Ask how the client feels about quitting.
- Provide reassurance if they are worried, and reinforce the benefits of quitting.
- Measure CO in expired breath.
- Discuss medication issues.
- Varenicline and bupropion:
  - Check usage and answer any questions
  - Summarise again how it will help (reducing withdrawal)
  - Enquire about any side effects
- NRT:
  - Provide the rationale for using NRT (reduces withdrawal, increases success).
  - Ask the client to start using it, and advise on correct use and dosage.

- Reassure about initial unpleasant effects (they will get used to the taste), and any safety concerns (it does not cause cancer; provides less nicotine than cigarettes).
- Explain the importance of complete abstinence: having just a puff of a cigarette will put them right back to the beginning, while stopping completely will make it easier and they will get through the withdrawal phase more quickly.
- Advise on coping: suggest techniques such as distraction, avoiding difficult situations, taking exercise and using medication.
- Suggest where the client can obtain additional support.
- Summarise:
  - Not a single puff
  - Take it step by step
  - It will get easier over time
  - Importance of making a good start.

— 3. **Each week after the quit date**

- Discuss how the week went
- If they have been abstinent:
  - Congratulate and give praise
  - Reinforce the importance of 'not a single puff'.
- If they had a few slips:
  - Acknowledge the effort made, but reinforce the rationale of complete abstinence
  - Each slip puts them back to the quit date
  - Having the odd cigarette makes the withdrawal worse
  - They will find it much easier to stop smoking altogether.
- If they have cut down:
  - Acknowledge that cutting down might seem a good idea, but explain why it does not work
  - Explain the ability for smokers to compensate
  - Explain that they will eventually go back to smoking more
  - Explain that they are making it harder on themselves
  - Suggest setting a new quit date and reinforce the rationale of complete abstinence.
- Check for withdrawal discomfort: reassure the client that most of the withdrawal symptoms are short-lived.
- Measure breath CO to confirm abstinence and provide some motivation.

- Check on medication use:
  - Enquire about dosage and any problems with use
  - Reassure the client that he or she will become used to the unpleasant taste/sensation.

— 4. Staying stopped

At the end of treatment, it is important to give advice on preventing a relapse. There is limited evidence for any effective interventions, but a number of basic strategies can be communicated:

- Medication use:
  - Advise varenicline and bupropion users to complete the course
  - Advise NRT users that they should continue for up to 12 weeks; oral NRT or nasal spray can still be used opportunistically.
- Discuss potential relapse situations, e.g.:
  - Stress
  - Where people are smoking and cigarettes are available
  - Bereavement
  - Under the influence of alcohol
  - Holidays.
- Discuss possible coping strategies, e.g.:
  - NRT use
  - Distraction.
- Discuss any ongoing support, e.g.:
  - Returning for continued supply of NRT
  - Local stop smoking services may offer ongoing support
  - Suggest sources of additional support on line, by phone and face-to face/free NHS quit smoking app for mobile phone.

— Smoking cessation: considerations in this case

In this case, you would first explain the scientific principles that can affect the success of Mr RS's attempt to stop smoking if he does not receive support from a trained adviser. The primary reason is the smoker's dependence on nicotine. Nicotine is a psychoactive, highly poisonous drug that is very addictive, and regular smokers soon become used to the presence of nicotine in their system. Smoking an average cigarette delivers approximately 1 mg absorbed nicotine into the circulation, and 40–60 mg is fatal (note that children may become seriously ill if they accidentally ingest the nicotine contained in just one cigarette!). Stopping smoking usually brings on a withdrawal syndrome comprising a range of symptoms, including depressed mood, sleep disturbance, irritability, difficulty concentrating, increased appetite and weight, constipation and a strong craving. These symptoms, in particular, urge users to smoke, and can lead to relapse early in a quit attempt. Most withdrawal symptoms last no longer than 2–4 weeks, so assisting smokers through the first 4 weeks is important.

Mr RS is of south Asian origin and, judging by his medications, he is already at high risk of developing cardiovascular diseases which could exacerbate if he does not stop smoking. Cardiovascular disease is one of the most common causes of smoking-related mortality, accounting for over a quarter of all smoking-related deaths. The average smoker has approximately double the risk of developing heart disease prematurely compared with someone who has never smoked. Even light smokers have a substantially increased risk of cardiovascular disease.

You should explain to Mr RS that the smoking cessation clinic focuses on preventing relapse in the early stages of a quit attempt by providing intensive support when withdrawal symptoms are at their worst, supervising medication use closely and emphasising the importance of complete abstinence. The structure of a smoking cessation programme includes: a pre-quit appointment for preparation; a quit date after which 'not even one puff' on a cigarette is permitted; and up to four weekly appointments for 4 weeks after the quit date. Services encourage the use of pharmacotherapies when appropriate.

— Biomarkers used in smoking cessation: their advantages and disadvantages

- A *biomarker* is a biological feature that can be used to measure the presence or progress of disease, or the effects of treatment. In smoking cessation, biomarkers are used to measure smoke intake or its consequences on physiological systems. They are also used in motivating smokers to become and remain abstinent.
- The two main biomarkers used in smoking cessation are expired air CO and salivary *cotinine.*
- CO is a poisonous gas contained in cigarette smoke that causes heart disease. Expired air CO is the standard biomarker for smoking in clinical practice and, when the smoker is enrolled in a smoking cessation programme, its level gets monitored routinely. The regular

monitoring of the expired CO level for a smoking quitter shows the client objective proof of improved health after they have stopped smoking completely, and to check whether they really have stopped smoking.

- CO is a good measure of smoke intake on the day, but it will not usually detect smoking the day before. The level of CO is built up over the course of the day, so its level is typically lower in the morning than the afternoon. The standard cut-off for detecting smoking is 10 p.p.m. but in practice it is rare to see levels >5 p.p.m. in non-smokers.

- Cotinine is a lactam (cyclic amide) metabolite of nicotine that is eliminated more slowly from the body than nicotine itself. Around 70–80% of nicotine undergoes metabolism in the liver (via CYP2A6, then cytoplasmic aldehyde oxidase) to give cotinine. It can be measured in urine, blood and saliva using laboratory analysis, with saliva collection being the most frequently used. It is by far the most accurate measure of smoking intake and also works very well for detecting exposure to environmental, so-called 'passive', tobacco smoke. However, the disadvantage of this method is that it cannot distinguish between actual smoking and NRT use, because nicotine absorbed from either means of administration will be metabolised in the same way. There are occasions when it is useful to measure cotinine in clinical practice, such as smoking cessation in pregnancy. It lasts for several days in the body so is better than CO at detecting intermittent or low levels of smoking; the optimal cut-off for detecting smoking is 13 ng/mL.

nicotine → (CYP2A6 then aldehyde oxidase) → cotinine

— **International perspectives and smoking**
Over 80% of the world's smokers live in low- and middle-income countries. As prevalence of smoking has declined in many of the high-income countries, there is concern that smoking rates may rise dramatically among populations where they were previously low. Contributory factors include tobacco companies seeking out new markets, increased availability and affordability, changing cultural perspectives and acceptability, and a lack of awareness of risks. Smoking is recognised as a major risk factor for many chronic diseases, which are becoming a main cause of premature death worldwide. Concerted action to contain smoking uptake, and promote quit rates, is an international priority. The World Health Organization advocates a broad strategy including enforcement of bans on smoking advertising, promotion and sponsorship, alongside public health initiatives to reduce uptake, support people to quit and protect people (especially children) from the risk of second-hand passive smoke in public places, cars and the home.

EXTENDED LEARNING

- What are e-cigarettes? How do they work and how useful are they as an effective method of NRT? Are they recommended clinically?

- How useful are herbal cigarettes, acupuncture and hypnosis as aids to giving up smoking?

- What is the role of NRT in pregnancy and breastfeeding?

- Smoking cessation advice is one of the many opportunities that pharmacists have for promoting public health. What other public health roles are available for pharmacists?

- Discuss the formulation, preparation and drug delivery of nicotine replacement from: chewing gum, patches, inhalers, tablets, lozenges, nasal sprays and mouth sprays.

References and further reading

DiClemente CC, Prochaska JO, Fairhurst SK, Velicer WF, Velasquez MM, Rossi JS (1991). The process of smoking cessation: An analysis of precontemplation, contemplation, and preparation stages of change. *J Consult Clin Psychol* 59:295–304.

Lancaster T, Stead LF. (2005). Individual behavioural counselling for smoking cessation. *Cochrane Database Syst Rev* 2:CD001292.

McRobbie H, McEwen A (2005). *Helping Smokers to Stop: Advice for pharmacists in England*. London: NICE, Royal Pharmaceutical Society of Great Britain and PharmacyHealthLink.

National Institute for Health and Clinical Excellence (2006). *Brief interventions and referral for smoking cessation (PH1).* London: NICE. Available at: www.nice.org.uk/PH1 (accessed 7 April 2014).

National Institute for Health and Clinical Excellence. (2008). *Smoking Cessation Services in Primary Care, Pharmacies, Local Authorities and Workplaces, particularly for Manual Working Groups, Pregnant Women and Hard to Reach Communities (PH10).* London: NICE. Available at: http://guidance.nice.org.uk/PH10 (accessed 7 April 2014).

National Institute for Health and Clinical Excellence (2010). *NICE Implementation Uptake Report: Smoking cessation drugs.* London: NICE. Available at: www.nice.org.uk/media/D79/42/UptakeReportSmokingCessationPublication.pdf (accessed 7 April 2014).

Case 13
Dementia/Alzheimer's disease

ANNETT BLOCHBERGER

LEARNING OUTCOMES

At the end of this case, you will be able to

- Outline the pathophysiology, signs, symptoms and diagnosis of dementia
- Describe the treatment options in different stages of Alzheimer's disease including monitoring parameters for effectiveness and side effects
- Describe the chemistry and mechanism of action of donepezil
- Recognise the importance of challenging antipsychotic prescribing in dementia
- Describe the type of help with medication that carers (family and friends) often provide, and some of the problems that they can encounter

Case study

Mr TS, an 85-year-old retired interpreter, was referred to the memory clinic at the local hospital by his GP. The referral was triggered by several incidents where Mr TS was found wandering the streets at night in his pyjamas because he had locked himself out of his house.

Mr TS attends the clinic with his wife who complains that her husband has become increasingly forgetful. On several occasions, he mistook the television remote control for the telephone, put the keys into the freezer and did not seem to recognise his grown-up children when they visited. Mr TS's skill of being fluent in five different European languages is being compromised by word-finding difficulties; however, he enjoys visits from former colleagues who engage him in conversations about the past.

After several tests and full examination, the consultant considers a probable diagnosis of Alzheimer's disease of moderate severity.

❓ How is the diagnosis of Alzheimer's disease confirmed?

❓ What other forms of dementia exist? Consider pathophysiology, signs and symptoms

❓ What are the treatment options at this stage?

Mr TS is started on the acetylcholinesterase inhibitor donepezil – 5 mg daily. Two weeks later, Mr TS's wife hands in a prescription for 10 mg daily. On questioning, Mrs S complains that she does not see any improvement in her husband. She also expresses concerns about his recent stomach problems and nausea.

❓ Draw the structure of donepezil. Which structural features and physicochemical properties are important in its clinical use?

❓ What is the rationale behind the choice of treatment?

❓ How should the treatment be monitored?

❓ What would your response be to the concerns raised by Mrs S?

A couple of months later, Mrs S presents a prescription for quetiapine for her husband and a prescription for citalopram for herself. You notice that the addresses on the prescriptions are different. Mrs S explains that she was initially very keen to look after her husband at home but the decision was made to move him into a care home after a fire incident at home. Since the move, Mr TS seems more confused and aggressive, especially when Mrs S is leaving after visiting hours. The carers told her the medication is necessary to calm him down as Mr TS wanders around a lot and does not seem to settle during the night. Mrs S asks you about the medication for her husband because she is not sure what 'it will do to him'.

- ❓ What are the social pharmacy issues in this case?
- ❓ What would you advise Mrs S?
- ❓ What other steps could you take to support Mr TS and his family?

Case discussion

— Dementia: signs, symptoms and differential diagnosis

The term 'dementia' describes a group of progressive neurodegenerative brain diseases that result in a decline in cognitive functions (such as memory, thinking, orientation, comprehension, calculation, learning capability and judgement) with an effect on the ability to execute activities of daily living. Non-cognitive symptoms such as impaired emotional control, social behaviour and motivation may also be present. Dementia is mainly a disease of the elderly, with a disproportionate increase after the eighth decade of life.

The most common cause of dementia is Alzheimer's disease (AD), followed by vascular cognitive impairment (VCI), dementia with Lewy bodies (DLB) and frontotemporal dementia (FTD). Dementia is also commonly seen as part of several neurological disorders such as Parkinson's disease (Parkinson's disease dementia – PDD) and Huntington's disease. Severe depression can also sometimes cause a 'pseudo-dementia'.

There is no definitive laboratory or imaging test available to confirm the diagnosis of dementia before death. Accurate diagnosis therefore relies on clinical examination, history taking and cognitive tests. Screening blood tests are undertaken to rule out reversible causes of cognitive impairment such as dehydration, thyroid abnormalities, malignancies, as well as renal, cardiac and liver disease. Brief cognitive tests, such as the Mini-Mental State Examination (MMSE), Abbreviated Mental Test Score (AMTS) and Addenbrooke's Cognitive Examination (ACE) are useful to support diagnosis and determine the severity of the disease. Some patients require more detailed neuropsychological assessment, especially in very mild or atypical cases, and where

depression or other mood symptoms are present. Brain imaging with CT or MRI is indicated in all patients with a suspected organic cause of dementia. Other tests sometimes used in the diagnosis include cerebrospinal fluid (CSF) examination and functional neuroimaging (e.g. positron emission tomography [PET] or single photon emission computed tomography [SPECT]).

Due to the lack of definitive screening tools, the diagnosis should always be made by a specialist skilled in cognitive assessments. Referral to the local memory clinic or dementia clinic is advisable.

— Types of dementia

Alzheimer's disease: a postmortem examination of the brain would show characteristic changes of the brain morphology with the presence of amyloid plaques between nerve cells and neurofibrillary tangles within neurons, both of which are thought to contribute to the progressive neuronal degeneration. β-Amyloid is a protein fragment found normally in the brain, which is derived from a longer amyloid precursor protein (APP). In healthy brain, β-amyloid is broken down and eliminated, but, in Alzheimer's disease, these fragments accumulate to form insoluble amyloid plaques. Neurofibrillary tangles are also insoluble twisted fibres of tau protein, coded by the MAPT (microtubule-associated protein tau) gene, which, together with tubulin, normally forms part of the intracellular axonal microtubule network involved in transporting nutrients from one part of the neuron to another. In AD, this tau protein becomes abnormal (hyperphosphorylated), so the microtubule structures do not assemble correctly and collapse and aggregate to form tangles.

The onset of AD is usually insidious over several months if not years. Profound short-term memory loss is usually an early feature with progression to global cognitive dysfunction. Recently learned information cannot be retained. Non-amnesic features such as deficits in word finding, impaired ability to identify objects or recognise faces (visuospatial), impaired reasoning, judgement and problem solving (executive dysfunction) are also present. Behavioural changes are common during the later stages of the disease, but can sometimes precede cognitive symptoms.

The cause of AD is largely unknown; several risk factors such as advancing age, head trauma, metabolic syndrome, diabetes, hypertension and genetics have been postulated. A small proportion of patients develop AD due to dominant mutations in genes involved in amyloid processing (presenilins I and II, APP). These are typically of early onset (aged <60 years).

Vascular cognitive impairment: is caused by cell death, which is attributable to ischaemic events (stroke, hypertension) and can be attributed to vascular risk factors (smoking, diabetes, atrial fibrillation). Onset is usually more sudden with a stepwise decline (e.g. after a stroke). Cell death can be observed on a brain scan. Patients may present predominantly with emotional instability followed by cognitive deficits during the course of the disease. Cognitive impairment depends on the affected brain area. A common pattern is diffuse small vessel disease, which typically causes cognitive slowing and executive dysfunction.

Dementia with Lewy bodies and Parkinson's disease dementia: may be considered as the same disease at opposite ends of the spectrum. Both are characterised pathologically by the presence of Lewy bodies in the brain, which contain abnormal deposits of a protein called α-synuclein. Which term is applied depends largely on time of onset of cognitive impairments in relation to the onset of motor symptoms. Both dementias present with visual hallucinations, a fluctuating picture of cognition and a high incidence of falls.

Frontotemporal dementia: also follows an insidious and slowly progressive pattern. Onset is usually earlier in life. First signs include behavioural changes (disinhibition, self-neglect, poor judgement) and difficulties with language. Memory loss is not usually a feature of early disease. Cognitive function tests may yield 'normal' cognition in pure behavioural cases because they do not test frontal lobe function. In most cases of FTD, brain pathology demonstrates abnormal deposits of either tau protein (so-called 'tauopathies') or transactivation response (Tar) DNA binding protein of 43 kDa (TDP-43) (so called 'TDP-43-opathies').

— **Treatment options for AD**

There is currently no cure for AD (or any other neurodegenerative form of dementia). However, several strategies (pharmacological and non-pharmacological) are available to influence and improve the situation for patients and carers affected by AD.

Pharmacological treatment options include the acetylcholinesterase inhibitors (AChEIs) donepezil, rivastigmine and galantamine, and the NMDA-receptor antagonist, memantine. The rationale behind using AChEIs is based on the cholinergic deficit found in AD and DLB/PDD, whereas NMDA-receptor inhibition is thought to influence glutamate-mediated destruction of cholinergic synapses.

AChEIs are licensed for treatment of mild-to-moderate AD. However, it is important to understand that the drugs affect only cognitive symptoms (comparable to stepping back in time once). The underlying neurodegenerative disease continues to progress at the same rate during treatment. The response to the drugs varies considerably among patients: the scale ranges from no response at all to substantial improvement for a minority. It should be borne in mind that even a small improvement leading to better function could reduce the burden of a carer. It is controversial whether drug treatment delays admission to care home facilities. A regular review of the patient is important to ensure ongoing clinical need and monitor for adverse reactions.

Initiation of AChEIs is not recommended during acute hospital or rehabilitation admissions. The impact of the change in environment on a person with dementia is profound and a true assessment of the treatment effect is impossible.

— **Chemical structure and properties of donepezil**

donepezil

Donepezil is a low polarity drug. The structure consists primarily of non-polar C–H and C–C bonds, and contains only a few electronegative atoms, with four hydrogen-bond acceptors and zero hydrogen-bond donors. On the basis of this low polarity, one might expect the drug to diffuse passively across the blood–brain barrier (BBB) in order to exert its central effects. However, the drug also contains a basic tertiary amino group (pK_a of the conjugate acid is around 9.1), which would be >90% protonated, and therefore ionised, at physiological pH. Protonated donepezil is considerably more polar and much less likely to diffuse across the BBB, but there is sufficient unionised (deprotonated) drug present at equilibrium to allow some penetration into the CNS. There is also evidence that some protonated donepezil undergoes active transport across the BBB via organic cation transporters (OCTs).

Donepezil also contains a chiral centre. The drug is manufactured and administered as a racemic mixture. Unusually, both *R* and *S* enantiomers seem to be equally active as AChEIs. The two enantiomers also rapidly interconvert in plasma through conversion of the ketone functional group to an enol and back again.

— Rationale for treatment choice

There are no clinical trials comparing the effects of different AChEIs in AD directly. Choosing an agent will therefore depend on co-morbidities, tolerability, choice and cost, because all three agents are similar with regard to their effects on symptoms. Common side effects, mediated by an increase of peripheral acetylcholine levels, are mainly of a GI nature (e.g. diarrhoea, nausea, vomiting, stomach cramps, dyspepsia). They can be reduced by slow dose titration in monthly increments, e.g. in the case vignette above, it would normally be recommended to increase donepezil from 5 mg daily to 10 mg daily after a minimum of 4 weeks. If intolerable side effects occur, slower titration or switching to another agent may be indicated.

After an initial treatment period of up to 3 months, an assessment of the effect should be undertaken (cognitive tests, carer's view). Treatment should be discontinued if there is no effect on the maximum tolerated dose. Switching to another agent is not recommended at this stage.

— NMDA-receptor antagonist

Memantine is considered as a treatment option in severe AD, or if AChEIs are not tolerated or contraindicated in patients with moderate AD. Titration should be undertaken slowly in order to minimise the risk of side effects (hallucinations, increasing confusion, dizziness and tiredness). It is available as a liquid to aid titration and administration in swallowing difficulties. The effect of the drug should be monitored regularly and discontinued if deemed ineffective. Again, the view of the carer needs to be taken into account

because assessment of the patient will become increasingly difficult with advanced dementia.

— Treatment options of behavioural symptoms

Non-drug management is preferred; methods include music therapy, aromatherapy, massage, changes in environment, avoidance of precipitating factors and appropriate activities. Precipitating factors such as pain, anxiety and acute illness (infection) must be ruled out and addressed. Pharmacological treatment should be considered as a last resort.

Neuroleptic drugs for management of non-cognitive symptoms are indicated only for a minority of patients with dementia. The higher risk of stroke, an increased mortality and increased side effects have to be balanced against potential benefit. Although risperidone is the only licensed antipsychotic for this indication, quetiapine is used as well. If use is unavoidable, the lowest effective dose should be prescribed with very frequent reviews.

— The role of carers: pharmacy and wider considerations

Many patients with memory problems will depend on carers (family members and friends) for assistance with many aspects of daily living. This often includes help with medicines. Older people can be taking a large number of medicines, including different formulations, which may require dosing at different times throughout the day, and sometimes the night. Carers may be checking when new supplies are needed, ordering and collecting them from a surgery or pharmacy. They may help in the administration of medicines, e.g. reminding, opening containers, ensuring the correct dose and timing, administering liquids, eyedrops, topical formulations, assisting with inhalation devices. As well as these everyday tasks, carers sometimes have concerns about the appropriateness of a medicine or possible side effects.

Pharmacists, who often have contact with carers when supplying medicines, may be able to help and advise, e.g. they can undertake medication reviews and make recommendations in terms of rationalising regimens. In discussion with the carers, the timing or formulations of the medication can be adapted to ensure that the needs of all parties are addressed. Pharmacists can ensure that the carer is informed about and understands any changes to medicines or regimens. They may also be able to signpost other agencies such as support groups, respite care, social services or community organisations.

EXTENDED LEARNING

- Outline the pharmacology of acetylcholinesterase inhibitors
- Describe the treatment of severe AD with memantine
- What are the treatment options for other forms of dementia?

References and further reading

Banerjee S (2009). *The Use of Antipsychotic Medication for People with Dementia: Time for action.* London: Department of Health.

Birks J (2006). Cholinesterase inhibitors for Alzheimer's disease. *Cochrane Database Syst Rev* 1:CD005593.

Birks J, Harvey RJ (2006) Donepezil for dementia due to Alzheimer's disease. *Cochrane Database Syst Rev* 1: CD001190.

Birks J, Grimley Evans J, Iakovidou V, Tsolaki M (2009). Rivastigmine for Alzheimer's disease. *Cochrane Database Syst Rev* 2:CD001191.

Kolarova M, García-Sierra F, Bartos A, Ricny J, Ripova D (2012). Structure and pathology of tau protein in Alzheimer disease. *Int J Alzheimer's Dis* Article ID 731526, doi:10.1155/2012/731526.

Loy C, Schneider L (2006). Galantamine for Alzheimer's disease and mild cognitive impairment. *Cochrane Database Syst Rev* 1:CD001747.

Mullane K, Williams M (2013). Alzheimer's therapeutics: continued clinical failures question the validity of the amyloid hypothesis – but what lies beyond? *Biochem Pharmacol* 85:289–305.

National Institute for Health and Clinical Excellence (2006). *Dementia: Supporting people with dementia and their carers in health and social care.* Clinical Guideline 42. Available at: www.nice.org.uk/guidance/cg42 (accessed 30 September 2013).

National Institute for Health and Clinical Excellence (2011). *Donepezil, Galantamine, Rivastigmine and Memantine for the Treatment of Alzheimer's Disease.* Technology Appraisal 217. Available at: www.nice.org.uk/guidance/TA217 (accessed 30 September 2013).

Case 14
Dementia and its pharmacotherapy

NELA RONČEVIĆ ASHTON AND SAMIR VOHRA

LEARNING OUTCOMES

At the end of this case, you will be able to:

- Outline the differences between different types of dementia
- Explain the mechanism of action of the drugs used to treat Alzheimer's disease and how this affects their use
- Explore the various formulations of the drugs used in the treatment of Alzheimer's disease

Case study

Mrs OL is 73 years old and lives with her 70-year-old husband. Over time, her husband noticed that she was always losing her keys or purse. Her husband realised that something serious was wrong when his wife went to the toilets at the airport and disappeared. She was found wandering around the terminal building, by the airport security officer.

❓ List and describe the different types of dementia with reference to their pathology

After being referred to a specialist, Mrs OL is diagnosed with Alzheimer's disease with an MMSE score of 24/30.

❓ What is an MMSE?
❓ What does an MMSE score of 24/30 signify?

You are the practice pharmacist and the GP has referred Mrs OL to you for a medication review. She is prescribed the following medications:

Simvastatin 40 mg at night (for post-myocardial infarction)

Bendroflumethiazide 2.5 mg (for high blood pressure)

Promethiazine 25 mg at night (to help her sleep)

Salbutamol 100 micrograms one or two puffs when required (for asthma)

❷ Would you change any of Mrs OL's existing medication?

Mrs OL is prescribed donepezil 5 mg at bedtime. She is asthmatic and has had a heart attack in the past. She has also previously been treated with Helicobacter pylori *eradication treatment.*

❷ Is donepezil a good choice for Mrs OL?

Answer this by considering:

- *The mechanism of action of the different drugs currently used to treat Alzheimer's disease and why some of these drugs need to be used with caution in asthma and chronic obstructive pulmonary disease (COPD), some types of cardiovascular disease (CVD) and peptic ulcer disease*
- *NICE (National Institute for Health and Care Excellence) and the issue of cost.*
- *Were there other non-drug treatments that should have been tried first?*

Mrs OL has been feeling nauseous and dizzy since starting donepezil.

❷ What would you do to assist Mrs OL in tolerating upward titration of the medication?

Around 10 months later, Mrs OL's cognition deteriorates further. Her MMSE score drops to 12/30. Her husband, who cares for her and assists her with medicines, wishes to support her at home for as long as possible.

❷ What would be the next step in her treatment?
❷ What medication activities may her husband be undertaking? What challenges might these present?

One year later, Mrs OL is in a care home. Her husband could not cope with her care any more and had to make this difficult decision. Mrs OL's memory has deteriorated dramatically. She has started to display some agitation and this disturbs other residents.

❷ Would it be appropriate to prescribe an antipsychotic drug for Mrs OL?
❷ What factors need to be considered before starting an antipsychotic? Think about the choice of drugs available, dose, monitoring required and the timescale for review

Some time later, the staff report that Mrs OL is regularly spitting her tablets out and so is not really taking her medication.

❷ Can Mrs OL's tablets be crushed? Consider the legal issues with regard to this
❷ Describe the advantages and disadvantages of the different formulations of the drugs used in the treatment of Alzheimer's disease

Case discussion

— Different types of dementia and differences in their pathology

Dementia involves memory loss, personality changes and difficulty in carrying out daily activities, progressing into self-neglect. It becomes particularly distressing for the families when it develops into eating problems, incontinence, delusions and behavioural changes, including aggression.

The dementia diagnosis requires involvement of a specialist. There are generally four types of dementia with different pathologies, but can present as mixed:

- Alzheimer's disease: the most common type of dementia, characterised by memory loss progressing to cognition loss with appearance of neurofibrillary tangles and amyloid plaques in the brain tissue
- Lewy body dementia: differs from AD in the pattern of symptoms and appearance of amyloid plaques in subcortical and cortical regions; seems to lie somewhere between Parkinson's disease and dementia
- Vascular dementia: characterised by ischaemic or haemorrhagic lesions, the risk factors for vascular dementia largely overlap with risks for CVD
- Frontotemporal dementias: earlier onset dementias, often characterised by changes in personality and language disturbances rather than memory or intellect loss
- Other: atypical dementia, Parkinson's disease dementia, HIV dementia, Creutzfeldt–Jakob disease.

— Assessing disease progression: MMSE test

The most commonly used way of assessing progression of the disease is the MMSE score (or Folstein's test), which is expressed out of 30, stratifying the dementia into mild, moderate or severe. The test involves a series of simple questions to assess basic abilities in arithmetic,

donepezil   galantamine   rivastigmine   memantine

memory recall and orientation (to time/place). A score $\geq 25/30$ generally indicates normal cognition. Lower scores would then be suggestive of mild (19–24), moderate (10–18) or severe (≤ 9) cognitive impairment. It is important to note that the outcome of the MMSE test is not absolutely diagnostic of dementia, because other mental disorders and/or physical disabilities could also affect the score outcome. Mrs OL's score appears to drop from near normal to moderate impairment as her condition slowly progresses.

— Choices and effectiveness of treatment for cognitive function and when to start them

There is a lot of public pressure in dealing with this highly emotive patient condition. Addressing the social care of an increasing number of patients is probably more important and realistic rather than the expectation of a 'miracle cure'.

Currently licensed treatments for dementia in the UK include AChEIs: donepezil, galantamine and rivastigmine and the glutamate N-methyl D-aspartate (NMDA)-type receptor antagonist, memantine. Modest but consistent effectiveness has been shown by improvement in MMSE scores in clinical trials.

AChEIs prolong the action of acetylcholine (ACh) at central synapses. Their use in the symptomatic treatment of Alzheimer's dementia is based on the so-called 'cholinergic hypothesis' wherein decreased cholinergic transmission and impaired memory are associated with the progressive loss of cholinergic projection neurones in the basal forebrain. Enhancing the action of released ACh from intact cholinergic neurones is thus a form of replacement therapy akin to the use of L-dopa as a synthetic precursor to replace deficient dopamine in the treatment of Parkinson's disease. As might be expected, AChEIs cause mostly cholinergic side effects, i.e. nausea, vomiting, diarrhoea and anorexia, but tolerance

often develops during titration. They are licensed for use in mild-to-moderate dementia; however, such therapy affords only palliative relief of AD symptoms and does not slow down or reverse the underlying progressive neurodegeneration of the disease. Interestingly, rivastigmine inhibits both acetylcholinesterase (AChE) and butyrylcholinesterase (BuChE), which can also hydrolyse ACh and therefore play a role in cholinergic neurotransmission. Apparently, BuChE can compensate for decreased levels of AChE in the AD brain so a dual inhibition of both cholinesterases should provide a better improvement in cholinergic function and cognition in AD, as appears to be the case in more recent clinical trials.

Memantine has been licensed for use in moderate-to-severe dementia, based on the hypothesis that an excess of central glutamatergic neurotransmission, resulting in neuronal excitotoxicity, is also involved in AD pathology. Memantine acts as a low-affinity, voltage-dependent, uncompetitive antagonist at glutamatergic NMDA-receptor/ion channels, thereby blocking their activity in a 'use-dependent' manner. It is generally well tolerated: side effects include dizziness, headache, hypertension, sleepiness and balance disorders. Seizures and psychosis have also been reported, suggesting a need for caution when using this drug for long-term AD treatment or in combination with other drugs.

In 2011, NICE Technology Appraisal 217 amended the previous recommendation to include AChEIs as an option for the management and treatment of mild AD and memantine as an option for people who cannot take AChEIs and in severe AD. The drug of lowest acquisition cost should be started by a specialist and in consultation with carers, but also reviewed regularly for benefit and risk assessment in terms of behavioural, psychiatric and cognitive changes. Other AChEIs may be considered, based on their side-effect profiles and dosage forms.

There is also a range of non-pharmacological psychosocial interventions with evidence to improve patients' cognitive and behavioural symptoms also recommended by NICE for all types of dementia, such as cognitive–behavioural therapy, reminiscence therapy, cognitive stimulation, music, life review recreational activity or sensory stimulation. However, availability of these interventions varies across the country.

Trials with vitamin E and *Gingko biloba* have yielded no evidence to support their usage.

— **Medication review issues in dementia**

Medication review is an important aspect of patient care in chronic conditions and especially so in older people. In the early stages of dementia, medication with sedative and anticholinergic action may worsen the cognitive symptoms, and alternatives should be considered. Untreated or inadequately treated depression can be misdiagnosed as dementia.

It is important to remember that a patient with dementia has got the same rights as other patients to be assessed and treated for cardiovascular risk with drugs such as statins, antiplatelets and antihypertensives, and their families should be consulted about such treatments.

As the patient's condition deteriorates, we may consider that the benefit of prevention of cardiovascular disease (CVD) is outweighed by the risk, e.g. a bed-bound patient struggling to take tablets may not get much benefit from CVD prevention treatment.

— **Behavioural issues in dementia and treatment**

Some distressing behavioural changes may develop in progressed disease, including depression, anxiety, shouting, aggression and wandering. Non-drug approaches including early assessment and individual care plans that address the patient's behaviour should be attempted as per NICE guidance. Pain relief assessment may be appropriate and medication should be adjusted accordingly. Other co-morbid conditions such as depression should be identified and treated, although the most recent trials suggest that use of some established antidepressants such as sertraline or mirtazapine offer no significant clinical advantage over placebo, in treating depression in AD patients.

Behavioural symptoms such as agitation, aggression and delusion are also commonly experienced by people with dementia. Although in some cases antipsychotic medication may be helpful, the overall benefits of these drugs are questioned. The high level of inappropriate prescribing of these agents to dementia patients has been challenged and recent policy documents across the UK have called for a review and reduction in their use. In some cases, they may be considered and tried, but this should not be a first resort and the effects should be carefully monitored and patients regularly assessed.

Two issues arise with regard to the adverse effects of these drugs. First, antipsychotics increase the risk of causing stroke and transient ischaemic attack (TIA) and therefore sudden death. As part of any prescribing decision that includes an assessment of risks and benefits, patients and carers should be aware of these potential problems. Second, these drugs can have a side-effect profile that can impact significantly on these patients' quality of life. Some of these side effects are behavioural symptoms not dissimilar from those that are typical of the disease, e.g. restlessness, agitation, irritability, social withdrawal. Side effects are often marked; it should not be assumed that they are signs of disease progression. Others include excessive sedation, Parkinson's disease-like symptoms and GI tract disturbances.

Thus, antipsychotics should not be considered as a first-line therapy for behavioural symptoms. If they are to be prescribed for a trial period, starting doses should be low and duration of therapy limited.

— **Medicine taking by patients with swallowing difficulties (dysphagia)**

In the later stages of dementia, patients may lose the swallowing function and, therefore, taking tablets becomes impossible. However, it cannot be assumed that they are not refusing consent to take medication, and therefore mixing their medication with food is against the code of ethics of the Nursing and Midwifery Council and is classified as deception.

Licensed liquids or alternative licensed preparations such as soluble tablets or patches are available for many medicines. Crushing licensed tablets, provided that there are data to support this 'off-licence' usage (e.g. enteric-coated formulations would not be crushed because this would modify the release profile of the drug), is preferred rather than the use of unlicensed liquids, which, in addition, can be very expensive. Donezepil is available as a small film-coated tablet or an orodispersible tablet. The latter is taken by placing on the tongue and being allowed to disintegrate before swallowing, either with or without water.

Liquid nutritional supplements may be required with essential dietician input and review.

— Looking to the future

As a consequence of many complex political, social and economic factors, changing fertility and mortality rates, populations throughout the world are ageing. This process is referred to as a *demographic transition*. Rising proportions of older people in the population have an impact on total disease burden. Older people are more likely to have long-term illness and co-morbidities, thus leading to greater demand for healthcare. Alongside this demographic transition is an epidemiological transition, i.e. changing patterns of disease. The most marked have been shifts from mortality from infectious disease to chronic diseases (especially CVD, diabetes, respiratory disease and cancer). However, partly as a consequence of ageing populations, rising neurological disease (especially the dementias and Parkinson's disease) is becoming a public health priority. Supporting these patients and their carers requires huge and increasing resources across medical and social care.

Research into AD and other dementias is recognised as a huge priority. Preventive and therapeutic options at present are so limited. An important focus of current research is exploration of pathophysiological mechanisms that contribute to different types of dementia so that potential new therapies can be identified.

Current AD research is tending towards an earlier identification and treatment of the disease in the hope that this will produce a more positive long-term clinical outcome. The main strategies are focused on reducing the production and aggregation of insoluble amyloid-β (Aβ) peptides identified as 'amyloid plaques' between nerve cells in the AD brain, and also the formation of intracellular neurofibrillary tangles due to deposition of abnormal hyperphosphorylated tau protein; both of these changes are believed to contribute to the progress of neuronal

degeneration in AD dementia. Novel drugs being developed include inhibitors of β-secretase (involved in the production of Aβ peptide fragments from the amyloid precursor protein [APP]), drugs that inhibit Aβ aggregation or disrupt aggregates, drugs that promote Aβ clearance and drugs aimed at preventing tau protein phosphorylation or fibrillisation. Whether these strategies will lead to a new, safe and clinically effective therapy for AD in the near future remains to be seen.

Alternatively, a different therapeutic approach may be required, which considers the fact that AD, similar to a number of other serious neurodegenerative disorders (e.g. Parkinson's disease, amyotrophic lateral sclerosis and multiple sclerosis), has a significant uninhibited neuroinflammatory component that may be contributing to the pathology. Chronic treatments with anti-inflammatory drugs have, however, so far proved ineffective in halting the progress of AD; thus a more specific targeting of the harmful versus the protective inflammatory pathways in the brain may be necessary.

EXTENDED LEARNING

- What is the pathophysiology of different types of dementia?

- What are the side-effect profiles for each inhibitor? How will these impact on patient tolerability and how will you address any compliance issues?

- What are the benefits of non-pharmacological therapy and the socioeconomic issues affecting their provision?

References and further reading

Enciu AM, Popescu BO (2013). Is there a causal link between inflammation and dementia? *Biomed Res Int* **316**:495.

Husband A, Worsley A (2006). Different types of dementia. *Pharm J* **277**:579–82.

Husband A, Worsley A (2006). Understanding Alzheimer's disease. *Pharm J* **277**:643–6.

National Institute for Health and Clinical Excellence (2006). *Dementia: Supporting people with dementia and their carers in health and social care.* Clinical Guideline 42. Available at: www.nice.org.uk/guidance/cg42 (accessed 30 September 2013).

Nordberg A, Ballard C, Bullock R, Darreh-Shori T, Somogyi M (2013). A review of butyrylcholinesterase as a therapeutic target in the treatment of Alzheimer's disease. *Prim Care Companion CNS Disord* **15**(2):ii.

Obulesu M, Jhansilakshmi M (2013). Neuroinflammation in Alzheimer's disease: An understanding of physiology and pathology. *Int J Neurosci* **124**:227–35.

Rafii MS (2013). Update on Alzheimer's disease therapeutics. *Rev Recent Clin Trials* **8**:110–18.

Rampa A, Gobbi S, Belluti F, Bisi A (2013). Emerging targets in neurodegeneration: new opportunities for Alzheimer's disease treatment? *Curr Top Med Chem* **13**:1879–904.

5

Infections cases

INTRODUCTION

This section contains 14 cases that are based primarily on patients presenting with bacterial or viral infections affecting a variety of body systems. Different types of pathogens, and the anti-infective therapeutic regimens to manage infections caused by them, are discussed. Many cases deal with factors relating to the prevention, diagnosis and treatment of infections, including surgical antibiotic prophylaxis, screening for *Chlamydia* sp., antibiotic-associated diarrhoea and travel immunisation.

typhoid are discussed, together with potential differential diagnoses for an unwell patient who has recently visited a tropical region. The case details the investigations carried out after admission and the consequences that the results have for management of the patient. The chemistry and mode of action of the fluoroquinolone and cephalosporin classes of antimicrobials are also discussed, alongside potential alternative anti-infective drugs. Finally, the structural differences between Gram-positive and Gram-negative microorganisms, and advice that should be given to patients travelling to countries in which typhoid is endemic, are outlined.

Case 1
Cellulitis and MRSA ► 173

This case concerns a patient admitted to hospital after worsening of cellulitis for which flucloxacillin and ampicillin had already been prescribed. The possible presentations, causes and management of cellulitis are discussed, along with the influence that a patient's weight, and renal and hepatic function may have on antibiotic chemotherapy. The evolution of the patient's treatment plan is described, moving from intravenous penicillins to vancomycin when microbiological sensitivities become known. Additional issues considered include the chemistry of the penicillins, patient-specific dosing of vancomycin, infection control practices with MRSA infections, intravenous-to-oral switching of antibiotics and bacterial resistance in general.

Case 2
Typhoid ► 178

This case describes a patient presenting to the hospital accident and emergency department (A&E) with a history of recent travel to Africa and symptoms suggestive of infection by *Salmonella typhi*. The signs and symptoms associated with

Case 3
Community-acquired pneumonia ► 183

This case is focused on the diagnosis and treatment of a patient with pneumonia. The signs and symptoms typical of pneumonia are presented, and the investigations most commonly conducted to confirm its diagnosis described. This case includes a summary of the common causative organisms of community-acquired pneumonia, along with some of those that are less common. Clinical management is based on an assessment of the severity of the infection and the results of microbiological sensitivity testing. *Streptococcus pneumoniae* sensitive to penicillins and macrolides is implicated in this case, and the chemical properties of erythromycin and clarithromycin are compared, together with a discussion of the general factors involved in the decision of when to switch from parenteral to oral antibiotics.

Case 4
Urinary tract infection ▶ 187

This case is centred on a pregnant patient presenting in a community pharmacy to request treatment for cystitis. The signs, symptoms and likely causative organisms of cystitis are considered, as well as potential non-bacterial causes. The increased susceptibility in pregnancy is also discussed, along with the implications for treatment. Uncomplicated urinary tract infections (UTIs) in most patients are self-limiting and require no antibiotic therapy, but a pregnant patient requires referral to her GP. The antibiotics of choice in cystitis are considered, and the chemistry and possible mechanism of action of nitrofurantoin are detailed. The evidence behind any likely benefit of consuming cranberry juice is briefly evaluated, and general considerations about the use of medicines in pregnancy and breastfeeding are also summarised.

Case 5
Uncomplicated genital *Chlamydia trachomatis* infection ▶ 189

This case is based on a patient presenting in the community pharmacy to make use of an established chlamydia screening and treatment service. The characteristics and potential complications of *Chlamydia trachomatis* infection are described together with the role of screening in promotion of population health. The role of the pharmacist in both screening and treatment is detailed, and the most common antibiotic therapies (doxycycline and azithromycin) are explained.

Case 6
Surgical antibiotic prophylaxis ▶ 193

This case focuses on patient-centred and procedure-centred risk factors that may predispose a patient towards developing a surgical site infection (SSI). These risk factors are illustrated using a case that compares the need for antibiotic prophylaxis in two patients undergoing different surgical procedures. The length of expected antibiotic prophylaxis and the circumstances under which additional doses may be given are explored. Finally, consideration is given to which anatomical sites should be sterile and which are colonised with bacteria, together with the main

Gram-positive and Gram-negative pathogens that must be covered when prescribing surgical antibiotic prophylaxis, with a particular emphasis on gastrointestinal (GI) surgery.

Case 7
Diarrhoea and antibiotic treatment ▶ 196

This case presents a patient with watery diarrhoea that started on discharge from hospital after treatment (with co-amoxiclav and erythromycin) for severe community-acquired pneumonia. The components of co-amoxiclav and the rationale for their combination in therapy are detailed. The potential for antibiotic therapy to cause diarrhoea is discussed, as are the options for its management. In the case described, stool cultures indicate *Clostridium difficile* as the causative organism associated with the diarrhoea, and the treatment options are presented, including precautions to minimise the risk of transmission and the contraindication of anti-diarrhoeal medication such as loperamide.

Case 8
'Fever with no focus' in a young infant ▶ 198

This case concerns an infant who presents to the hospital A&E with fever and a rash, prompting concerns about possible sepsis. The most common pathogens associated with meningococcal disease/sepsis in the first few months of life are considered, along with empirical antibiotic therapy for their management. Infants and children have specific daily fluid requirements when receiving enteral or intravenous fluids, and the principles concerned with the calculation of fluid requirements are detailed. The means by which intravenous fluids are sterilised are also discussed. Urine cultures in this case indicate the presence of *Escherichia coli* and appropriate oral antibiotic therapy is considered. Finally, the national immunisation programme is outlined, together with the types of studies that can identify and monitor potential adverse drug reactions.

Case 9
Management of tuberculosis and its complications ▸ 202

This case is based on a patient with recently diagnosed pulmonary tuberculosis (TB). The pathophysiology, signs and symptoms of TB are presented, in addition to the diagnostic tests used to confirm suspected TB infection. TB treatment options are discussed in the initial and continuation phases of the disease, and the mechanism of action and chemistry of isoniazid are considered in detail. The role of directly observed therapy (DOT) in TB management is also detailed, along with a consideration of potential complications that may arise with infection, and how management may be altered accordingly. An international perspective on TB prevalence is presented at the conclusion of the case.

Case 10
Management of latent TB infection and pharmacy interventions ▸ 205

This case follows on from the preceding case and is centred on the diagnosis of latent TB infection in the 6-year-old son of the patient being treated for pulmonary TB. The definition, diagnosis, treatment and monitoring of latent TB infection are outlined, followed by considerations for its recommended treatment. Adherence and counselling points in relation to latent TB infection are discussed in detail, together with the monitoring required for patients taking anti-TB medications long term. The young patient in this case is also having difficulties taking his medication, and potential alternatives are considered, identifying differences between licensed medicines, 'specials' and extemporaneously prepared medicines.

Case 11
Influenza ▸ 207

This case considers a patient with asthma who presents with suspected influenza. The common symptoms and their treatment are discussed, including the use of the neuraminidase inhibitors oseltamivir and zanamivir, their mechanism of action, and the relationship between their physicochemical properties and clinical use. Influenza may present an additional risk in patients with asthma, and further consideration is given in this case to the patient's asthma medication, including the use of pMDIs and associated spacer devices for delivery of drugs to the lungs. Finally, seasonal influenza is considered, along with the guidance and recommendations for influenza immunisation programmes.

Case 12
Chronic hepatitis C ▸ 210

This case concerns a patient who presents with abnormal liver function tests, further investigation of which leads to a diagnosis of chronic hepatitis C infection. The routes of hepatitis C viral transmission and the phases of infection progression are discussed. The means by which hepatitis C is diagnosed is also explained, including a detailed description of the use of PCR (polymerase chain reaction) to amplify viral DNA for diagnosis. Current antiviral treatments are outlined, including ribavirin, interferon and its pegylated derivatives, and the newer protease inhibitors boceprevir and telaprevir. A perspective on future treatment options is given at the end of the case, including new drugs in various stages of clinical trials. The phases of clinical trials used in new drug development are also described here.

Case 13
Primary HIV infection ▸ 215

This is a detailed case describing the presentation of a patient with a variety of symptoms including general malaise, headache, additional flu-like symptoms, oral thrush and perianal ulceration. After empirical treatment to cover bacterial meningitis, a diagnosis of primary HIV infection is made. HIV seroconversion is defined and the symptoms typical of seroconversion illness are described. The diagnostic processes to confirm suspected HIV infection are also detailed, along with some of the limitations of HIV antibody tests. Current UK recommendations for the treatment of primary HIV are described, including a consideration of the different classes of antiretroviral agents, their suitability in this case and the potential long-term complications associated with their use. The management (and prevention) of other co-morbidities specific to the case is also considered.

Case 14
Immunisations against infectious diseases and malaria chemoprophylaxis ► 221

This case considers a prospective visitor to South America and the necessary travel immunisations and prophylactic antimalarial treatment likely to be required. The health risks that may be encountered by travellers are considered, along with sources from which to obtain the most up-to-date information. Common travel immunisations (including hepatitis, typhoid, tetanus, yellow fever, rabies, diphtheria and TB) are all discussed, in general and in the context of the case, along with potential cautions and contraindications. The options for antimalarial chemoprophylaxis and additional precautions to limit exposure are also considered, together with some international perspectives on malaria prevalence and management strategies.

Case 1
Cellulitis and meticillin-resistant *Staphyloccocus aureus*

LISA BOATENG

LEARNING OUTCOMES

At the end of this case, you will be able to:

- Describe the possible presentation, cause and management of cellulitis
- Outline how patient characteristics, e.g. body weight, renal and liver function, may impact on the dosing regimens of a range of antibiotics
- Outline the chemistry and properties of penicillins
- Recognise how co-morbidities and complexities of a presenting complaint may impact on investigations and the treatment plan
- Indicate approaches to the management of MRSA infection

Case study

— Day 1

Mr RA, a 73-year-old obese man, is referred to A&E by the district nurse, with worsening cellulitis of his right leg. Five days earlier, he had received a prescription for co-fluampicil 250/250, one capsule four times daily from his GP for cellulitis in his right leg. However, the cellulitis in his leg had become worse and he was now systemically unwell.

CASE NOTES

History of presenting complaint (HPC)

- Mr RA suffers from heart failure and was recently admitted to hospital for management of worsening heart failure. He was discharged 12 days ago. He had also been diagnosed with atrial fibrillation (AF). His heart failure treatment was optimised and he was initiated on digoxin and aspirin for AF.
- Mr RA lives by himself and had previously been self-caring. However, due to worsening heart failure and newly diagnosed AF he had been referred for a district nurse visit as a follow-up on discharge from hospital. On the district nurse's visit, she noticed cellulitis on Mr

RA's right leg. Mr RA described how he had obtained insect bites around his ankles and shins since discharge from hospital. He had been frantically scratching his legs, in particular his right leg. The nurse contacted the GP to initiate antibiotics for Mr RA and he was prescribed co-fluampicil 250/250, one capsule four times a day for 7 days.

- Five days later, the district nurse revisited Mr RA and observed that his cellulitis was worsening and on examination found him to be pyrexial (temperature 37.8 °C) and generally unwell, and so referred him to the accident & emergency department of his local hospital.

Medical history

- Heart failure
- Atrial fibrillation

Current medication

- Furosemide 40 mg daily
- Spironolactone 25 mg daily
- Ramipril 10 mg daily
- Digoxin 125 micrograms daily
- Aspirin 75 mg daily
- Simvastatin 40 mg daily
- Lansoprazole 30 mg daily
- Paracetamol 1 g four times daily
- Co-fluampicil 250/250, one four times daily started 5 days ago

On examination

- Grossly intact, weight = 90 kg, height = 5 feet 8 inches
- Chest: basal crackles, chest X-ray – no new shadowing on chest X-ray
- Abdomen: soft, non-tender
- Both legs oedematous with pitting oedema
- Right leg: cellulitis from base of shin rising to knee
- Temperature: 37.9 °C
- BP: 105/46 mmHg
- Pulse: 90 beats/min

173

- SOB (shortness of breath); RR (respiratory rate) = 25; Sat (Hb saturation) = 98% on 2 L oxygen
- Urine dipstick: protein +ve, nitrite −ve, blood −ve, leukocytes −ve, ketones +ve, glucose −ve
- Blood cultures taken

Mr RA's blood results are as shown in Table 5.1.

▼ TABLE 5.1
Mr RA's blood results

Haemoglobin (Hb) (g/dL) Normal range: 11.5–16.5	11	Bilirubin (μmol/L) Normal range: 1–17	5
White cell count (WCC) ($\times 10^9$) Normal range: 4–11	14	ALT (units/L) Normal range: 7–35	22
C-reactive protein (CRP) (mg/L) Normal range: <5	30	ALP (units/L) Normal range: 35–104	90
Serum creatinine (μmol/L) Normal range: 44–80	150	GGT (units/L) Normal range: 5–39	15
Urea (mmol/L) Normal range: 2.5–6.1	9.9		
Sodium (mmol/L) Normal range: 136–140	136		
Potassium (mmol/L) Normal range: 3.5–5.1	4.7		

Liver function tests (LFTs): ALT, serum alanine aminotransferase; ALP, serum alkaline phosphatase; GGT, serum γ-glutamyl transferase.

Mr RA's antibiotics are changed. The co-fluampicil is stopped and intravenous (i.v.) benzylpenicillin 1.2 g 6-hourly and i.v. flucloxacillin 1 g 6-hourly are prescribed.

- ❷ What is cellulitis and what are its causes?
- ❷ You review Mr RA's medication on the medical ward. Comment on the above clinical history, results and empirical choice of antibiotics
- ❷ Draw and compare the structures of the two penicillins now prescribed. How do their structural differences impact on their clinical use?

— **Day 3**

On day 3, Mr RA's microbiology results are available.

On admission, Mr RA had been swabbed from the nose, throat and perineum for MRSA as per the protocol in the hospital. A wound swab should have also been taken as part of the screen but was accidently omitted.

The MRSA swab results are reported to be positive in the perineum and nose. These were the sensitivities of the organism to the following antibiotics:

Mupirocin – sensitive
*Flucloxacillin – **resistant***
Vancomycin – sensitive
Rifampicin – sensitive
Sodium fusidate – sensitive
Blood cultures: no growth to date

- ❷ Review Mr RA's antibiotic medication in the light of these microbiology results
- ❷ What implication does the MRSA result have for infection control practice?

Mr RA is started on i.v. vancomycin 1 g twice a day by the house officer for the treatment of the MRSA infection. The house officer asks you how often he should request vancomycin levels to be taken.

- ❷ Comment on the appropriateness of this antibiotic regimen and the necessary therapeutic drug monitoring

— **Day 4**

A maintenance dose of 1 g vancomycin every 24 h is recommended and you advise for a first trough level to be taken at steady state, which is before the third dose for Mr RA. However, a vancomycin level is taken on the second day by the phlebotomist. The level is reported in the afternoon as 8.8 mg/L. You are aiming for a target trough level of 10–15 mg/L.

- ❷ The doctor asks if, in the light of this vancomycin level being low, the dose should be increased back to 1 g twice a day. How would you respond?

— Day 7

Mr RA's cellulitis is healing well.

The medical team ask if there are any oral antibiotics with which Mr RA can be discharged home for a further 7 days

Case discussion

— Reviewing antibiotics
When reviewing antibiotics, pharmacists should not assume the clinical indication being treated but fully review the patient's history, clinical symptoms and diagnosis. In this case, from the history of events, and examination, the suspected clinical infection is cellulitis. However, the full medical review on presentation to A&E suggests that the possibility of chest infection or urinary tract infection may be added to this.

— Causes and symptoms of cellulitis
Cellulitis is a common skin infection caused by bacteria, with severe inflammation of dermal and subcutaneous layers of the skin. The skin in the infected area becomes inflamed, irritated and painful. Cellulitis can be caused by endogenous bacteria on the skin or by exogenous organisms, with staphylococci and streptococci bacteria being the most common causes.

In this case, the cellulitis is likely to have arisen as a result of the insect bite to Mr RA's leg, followed by the subsequent abrasion of the skin from scratching. This would have allowed pathogens colonising the skin and possibly other sites of the body (such as *Streptococcus pyogenes* from the nose) to enter the dermis and cause a clinical infection. This is a common cause of cellulitis.

— Possibility of chest infection
The basal crackles on Mr RA's chest accompanied by shortness of breath (SOB), fast respiratory rate (RR) and elevated temperature could indicate a chest infection. However, in the absence of mucopurulent sputum and no new shadowing on the chest radiograph, the respiratory symptoms are likely to be due to pulmonary oedema secondary to heart failure. The elevated temperature is likely to be due to the cellulitis.

— Possibility of urinary tract infection
The urine dipstick tested negative for nitrites and negative for leukocytes, which indicates that a UTI is unlikely. Nitrites are produced in the urine by the metabolism of some bacteria that convert nitrate to nitrite. Leukocyte esterase is present in white blood cells, which are produced in response to infection or contamination. A urine specimen should be sent to microbiology only for microscopy, culture and sensitivities (MC&S) if there are clear clinical signs such as dysuria, frequency and urgency. These are absent for Mr RA.

— Treatment of cellulitis by the GP
The most common causative organisms for cellulitis are *Staphylococcus aureus* and *Streptococcus pyogenes*. The GP's choice of co-fluampicil consists of flucloxacillin 250 mg and ampicillin 250 mg. These two antibiotics are generally active against sensitive strains of *Staph. aureus* and *Strep. pyogenes*, respectively, in the community. However, the dose of co-fluampicil one capsule four times a day is too low for an obese patient with cellulitis without end-stage renal failure.

Mr RA's weight is given as 90 kg with a height of 5 feet and 8 inches (ideal body weight, IBW = 68.4 kg). IBW = 50 kg + 2.3 kg for each inch over 5 feet.

Based on his actual weight of 90 kg, he is more than 30% above his IBW and therefore would be classified as clinically obese.

Mr RA's creatinine clearance (CrCl) is 30 mL/min, as calculated using the Cockcroft–Gault formula. No dose reduction of these antibiotics is required above a CrCl of 10 mL/min.

The LFTs for ALT, ALP and GGT are normal. The antibiotic route and dose should be assessed according to the severity of the infection, the site of the infection, the patient's age, weight, renal and hepatic function, and the ability of the patient to receive intravenous or oral antibiotics.

The treatment failure of co-fluampicil for Mr RA's cellulitis may have been caused by the low dose prescribed, resulting in subtherapeutic concentrations at the site of infection (i.e. below the minimum inhibitory concentration [MIC] of the causative organism). Inappropriate antibiotic dosage can result is treatment failure and encourage the development of antibiotic resistance.

Mr RA's recent admission to hospital may also mean that he is colonised with hospital-associated organisms or resistant strains of *Staph. aureus*. It would have been prudent for the GP to check Mr RA's hospital discharge records for any record of

MRSA colonisation or resistant organisms before starting on empirical antibiotics.

— Intravenous antibiotics for cellulitis: on admission

Intravenous benzylpenicillin and flucloxacillin have activity against sensitive strains of *Strep. pyogenes* and *Staph. aureus* respectively. However, due to recent inpatient admission, microbiology results should be checked before commencing these.

In the absence of positive microbiology results indicating that Mr RA is colonised with resistant organisms, i.v. benzylpenicillin and i.v. flucloxacillin are the appropriate antibiotics. The dose and route are appropriate. No dose reduction is required for these antibiotics if CrCl >10 mL/min. A switch from i.v. to oral should be anticipated at 5–7 days, depending on clinical response.

— Chemistry and properties of benzylpenicillin and flucloxacillin

The structures of benzylpenicillin (penicillin G) and flucloxacillin are shown in the diagram. Both drugs are examples of β-lactam antibiotics. The term 'β-lactam' is used to describe a cyclic amide that is part of a four-membered ring – the characteristic structural feature of both penicillins and cephalosporins.

Each penicillin has the same core fused ring system with the same stereochemical configuration. Note also the same substituents, essential for antibacterial activity, attached to the rings – a carboxylic acid, two methyl groups and a secondary amide.

The key difference between benzylpenicillin and flucloxacillin is the side chain of the secondary amide substituent and this accounts for the differences in their use, as well as the susceptibility of the microorganisms for which they are used to treat. Benzylpenicillin has poor oral bioavailability and is only used parenterally. All β-lactams show poor stability in acidic environments because they are readily hydrolysed, as well as often being susceptible to enzymatic degradation. This lability in acidic conditions is the reason that orally administered penicillins should be taken on an empty stomach, because gastric pH is lower after eating. An electron-withdrawing amide side chain reduces susceptibility to hydrolysis so flucloxacillin is available for oral use. The very large size of the side-chain group in flucloxacillin also inhibits its recognition by β-lactamases due to steric hindrance. Unlike benzylpenicillin, flucloxacillin is not inactivated by microorganisms that express β-lactamase enzymes.

— Reviewing the antibiotic prescription in this case

In Mr RA's case, the prescribing of flucloxacillin and benzylpenicillin is not appropriate due to resistance, so a switch to i.v. vancomycin should be considered. However vancomycin interacts with the loop diuretic (furosemide) and increases the risk of ototoxicity; the patient should be counselled and monitored. If vancomycin is considered inappropriate due to the interaction, then teicoplanin may be considered as an alternative glycopeptide antibiotic.

— Intravenous vancomycin for the treatment of MRSA

Vancomycin is a glycopeptide antibiotic that interferes with cell-wall synthesis in Gram-positive bacteria. It is not active against Gram-negative organisms. According to the Infectious Diseases Society of America (IDSA) and the vancomycin dosage guidelines of North Glasgow University Hospitals, a loading dose of vancomycin is recommended to rapidly obtain therapeutic levels of the drug.

An initial loading dose of 25 mg/kg is recommended according to actual body weight. A maximum dose of 2 g is used in the North Glasgow University guidelines.

benzylpenicillin

flucloxacillin

▼ TABLE 5.2

Maintenance dose of vancomycin for creatinine clearance (CrCl)

CrCL (mL/min)	Dose (mg)	Interval (h)
<20	500	48
20–29	500	24
30–39	750	24
40–54	500	12
55–74	750	12
75–89	1000	12
90–110	1250	12
>110	1500	12

The maintenance dose of vancomycin would be calculated according to the patient's renal function as shown in Table 5.2.

According to the protocol above, Mr RA would receive a dose of 750 mg every 24 h as a maintenance dose. However, due to his obesity, a higher maintenance dose of 1 g every 24 h is recommended.

The target trough level of 10–15 mg/L is required. The first trough level should be taken at steady state, which is before the third dose for Mr RA. Subsequent levels should be taken approximately once a week (depending on the length of treatment) if the level is within the therapeutic range. If the level is not within the therapeutic range, then levels will need to be taken more often.

Drug levels need to be taken when the drug has reached steady state. In Mr RA's case, the vancomycin levels were taken before the drug had reached steady state, so the vancomycin level will continue to rise. The current dose of 1 g daily should be continued.

— Infection control practice with MRSA

Due to the MRSA result in this case, the patient requires isolation. Apron and gloves need to be worn by all healthcare workers, including the pharmacist reviewing the patient. An MRSA eradication protocol needs to be started: Bactroban (mupiricin) nasal ointment three times a day for 10 days, plus an antiseptic wash daily.

— Changing intravenous antibiotics to oral medication

Full sensitivities should be checked with the microbiology department. The British Society of Antimicrobial Chemotherapy (BSAC) guidelines offer oral options according to sensitivities. In this case they are: rifampicin, sodium fusidate, doxycyline and co-trimoxazole.

Rifampicin and sodium fusidate should not be used alone (monotherapy) due to the rapid development of resistance.

A possible combination of antibiotics for Mr RA on discharge would be doxycyline 200 mg daily and sodium fusidate 500 mg three times daily for 7 days.

— Antimicrobial resistance as an international issue

Antimicrobial resistance (AMR) is a global health problem. Increases in the prevalence of resistant strains of bacteria, together with the decline in the discovery and development of new antibiotic drugs, are the result of years of worldwide misuse and over-prescription of antibiotic medicines. A number of issues have been identified as particular areas of concern:

- There are few new drugs being developed, especially for Gram-negative organisms
- The development of new drugs to fight resistant microorganisms takes time
- Infection prevention and control need to be optimised worldwide.

Coordinated strategies will be needed to promote the development of diagnostics and new drug therapies. Key points identified for action are:

- Improved antibiotic prescribing through good clinical practice
- Containment of the transmission of infections acquired at home and abroad
- Antimicrobial stewardship – where antibiotics are used only when needed, in the right way, at the right dose for the right duration.

EXTENDED LEARNING

- How are bacteria classified?
- Classify the different classes of antibiotics according to their modes of action
- What are the most common hospital-acquired infections and how are they managed?

References and further reading

Davies SC (2011). Chief Medical Officer's summary. In: *Annual Report of the Chief Medical Officer*, Vol 2: Infections and the rise of antimicrobial resistance. London: Department of Health, 11–26.

Editorial (2013). The antibiotic alarm. *Nature* **495**:141.

Rybak M, Lomaestro B, Rotschafer JC et al. (2009). Therapeutic monitoring of vancomycin in adult patients: a consensus review of the American Society of Health-System Pharmacists, the Infectious Diseases Society of America, and the Society of Infectious Diseases Pharmacists. *Am J Health-System Pharmacy* **66**:82–98.

Thomson AH, Staatz CE, Tobin C, Gall M, Lovering AM (2009). Development and evaluation of vancomycin dosage guidelines designed to achieve new target concentrations. *J Antimicrob Chemother* **63**:1050–7.

Case 2
Typhoid

LISA BOATENG

LEARNING OUTCOMES

At the end of this case, you will be able to:

- Describe the symptoms and signs of typhoid
- Consider possible differential diagnoses in an unwell patient who has recently visited a tropical region
- Comment on the treatment of infections with antibiotics, both empirically and after culture
- Outline the chemistry and modes of antimicrobial action of cephalosporin and fluoroquinolone antibiotics
- Outline the structural differences between Gram-positive and Gram-negative bacteria

Case study

— Day 1

A 22-year-old student, Ms AB, presents to A&E with symptoms of headache, fever (temperature 39.5 °C) and feeling generally unwell.

Ms AB had been on holiday to Nigeria for 3 weeks after completing her final degree examinations in business studies. She presented in A&E within 24 hours of arriving back in the UK.

CASE NOTES

History of presenting complaint (HPC)
- 7-day history of headache, fever, malaise and lethargy
- No history of sore throat, cough or sputum production
- No history of neck stiffness or photophobia
- No urinary symptoms
- No vomiting or diarrhoea but some generalised abdominal pain
- Doxycycline had been taken for malaria prophylaxis with the omission of a few doses

Medical history
- Sickle cell disease (homozygous)
- Splenectomy
- Penicillin allergy – mild itchy rash as a child, which developed over a few days

Current medication
- Doxycyline 100 mg daily for malaria prophylaxis
- Erythromycin 250 mg twice daily (prophylaxis for pneumococcal disease)
- Hydroxycarbamide (hydroxyurea) 1.5 g daily
- Folic acid 5 mg daily

On examination

- Pupils equal and reactive to light (PEARL), no photophobia
- No objective neck stiffness
- Chest – occasional crackles
- Abdomen – generalised tenderness, marked right-upper quadrant pain, no distension

? What further information would you like to obtain to determine the possible causes for Ms AB's symptoms?

The clinical team request the following haematology and biochemical tests to be conducted:

- *Full blood count, liver function tests, urea and electrolytes and C-reactive protein.*

A chest radiograph and abdominal CT scan are also arranged.

Diclofenac 50 mg three times daily regularly, paracetamol 1 g four times daily regularly and oxycodone 10 mg when required are prescribed for pain relief.

The duty medical microbiologist recommends a request for malarial parasite screening to be conducted in addition to blood cultures, viral serology, stool culture and a urine specimen.

Ms AB's laboratory results on day 1 are as shown in Table 5.3.

The relevant microbiology specimens are taken and Ms AB is started on i.v. ceftriaxone 2 g daily and i.v. metronidazole 500 mg three times daily for the empirical treatment.

- Comment on the laboratory results and the choice of antibiotics in relation to the treatment of possible tropical disease and the patient's allergy status

▼ TABLE 5.3

Ms AB's laboratory results on day 1

Haemoglobin (Hb) (g/dL) Normal range: 11.5–16.5	8	Bilirubin (μmol/L) Normal range: 1–17	18
White cell count (WCC) (×10⁹) Normal range: 4–11	15	ALP (units/L) Normal range: 35–104	77
C-reactive protein (CRP) (mg/L) Normal range: <5	60	ALT (units/L) Normal range: 7–35	212
Serum creatinine (μmol/L) Normal range: 44–80	40	GGT (units/L) Normal range: 5–39	117
Urea (mmol/L) Normal range: 2.5–6.1	2.0		
Sodium (mmol/L) Normal range: 136–140	140		
Potassium (mmol/L) Normal range: 3.5–5.1	3.8		

- Review the admission medication Ms AB is taking in relation to initiating these new antibiotics

— **Day 2**

The next morning, the microbiology department report that Gram-negative rods have grown in two out of four blood culture bottles.

There are no malarial parasites seen on the malarial blood films.

- What is Gram staining of bacteria?
- What determines whether an organism is Gram positive or Gram negative?

The duty microbiologist recommends the addition of ciprofloxacin to the ceftriaxone for the treatment of possible *Salmonella sp.* because certain species may be resistant to ceftriaxone but sensitive to ciprofloxacin, and vice versa. The junior doctor looking after Ms AB asks you, as the clinical pharmacist, whether the ciprofloxacin should be given orally or intravenously and what the dose should be.

- What factors need to be taken into account in determining the route and dose of ciprofloxacin for Ms AB?

Mrs AB's temperature is now 36.9 °C, her blood pressure 105/58 mmHg and pulse rate is 80 beats/min. She is able to take oral medication and fluids and has no reports of diarrhoea. After taking these factors into account, oral ciprofloxacin 500 mg twice daily is prescribed.

— **Day 3**

On day 3, the Gram-negative rods grown from Ms AB's blood cultures have been confirmed to be *Salmonella sp.* – suspected *Salmonella typhi*. However, this is to be confirmed with the microbiology reference laboratory. Full sensitivities for this organism are pending.

- Which species of *Salmonella* are associated with typhoid (enteric) fever?
- How does this differ from enterocolitis caused by *Salmonella* sp.?

— **Day 4**

The microbiology department have contacted the clinical team and confirm that the *Salmonella sp.* is sensitive to ceftriaxone, resistant to ciprofloxacin and sensitive to azithromycin. The duration of treatment differs depending on the antimicrobial *agent used for treatment. The recommended durations are as follows: ceftriaxone for 14 days, ciprofloxacin for 10 days and azithromycin for 7 days.*

❷ What are the modes of antimicrobial action of ceftriaxone and ciprofloxacin?
❷ Draw the structures of ceftriaxone and ciprofloxacin. To which classes of antibiotics do these two drugs belong?
❷ In the light of ciprofloxacin resistance, which other antibiotics could Ms AB be given?

Case discussion

When a presenting patient has recently returned from travel abroad, it is important to determine:

- Vaccine status before travel
- Full travel history, e.g. in relation to this case:
  - Did she only visit Nigeria or did she travel to other parts of Africa?
  - Where in Nigeria did she stay: city or rural areas?
  - Was there any exposure to mosquito bites?
  - Possible intake of contaminated food/water: where did she eat and drink?
  - Were other members of her family/friends unwell during her stay in Nigeria?

In addition, where patients have a history of splenectomy, it is also important to determine their vaccine status: pneumococcal, *Haemophilus influenzae* type b, influenza virus and meningococcal.

— Consideration of the laboratory results in this case

Ms AB's Hb is low, which is likely to be caused by the sickle cell anaemia. A comparison with previous FBC results will help to determine if this Hb is within the regular range for her.

Her WCC is raised – characteristic of a systemic infection.

Her CRP (a non-specific marker of inflammation) is raised, which is characteristic of chronic inflammation or acute infection. Her underlying sickle cell disease and possible crisis make the CRP difficult to interpret as a marker for infection alone.

The U&Es indicate that there is no renal impairment.

Ms AB's LFTs are elevated. This could be caused by cholecystitis, typhoid fever and/or an inflamed gallbladder secondary to sickle cell disease.

From Ms AB's history the possible differential diagnoses are:

- Malaria
- Typhoid fever (caused by *Salmonella typhi* or *S. paratyphi*)
- Tropical viruses
- Viral hepatitis
- Cholecystitis
- Sickle cell disease.

The abdominal symptoms and pain in the right upper quadrant could be cholecystitis unrelated to her travel or sickle cell crisis. Empirical antibiotic therapy should cover *Salmonella typhi* and organisms associated with cholecystitis. Cholecystitis is caused by organisms normally found in the GI tract, including Gram-negative organisms (Enterobacteriaceae), anaerobes and *Streptococcus pneumoniae*.

— Gram staining and bacterial cell wall structure

Bacteria can be classified into two groups, based on differences in the structure of their cell walls. The classification is based on whether bacterial cells retain the dye methyl violet after washing with a decolorising agent, such as absolute alcohol. Gram-positive cells retain the stain, whereas Gram-negative cells do not. The Gram-positive bacterial cell wall is a relatively simple structure, containing peptidoglycan (a polymer, comprising sugars and amino acids) and teichoic acid polymers. The walls of Gram-negative bacteria are more complex, comprising peptidoglycan and a bilayered membrane, which makes Gram-negative organisms less sensitive to antimicrobial agents. In general, most small rod-shaped bacteria are Gram negative, whereas most large rod-shaped bacteria, e.g. Bacillaceae, lactobacilli and actinomycetes, and most cocci are Gram positive.

— Hypersensitivity to penicillin

Due to the penicillin-allergic reaction as a child, all penicillins would be contraindicated. The severity of the reaction would determine the appropriateness of using other β-lactam antibiotics. Patients with a history of immediate hypersensitivity to penicillin (which is characteristic of type 1 penicillin hypersensitivity) should not receive a cephalosporin. The cross-allergenicity of cephalosporins to penicillins is more recently reported to be 0.5–6.5%, rather than the 10% commonly stated in the past. The first-generation cephalosporins have a cross-allergenicity to the penicillins closer to 0.5%. The second- and third-generation cephalosporins, such as ceftriaxone, are unlikely to be associated with cross-reactivity because they have different side chains to penicillin and so are the safest cephalosporins to prescribe in patients with a history of penicillin allergy where there is no suitable alternative.

Ceftriaxone is a broad-spectrum antibiotic and would be suitable for treating Gram-negative and Gram-positive causes of cholecystitis. Metronidazole is a nitroimidazole antibiotic that would be used for treating infection by any anaerobic organisms.

— **Chemistry and modes of antimicrobial action of ceftriaxone (cephalosporin) and ciprofloxacin (quinolone)**

The substituted β-lactam ring system, common to all cephalosporins, is highlighted in red in the structure of ceftriaxone. In a similar manner to the penicillins, cephalosporins act via the selective, irreversible inhibition of peptidoglycan biosynthesis in bacterial cell walls. As a consequence of their similarity to the native substrate, cephalosporins covalently modify the active site of the transpeptidase enzyme responsible for peptidoglycan cross-linking. This results in defective cell walls, and eventually cell lysis.

Ciprofloxacin is a second-generation fluoroquinolone antibiotic. It is used to treat a wide range of infections, but is particularly useful against Gram-negative organisms. The core structure of 4-quinolone is highlighted in red in the structure of ciprofloxacin. Ciprofloxacin and other quinolone antibiotics act through inhibition of bacterial DNA gyrase and topoisomerase IV. These enzymes are responsible for the winding

and unwinding of supercoiled bacterial DNA – steps that are essential in bacterial replication.

The suspicion of *Salmonella* sp. is high due to the clinical symptoms, elevated LFTs and sickle cell status. Sickle cell patients have a greater incidence of salmonella infections due to a dysfunctional spleen or asplenia, predisposing them to infections caused by encapsulated organisms. Possible damage to the GI tract from sickle cell infarcts may also increase the GI acquisition of this organism.

For Ms AB's differential diagnosis, ceftriaxone would be a good broad-spectrum choice for both efficacy and safety in non-type 1 penicillin allergy. For the specific treatment of typhoid fever, alternative antibiotic choices to ceftriaxone would be ciprofloxacin or azithromycin.

— **Alternative treatments in cases of ciprofloxacin resistance**

Ciprofloxacin is considered the treatment of choice for susceptible strains of *S. typhi* and *S. paratyphi*. However, there is a high level of resistance, particularly in Asia, and for this reason ceftriaxone should be used first line empirically. The Health Protection Agency (now part of Public Health England) reported 48% low-level *S. typhi* resistance to ciprofloxacin in December 2005.

Azithromycin is unlicensed for the treatment of typhoid fever, but is established within national guidelines and in clinical practice as an alternative for the treatment of mild and moderate typhoid in antibiotic resistance.

Chloramphenicol was widely used to treat typhoid fever from 1948 until the 1970s, but the development of resistance and serious haematological side effects preclude chloramphenicol from routine use in clinical practice. In light of Ms AB's sickle cell and chronic anaemia, this drug would be considered only after

ciprofloxacin

ceftriaxone

alternative treatment options and with confirmation of laboratory susceptibility.

Although malaria is among the differential diagnoses, treatment for this would not be initiated until parasites are confirmed in the blood films and based on the clinical signs and symptoms.

Treatment for tropical viral disease or viral hepatitis would not be initiated until confirmation of viral serology tests.

— Review of admission medication

The initiation of ceftriaxone will negate the need for erythromycin prophylaxis because ceftriaxone will provide antibiotic cover for *Streptococcus* sp.

The doxycyline 100 mg daily should continue until further confirmation of malarial parasites has been received. The hydroxycarbamide and folic acid are to continue as normal.

Intravenous antibiotics should be initiated only in patients with severe symptoms, or where no equivalent oral antibiotics are available or where the oral administration is contraindicated/compromised. An intravenous-to-oral switch should be considered in a patient who has shown clear evidence of improvement with the following features:

- Resolution of fever for >24 h
- Pulse rate <100 beats/min
- Resolution of tachypnoea
- Clinically hydrated and taking oral fluids
- Resolution of hypotension
- Absence of hypoxia
- Improving WCC
- Non-bacteraemic infection
- No concerns over GI absorption.

Once Ms AB is clinically stable and ready for discharge the prescription can be switched to azithromycin orally 500 mg daily for 7 days.

— Guidance for travellers to countries where typhoid is endemic

Immunisation is recommended for those travelling to parts of the world where typhoid fever is present, particularly if individuals are planning to work or live with local people. Typhoid is found throughout the world, but is more likely to occur in areas where there is poor sanitation and hygiene. Travellers are advised to take basic precautions when travelling in countries where

typhoid fever might be present. These include attention to personal hygiene and food preparation methods. In particular, advice often includes:

- Drink only bottled water from a bottle that is properly sealed
- Don't eat ice cream, ice cubes or fruit juice from street vendors
- Eat only food that has been freshly prepared and hot (do not eat uncooked vegetables or salads)
- Eat only fruit that can be peeled.

When travelling from the UK, the latest information on immunisation requirements and precautions for avoiding diseases may be found at the National Travel Health Network Centre (www.nathnac.org). Current immunisation requirements for any particular country may also be obtained from the embassy of the appropriate country. Refer to Case 14 below.

EXTENDED LEARNING

- What are the distinguishing features of prokaryotic and eukaryotic organisms?
- Compare the morphology of different types of microorganisms, including viruses, bacteria and fungi
- What are the principal classes of antimicrobial agents and their modes of action?
- What are the mechanisms whereby bacteria become resistant to antibiotics?
- How common is penicillin allergy? What would be the symptoms and how would they be treated?
- What are the public health implications for confirmed cases of typhoid fever? How are the risks of secondary transmission reduced?

References and further reading

Denyer SP, Hodges NA, Gorman SP, Gilmore BF (2011). *Hugo and Russell's Pharmaceutical Microbiology*, 8th edn. Oxford: Blackwell Publishing.

Hanlon GW (2013). Fundamentals of microbiology. In: Aulton ME, Taylor KMG (eds), *Aulton's Pharmaceutics: The design and manufacture of medicines*, 4th edn. London: Elsevier, 200–24.

Case 3
Community-acquired pneumonia

NEIL POWELL

LEARNING OUTCOMES

At the end of this case you will be able to:

- Outline the pathophysiology, signs, symptoms and diagnosis of pneumonia
- Identify the common causative organisms of community-acquired pneumonia, and the less common causative organisms
- Describe antibiotic regimens and appropriate course lengths
- Outline the chemistry of macrolide antibiotics
- Discuss the appropriate switching from intravenous to oral antibiotics

Case study

Mr TD, a 58-year-old welder, presents to A&E with a 2-day history of haemoptysis (coughing up blood) and feeling unwell. On presentation, he is feverish with an oral temperature of 37.8 °C, short of breath, has pleuritic chest pain and dark urine. He has a past medical history of hypertension for which he takes losartan 100 mg once daily and amlodipine 10 mg once daily. He has no known drug allergies.

On examination:

- Heart sounds normal with a pulse of 120 beats/min
- Blood pressure 108/70 mmHg
- Abdominal and neurological examinations normal
- Crepitations (chest 'crackles') and pleural friction rub audible at the base of the right lung
- Respiratory rate 30 breaths/min
- Oxygen sats on air 93%

▼ TABLE 5.4
Blood test results

Total WCC 27.2 × 10^9/L (normal: 3.7–9.5 × 10^9/L)
Neutrophil count 23.8 × 10^9/L (normal: 1.7–7.5 × 10^9/L)
CRP 408 mg/L (normal: <5 mg/L)
Urea 11.7 mmol/L (normal: 2.5–7.8 mmol/L)
Creatinine 165 μmol/L (normal: 62–106 μmol/L)
Bicarbonate 21 mmol/L (normal: 22–29 mmol/L)
LFTs normal
Urine dip clear (i.e. not indicative of a UTI)

ABG analysis on 10 L/min O_2:

pH 7.33 (normal 7.35–7.45)
PCO_2 5.5 kPa (normal 4.5–6.1 kPa)
PO_2 14.4 kPa (normal 12–15 kPa)
Base excess −4 (<−3 indicates metabolic acidosis)
Arterial blood lactate 3 mmol/L (resting plasma lactate >2 mmol/L indicates hyperlactaemia)
(Base excess is a calculated figure providing an estimate of the metabolic component of the acid–base balance)
CURB-65 severity score for community-acquired pneumonia = 2 (raised respiratory rate and raised blood urea)
(The CURB-65 scoring system assigns 1 point for each of five clinical features – see below)

❓ What is pneumonia?
❓ What signs of pneumonia does this patient have?
❓ What further investigations are needed?
❓ What are the likely organisms causing this infection?
❓ What antimicrobial therapy should be initiated?

Mr TD is initiated on a broad-spectrum empirical intravenous antibiotic regimen (co-amoxiclav plus clarithromycin). His chest radiograph shows consolidation (a region of hardening of lung tissue, most probably the result of the accumulation of fluid, which may be pulmonary oedema, inflammatory exudate, pus or blood) in the right lower lobe. The urine antigen tests and blood cultures are negative for growth but the sputum culture indicates the presence of Streptococcus pneumoniae, *with sensitivity to both penicillins and macrolides.*

- ❷ Can Mr TD now be switched to a narrower-spectrum antibiotic?
- ❷ When should he be switched from intravenous antibiotics to oral antibiotics?
- ❷ What are the benefits of switching from intravenous to oral antibiotics?
- ❷ When should his antibiotics be stopped?

Case discussion

— Pneumonia
Pneumonia is inflammation of the lung alveoli. Most cases are due to inhalation of the offending organism. In hospital, pneumonia is diagnosed clinically on the basis of suggestive signs and symptoms of pneumonia plus new unexplained chest radiograph shadowing.

— Signs and symptoms of pneumonia
- Malaise, fever, rigours
- Vomiting, diarrhoea
- Confusion (especially in elderly people)
- Dyspnoea, cough
- Sputum (there may be no sputum, it may be blood stained, and it may be viscid and difficult to expectorate)
- Pleuritic pain
- High fever (often absent in elderly people)
- Tachycardia
- Tachypnoea
- Localised crackles on auscultation
- Bronchial breathing (in about a third of hospital admissions)
- Reduced oxygen saturation
- Chest signs may be absent or masked by other respiratory signs, e.g. COPD

— Investigations required for patients with suspected pneumonia
All patients admitted to hospital with suspected pneumonia should have the following tests performed: chest radiograph; FBC, blood urea, electrolytes and LFTs; CRP; oxygenation assessment.

Blood cultures and sputum samples from patients able to expectorate sputum need to be sent urgently to the microbiology laboratory for culture and sensitivity testing. These samples need to be obtained before the administration of antibiotics. It is also recommended that pneumococcal and legionella urine antigen tests be performed on all patients with severe community-acquired pneumonia.

In this case, a chest radiograph is requested and sputum and blood samples are sent to the microbiology laboratory for culture and sensitivity testing. Pneumococcal and legionella urine antigen tests were also sent.

— Causative organisms
The most common cause of community-acquired pneumonia is *Streptococcus pneumoniae* which is grown in roughly 40% of cases, with *Haemophilus influenzae* being the second most common bacterial cause, grown in approximately 10% of cases. Other less common organisms include *Staphylococcus aureus*, Gram-negative enteric bacilli, and the atypical organisms (termed 'atypical' due to their cell wall structure) *Legionella pneumophila, Mycoplasma catarrhalis, Mycoplasma pneumoniae, Chlamydia psittaci* and *Coxiella burnetii*. Viruses account for approximately 10% of cases.

— Treatment
Management is based on an assessment of the severity of the pneumonia. This should be determined by clinical judgement. The CURB-65 score is an aid to clinical judgement, and is based on a 5-point score, 1 point for each of the following clinical symptoms (www.qxmd.com/calculate-online/respirology/curb-65):

Confusion of recent onset
Blood **u**rea nitrogen ≥7 mmol/L
Respiratory rate ≥30 breaths/min
Systolic **B**P <90 mmHg or diastolic BP ≤60 mmHg
Age ≥**65**

In a prospective trial in which patients were stratified according to their CURB-65 score on admission to hospital, the risk of mortality or need for intensive care was 0.7% in those scoring 0. As

erythromycin   clarithromycin

the CURB-65 score increased so did their risk of mortality or need for intensive care as shown:

Score 1: 3.2%

Score 2: 13%

Score 3: 17%

Score 4: 41.5%

Score 5: 57%

- Patients with a CURB-65 score of 0 and no other coexisting chronic illnesses could be considered for outpatient management.
- Patients with CURB-65 scores of 1 or 2 will require clinical judgement in deciding where best to manage them, i.e. in hospital or at home, and the level of treatment that is appropriate.
- Patients with a CURB-65 score of ≥ 3 should be managed in hospital as cases of severe community-acquired pneumonia.

It is not uncommon for clinicians to diagnose patients as severe despite CURB-65 scores of ≤ 2. The CURB-65 score is a tool to aid diagnosis but does not replace clinical acumen. In this case, Mr TD's WCC is very high and his blood pressure is low, which may lead clinicians to be more concerned and diagnose Mr TD with severe community-acquired pneumonia.

If the sputum and/or blood cultures grow an organism consistent with pneumonia then the organism will be sensitivity tested. This usually takes 48 hours from sending the sample to the laboratory.

Mr TD's sputum grew *Streptococcus pneumoniae* which was sensitive to penicillins and

macrolides, so the co-amoxiclav could be de-escalated to a penicillin with a narrower spectrum, such as amoxicillin, or to a macrolide, such as clarithromycin, as a sole agent.

— **Chemical properties of clarithromycin**
The macrolide antibiotic clarithromycin is almost structurally identical to erythromycin. The important difference (highlighted in red on the structure in the diagram) is the synthetic conversion of the hydroxyl group at C6 to the corresponding methyl ether. This small change results in clarithromycin being significantly more acid stable than erythromycin. Under acidic conditions, such as in the stomach, the ketone group in erythromycin can be protonated and is then susceptible to attack by the C6 hydroxyl, resulting in a rearrangement reaction that inactivates the antibiotic. The eventual products of this rearrangement are also implicated in gastric disturbance. For this reason, erythromycin needs to be formulated as enteric-coated tablets for oral administration. Clarithromycin lacks the nucleophilic hydroxyl group and is hence more acid stable and less prone to cause gastric upset.

— **Switching from intravenous to oral antibiotics**
Patients requiring intravenous antibiotics should have the route of administration switched to oral when they show signs of clinical improvement. The features outlined above may be helpful in making this decision.

- Resolution of fever for >24 hours
- Pulse rate <100 beats/min
- Resolution of tachypnoea
- Absence of hypotension

- Absence of hypoxia
- Improving WCC
- No concerns over GI absorption

There are the following benefits when switching from intravenous to oral antibiotics:

- Cost: intravenous antibiotics usually cost more than oral antibiotics
- Narrow the spectrum of antibiotic cover: broad-spectrum antibiotics have a greater potential to cause *Clostridium difficile*-associated diarrhoea and a greater driver for antimicrobial resistance
- Removing a portal for infection: cannulae breach the skin, which is a natural barrier to infection
- Convenience and safety of drug dosing: administration of intravenous drugs takes more time than oral medication and their administration comes with a greater risk of administration error compared with oral administration
- Aiding discharge home: administration via the oral route may allow the patient to go home.

The precise duration of antibiotic therapy is not supported by robust evidence. The aim of antibiotic therapy is to ensure elimination of the target pathogen in the shortest time. In uncomplicated infections this may occur rapidly, e.g. within 3 days for many common respiratory pathogens, such as *Streptococcus pneumoniae*. There is evidence, however, that infections caused by atypical bacteria such as *Legionella* sp. may require 14–21 days of antibiotic therapy. Staphylococci and Gram-negative bacilli may also need these longer courses.

— Duration of antibiotic therapy

Until more evidence becomes available, the duration of antimicrobial therapy will remain subject to clinical judgement and will vary with the individual patient, disease severity and speed of resolution.

In this case, if Mr TD's symptoms had improved so that by day 2 he could be switched to oral antibiotics and, as it was known to be *Streptococcus pneumoniae* sensitive to the current treatment causing the pneumonia, one would expect him to be on antibiotic therapy for a total of 7 days.

EXTENDED LEARNING

- What do you understand by the term 'antibiotic resistance'?
- How would you expect a child with community-acquired pneumonia to be treated?
- What influence has immunisation had on pneumonia and child survival worldwide?

References and further reading

British Thoracic Society (2009). Guidelines for the management of community acquired pneumonia in adults: update 2009. *Thorax* **64**(Suppl 3):1–55.

Kumar P, Clark M (2009). *Clinical Medicine*, 7th edn. Philadelphia, PA: Elsevier.

Robb A, Berrington AW (2012). Respiratory infections. In: Walker R, Whittlesea C (eds), *Clinical Pharmacy and Therapeutics*, 5th edn. London: Churchill Livingstone, 545–60.

Case 4
Urinary tract infection

KIRSTY WORRALL

LEARNING OUTCOMES

At the end of this case, you will be able to:

- Describe the signs and symptoms of cystitis
- State the likely cause of cystitis in pregnant women
- Outline the treatment options for a pregnant women with an uncomplicated UTI
- Discuss general considerations about the use of medicines in pregnancy and breastfeeding

Case study

You're working in a busy community pharmacy and are approached by a woman who asks to have a quiet word with the pharmacist. She looks to be about 30 years old and seems embarrassed. She asks for something to treat cystitis.

❓ What symptoms may she be experiencing?

After further questioning you learn that she has had the symptoms since last night, is not taking any other medication, either from the doctor or over the counter, and is 4 months' pregnant with her first child.

❓ What would be your course of action? Why?

She asks you what has caused the cystitis.

❓ How do you respond?

The patient's GP diagnosed an uncomplicated lower UTI and the patient returns with a prescription for:

Nitrofurantoin 50 mg four times daily for 7 days

❓ What is the likely causative organism in this patient?
❓ Draw the structure of nitrofurantoin and comment on its mechanism of action
❓ Is this prescription appropriate for this patient?

When you hand her the medication she tells you that her friend has recommended drinking cranberry juice.

❓ What do you think of this recommendation?

Case discussion

— Cystitis

Cystitis is inflammation of the bladder. It is estimated that up to half of all women will experience at least one episode of cystitis during their life. In more than 60% of cases, cystitis is caused by a bacterial infection, with the most likely causative organism being *Escherichia coli*.

Non-bacterial (interstitial) cystitis may have a number of causes: irritation and bruising caused by sexual intercourse, irritation from chemicals in soaps and bubble baths, etc., dehydration, oestrogen deficiency, or medications such as cyclophosphamide, allopurinol, danazol and tiaprofenic acid.

— Symptoms of cystitis

Symptoms of cystitis may include bad smelling or cloudy urine, increased frequency, dysuria, urgency and haematuria (blood in the urine). Additional symptoms that may indicate a more complicated infection, such as pyelonephritis (acute infection of the kidney), are loin pain and fever.

Pregnant women are more prone to UTIs than non-pregnant women. This is due to hormonal changes and physical changes in pregnancy that affect the urinary tract, slowing down the flow of urine and thus allowing bacteria to multiply.

— Treatment options

For most patients with an uncomplicated UTI, antibiotic treatment is unnecessary, because symptoms will normally resolve in 4–9 days. Pregnant women are more likely to have complications, which could lead to low-birthweight infants and premature birth. For this reason they should be given antibiotic treatment, usually a 7-day course.

In this case, the patient should be referred to her doctor because she is pregnant. Products containing urine-alkalinising agents such as potassium or sodium citrate are available for symptomatic relief, but should not be recommended. However, you could recommend paracetamol for analgesia.

With increasing bacterial resistance to antibiotics, particularly amoxicillin and trimethoprim, the choice of antibiotic should be determined by the culture results and the organism susceptibility. Amoxicillin should be used only if the pathogen is reported to be susceptible.

Local antibiotic prescribing guidelines may be in place; usually nitrofurantoin, trimethoprim or cefalexin is the antibiotic of choice.

— Chemistry and mechanism of action of nitrofurantoin

Nitrofurantoin has been in use for over 60 years, primarily for UTIs, with little evidence of the development of clinically significant resistance. The structure of the drug includes a nitrated furan ring (a five-membered, oxygen-containing, aromatic heterocycle) and a hydantoin ring system (highlighted in red in the diagram), from which the drug's name is derived. Its mechanism of action is still not fully understood, but it is thought to undergo selective enzymatic (nitrofuran reductase) reduction of the nitrofuran within bacterial cells, producing highly reactive electrophilic metabolites that damage bacterial ribosomal proteins non-specifically, inhibiting protein synthesis. It is likely that the same metabolites also cause damage (through covalent modification) to other bacterial macromolecules, including DNA.

nitrofurantoin

— Cranberry juice in cystitis

A Cochrane systematic review found no good evidence to support the use of cranberry juice or other cranberry products for treating acute UTIs (Jepson et al., 2012). So, in this case, it would not be appropriate to recommend cranberry juice. However, it is unlikely to cause harm (cranberries are quite acidic so could cause some gastric upset), so the patient could have it should she wish. Further trial data are required to determine if cranberry juice has any protective properties against recurrent UTIs.

— Medicines in pregnancy and breastfeeding

Special consideration about the use of medicines in pregnancy is required because of the potential to harm the embryo or fetus. Pregnancy is commonly viewed as three trimesters and, although harm can occur at any time, the types of risk from medicines are often determined by the stage of the pregnancy. Thus, information on the possible safety risks is often presented in relation to particular trimesters.

The first trimester is the time of organogenesis, when the organs and limbs are forming and the neural tube is closing. This is the period of greatest risk, when drugs can interfere with these structural developments and cause congenital malformations (teratogenesis). All drugs should be considered as potentially posing a risk to the fetus if taken in the first trimester and should be avoided if possible. In the second and third trimesters, the fetus grows and matures and, although risks of congenital malformations are fewer, drugs taken at these later stages can affect the growth and functional development of the organs of the fetus. Drugs taken shortly before delivery may have an effect on the neonate.

Most drugs (except the largest molecules, e.g. insulin) are able to pass through the placenta to the fetus. In cases in which drug therapy is essential for the health of the mother, drugs that have been extensively used with no reports of problems should be preferred over newer agents. The lowest effective doses should be taken, single agents rather than combination therapy, and choice governed by the most up-to-date and robust evidence. Some drugs that have been used extensively over many years are believed not to be harmful in pregnancy. However, no drug should be assumed to be completely safe in early pregnancy, and the possible risks of adverse effects should be carefully considered at all stages.

Drugs can also appear in the breast milk from which they may be passed on to the infant. It should be assumed that any drug can enter the breast milk, although in general only small amounts of any drug would be transferred in this way. The potential clinical significance of ingestion of drug by an infant needs to be assessed for each drug. The *BNF* identifies drugs that:

- Are contraindicated because of actual or theoretical risks
- Can be given because the amounts in breast milk are believed to be too small to cause harm
- Might be present in breast milk but are not known to be harmful.

No evidence of congenital abnormalities has so far been reported for nitrofurantoin during pregnancy but the *BNF* recommends avoidance of using it near term (38–42 weeks' gestation) and during labour/delivery due to the risk of inducing neonatal haemolysis. Trimethoprim being a dihydrofolate reductase inhibitor carries a teratogenic risk in the first trimester (4–12 weeks) and is best avoided, whereas cefalexin is not known to be harmful in pregnancy.

EXTENDED LEARNING

- What are the potential underlying causes of recurrent cystitis?
- How are complications such as pyelonephritis managed?
- What are the mechanisms whereby microorganisms acquire resistance to antibiotics?
- What can pharmacists do to reduce the development of antibiotic resistance?
- What are the symptoms and treatment for an upper UTI?

- What physiological changes take place in pregnancy that can impact on drug distribution in the body?

ADDITIONAL PRACTICE POINTS

- What counselling advice would you give to a patient with cystitis?
- What steps may be taken to reduce an individual's risk of developing a UTI?

References and further reading

Gupta K, Trautner BW (2013). Diagnosis and management of recurrent urinary tract infections in non-pregnant women. *BMJ* **346**:f3140.

Jepson RG, Williams G, Craig J (2012). Cranberries for preventing urinary tract infections. *Cochrane Database Syst Rev* **10**:1–65.

Litza JA, Brill JR (2010). Urinary tract infections. *Primary Care* **37**:491–507.

National Institute for Health and Clinical Excellence (2009). *Urinary Tract Infection (Lower) – women – NICE Clinical Knowledge Summaries.* Available at: http://cks.nice.org.uk/urinary-tract-infection-lower-women (accessed 14 March 2014).

Walker R, Whittlesea C (2011). *Clinical Pharmacy & Therapeutics*, 5th edn. London: Churchill Livingstone.

Case 5
Uncomplicated genital *Chlamydia trachomatis* infection
KATE SHARDLOW AND SALLY-ANNE FRANCIS

LEARNING OUTCOMES

At the end of this case, you will be able to:

- Describe the role of screening in promoting the health of a population
- Explain the concepts of prevalence, false positives, false negatives, specificity and sensitivity
- Outline the process of screening for chlamydia infection
- Understand the presentation and treatment for uncomplicated *Chlamydia trachomatis* infection

Case study

A young woman, Ms EF, visits your community pharmacy on the university campus and asks to speak to the pharmacist. She asks to go to a quiet area and have a confidential conversation with you. She explains that she has had a new boyfriend for the past month but they have not been using condoms when having sex, and she would like to be tested for Chlamydia *sp. You are authorised to provide a screening and treatment service for chlamydia infection through a patient group direction (PGD).*

- What is *Chlamydia*?
- Why may chlamydia infection be an appropriate condition for a public health screening programme?
- What is a patient group direction?
- What questions might you wish to ask before issuing a chlamydia screening test?

Ms EF returns to your pharmacy 10 days later, having received notification that her chlamydia test was positive. Ms EF asks if the test result could be inaccurate, because she is not experiencing any symptoms.

❓ How would you respond?

❓ What questions might you wish to ask Ms EF before deciding that a pharmacy-based treatment is the most appropriate course of action?

After further discussion with Ms EF, you determine that you are able to offer treatment with azithromycin for her chlamydia infection, in accordance with the PGD.

❓ What further information would you wish to discuss with Ms EF and what would be your advice?

Case discussion

— Key features of *Chlamydia trachomatis* infection

Chlamydia trachomatis infection is the most common curable sexually transmitted infection (STI) in the UK, with the highest incidence in young adults (see the Health Protection Agency website for the latest infection rates in the UK: www.hpa.org). Approximately two-thirds of sexual partners of *Chlamydia*-positive individuals will also test positive for *Chlamydia*. It is caused by a bacterium called *Chlamydia trachomatis*. *C. trachomatis* is an obligate intracellular pathogen with a lifecycle of 48–72 hours. Risk factors for genital chlamydia infection are: aged <25 years, more than one sexual partner in the last year, or a recent new sexual partner and lack of consistent use of condoms. Untreated infections may persist for longer than 1 year.

Frequently, uncomplicated genital chlamydia infection is asymptomatic; approximately 70% of infected women and 50% of infected men do not exhibit any obvious symptoms. Women who go on to experience symptoms associated with *C. trachomatis* infection may present with a change in vaginal discharge, lower abdominal pain, bleeding after sex and/or in between periods, and discomfort on passing urine. In men, symptoms can include a urethral discharge or discomfort on passing urine.

Chlamydia infection can be associated with a number of complications in some cases: women can develop pelvic inflammatory disease (PID). which is associated with infertility, ectopic pregnancy and chronic pelvic pain; men can go on

to experience painful inflammation in the testicles, which can also be associated with decreased levels of fertility. The risk of complications with chlamydia infection increases with repeated untreated infections.

— Screening for promoting the health of the population

Screening is a process of identifying apparently healthy people who may be at increased risk of a disease or condition. They can then be offered information, further tests and appropriate treatment to reduce their risk and/or any complications arising from the disease or condition. Screening can reduce the risk of developing a condition or its complications but it cannot offer a guarantee of protection. In any screening programme, there is a minimum of false-positive and false-negative results (Public Health England, 2013).

— False-positive and false-negative results

To explain these terms, you start with the population for whom screening for a particular condition is relevant. The false-positive result is the proportion of individuals identified as having the condition according to the screening criteria, when they do not. Conversely, the false-negative result is the proportion of individuals identified as not having the condition according to the screening criteria, when they do in fact have the condition.

A seminal report published by Wilson and Jungner for the World Health Organization in 1968 listed 10 principles, which they offered for reflection and debate when considering which conditions are suitable for screening:

1 The condition should pose an important health problem
2 The natural history of the disease should be well understood
3 There should be a recognisable early stage
4 Treatment of the disease at an early stage should be of more benefit than treatment started at a later stage
5 There should be a suitable test
6 The test should be acceptable to the population
7 There should be adequate facilities for the diagnosis and treatment of abnormalities detected
8 For disease of insidious onset, screening should be repeated at intervals determined by the natural history of the disease

9 The chance of physical or psychological harm to those screened should be less than the chance of benefit

10 The cost of a screening programme should be balanced against the benefit that it provides.

Many variations on the classic criteria of Wilson and Jungner are used today. However, there are international differences in the adoption of screening programmes with different countries having different approaches, including the amount of screening offered and the involvement of public and private health providers.

In response to evidence of high and increasing rates of chlamydia infection and the benefits of subsequent treatment, many countries have introduced national chlamydia screening programmes. However, the efficacy and cost-effectiveness of such programmes remain debateable due to disagreements about the true prevalence in the population, patterns of transmission and the rates of progression to serious complications.

— **Prevalence**
Prevalence is the proportion of individuals in a defined population who have a condition. There are three measures of prevalence:

1 Point prevalence is a cross-sectional measure that states the proportion of people with a condition at a single point in time.

2 Period prevalence states the proportion of people with a condition at any point in time during a defined period.

3 Lifetime prevalence states the proportion of the population that experiences a condition during their lifetime.

— **Pharmacists and chlamydia screening**
In the UK, chlamydia screening is offered to sexually active men and women aged <25 years. Screening can be offered to individuals aged <16 years if 'Fraser competent'. Fraser guidelines were developed following the famous 'Gillick case' in which a mother contested whether a health professional should be able to give contraceptive advice or treatment to an under 16 year old without parental consent. The guidelines are now used to help assess whether a child has the maturity and understanding to make independent decisions about his or her treatment.

Chlamydia samples are a self-taken vaginal swab or first-pass urine. Samples are sent to a testing laboratory. Chlamydia screening offices

coordinate the service locally and individuals are informed of their results. Treatment is offered to people who screen positive.

Some community pharmacists provide a chlamydia screening service and are able to supply treatment for *Chlamydia trachomatis* infection via a patient group direction (PGD) if the test is positive.

Nucleic acid amplification tests (NAATs) are currently used in the screening programme. These tests are designed to amplify nucleic acid sequences that are specific for the organism being detected and do not require viable organisms. These tests have the ability to produce a positive signal from as little as a single copy of the target DNA or RNA.

NAAT samples are still suitable for testing several days after collection. NAATs can detect chlamydia in urine and swabs with >90% sensitivity and >95% specificity. However, as they are not 100% sensitive or specific, confirmation of a reactive test is currently recommended.

— **Sensitivity and specificity**
These are measures of test performance. High sensitivity means that the test identifies as many people with the condition as possible. It is measured as the proportion of those with the condition, who have a positive test result. It is the same as the detection rate. High specificity means that the test has as few false positives as possible. It is measured as the proportion of those without the condition, who have a negative test result.

Current opinion suggests a 2-week window period after exposure to genital chlamydia infection before reliable detection when using NAAT sampling. Individuals who are concerned about risk of chlamydia infection after recent sexual exposure are currently advised to have a screening test when they first present, but to return for repeat testing 2 weeks after the last sexual exposure (BASHH, 2008).

If an individual wishes to be retested for chlamydia infection following treatment this should be deferred for 5 weeks after treatment is completed (6 weeks if azithromycin is prescribed). This is because the NAAT screening test used may remain positive for several weeks following treatment. This does not necessarily mean active infection, however, as it may represent the presence of nucleic acid from non-viable organisms resulting in a false-positive test result.

Individuals with a positive test need to be advised of the importance and need for sexual partner(s) to be treated. Contact tracing should be conducted with positive results. Clear testing and referral pathways exist for individuals where further clinical assessment in a sexual health service is needed, for example in symptomatic chlamydia infection. All individuals with a positive chlamydia screening test should be advised about testing for other sexually transmitted infections. Privacy and confidentiality are key issues that pharmacists need to consider when offering the service. Pharmacists providing the service also need to be aware of local and national guidance on safeguarding children and vulnerable adults.

— **The role of the pharmacist in treating uncomplicated genital *Chlamydia trachomatis* infection**

Individuals diagnosed with a chlamydia infection should be given a full explanation of the condition and its treatment, with written information.

Treatment should be offered in line with local and national treatment guidelines and patient group directions. A PGD is a written instruction for the supply or administration of a named medicine, for a defined clinical condition, to a group of patients who may not be individually identified before presentation for treatment.

Chlamydia infection can be effectively treated with antibiotics. First-line treatment is either with the tetracycline antibiotic doxycycline 100 mg twice a day for 7 days (contraindicated in pregnancy) or the macrolide azithromycin 1 g single oral dose (useful where prescription compliance may be a problem). Alternative antibiotics such as erythromycin may also be used to treat chlamydia infection.

Individuals should be advised to allow time for the treatment to work and avoid any sex (including vaginal, oral, anal and genital contact) even using condoms until they and their partner(s) have completed treatment (or have waited 7 days if treated with single-dose azithromycin), otherwise there is a risk or reinfection.

When treating female individuals for chlamydia infections with antibiotics (non-enzyme inducing) no additional precautions are routinely required if they are using hormonal contraceptives. The only proviso would be if antibiotics caused vomiting or diarrhoea, and then advice on the potential effect on oral contraception should be given, and additional precautions observed.

It is very important that the sexual partners of *chlamydia*-positive individuals are evaluated and treated. Treatment for chlamydia infection should be offered to all sexual partners. If declined, individuals must be advised to abstain from sex until they have received a negative result.

Individuals should be advised of the availability of a full sexual health check at the local sexual health clinic. Routine testing to check whether chlamydia infection has resolved should be performed in pregnancy and if non-compliance or re-exposure is suspected. The national chlamydia screening programme recommends re-testing to individuals with a positive chlamydia result 3 months after treatment has been completed. Repeat testing after a few months should also be considered, when individuals have just started a new sexual relationship.

Pharmacists have an important role in sexual health including advice about safer sex and promoting condom use. There are opportunities to discuss chlamydia screening when offering pregnancy testing, dispensing prescriptions for contraception and supplying emergency contraception, for example.

EXTENDED LEARNING

- What factors may lead to treatment failure when treating individuals for chlamydia infection?
- How is *Fraser competency* defined?
- What are the wider debates about screening for genetic conditions?

References and further reading

Andermann A, Blancquaert I, Beauchamp S, Déry V (2008). Revisiting Wilson and Jungner in the genomic age: a review of screening criteria over the past 40 years. *Bull WHO* **86**:241–320. Available at: www.who.int/bulletin/volumes/86/4/07–050112/en/# (accessed 3 October 2013).

BASHH (2006). UK *National Guideline for the Management of Genital Tract Infection with* Chlamydia trachomatis. Available at: www.bashh.org/documents/65.pdf (accessed 3 October 2013).

BASHH Clinical Effectiveness Group (2008). *Testing for Chlamydia – the 'window period'*. Available at: www.bashh.org/documents/1686.pdf (accessed 3 October 2013).

Faculty of Sexual and Reproductive Healthcare (2012). *Drug Interactions with Hormonal Contraception*. Available at:

www.fsrh.org/pdfs/CEUGuidanceDrugInteractionsHormonal.
pdf (accessed 3 October 2013).

Flavell G (2010). *Sexual Health in Pharmacies: Developing your
service.* Manchester: Centre for Pharmacy Postgraduate
Education.

Health Protection Agency (2014). National Chlamydia
Screening Programme (NCSP) Standards, 7th edn. Available
at: www.chlamydiascreening.nhs.uk/ps (accessed 20 February
2015).

Lazaro N (2013). *Sexually Transmitted Infections in Primary
Care 2013.* Available at: www.rcgp.org and www.bashh.org/
guidelines (accessed 3 October 2013).

National Institute for Health and Clinical Excellence (2009).
Chlamydia – uncomplicated genital. Clinical Knowledge
Summaries. Available at: http://cks.nice.org.uk/chlamydia-
uncomplicated-genital (accessed 3 October 2013).

Public Health England (2013). National Chlamydia Screening
Programme. Available at: www.chlamydiascreening.nhs.uk
(accessed 3 October 2013).

Wilson JMG, Jungner G (1968). *Principles and Practice of
Screening for Disease.* WHO Public Health Paper No. 34.
Geneva: WHO. Available at: www.who.int/bulletin/volumes/
86/4/07–050112BP.pdf (accessed 3 October 2013).

Case 6
Surgical antibiotic prophylaxis

TRACY LYONS

LEARNING OUTCOMES

At the end of this case you will be able to:

- Describe the patient-centred risk factors
  that may predispose a patient towards
  developing a surgical site infection (SSI)

- Describe the different types of surgery to be
  considered when prescribing surgical
  antibiotic prophylaxis, i.e. procedure-
  centred risk factors for the development of
  an SSI

- Understand for how long antibiotic
  prophylaxis should continue

- Identify which parts of the body should be
  sterile and where bacteria may be expected
  to be found

- List some of the main pathogens that
  prophylaxis must cover for GI surgery

Case study

*You are a pharmacist working on a general surgery
ward and a patient, Mr WD, asks you why he has
been prescribed antibiotics for his surgery when his
neighbour, Mr NT, has not. He is concerned that
patients are being treated differently.*

*You investigate and notice that Mr WD is an obese
72-year-old patient with type 2 diabetes and severe
asthma, but that Mr NT is a 38-year-old patient
who has no other concurrent medical problems.*

❓ Explain the potential patient-centred risk
factors that can predispose patients to the
development of an SSI. Relate these to both of
your patients, considering their existing health
characteristics and the medication that they
may take for concurrent medical issues

*Mr WD thanks you for your explanation but says
that he has also asked the doctor on the ward the
same question and was told it was due to the
difference in the operations that both patients were
due to have. He also asks why, if antibiotics are
needed, he hasn't been given a 'proper' course
rather than just a few doses. On reading through
the surgical notes you discover that Mr WD is
in hospital for colorectal surgery, whereas
Mr NT is due for a procedure to correct his
varicose veins.*

❓ Explain the difference between clean, clean–
contaminated, contaminated and dirty surgery,
i.e. procedure-related risk factors for the
development of an SSI

❓ Describe how you would reassure the patient
(with reasons) why only a short course of
antimicrobial therapy is needed for most
surgical prophylaxis. Describe the
circumstances in which you would give
additional doses of antibiotic prophylaxis

*A pre-registration pharmacist is on the ward with
you listening to these conversations. He does not
understand why some body sites are considered
sterile and some are not. He asks for help in
understanding which areas might normally be free*

of bacteria. He is also concerned that there are too many bacteria for him to remember, and asks if there is a simple way to remember against which pathogens patients might need prophylactic protection for GI surgery.

❓ How would you describe to the student an easy way of remembering which body sites would normally be sterile?

❓ Outline the bacteria that are likely to be encountered during GI surgery so that the student can understand the bacterial coverage needed for surgical prophylaxis

Case discussion

Surgical site infections (SSIs) are an important source of hospital-acquired infections (HAIs). It has been estimated that approximately 5% of all patients who undergo surgery will develop a postoperative infection, although this can vary from localised and superficial infections to severe, deep-seated and life-threatening conditions that put patients' lives at risk and require prolonged hospital stays or readmission to hospital for further therapy. Consequently, SSIs can become distressing to patients and costly to hospitals and their prevention is a significant clinical and economic objective.

— Patient-centred risk factors for the development of SSIs

Patients are more likely to develop an SSI if:

- Their immune response is less than ideal, i.e. due to drug therapy (e.g. steroids, immune suppressants) or disease (e.g. HIV or obesity)
- They have impaired blood circulation, i.e. due to vascular pathologies or diabetes
- They are at risk of additional bacterial exposure, i.e. having catheters or implants *in situ* that will quickly become colonised with bacteria.

The National Institute for Health and Care Excellence (NICE) and the Scottish Intercollegiate Guidelines Network (SIGN) both list patient risk factors that may contribute to the development of an SSI such as:

- Age: risk increases with age
- Concurrent illness: the more severe it is, the more likely a patient will develop an infection
- Diabetes
- Malnourishment
- Low serum albumin
- Chemotherapy

- Radiotherapy
- Steroid use
- Obesity
- Smoking.

In this case, when comparing Mr WD and Mr NT, four of these factors probably apply to Mr WD (older age, diabetes, long-term steroid therapy for asthma and obesity), whereas none applies to Mr NT.

— Procedure-related risk factors for the development of an SSI

When considering antibiotic prophylaxis, surgery is typically described in one of four ways:

1 *Clean*: elective (non-emergency), non-traumatic surgery with no acute inflammation, no break in surgical aseptic technique, no involvement of the respiratory, GI, biliary or genitourinary tracts

2 *Clean–contaminated*: urgent or emergency cases that are otherwise clean; when there is elective opening of respiratory, GI, biliary or genitourinary tract with minimal spillage (e.g. appendectomy) but not encountering infected urine or bile; surgery with minor breaks in surgical aseptic technique

3 *Contaminated*: non-purulent inflammation; gross spillage from GI tract; entry into biliary or genitourinary tract in the presence of infected bile or urine; major breaks in aseptic surgical techniques; penetrating trauma <4 hours old; chronic open wounds to be grafted or covered

4 *Dirty*: purulent inflammation and active infection (e.g. abscess); preoperative perforation of respiratory, GI, biliary or genitourinary tract; penetrating trauma >4 hours old.

It is important to note that 'clean' surgery may not need antibiotic prophylaxis at all if proper aseptic technique is employed, because exposure to bacteria is low for this type of procedure.

If surgery involves areas of the body more heavily colonised with bacteria or takes place in the presence of existing inflammation, the chances of an SSI increase.

'Clean–contaminated' and 'contaminated' operations will need short courses of antibiotics to cover the procedures and prevent infection developing.

'Dirty' surgery involves a patient with existing, active infection and therefore the patient will get a 'treatment' course of antibiotic therapy rather than antibiotic prophylaxis.

Mr WD is in hospital for colorectal surgery, which will involve opening of the GI tract and hence will need a short course of antibiotic prophylaxis. Mr NT is due to undergo a procedure to correct his varicose veins which is considered 'clean' surgery and, as such, he does not need to be prescribed prophylactic antibiotics.

— Length of surgical antibiotic prophylaxis
Antibiotic prophylaxis is normally started shortly before the operation, allowing sufficient time for the drug to reach therapeutic plasma concentrations before surgery begins ('knife-to-skin' time). The exact timing will depend on the way in which the antimicrobial must be administered (i.e. as an intravenous bolus or infusion) and if a surgical tourniquet is to be used (tourniquets are designed to reduce blood flow to limbs and will therefore prevent drug distribution to them as well).

However, studies have shown that the optimal time is 30–60 min pre-surgery for most i.v. prophylaxis. Administration too late or too early reduces the efficacy of the antibiotic and will increase the risk of SSI.

Antibiotic prophylaxis is continued only long enough to maintain therapeutic serum antibiotic concentrations while the surgery continues. This is normally just a small number of doses and, in fact, single doses are sufficient cover for many procedures (particularly if the antibiotic has a long half-life). Extended courses of antibiotics do not provide additional benefit to patients; rather they place the patient at increased risk of antibiotic-associated side effects, such as *Clostridium difficile* infection or the development of bacterial resistance.

— Additional doses of antibiotic prophylaxis
If for some reason surgery is prolonged (i.e. due to complications) and continues for more than two half-lives of the prophylactic antibiotic, additional doses of prophylaxis may be considered

In addition, if there is excessive blood loss (>1500 mL), which would reduce plasma antibiotic concentrations to subtherapeutic levels, additional doses may be administered.

— Expected bacterial colonisation at different body sites
Internal anatomical sites that are naturally colonised with bacteria are those that are linked by a mucous membrane to the external environment, i.e. the respiratory, GI (including biliary) and genitourinary tracts. The skin is also colonised with bacteria, which must be taken into account for surgical antibiotic prophylaxis, because for most operations the skin is incised, allowing skin pathogens access to blood in the circulatory system and locations that are otherwise sterile. Other internal sites and organs such as the blood and brain should be sterile and free of bacteria.

As a general rule, bacteria associated with the skin tend to be Gram-positive bacteria such as staphylococci and streptococci:

- *Staphylococcus aureus* (both meticillin-sensitive *S. aureus* [MSSA] and meticillin-resistant *S. aureus* [MRSA])
- *Staphylococcus epidermidis* (also called coagulase-negative staphylococci or CNS)
- *Streptococcus pyogenes* (also called group A streptococci or GAS).

The gastrointestinal tract may be thought to be colonised with more Gram-negative bacteria, as well as Gram-positive enterococci and anaerobic bacteria such as *Bacteroides* spp.:

- *Escherichia coli*
- *Pseudomonas aeruginosa* } Gram-negative bacteria
- *Klebsiella* spp.
- *Enterobacter* spp.
- *Enterococcus* spp. – Gram-positive bacteria
- *Bacteroides* spp. – Anaerobic bacteria

EXTENDED LEARNING

- What is Gram staining of bacteria, and what are the structural differences between Gram-positive and Gram-negative bacteria?

- What other types of healthcare-associated infections (HCAIs) can you think of and what are the risk factors for developing them?

References and further reading
National Institute for Health and Clinical Excellence (2008). *Surgical Site Infection: Prevention and treatment of surgical site infection.* NICE Clinical Guideline 74. London: NICE. Available at: www.nice.org.uk/CG74 (accessed 22 August 2013).

Scottish Intercollegiate Guidelines Network (2008). *Antibiotic Prophylaxis in Surgery.* SIGN Guideline 104. Edinburgh: SIGN. Available at: www.sign.ac.uk/pdf/sign104.pdf (accessed 22 August 2013).

Talbot TR (2010). Surgical site infections and antimicrobial prophylaxis. In: Mandell GL, Bennett JE, Dolin R (eds), *Mandell, Douglas and Bennett's Principles and Practice of* *Infectious Diseases,* 7th edn. Philadelphia, PA: Churchill Livingstone, 3891–904.

Case 7
Diarrhoea and antibiotic treatment
TIM HILLS

LEARNING OUTCOMES

At the end of this case, you will be able to:

- Describe the role of antibiotics as a possible cause of diarrhoea
- Outline approaches in the management of diarrhoea
- Outline the rationale for combining clavulanic acid and amoxicillin for antibiotic therapy

Case study

Mr JD, an 80-year-old man, was discharged from hospital 2 days ago after treatment for pneumonia. He phones his GP's practice for advice. He is complaining of watery diarrhoea, which started on the day that he was discharged. His drug history is as follows in the box.

CASE NOTES

Drug history
- Salbutamol nebuliser 2.5 mg q.d.s.
- Ipratropium nebuliser 500 micrograms q.d.s.
- Symbicort 200/6 two puffs b.d.
- Prednisolone 30 mg o.m. for 7 more days
- Co-amoxiclav 625 mg t.d.s. for 7 more days
- Erythromycin 500 mg q.d.s. for 7 more days

On further questioning, Mr JD says that he is opening his bowels three or four times a day, but apart from that he feels relatively well, and is eating and drinking okay.

From his discharge letter, you learn that he was diagnosed with severe community-acquired pneumonia. He was treated with i.v. co-amoxiclav 1.2 g three times daily plus i.v. clarithromycin 500 mg twice daily for 5 days, then transferred on to oral co-amoxiclav 625 mg three times daily plus *erythromycin 500 mg four times daily for a further 4 days before discharge.*

- What is the most likely cause of Mr JD's diarrhoea?
- Describe how this would have happened
- How should the condition be managed?
- What are the two components of co-amoxiclav and what amount of each is present in the combination preparation? What is the rationale for their combined use?

Stool results show positive for Clostridium difficile *toxin. Telephoning Mr JD, you discover that his diarrhoea is not ceasing and he is now going to the toilet about four or five times a day. His daughter has given him some Imodium capsules left over from when she was on holiday. (Each capsule contains loperamide hydrochloride 2 mg, which is the active ingredient.) He asks if he can take them.*

- How do you respond?
- Is there anything else that should be added to his treatment now?
- If the diarrhoea continues what else can be tried?

Case discussion

— **Causes and symptoms of diarrhoea**

Diarrhoea may occur as a result of food poisoning, a gastric virus or a side effect of medication prescribed for another indication. Erythromycin and related antibiotics are motilin agonists and are sometimes prescribed as gastric prokinetic agents for patients on the AICU (adult intensive care unit). Antibiotic-associated diarrhoea occurs as a result of disruption to the GI tract's microbial flora. Disruption of normal GI flora allows overgrowth and superinfection of the resistant organisms. This overgrowth may cause diarrhoea.

In this case, however, erythromycin is unlikely to be the cause of Mr JD's diarrhoea, because the onset of symptoms is 4 days post-initiation of the

amoxicillin

clavulanic acid

reduced relapse rates compared with oral vancomycin but is very expensive.

C. difficile is one of a number of organisms frequently acquired by patients while in hospital (hospital-acquired or nosocomial infection). It is spread via faeces, and the organism can survive in spore form for prolonged periods on contaminated surfaces. Infection is best prevented by regular cleaning and disinfection of surfaces, wearing gloves and hand washing. Bacterial spores are not inactivated by the alcohol hand gels frequently encountered in hospitals. Rather, they have to be physically removed from the hands using soap and water.

Anti-diarrhoeal medication is contraindicated in *C. difficile*-positive diarrhoea because it may cause toxic megacolon.

erythromycin. Mr JD is well and only passing stools three or four times a day so it would be prudent to hold off antibiotic therapy for the diarrhoea, and review treatment once stool cultures have been obtained and reviewed by the microbiology department.

— **Management of diarrhoea**

In the meantime, Mr JD should drink plenty of liquids, eat sensibly and be advised to stop taking the co-amoxiclav and erythromycin.

Mild *C. difficile* diarrhoea is often a self-limiting condition requiring only supportive treatment and removal of the causative antibiotic. However, patients who are having more than four stools/day and/or are systemically unwell require treatment with either oral metronidazole or oral vancomycin. Both are similarly effective, but due to vancomycin's increased cost and worries about vancomycin-resistant enterococci (VREs), metronidazole should be used as first-line therapy in mild-to-moderate infection. In patients with severe *C. difficile* infection, oral vancomycin is more effective and should be used. Intravenous vancomycin therapy is not useful because it is not excreted into the GI tract. Fidaxomicin is a new antibiotic licensed for the treatment of *C. difficile*. It is a complex macrocyclic natural product isolated from the fermentation of the producing organism, the actinomycete *Dactylosporangium aurantiacum*. It has the advantage of significantly

— **Co-amoxiclav: rationale for this combination preparation**

Co-amoxiclav 625 mg contains 500 mg amoxicillin (as the trihydrate) and 125 mg clavulanic acid (as the potassium salt). The structures of the two drugs are shown in the diagram above.

Amoxicillin is a broad-spectrum β-lactam antibiotic of the penicillin class. It has improved acid stability compared with other penicillins and shows good oral bioavailability. Amoxicillin is, however, sensitive to hydrolysis catalysed by bacterial β-lactamases. β-Lactamases are proteolytic enzymes produced by a variety of different microorganisms as a defence mechanism, conferring a degree of drug resistance. These enzymes hydrolyse the β-lactam ring of many penicillins, leading to abolition of anti-bacterial activity. Clavulanic acid is also a substrate for β-lactamase but results in irreversible covalent modification of the active site, inactivating the enzyme. When co-administered with amoxicillin, clavulanic acid competes for the β-lactamase active site, resulting in enzyme inactivation and enhancing the potency of amoxicillin against strains that express the enzyme.

EXTENDED LEARNING

- How could the management and control of HAIs be improved?
- What roles do the normal microbial flora of the GI tract perform?

- What is the role of oral rehydration therapies in the management of diarrhoea?
- What infection control practices should be adopted when involved in the care of someone with *C. difficile*-associated diarrhoea?

- How do bacteria form spores and how do the properties of the spore form differ from vegetative bacteria?

Reference/further reading

Hanlon G, Hodges N (2013). *Essential Microbiology for Pharmacy and Pharmaceutical Science*. Oxford: Wiley-Blackwell.

Case 8
'Fever with no focus' in a young infant

NEIL TICKNER

LEARNING OUTCOMES

At the end of this case, you will be able to:

- Define empirical antibiotic therapy for paediatric sepsis
- Calculate the fluid requirements for infants and children
- Outline how aqueous injections, such as intravenous fluids, are sterilised
- Outline the components of the national immunisation programme
- Outline the designs and types of study that can be applied to identify and monitor potential adverse drug reactions.

Case study

Alfie is a 66-day-old boy who has presented to A&E as generally unwell, not feeding, with a small petechial (non-blanching) rash and a temperature of 38.9 °C. He was born at term and has recently had his first immunisations. His current weight is 4.7 kg. The paediatric consultant is concerned that this may be sepsis and wishes to start immediate antibiotic therapy and maintenance i.v. fluids.

You are the paediatric pharmacist for your hospital and one of the junior doctors asks you what antibiotics and fluids to prescribe.

- What are the potential bacterial pathogens in this age group and what i.v. antibiotic(s) would you advise to cover them?
- What would you advise for maintenance fluids in terms of fluid selection and volume?

After 2 days, Alfie has improved significantly and looks back to his normal self. He hasn't had any further high temperatures and is now feeding well so the fluids have been stopped. Blood cultures were negative at 48 hours and a urine culture taken on admission has grown Escherichia coli *but with no sensitivities reported yet. The team are keen to discharge him today.*

- What oral antibiotic and dose could you recommend?
- What immunisations will Alfie have had at 2 months and what should he also receive throughout childhood?

Case discussion

— Potential pathogens for sepsis

The common pathogens for meningococcal disease and sepsis in infants may depend on age. Immediately after delivery, the baby (neonate) is covered by the flora of the maternal birth canal. Possible bacteria found in the birth canal are:

- Group B streptococci
- *E. coli*
- *Listeria monocytogenes*.

Mothers may be tested for these pathogens during pregnancy and prophylactic antibiotics administered to prevent spread to the baby at birth.

In the first few months of life, a baby will gradually develop the normal flora that you would expect in an adult through contact with family members and surroundings. The most common pathogens for sepsis beyond 1 month are:

- *Neisseria meningitidis*

- *Streptococcus pneumoniae*
- *Haemophilus influenzae* type b (Hib)
- *E. coli* and other coliforms.

— **Treatment of meningococcal disease/sepsis**

Recommended empirical treatments for meningococcal disease (NICE 2010) and sepsis in secondary care are based on age: infants aged <3 months should receive a third-generation cephalosporin AND amoxicillin. Those aged >3 months should receive a third-generation cephalosporin as a single agent.

The most recent edition of the *BNF for Children* should be consulted for appropriate doses.

Amoxicillin is required in the under 3-month group to cover the potential for listerial meningitis, which, although rare, is a potential pathogen in this age group. Amoxicillin can be stopped at 48 hours if blood cultures are negative or fail to isolate *Listeria*.

Third-generation cephalosporins are broad-spectrum antibiotics with extended spectra against Gram-negative bacteria, suitable for most pathogens implicated in sepsis. The choice of a third-generation cephalosporin depends on age and contraindications related to each drug; however, NICE recommends the use of cefotaxime as the first-line treatment in the under 3-month age group because there have been case reports of fatalities in neonates given concomitant ceftriaxone and calcium intravenously. Patients with confirmed meningococcal disease often have deranged plasma calcium levels requiring i.v. calcium correction, so starting on cefotaxime is usually the safest option. Ceftriaxone can be substituted if clinically appropriate in the absence of contraindications (see *BNF for Children*) or, for patients >3 months, it can be used first line.

For the patient presented in this case, an example of appropriate empirical therapy would be:

- Cefotaxime 235 mg three times daily (50 mg/kg)
- Amoxicillin 235 mg four times daily (50 mg/kg).

— **Intravenous fluid requirements for children**

Unlike adults, infants and children have specific daily fluid requirements when administering enteral or intravenous fluids; the approximate daily requirement should be calculated using the information in Table 5.5.

▼ TABLE 5.5

Daily requirement of fluid for children

Body weight (kg)	24-hour fluid requirement
<10	100 mL/kg
10–20	100 mL/kg for the first 10 kg (i.e. 1000 mL)
	+ 50 mL/kg for each 1 kg body weight >10 kg
>20	100 mL/kg for the first 10 kg (i.e. 1000 mL) + 50 mL/kg for each 1 kg body weight between 10 and 20 kg (i.e. 500 mL) + 20 mL/kg for each 1 kg body weight >20 kg (maximum 2 L in females, 2.5 L in males)

For i.v. fluids, this should be expressed on the prescription as a rate in millilitres per hour, simply because this is the default setting for fluid administration pumps.

Choice of fluids to give is more complex and the *BNF for Children* gives little guidance on this; however, the National Patient Safety Agency (NPSA) issued guidance in 2007. The golden rule is that previously well children aged >1 month who are admitted to hospital with illness or for surgery should never be given hypotonic fluids in the form of 0.18% sodium chloride. Neonatal fluid requirements are different and are beyond the scope of this case study.

Historically, 0.18% sodium chloride was the fluid of choice in paediatrics because it combined the daily fluid volume with the daily requirement for sodium chloride (approximately 3 mmol/kg). However, under stress (i.e. illness or surgery), the body increases the secretion of non-osmotic antidiuretic hormone (ADH or vasopressin), leading to water retention and a dilutional hyponatraemia – in severe cases leading to brain swelling, coma and death.

To avoid this risk, fluid choice is therefore recommended as 0.45% or 0.9% sodium chloride (physiological saline) depending on plasma sodium concentration or severity of illness. Glucose at a concentration of 2.5% or 5% is frequently combined in these bags to add calorie content for patients who have little or no milk/food intake. These fluid bags may also come with either 10 or 20 mmol potassium per 500 mL to supplement dietary intake while fluids are running, or to replace potassium if the plasma level is low.

For this patient, appropriate initial i.v. fluid therapy would be:
0.45% or 0.9% sodium chloride + 5% glucose (with or without potassium) run at a rate of 19.6 mL/h (470 mL/day).

— Intravenous fluid sterilisation

As parenteral routes of drug administration (including intravenous administration) bypass the body's first line of defence against pathogens, namely the skin, it is essential that they are sterile, i.e. free from viable organisms. There are five main methods of sterilisation listed in international pharmacopoeias, namely: steam sterilisation, dry heat sterilisation, ionising radiation sterilisation, gaseous sterilisation and sterilisation by filtration. For aqueous preparations, such as i.v. fluids, sterilisation using saturated steam under pressure (using an autoclave) is the preferred method. Saturated steam is highly efficient as a steriliser, as on contact with a cooler object it gives up its latent heat of vaporisation. Steam sterilisation is a terminal method of sterilisation, with the product sterilised in its final container, which is preferred over a non-terminal sterilisation process, such as filtration. The standard conditions for sterilisation using this method are a minimum of 121 °C for 15 min, which provides a good safety margin. Other combinations may be used, provided they have been adequately validated.

Intravenous fluids must also be free from pyrogens. These are materials that cause an increase in temperature if injected into the body. The most commonly encountered pyrogens are the endotoxins produced by Gram-negative bacteria, comprising cell-wall lipopolysaccharides. Pyrogens are not inactivated at the temperatures employed in steam sterilisation, so high quality water for injections, prepared in such a way as to exclude pyrogens, must be used to manufacture sterile pharmaceutical products.

— Appropriate oral antibiotics for UTIs in children

Oral antibiotics for children are a cornerstone of paediatric pharmacy and are used to treat the common ailments of childhood. An ideal antibiotic for children should:

- Have a pleasant taste
- Be given as few times a day as possible (long half-life)
- Not cause resistance
- Not require monitoring (non-toxic to humans)
- Have a good stability profile in liquid form
- Have a good spectrum of action against expected pathogens
- Be cost-effective
- Not have absorption affected by milk/food.

In this case, Alfie has grown *E. coli* in his urine culture and antibiotic sensitivities won't be available for another 24 hours. Empirical antibiotic therapy for UTIs should always be guided by local policy and resistance patterns, then by culture sensitivities once available. Options for treatment would include antibiotics that are broad spectrum but with good activity against Gram-negative organisms and excreted renally (so that they are concentrated in the urine). Possible antibiotics that fit this profile are:

- Trimethoprim
- Nitrofurantoin
- Amoxicillin
- Co-amoxiclav
- Second-generation cephalosporins (e.g. cefadroxil).

— Immunisation schedule

The national immunisation schedule has evolved to incorporate pathogens common in childhood for which a safe and effective vaccine has been developed. By 13 months of life, a child should have had a set of comprehensive vaccines protecting against most of the known causes of meningococcal disease as well as other serious diseases such as diphtheria, tetanus, pertussis, polio, measles, mumps and rubella. Recommended schedules are continually updated by health departments.

Huge efforts go into promoting comprehensive delivery of national immunisation programmes, because high population coverage is essential to ensure maximum health benefits ('herd immunity'). In the early 2000s, after the publication of a study that suggested a possible link between MMR immunisation and autism, the uptake of MMR immunisation dropped. As a consequence there have been outbreaks of disease, particularly measles, among certain populations. The research that suggested a possible link between MMR immunisation and autism has since been discredited and removed from public record. A number of subsequent large epidemiological studies have found no scientific evidence of any link. However, this case highlights the importance of rigorous scientific methodology in research as well as the critical review that is required in the interpretation of findings.

The more recent studies employed epidemiological approaches, which examine associations between variables (e.g. autistic spectrum disorders [ASDs] and MMR immunisation) in population data. The research is often based on very large datasets and the application of probability statistics. Such studies involved looking at trends in both MMR uptake and ASDs at crucial time periods, to establish whether there was any likelihood of a causal relationship.

Case–control studies have also been employed. These studies identify individuals who have a particular characteristic (e.g. in this case an ASD) and compare them with 'controls', who are similar in other respects but do not display the characteristic of interest. The researcher then examines exposure to potential causative events in the two groups to establish any differences.

EXTENDED LEARNING

- What features distinguish bacterial and viral meningitis?
- How do neonatal fluid requirements differ from those of older infants?
- What are the applications, advantages and disadvantages of the pharmacopoeial sterilisation processes?

- How are pharmaceutical products tested for sterility and how are endotoxins tested for or quantified?
- Outline the structure, properties, activity and therapeutic uses of penicillins and cephalosporins.
- What different types of study are employed by pharmacoepidemiologists to identify, monitor and confirm the incidence of adverse drugs reactions? What are their strengths and limitations?

ADDITIONAL PRACTICE POINTS

- What are the symptoms of meningitis to which parents and health professionals should be alert?
- Investigate the current immunisation schedules for children and adults. How are these programmes delivered locally?

References and further reading

National Institute for Health and Clinical Excellence (2007). *Urinary Tract Infection in Children*. NICE Clinical Guideline 54. London: NICE. Available at: http://guidance.nice.org.uk/CG54 (accessed 2 October 2013).

National Institute for Health and Clinical Excellence (2010). *Bacterial Meningitis and Meningococcal Septicaemia in Children*. NICE Clinical Guideline 102. London: NICE. Available at: http://guidance.nice.org.uk/CG102/Guidance (accessed 2 October 2013).

National Patient Safety Agency (2007). *Reducing the Risk of Hyponatraemia when Administering Intravenous Infusions to Children*. London: NPSA. Available at: www.nrls.npsa.nhs.uk/resources/?entryid45=59809 (accessed 2 October 2013).

Case 9
Management of tuberculosis and its complications
TIM RENNIE

LEARNING OUTCOMES

At the end of this case, you will be able to:

- Outline the pathophysiology, signs, symptoms and diagnosis of TB
- Describe the treatment options for TB
- Describe the complications of TB and how treatment management options may be altered
- Describe the structure and mechanism of action of isoniazid

Case study

Mrs AB, aged 32 years, was born in Bangladesh and moved to the UK 7 years ago. She visited her GP when she started having non-specific symptoms – cough and fever – and she was prescribed broad-spectrum antibiotics. However, her condition worsened and after several months of repeat GP visits she was eventually referred to the local A&E with haemoptysis. After examination, she was admitted to hospital and put into a negative pressure room, with a preliminary diagnosis of pulmonary TB (PTB).

- What are the typical symptoms of PTB?
- How else might TB present?
- How is TB diagnosed?

Mrs AB was started on a standard anti-TB regimen, discharged from hospital after 2 weeks and referred to the outpatient TB clinic for follow-up. Mrs AB showed initial improvement and her symptoms subsided. However, culture results established that her TB was isoniazid resistant.

- What standard medicines regimen is Mrs AB likely to have been prescribed?
- What are the implications of isoniazid resistance for her management?
- What is the chemical structure and mechanism of action of isoniazid and how is this related to the development of resistance?

As a precaution, Mrs AB was started on 'DOT' (directly observed therapy). In addition, close

contacts of Mrs AB (in this case just her family and close friends) were screened for TB.

- What is 'DOT' and when is it used in the UK?

Case discussion

— TB and its pathophysiology

TB is an infectious disease most commonly of the lungs (PTB) caused by the rod bacillus *Mycobacterium tuberculosis*. The disease can be described as 'chronic' due to the usually slow onset of symptoms, dormancy as a result of the immune response and long duration of treatment. The prolonged treatment is due to the slow growth of the organism and the thick cell wall that makes it impenetrable to conventional antibiotics. Primary infection is almost exclusively in the lungs, and is spread by the coughing of an individual with infectious pulmonary disease (although it is theoretically possible by other means). However, the likelihood of transmission is relatively low. Only those individuals exposed to disease over a prolonged period of time ('close contacts') generally require initial medical investigation. For people who are infected, approximately a third of the global population, progression to disease is also unlikely, with about a 10% lifetime risk. However, this is increased in those with immune insufficiency (especially in HIV-positive patients, see below). Nevertheless, TB can lie latent in the lungs, or in virtually any part of the body to which it has spread, where reactivation may occur later in life. In the UK, over half of TB patients have extrapulmonary TB, with or without pulmonary disease (Health Protection Agency, 2009).

— Signs, symptoms and diagnosis of TB

Symptoms of TB disease depend on the site of infection, but typically PTB could present with cough, fever, night sweats, sputum production, haemoptysis (coughing up blood), weight loss and lethargy.

TB infection stimulates an immune response, the mechanism for which is utilised in both diagnostic testing and primary prevention. Tuberculin skin tests (TST: Mantoux and the now obsolete Heaf test) work on the principle of injection into the skin of a small amount of purified protein derivative (PPD), eliciting an immune response in those who have previously encountered this 'pathogen'. By the same principle, BCG immunisation (primary TB prevention) involves subcutaneous injection of a live attenuated *Mycobacterium bovis* strain to prime the immune system against TB infection. Studies of this vaccine suggest that it exhibits between 0% and 80% efficacy, depending on geographical location.

There is no single 'gold-standard' TB diagnostic test; diagnostics are used in concert and vary in terms of specificity and sensitivity. Generally, depending on the site of TB infection, diagnosis will be based on clinical judgement considering: symptoms, radiography for chest abnormalities or MRI on parts of the body besides the lungs, and smear microscopy of sputum or biopsies with follow-up rapid culture techniques to confirm disease microbiology and sensitivities (bacterial resistance).

— **Treatment options**

Treatment of TB is a specialist area and is usually initiated and managed in the acute healthcare setting. Patients may be admitted to hospital initially, but will generally attend outpatient clinics in follow-up appointments. Aspects of their treatment, such as DOT and TB screening, may be managed in the community, including community pharmacy settings where such services are offered.

First-line recommendations for treatment of PTB utilise standard combination regimens (see the latest *BNF*). Therapy is complex, comprising two phases: an initial phase and a continuation phase. Both involve concurrent use of a combination of different drugs to prevent the development of drug resistance and increase the effectiveness of therapy.

Initial phase: concurrent use of four drugs – isoniazid, rifampicin, ethambutol and pyrazinamide – for 2 months to reduce the burden of infection and render the patient non-infectious. *Continuation phase*: isoniazid and rifampicin for a further 4 months to sterilise the lungs of residual infection.

— **Structure and mechanism of action of isoniazid**

Isoniazid is the hydrazide of an isomer of nicotinic acid.

It has only recently become well established. An enzyme specific to *Mycobacterium tuberculosis*, KatG, oxidises isoniazid to give a highly reactive radical intermediate. This intermediate then reacts with NAD(H) to generate adducts that inhibit mycobacterial synthesis of mycolic acids, essential for cell-wall assembly. Isoniazid resistance can arise in mycobacteria that do not produce KatG or produce KatG mutants. Other isoniazid-resistant mycobacteria over-express the enzyme(s) involved in mycolic acid biosynthesis, partially bypassing the effects of the drug.

isoniazid

Rifamycin antibiotics inhibit bacterial RNA synthesis by inhibiting DNA-dependent RNA polymerase. Acquired resistance is often due to a mutation in the DNA-dependent RNA polymerase. As a consequence of the potential for resistance development, these agents are always used in combination with other types of antibiotic.

Dose and frequency of administration depend on three predominant factors: (1) the patient's weight; (2) whether combination regimens or single-drug formulations are used; and (3) whether the treatment is supervised (DOT) or 'self-supervised'.

TB treatment may deviate from standard regimens if mycobacterial resistance is identified or therapy is not tolerated by the patient (adverse drug reactions), or for the treatment of extrapulmonary TB (e.g. TB meningitis).

Unlike in countries of high TB prevalence, DOT is recommended only where an adherence risk assessment has identified those at greater risk of non-adherence, including street- or shelter-dwelling homeless people with active TB, and those with a history of non-adherence. Bacterial resistance may be suggestive of previous poor adherence, but DOT may also be advocated as second-line regimen – often less efficacious and less well tolerated.

— **Latent TB**

Follow-up radiographs or BCG immunisation may be utilised to rule out or prevent TB disease (see NICE guidance). As adherence, especially to preventive treatments, presents a challenge, the shorter 3-month regimen may be favoured, although monotherapy with isoniazid can be utilised when rifampicin resistance presents, or if the combined regimen is not tolerated. See also Case 10 below.

— **Prevalence of TB: international perspectives**
This patient is of Bangladeshi origin and prevalence of TB is high in many countries in Asia. TB, which was very prevalent in the UK and declined significantly in the second half of the twentieth century, is now rising again. Movement of people from regions where TB has remained prevalent is a major factor in this resurgence, and rates are higher among certain immigrant population groups. Infectious disease (especially TB, malaria, HIV, pneumonia and diarrhoeal disease) still account for high levels of morbidity and mortality in many of the poorest countries, TB being one of the world's leading causes of death from a single disease. A high proportion of cases and deaths from TB are among people who are HIV positive, and thus immunocompromised. TB is the single biggest cause of mortality in this group.

Notwithstanding the importance of measures to prevent, diagnose and effectively treat TB and other infectious diseases, patterns of disease are changing. Chronic diseases (including cardiovascular disease, diabetes, respiratory disease and cancers), once associated with more affluent nations, are now an increasing burden in low- and, especially, middle-income countries. These changes in population disease patterns, which are to a large extent the consequence of complex social, economic and political factors, as well as globalisation and population age structures, are referred to as the 'epidemiological transition'. The

ageing of populations across most parts of the world is sometimes referred to as a 'demographic transition'. This also has implications for changing patterns of morbidity, mortality and healthcare.

EXTENDED LEARNING

- What are second-line options for TB treatment?
- What are the mechanisms of action of the different classes of antibiotics?
- What are the mechanisms and causes of antibiotic resistance?
- Distinguish the different types of immunity and vaccines.
- How are the prevalence rates of TB changing in the UK and globally?

References and further reading

Capstick TGD (2013). Tuberculosis: clinical features and diagnosis. *Clin Pharmacist* 5:161–6.

Gothard A, Millington K, Capstick TGD (2013). Tuberculosis management. *Clin Pharmacist* 5:167–70.

Health Protection Agency (2009). *Tuberculosis in the UK: Annual report on tuberculosis surveillance in the UK.* Available at: www.hpa.org.uk/Publications/ InfectiousDiseases/Tuberculosis/0912TuberculosisintheUK/ (accessed 2 October 2013).

National Institute for Health and Clinical Excellence (2011). *Tuberculosis: Clinical diagnosis and management of tuberculosis, and measures for its prevention and control.* NICE Clinical Guideline 117. London: NICE. Available at: http://guidance.nice.org.uk/CG117 (accessed 2 October 2013).

Rennie TW (2008). Historical non-involvement and future opportunities: pharmacy and TB. *Int Pharmacy J* 23:36–44.

Rennie TW, Bothamley GH, Engova D, Bates IP (2007). Patient choice promotes adherence in preventive treatment for latent tuberculosis. *Eur Respir J* 30:728–35.

Case 10
Management of latent TB infection and pharmacy interventions
TIM RENNIE

LEARNING OUTCOMES

At the end of this case, you will be able to:

* Outline the diagnosis, treatment and monitoring of latent TB infection (LTBI)
* Describe the main counselling points in relation to treatment of LTBI
* Identify ways in which licensed medicines, 'specials' and extemporaneously prepared medicines may differ

Case study

Mrs AB, aged 32 years, was born in Bangladesh and moved to the UK 7 years ago. She has a diagnosis of PTB which is isoniazid resistant. Mrs AB was started on 'DOT' and her family and friends were screened for TB.

No contacts of Mrs AB exhibited TB disease, but her 6-year-old son, MB, was diagnosed with latent TB.

❓ What is latent TB and how is it currently diagnosed?

❓ What are the treatment options for MB and what considerations will be made in relation to his treatment?

❓ When might other interventions besides treatment of LTBI be used to reduce the risk of development of TB disease and limit disease spread?

MB is started on preventive treatment for LTBI. He is referred to his local community pharmacy, from where his medicines will be collected on a weekly basis but he will need to return to the TB clinic for monthly checks.

❓ What monitoring is necessary during MB's treatment and why is it necessary for him to return to the TB clinic?

❓ What counselling points are necessary on initiation of treatment, and what might the pharmacist enquire about at the weekly visits to the pharmacy?

On one of the initial pharmacy visits, Mrs AB reports that MB is struggling to swallow his tablets (he is taking Rifinah tablets) and asks for help.

❓ Are there any options for changing MB's medicines?

❓ What is the importance of continuing to take preventive TB treatment?

Case discussion

— Symptoms and diagnosis of latent TB infection

By definition, there are no symptoms of latent TB infection (LTBI). The interferon-γ release assays (IGRA, including QuantiFERON-TB and T-SPOT. TB) essentially identify interferon-γ – the immune cascade 'communicator' cytokine – through blood tests to identify previous infection. All commercial IGRA tests are currently licensed for LTBI diagnosis only; the Mantoux test is unlicensed but is routinely used for LTBI diagnosis.

— Treatment options

Treatment of LTBI is a specialist area and is usually initiated and managed in the acute healthcare setting; patients may be admitted to hospital initially but will generally attend outpatient clinics for follow-up appointments. Aspects of their treatment, such as DOT and TB screening, may be managed in the community, including community pharmacy settings where such services are offered.

From a healthcare perspective, latent TB treatment is essentially an exercise in ensuring adherence for maximum public health benefit and identifying any adverse drug reactions; this makes it an ideal potential service that pharmacists can offer. Two regimens are recommended in the UK for treatment of LTBI:

1 Daily isoniazid for 6 months' duration
2 Combined rifampicin + isoniazid for 3 months' duration

Chemotherapy for LTBI is not offered in those aged >35 years in the UK, because the risk of adverse drug reactions (ADRs) outweighs any benefit derived from treatment.

— **Adherence and counselling points**

The theoretical risk of bacterial TB resistance occurring to four first-line medicines used in combination is negligible. Multidrug therapy decreases the chance that the infecting strain(s) will be resistant to all of the antibiotics used, increasing efficacy. The likelihood of the infecting strain(s) acquiring resistance (through random genetic mutation) to multiple agents simultaneously is also very low. However, as resistance is relatively common, it must be assumed that a degree of non-adherence occurs on the part of the healthcare establishment as well as the patient. The question to ask is: faced with a potentially life-threatening and unpleasant disease, why would anyone be non-adherent? A possible answer is that adherence to treatment may lie beyond the patient's control; non-adherence may be unintentional or there may be other factors, such as drug addiction or homelessness, that take greater priority.

As such, pharmacists should do everything in their power to aid adherence including: 'educating' patients about side effects and possible ADRs:

- Rifampicin will stain bodily fluids red/orange, including tears (think: contact lenses), sweat (think: wearing white shirts), urine, saliva, semen, etc. Rifampicin contains an extensive system of conjugated π bonds and is consequently intensely coloured (similar to a dye) through interaction with visible light. Even small concentrations of drug present in body fluids will impart a red–orange coloration. Rifampicin is also a very powerful enzyme inducer and, as such, will interact with many drugs, in particular oral contraceptives: make sure that your patient is aware of this. Do they need to use other contraceptive methods if they are female?
- Ethambutol can affect eyesight. Has the patient had baseline/ongoing visual acuity tests?
- Rifampicin/isoniazid/pyrazinamide can cause liver damage. Is the patient aware of the signs/ symptoms of hepatotoxicity and do they know what to do (i.e. seek immediate medical attention) if they experience such signs/ symptoms? Existing hepatitis and alcoholism are risk factors.
- As an aminoglycoside, streptomycin should never be given to children or pregnant/ breastfeeding mothers.

— **The importance of adherence**

- The minimum duration of treatment of TB with these very unpleasant drugs is 6 months and often exceeds this. However, symptoms (of TB disease) often subside after a few weeks. Treatment of latent TB may continue for 3–6 months but, as a preventive treatment, adherence is likely to be worse.
- Patients will need motivation and social support in completing their treatment: consider the sheer volume/size of medicines that have to be consumed every day.
- There is a great deal of stigma associated with this communicable disease that may impact on adherence, and it is important to try to normalise the disease, e.g. by emphasising that patients will be non-infectious for the large part of their treatment and that most anti-TB drugs are safe to use in pregnancy.
- There is a variety of TB preparations available that can be tailored to a patient's needs. Some patients may find it difficult to swallow some combined preparations or struggle with the sheer volume of medicines to take with single preparations. Although only a few liquid preparations are manufactured (notably isoniazid and rifampicin) these can be ordered, at some expense, from 'specials' manufacturers.

— **Extemporaneously prepared medicines and 'specials'**

Be aware that there are differences between licensed medicines (those having a marketing authorisation), those prepared extemporaneously in a pharmacy (for a single patient) and specials, produced by licensed specials manufacturers (Table 5.6).

— **Monitoring**

- Eye tests: (ethambutol) before treatment (baseline) and during treatment.
- Liver function blood tests: (e.g. isoniazid) AST: ALT ratio, liver transaminase levels. This is also a requirement for latent TB treatment because patients will normally be prescribed isoniazid and rifampicin.
- Symptoms: rash, itchiness, joint aches, visual changes, jaundice, nausea and vomiting, peripheral neuropathy.
- Adherence: indicators of adherence used in concert, including self-report (e.g. 'How many pills have you missed in the last week?'), attendance at scheduled appointments, pill

▼ TABLE 5.6
Differences between licensed, extemporaneously prepared and 'special' medicines

Preparation	Licensed	Special	Extemporaneously prepared
Method of preparation	GMP	GMP	Often not under GMP
Product quality	Best	Intermediate	Good (less strictly controlled)
Quality control	Extensive tests	Minimal	Very limited, if at all (single product for one patient)
Risk	Low	Higher	Highest
Shelf-life	Long	Medium	Short
Responsibility for quality	Manufacturer (pharmaceutical company)	Pharmacist/clinician	Pharmacist

GMP is Good Manufacturing Practice: a system for ensuring that products are consistently produced and controlled in accordance with standards appropriate to their intended use and the product specification.

counts and a simple urine colour check can be used as a blunt tool to check adherence for patients taking rifampicin.

EXTENDED LEARNING

- Identify any new developments for the diagnosis, prevention and treatment of TB and LTBI
- Describe the place and operation of DOT programmes in the management of TB
- Outline the strategies and recommendations of the World Health Organization for the prevention and management of TB
- What is Good Manufacturing Practice and how is the quality of a pharmaceutical product assured?

- How are medicines and medical devices regulated and licensed?

References and further reading

Capstick TGD (2013). Tuberculosis: clinical features and diagnosis. *Clin Pharmacist* 5:161–6.

Furniss D, Barber N, Lyons I, Eliasson L, Blandford A (2013). Unintentional non-adherence: can a spoon full of resilience help the medicine go down? *BMJ Qual Saf* 23:95–8.

Gothard A, Millington K, Capstick TGD (2013). Tuberculosis management. *Clin Pharmacist* 5:167–70.

Rennie TW (2008). Historical non-involvement and future opportunities: pharmacy and TB. *Int Pharmacy J* 23:36–44.

Rennie TW, Bothamley GH, Engova D, Bates IP (2007). Patient choice promotes adherence in preventive treatment for latent tuberculosis. *Eur Respir J* 30:728–35.

Case 11
Influenza
TIM HILLS

LEARNING OUTCOMES

At the end of this case, you will be able to:

- Summarise the symptoms and treatment of influenza
- Outline the chemistry and mode of action of oseltamivir and zanamivir
- Describe the advantages and disadvantages of the pressurised metered dose inhaler as an inhalation drug delivery device
- Outline the use of spacers with inhalation devices
- Outline the guidance for seasonal influenza immunisation programmes

Case study

Ms FC is a 40-year-old woman who presents to your practice saying that she feels 'hit by something nasty'. On further questioning, you discover that she has been having symptoms of fever, malaise, headache and cough since yesterday; she has not noticed any changes in the nature of her sputum.

CASE NOTES

Past medical history:
- Asthma

Drug history
- Salbutamol pMDI two puffs p.r.n.
- Beclometasone pMDI 100 micrograms/puff two puffs b.d. via spacer
- AeroChamber Plus

On examination

- Alert
- SOBOE (shortness of breath on exertion) with intermittent coughing
- Temp: 39°C
- PEFR (peak expiratory flow rate): 280 L/min (normal for her: 400 L/min)
- Mild wheeze
- No creps (respiratory crepitation: dry, crackling sound)

- What are the possible diagnoses?
- What is a pMDI? What are the advantages and disadvantages of pMDIs compared with other devices for delivering drugs to the lungs?
- What is an AeroChamber Plus? What advantages does such a device offer when used with a pMDI?

Influenza A is currently circulating in the local area and this year the vaccine is considered to offer adequate cover for the circulating strain. Looking on the practice database, you discover that Ms FC did not receive an influenza vaccine this year.

- What treatments are available for treating likely/proven influenza infection?
- What restrictions are there on the use of these drugs?
- What do you recommend for Ms FC?

Case discussion

— Signs, symptoms and diagnosis of influenza

Common symptoms of influenza may include sudden fever, chills, headache, tiredness, loss of appetite, aching muscles, limb/joint pain, difficulty sleeping and an upset stomach, in addition to respiratory symptoms such as a dry, chesty cough, sneezing, runny or blocked nose and sore throat. In this case, possible diagnoses may include a respiratory virus, an atypical pneumonia or an influenza virus. It is important to be aware of the influenza viral strains circulating in a community and the relationship between this and those included in the seasonal immunisation programme.

— Treatment of influenza

In general, patients experiencing flu symptoms may be advised to rest, keep warm and drink plenty of water to avoid dehydration. Paracetamol or ibuprofen may be appropriate, depending on the individual's medical history and if symptoms of fever are being experienced. For specific groups of 'high-risk' patients, antiviral medication may be prescribed.

Oseltamivir and zanamivir can be effective antiviral treatments for influenza if started within a few hours of the first symptoms. NICE guidance (2009) states the conditions under which these drugs are licensed and may be effectively prescribed.

Oseltamivir and zanamivir are inhibitors of viral neuraminidase, an enzyme required to cleave terminal sialic acid carbohydrate residues from host cell glycoproteins, enabling release of new viral particles from infected cells. Inhibition of neuraminidase inhibits the release of new viral particles and can help limit the spread of the influenza virus to other cells.

Structurally, both oseltamivir and zanamivir resemble the transition state that sialic acid goes through during cleavage. Zanamivir is considerably more polar than oseltamivir and consequently is not orally bioavailable. This very high polarity results from the presence of multiple hydroxyl groups and both an acidic (carboxyl) and basic (guanidine) group, which would be predominantly charged in the small intestine. Zanamivir is generally administered as a dry powder for inhalation. Oseltamivir is a prodrug (ethyl ester) that is readily absorbed after oral administration. After absorption, the ester is hydrolysed during first-pass metabolism to give the active carboxylic acid metabolite.

— Pressurised metered-dose inhalers for drug delivery to the lungs

Pressurised metered-dose inhalers (pMDIs), sometimes called metered dose inhalers (MDIs), are the most commonly used inhalational drug oseltamivir

zanamivir

delivery devices. In pMDIs, the drug is dissolved or suspended in liquefied propellant(s), usually a hydrofluoroalkane (HFA), together with other excipients. The formulation is contained in a pressurised aluminium canister fitted with a metering valve, which permits the reproducible delivery of small volumes (25–100 μL) of product.

The pMDIs may be formulated as either solutions or suspensions of drug in the liquefied propellant. Most formulations are suspensions, in which case the particle size of the solid (usually micronised to between 2 and 5 μm) is important to ensure deep lung drug deposition. Surfactants may be included as suspending agents, but sometimes have very poor solubility in HFAs (e.g. propellants HFA 134a and HFA 227) and so ethanol is often included as a co-solvent. On expulsion from the canister, propellant rapidly evaporates (flashes) from the emitted aerosol droplets, such that the drug is available as fine particles. Evaporation of HFA propellant from solution formulations of drugs, such as some formulations of beclometasone dipropionate, results in smaller particle sizes than with conventional suspension formulations of the same drug, changing pulmonary distribution and requiring adjustment of dose.

The major advantages of pMDIs are their portability, low cost and ability to store multiple doses. They are inefficient at drug delivery. On actuation, the large drug-containing propellant droplets exit at a high velocity, so that a lot of drug is lost by impaction in the oropharyngeal areas. Correct use of these devices by patients is vital for effective drug deposition and therapeutic action. The pMDI should be actuated as the patient takes a slow, deep inhalation, followed by a period of breathholding. The misuse of pMDIs through poor techniques can be significantly reduced with appropriate instruction and counselling.

— Use of spacers with pMDIs
Some of the disadvantages of pMDIs, particularly the need for inhalation/actuation coordination and the deposition of large droplets high in the airways, can be overcome by using 'spacers'. These devices allow the initial droplet velocity to decrease; large droplets are removed by impaction, propellant evaporation reduces the droplet size and the need for actuation/inhalation coordination is removed. Traditional spacers, though effective, have been large and cumbersome. However, smaller, medium-volume spacers, such as the AeroChamber Plus, are more patient acceptable.

— Seasonal influenza: preventing spread of disease and immunisation
Influenza viruses circulate worldwide and can affect anybody in any age group. Influenza spreads easily from person to person through droplets created when someone with the infection coughs or sneezes. The virus can also be spread by hands infected with the virus. To prevent spreading the virus, people should cover their mouth and nose with a tissue when coughing, and wash their hands regularly. Worldwide, annual flu epidemics result in about 3–5 million cases of severe illness, and about 250 000–500 000 deaths. Most deaths associated with influenza in industrialised countries occur among people aged $\geq$65 years. Seasonal influenza vaccines will not control epidemics.

Immunisation against seasonal flu is given annually to people who are at risk of developing complications from the flu virus. The highest risk of complications occurs among children aged <2 years, adults aged $\geq$65 years, and people of any age with certain medical conditions, such as chronic heart, lung, kidney, liver, blood or metabolic diseases (e.g. diabetes), or a poor immune system.

Furthermore, individuals may be offered immunisation if they are the main carer for an elderly or disabled person whose care may be at risk if the carer falls ill with flu, or if they are involved in direct patient care (including workers in nursing and care homes). It is recommended that all pregnant women receive the flu immunisation, even if they are otherwise healthy.

There are different strains of influenza virus. Influenza immunisation is most effective when circulating viruses are matched with vaccine viruses. Influenza viruses are constantly changing, and the WHO Global Influenza Surveillance Network (GISN), a partnership of national influenza centres around the world, monitors the influenza viruses circulating in humans. WHO annually recommends a vaccine composition that targets the three most representative strains in circulation. A new vaccine is formulated each year and at-risk groups need annual immunisation to remain protected.

Recommendations are constantly reviewed and pharmacists should ensure that they have the most up-to-date guidance for use in their practices, e.g. in England from September 2013, all 2-year-old children are offered a nasal influenza immunisation, available to all preschool and primary school-aged children from 2014. Secondary school-aged children will then be enrolled in pilots from 2014, extended to all from 2015 (Public Health England, 2013).

> **EXTENDED LEARNING**
>
> - What do you understand by the term pandemic influenza?
> - Not all healthcare workers choose to receive vaccination for influenza. Do you think it should be mandatory and why?

References and further reading

Caplan A (2011). Time to mandate influenza vaccination in health-care workers. *Lancet* **378**:310–11.

National Institute for Health and Care Excellence (2009). Influenza – zanamivir, amantadine and oseltamivir (review) – NICE Technology Appraisal 168. Available at: http://guidance.nice.org.uk/TA168 (accessed 8 July 2013).

Public Health England (2013). Influenza. In: *Immunisation against Infectious Disease (The Green Book)*. London: Public Health England, 185–218. Available at: https://www.gov.uk/government/uploads/system/uploads/attachment_data/file/239268/Green_Book_Chapter_19_v5_2_final.pdf (accessed 16 June 2013).

Taylor KMG (2013). Pulmonary drug delivery. In: Aulton ME, Taylor KMG (eds), *Aulton's Pharmaceutics: The design and manufacture of medicines*, 4th edn, London: Elsevier, 638–56.

World Health Organization (2013). *Influenza*. Geneva: WHO. Available at: www.who.int/influenza/en (accessed 16 June 2013).

Case 12
Chronic hepatitis C

JOYETA DAS

LEARNING OUTCOMES

At the end of this case, you will be able to:

- Discuss the phases and progression of chronic hepatitis C infection
- List the routes of hepatitis C virus transmission
- Describe the diagnosis process for hepatitis C
- Discuss the treatment options for the management of chronic hepatitis C
- Discuss the main parameters that should be monitored when a patient is taking treatment
- Outline the use of pegylation to modify the fate of a drug molecule in the body
- Describe the use of the PCR to amplify segments of DNA
- Describe the different phases of clinical trials

Case study

Mrs FK, a 34-year old woman, was found to have abnormal LFTs during investigation for diabetes mellitus. A viral screen was positive for hepatitis C virus (HCV) antibodies and she was referred to see a consultant hepatologist for further investigations.

❓ What is chronic hepatitis C viral infection?

During the consultation, it was established that Mrs FK had been a resident of the UK for all of her life apart from a 3-year period when she lived in Pakistan. During this time, she was involved in an RTA (road traffic accident) and received a blood transfusion.

❷ How can the hepatitis C virus be contracted?

Further investigations found Mrs FK to be PCR positive with a HCV RNA level of 289 000 copies/mL. A diagnosis of chronic HCV was confirmed.

❷ How is hepatitis C infection diagnosed?

The consultant hepatologist arranged for Mrs FK to have a FibroScan and submitted further blood samples to establish her genotype.

❷ Why is it important to establish the patient's genotype?

The results of the FibroScan showed inflammation. With a FibroScan score of 14.1 kPa, the results of genotypic testing indicate genotype 1. The consultant hepatologist informs Mrs FK of her diagnosis and recommends that she start treatment.

❷ What is a FibroScan?
❷ What are the treatment options?

Before starting treatment, Mrs FK mentions that she is considering starting a family.

❷ What advice should be given?

Case discussion

— Hepatitis C virus infection
Hepatitis C is a 'silent' infectious disease of the liver caused by the hepatitis C virus (HCV), which is a single-stranded RNA virus. It was first identified in 1989 and the ability of the virus to mutate has resulted in six recognised different genetic variations of HCV. These variations are known as genotypes and are numbered 1–6. These are linked largely, but not exclusively, to various parts of the world.

There are two main phases of infection: acute and chronic. Acute HCV infection refers to the period immediately after HCV infection, whereas chronic HCV infection is defined as infection persisting for >6 months.

Adults infected with HCV are often asymptomatic, but about 20% will develop acute hepatitis. Some of these people will experience non-specific symptoms including malaise,

weakness and anorexia. Approximately 80% of those exposed fail to clear the virus and go on to develop chronic hepatitis. Due to the common absence of symptoms, many people are unaware that they have hepatitis C infection until some time after initial infection.

Chronic HCV is categorised as mild, moderate or severe depending on the extent of liver damage. The rate of progression of the disease is slow but variable, taking about 20–50 years from the time of infection. About 20–30% of those infected develop cirrhosis within 20 years, and a small percentage of these people are at high risk of hepatocellular carcinoma (HCC). Some people with end-stage liver disease or hepatocellular carcinoma (HCC) may require liver transplantation.

— Transmission of the hepatitis C virus
HCV is a blood-borne virus and is primarily transmitted parenterally through percutaneous exposure to contaminated blood. The main routes of transmission are as follows:

- Blood transfusion with unscreened blood products; in the UK since September 1991, all blood and blood products are screened for blood-borne viruses; however, this is not the case in all other countries
- Reuse of needles and syringes that have not being adequately sterilised, e.g. by intravenous drug users
- Needle-stick injuries
- Tattooing
- Acupuncture
- Intranasal cocaine use
- Perinatal (mother to baby); the risk of transmission is approximately 5%
- Sexual (exposure to an infected partner or multiple partners).

— Diagnosis
The diagnosis process comprises two tests and involves assessment via serological tests. The first test detects antibodies to HCV; it can take up to 3 months for the antibodies to become detectable after infection with HCV. A positive antibody test does not mean that the patient has chronic HCV infection, because he or she may have spontaneously cleared the virus. Therefore, if an antibody test is positive, the second test is to check if the virus is still present, by using a qualitative PCR test. This test indicates the presence of viraemia (virus in the bloodstream). A

positive (detectable) PCR result means that the immune system did not clear the infection during the acute phase of infection and has progressed to the chronic phase.

— Polymerase chain reaction

PCR is a fast, inexpensive technique, widely used to copy (amplify) small segments of DNA. It is invaluable in a range of techniques, including DNA cloning for sequencing, functional analysis of genes, genetic fingerprinting and detection of bacteria or viruses.

Most PCR methods use thermal cycling, whereby a sample is alternately heated and cooled in a series of steps to physically separate the two strands of DNA. A heat-stable DNA polymerase enzyme, usually Taq polymerase, is employed to synthesise a new DNA strand from the nucleotides, by using single-stranded DNA as a template and DNA oligonucleotides (DNA primers), which initiate DNA synthesis.

This process duplicates the original DNA, with each of the new molecules containing one old and one new strand of DNA. Each of these strands can then be used to create two new copies, and so on. The cycle of denaturing and synthesising new DNA is repeated up to 40 times, such that the sequence of interest can be copied more than one million-fold.

PCR requires the following:

- DNA template that contains the DNA sequence to be amplified.
- Two primers that are complementary to the 3'-ends of each of the sense and anti-sense strand of the DNA target; these are short single-stranded DNA molecules.
- Taq polymerase (or other DNA polymerase) with a temperature optimum at approximately 70 °C.
- Deoxynucleoside triphosphates (dNTPs – nucleotides containing triphosphate groups).
- Buffer solution (for optimal enzymatic activity and stability).
- Monovalent and divalent cations, e.g. potassium, magnesium.

PCR usually comprises 20–40 temperature cycles, with each cycle having three discrete steps:

1 Denaturation (temperature >90 °C): the DNA double helix separates into two single strands.
2 Annealing (typically 40–60 °C): cooling, allowing primers to bind to single strands, without re-formation of the double helix.
3 Elongation (approximately 70 °C; 72 °C for Taq): the DNA polymerase copies the target sequence.

The cycling, carried out in a heating block, is often preceded and followed by holding at a temperature >90 °C. The temperatures and durations employed depend on a number of variables, including the enzyme used for DNA synthesis and the concentrations of ions and nucleotides. The entire PCR process is automated and can be completed in a few hours.

Reverse transcription PCR (rt-PCR) is a variation of the technique that can be used to quantify viral RNA.

Once diagnosis has been confirmed, it is necessary for HCV genotyping to be performed, because this guides treatment strategies and predicts response. Sustained virological response (SVR) is the indicator used to monitor treatment progression after a complete course of therapy. There are six genotypes and several subtypes of HCV. The prevalence of each genotype varies geographically, with genotype 1 being most prevalent in the western world.

Liver biopsies have traditionally been used to provide information on disease severity. However, rapid, non-invasive methods have now been developed to assess liver fibrosis, e.g. FibroScan, which uses ultrasound to determine the elasticity/stiffness of the liver; this is related to the degree of fibrosis.

— Drug treatment and properties

Antiviral therapy for the management of hepatitis C has improved significantly with the development of directly acting antiviral drugs. New therapeutic agents have recently been licensed, with more in the pipeline. Consequently, the management of hepatitis C is constantly evolving, with treatment strategies and guidelines evolving to keep up with the new drugs being licensed.

The primary aim of treatment is to clear the virus from the blood. Successful treatment is usually indicated by a sustained virological response, defined as undetectable serum HCV RNA 6 months after treatment ends.

Current guidance recommends combination therapy, with the antiviral drugs ribavirin plus either peginterferon-α-2a or peginterferon-α-2b as the backbone of therapy for all patients with hepatitis C. For those patients with genotype 1 infection (most common in the UK), current guidance recommends triple therapy by adding a protease inhibitor boceprevir or telaprevir.

Ribavirin is a nucleoside analogue that inhibits viral replication by inhibiting viral mRNA polymerase and disrupting intracellular nucleotides. When used in treatment on its own, ribavirin is not effective against HCV. Three forms of ribavirin (Rebetol, Copegus and Ribavirin Teva) are available, having recommended doses ranging from 800 mg to 1400 mg depending on bodyweight, taken orally each day in two divided doses.

ribavirin

Ribavirin is a very polar drug, containing many highly electronegative atoms and several –OH and –NH groups resulting in significant hydrogen-bonding potential. Similar to many highly polar drugs, the oral bioavailability of ribavirin is fairly poor because its ability to diffuse through the lipophilic cell membranes is limited. This high polarity also means that it has sufficient water solubility for formulation as an oral solution. Ribavirin should generally be avoided in patients with renal impairment because this is the primary means of clearance of the drug – another feature that is commonly seen with polar drugs.

Interferon is a manufactured drug that mimics the naturally occurring interferon produced as part of the body's immune response to a viral infection. The aim of the drug is to prevent the virus from multiplying and causing further liver damage. The addition of an inert polyethylene glycol (PEG) moiety to the interferon molecule alters metabolism and decreases renal clearance, thereby increasing the half-life of the interferon molecule, allowing for once-weekly dosing.

PEG is a polyether compound, which is commercially available in a range of molecular weights and has widespread use as a pharmaceutical excipient. The structure of PEG is:

$$\text{HO–CH}_2\text{–(CH}_2\text{–O–CH}_2\text{–)}_n\text{–CH}_2\text{–OH}$$

Pegylation involves the covalent attachment of PEG to a therapeutic agent, such as a drug or biopharmaceutical. This can shield the therapeutic agent from the immune system after injection, and increase the molecular size, prolonging its circulatory time by reducing renal clearance.

The recommended dose of peginterferon-α-2a (Pegasys) is 180 micrograms once per week, administered subcutaneously, for 16, 24, 48 or 72 weeks depending on genotype, baseline viral load, treatment response and prior therapies received. The recommended duration of peginterferon-α-2a monotherapy is 48 weeks.

Peginterferon-α-2b (ViraferonPeg) has a recommended dose of 1.5 mg/kg bodyweight once a week, administered subcutaneously for 24 or 48 weeks, depending on genotype, baseline viral load and treatment response.

Adverse effects are numerous, troublesome and mainly dose related. They include flu-like symptoms, anorexia, nausea, anaemia, myelosuppression, depression, skin reactions, alopecia and fatigue, to name but a few.

Boceprevir and *telaprevir* are relatively new drugs. They are first-generation protease inhibitors that inhibit replication of HCV genotype 1 organisms, but are much less active against the other genotypes. They specifically inhibit the HCV viral enzyme NS3/4A serine protease, which cleaves proteins. Inhibition of this enzyme consequently interferes with viral replication. Boceprevir is available as hard capsules (Victrelis), with a dose of 800 mg three times daily, whereas telaprevir is available as film-coated tablets (Incivo) with a dose of 750 mg three times a day. Monotherapy with these agents is not recommended, because resistance is likely to occur, and so they are used as triple therapy with ribavirin and peginterferon. Triple-therapy regimens including boceprevir are associated with higher incidence of neutropenia than those with telaprevir. Rash is a very common side effect with telaprevir.

The risk of vertical transmission is 5%. However, ribavirin has been found to be teratogenic, and is therefore contraindicated during pregnancy. Women of childbearing age and their male partners must use contraception during treatment and for a period after treatment due to the long half-life of ribavirin. Female patients need to use effective contraception during treatment and for 4 months after treatment. Male patients and their female partners must use an effective contraceptive during treatment and for 7 months after treatment.

— Future treatments

Greater understanding of the lifecycle of HCV in recent years has led to the clinical development of directly acting antivirals, including protease inhibitors, nucleoside and nucleotide polymerase inhibitors, non-nucleoside polymerase inhibitors, NS5A inhibitors, entry inhibitors and host-targeting drugs. Examples of directly acting antivirals that have undergone phase 3 clinical trials include sofosbuvir (a nucleotide polymerase inhibitor), simeprevir (a protease inhibitor) and daclatasvir (a NS5A inhibitor) (Knighton, 2013a,b) and some, or all, are likely to be licensed in the near future.

Future treatments are researched and developed for human use by the pharmaceutical industry, academia and practice-based researchers through different phases of clinical trials:

- A *phase 1* trial is when a new chemical entity is tested in humans for the first time. A small number of people (approximately 20–100), often healthy volunteers, take the medicine to identify whether it is safe to take and to examine what happens when it enters the human body. The trial starts with small doses, which are slowly increased to determine information about the correct dose and at what dose adverse effects occur.
- During a *phase 2* trial the medicine's efficacy is evaluated in patients with the disease (approximately 100–500) to monitor the effects against the disease in the short term.
- *Phase 3* trials test the new medicine in a greater number of patients with the disease (approximately 1000–5000) to determine the safety, efficacy, and overall benefits and risks. In these trials, the new medicine may be tested against a control, which may be an existing treatment or, if there is no current treatment, against a placebo medicine (an inactive substance). The data generated by a phase 3 trial may be used by a pharmaceutical company to apply to regulatory agencies for licensing approval.
- Once the new medicine has been licensed for use, it is available to patients on prescription. However, further consideration may be given to value, cost-effectiveness and local health budgets before routine prescribing may occur. *Phase 4* trials collect additional data on the safety and efficacy of the medicine while the medicine is in routine use (pharmacovigilance).

EXTENDED LEARNING

- Outline the classification, mechanisms of action and drug interactions of antiviral drugs
- Describe the immune response and the role of interferon
- Discuss the various uses of polyethylene glycols as pharmaceutical excipients
- What are hard capsules? How do they differ from soft capsules? Describe how both types of capsules are formulated and manufactured

ADDITIONAL PRACTICE POINTS

- What are the processes by which prescription medicines are licensed?
- What is meant by the 'off-label use' of a medicine?
- What is the post-marketing surveillance of prescription medicines?

References and further reading

Fletcher H, Hickey I, Winter P (2007). *Genetics*, 3rd edn. Abingdon: Taylor & Francis Group plc.

Ghany MG, Strader DB, Thomas DL, Seeff LB (2009). AASLD practice guideline. Diagnosis, management and treatment of hepatitis C: an update. *Hepatology* **49**:1335–74.

Knighton S (2013a). Hepatitis C: clinical features and diagnosis. *Clin Pharmacist* 5:100–2.

Knighton S (2013b). Hepatitis C: management. *Clin Pharmacist* 5:103–8.

Case 13
Primary HIV infection
JESS CLEMENTS

LEARNING OUTCOMES

At the end of this case, you will be able to:

- List the symptoms of HIV seroconversion illness and describe how these may be mistaken
- Describe what is meant by seroconversion and discuss the limitations of HIV tests
- Know where to find guidance about when to start antiretroviral therapy in relation to the stage of infection
- Discuss the long-term side effects of antiretroviral therapy

Case study

Mr JR, a 28-year-old man, has been admitted to the ward via the sexual health clinic. Six days ago he attended his GP with headaches, flu like symptoms and general malaise. His GP diagnosed flu and sent him home with the advice to rest, take paracetamol for his headache and fever, to drink plenty of fluid and to return if his symptoms got any worse.

He returned to the GP yesterday with an increased severity of his headache now accompanied with photophobia. He has also noticed some pain on defecation. The GP has known Mr JR since he was a child and is concerned that his behaviour is very out of character; he seems agitated and confused. He is aware that Mr JR is openly homosexual. During his examination of Mr JR, the GP noticed that he appears to have oral thrush and ulceration around the anus. The GP referred Mr JR urgently to the local sexual health clinic.

CASE NOTES

Past medical history
- Negative HIV test 3 months earlier
- Hepatitis B vaccination course completed

Social history
- Lives alone
- Works in media

- Sexually active although no regular partner, however, multiple casual male partners
- Occasional recreational drug use but denies intravenous drug use
- No recent travel or pets

Drug history
- Occasional recreational drugs use – ketamine, GBL, cocaine, marijuana
- No known drug allergies

Mr JR admits to attending a sex party 3 weeks ago when he used several recreational drugs (ketamine, GBL [γ-butyrolactone] and cocaine) and had several sexual partners; he is unsure how many. He usually uses condoms, but admits that he may have had unprotected penetrative anal intercourse on this recent occasion.

On examination
- Photophobia
- Nystagmus (repetitive, involuntary eye movements)
- No neck stiffness
- Submandibular lymphadenopathy
- Perianal ulceration
- Oral thrush
- Temperature 38 °C
- BP 130/78 mmHg
- Pulse 78 beats/min

Tests performed in clinic
Fourth-generation HIV Ab/Ag test
Full sexual screen
Swab of anal ulcers
Syphilis serology
Hepatitis B serology
Hepatitis C serology

> Tests ordered
>
> Lumbar puncture
> Cryptococcal antigen

- ❷ What does the term seroconversion mean?
- ❷ List the symptoms associated with HIV seroconversion
- ❷ List the factors that would make you suspect HIV infection in this case
- ❷ List the other differential diagnoses in this case

The patient is admitted to hospital from the clinic for further investigation.

> Lumbar puncture results
>
> - WBCs (white blood cells) 12 cells/mm³ (90% mononuclear cells)
> - RBCs (red blood cells) 31 cells/mm³
> - India ink negative
> - No organisms seen under direct microscopy
> - CSF glucose 2.4 mmol/L, serum glucose 4.8 mmol/L
> - CSF total protein 1.15 g/L

Mr JR is treated empirically for bacterial meningitis with 2 g ceftriaxone intravenously twice daily. He is started on i.v. aciclovir 10 mg/kg three times a day for viral encephalitis. He is prescribed fluconazole 100 mg daily for 7 days to treat oral Candida sp. *Mr JR is also prescribed regular analgesia for the headache and pain from the ulcers.*

Syphilis serology: negative
Hepatitis B serology: surface antigen negative (antibody positive)
Hepatitis C serology: immunoglobulin G negative
Cryptococcal antigen: negative
Perianal ulcer swabs: herpes simplex virus 2 positive
CSF: HSV negative, HIV viral load 10 000 copies/mL

— **Day 2 of admission**

The fourth-generation laboratory blood test had the following results: HIV antibody negative, but p24 viral antigen (a viral protein making up most of the HIV viral core) positive. A diagnosis of acute or primary HIV infection was made.

- ❷ Explain why the HIV antibody test is negative at this point

- ❷ What makes this likely to be an acute or primary HIV infection?

After 2 days of treatment Mr JR is a lot less confused and his headache is resolving. An additional confirmatory test is run and his HIV-positive diagnosis is discussed with him.

He wants to know about what happens next. He has some friends who are HIV positive but do not require treatment yet, a couple of friends who are on treatment and are doing well, but he is also aware of some horror stories about the treatments being really 'nasty'. He asks you to explain when he is likely to need treatment and what that treatment will be.

- ❷ Where would you be able to find information about when to start treatment?
- ❷ What are the current UK recommendations on primary HIV and how do these apply to Mr JR's case?
- ❷ If Mr JR was to start treatment, what are the long-term complications of antiretroviral treatment?
- ❷ If Mr JR was to start treatment, which antiretrovirals would you recommend?

Additional blood tests show:

CD4+ count 90 cells/mm³
Viral load: >1 000 000 copies/mL.

Case discussion

— **Seroconversion**
This is the process by which the body generates specific antibodies to an antigen. In this instance, the antigen is HIV and seroconversion is said to have taken place when an individual produces anti-HIV antibodies.

— **Symptoms of HIV seroconversion**
Seroconversion may be asymptomatic or accompanied by general non-specific transient symptoms (acute retroviral syndrome) often described as 'flu like'. The symptoms associated with seroconversion are:

- Malaise
- Lymphadenopathy
- Fever
- Rash
- Arthralgia
- Headache
- Sore throat
- Aseptic meningitis

- Diarrhoea
- GI upset
- Oral candidiasis (thrush)
- Mouth ulcers
- Ulceration of the genitals.

Not all patients experience symptoms, and often those who do may mistake these symptoms for a different condition, such as flu. However, some patients have a more serious combination of symptoms than others and some may even develop an opportunistic infection at this time.

— **When to suspect HIV infection**
In the UK, over a quarter of individuals infected with HIV are unaware of their infection. As the symptoms of HIV infection and primary HIV infection (PHI) can be very non-specific, it is always worth while considering HIV as a differential diagnosis.

In this case, Mr JR's lifestyle puts him at high risk of contracting HIV; he is a man who has sex with men, who has reported some recent high-risk sexual activity. A number of Mr JR's presenting complaints are also suggestive of HIV infection; it is unusual for a fit and healthy adult to develop oral thrush (unless he uses a steroid inhaler). Mr JR also has perianal herpes simplex virus (HSV); the presence of an STI (sexually transmitted infection) makes Mr JR at higher risk of having HIV.

Mr JR's symptoms suggest a number of differential diagnoses such as bacterial/viral/TB meningitis, Epstein–Barr virus, HSV encephalitis, tumour or space-occupying lesion, cerebral malaria, toxoplasmosis and cryptococcal meningitis. This means that HIV infection could be missed, especially if Mr JR's social history is not considered.

Current HIV testing guidelines recommend increased testing in all medical settings with some settings being specified as all patients being offered a test; these include sexual health clinics and antenatal clinics.

— **Explaining why the HIV antibody test is negative at this point**
Antibodies are normally produced by B cells (a type of lymphocyte) in the blood. When an antigen (in this case the HIV virus) is exposed to an antigen-receptive B cell it differentiates into either an antibody-secreting cell called a plasma cell or a memory cell. The activated plasma cells undergo rapid proliferation, which allows the

genetic sequence to undergo point mutations, which then produce changes in the antibody detection zone. When an antibody is produced that has a strong affinity for binding with the antigen, it sends a signal back to the producing cell; this allows that particular cell line to survive. This process can take some time (up to several weeks). Once antibody production has started, the levels then need to reach a level sufficient for detection. Usually, this takes another couple of weeks. Most people will develop antibodies to HIV 6–12 weeks after infection; however, in some rare cases it may take up to 6 months.

A laboratory test that can be performed early in the disease process, before antibodies may be detectable, is an assay for the p24 antigen, especially in acute infection. The antigen p24 is the protein expressed by the HIV virion which causes an immune response. In early infection, there is increased p24 production and this can be measured in the blood: p24 antigen may be detectable as early as 2 weeks after exposure. In established infection, the levels of this protein are not normally measurable. This could be due to antigen–antibody complexing in the blood. The fourth-generation HIV test used will test for either antigens or antibodies. In all cases of a positive result, a second venous sample is sent to confirm a positive HIV diagnosis

— **Indications that this could be an acute or primary HIV infection**
- Antibody test is negative
- The p24 antigen test is positive
- Mr JR had a negative HIV test 3 months ago
- Mr JR reports recent high-risk exposure.

— **Information sources for when to start treatment**
There are national guidelines for use in the UK produced by the British HIV Association (BHIVA). Guidelines are also produced by a number of other national and international agencies.

Guidance for primary infection differs from that of established infection. Due to the need to continue treatment once started in established infection and concerns about drug toxicity, treatment is not recommended until the patient's CD4+ cell count falls to a level associated with an increase in morbidity and mortality. As new data become available and as the drug treatments become less toxic, the point at which the benefit of starting treatment outweighs the risks changes.

Check current guidance on when to start treatment, for the most up-to-date CD4+ cell threshold in established infection.

— Current UK recommendations on primary HIV and application in this case

The rationale for treating with antiretroviral drugs in primary HIV infection is as follows:

1 Preservation of specific anti-HIV immune responses that would otherwise be lost, and which are associated with long-term non-progression in untreated individuals
2 Reduction in morbidity associated with high viraemia and CD4 depletion during acute infection
3 Reduction in the risk of onward transmission of HIV.

Multiple studies have produced varying results regarding the short- and longer-term benefits of early therapy in terms of immunological markers, viral load and CD4 lymphocyte count, e.g. the SPARTAC study, a large randomised controlled trial, found that 48 weeks of early treatment delayed the time to the patient needing long-term treatment, although this was only by a matter of weeks. This effect was apparent only in the people who received 48 weeks of treatment; a similar effect after 12 weeks of early treatment was not observed. The reasons are unclear, and further research is needed, but perhaps 48 weeks of treatment reduces the amount of hidden virus in the body (viral reservoir size). Importantly, there was no evidence of harm of early treatment in terms of deaths, adverse events and the effectiveness of long-term treatment later on.

However, treatment in primary infection (outside a prospective study) should only be routinely considered in those with:

- neurological involvement
- any AIDS-defining illness
- a CD4 cell count persistently (i.e. for 3 months or more) <200 cells/mm^3.

Mr JR should be offered antiretroviral treatment (ART). He has neurological involvement. Currently, his CD4+ cell count is 90 cells/mm^3 and viral load >1000 000 copies/mm^3. The CD4+ cell count of an uninfected individual is normally between 500 and 1500 cells/mm^3. Although it is usual for the CD4+ cell count to drop during primary HIV infection and then return to pre-infection levels, a

very low count or a persistently low count is now known to be indicative of a poor prognosis. Severe seroconversion illness, such as Mr JR has presented with, is associated with rapid disease progression. The aim of treatment at this point is to minimise the damage done to the immune system, to rapidly reduce the viral load and to reduce the size of the viral reservoirs. There are data to suggest that people are more infectious during primary HIV infection than later in established infections. This may be because of the high levels of uncontrolled viraemia during a primary infection compared with asymptomatic infection. This gives rise to an argument that ART should be offered in primary HIV infection (PHI) for public health benefits, in preventing onward transmission of HIV, as well as the benefits to individuals.

Treatment for PHI should be continued for at least 48 weeks; however many clinicians would be unlikely to stop HAART (highly active antiretroviral therapy) once started regardless of indication for starting. Mr JR may be in a vulnerable psychological state following his recent diagnosis and therefore ill-prepared for committing to long-term treatment. Time should be taken to discuss to the benefits and risks associated with starting treatment with Mr JR.

If Mr JR had asymptomatic seroconversion or very mild symptoms, then the case for offering treatment is less clear. The risk of toxicity and a possible risk associated with stopping treatment (some data have suggested that interruptions of ART may be associated with an increase in both morbidity and mortality) means that most guidelines currently don't recommend treatment in primary infections unless as part of a trial. These considerations demonstrate difficulties of interpreting evidence from different research studies to inform care guidelines and therapy decisions for individual patients. Evidence can be complex, inconclusive and subject to continual change.

— Long-term complications of antiretroviral treatment

The first antiretroviral drug became available in 1986. There are now over 20 antiretroviral drugs licensed in the UK from five different classes. Assessment of concurrent morbidities needs to be undertaken in all patients about to start antiretroviral therapy and this will affect the decision on what drugs to use. In addition, side effects and management need to be discussed with the patient, as well as the importance of long-term adherence to ART. Long-term toxicity data are not available for all of these drugs. The information below is not an exhaustive list of toxicity associated with antiretroviral therapy; for details of the adverse effects of individual drugs the reader should consult the summary of product characteristics for that drug.

— Lipodystrophy
Changes in body fat distribution have been associated with long-term use of some nucleoside reverse transcriptase inhibitors (NRTIs) and protease inhibitors (PIs). These changes include loss of peripheral body fat, known as lipoatrophy, characteristically from the face and legs, and fat accumulation resulting in the development of a 'buffalo hump' or an increase in abdominal fat or breast enlargement.

— Lipid abnormalities
PI use has been associated with hyperlipidaemia.

— Cardiovascular disease
Some observational cohort data suggest that abacavir and certain PIs may be associated with an increased risk of myocardial infarction. The data are conflicting and no mechanism of action has been identified.

— Renal impairment
Tenofovir is associated with Fanconi's syndrome (proximal renal tubule disease). Indinavir and atazanavir have both been shown to cause renal stones and crystalluria.

— Liver function
Non-nucleoside reverse transcriptase inhibitors (NNRTIs) and PIs may cause LFTs to become deranged. Didanosine is associated with the development of non-cirrhotic portal hypertension and non-alcoholic steatohepatitis (fatty liver disease) and is rarely used nowadays. A number of the antiretrovirals are potent inducers or inhibitors of the cytochrome P450 isoenzyme system and therefore are subject to numerous drug–drug interactions. Atazanavir is associated with a benign hyperbilirubinaemia; however, yellow discoloration of eyes and skin in some patients may require atazanavir to be switched to an alternative drug.

— Myelosuppression
Zidovudine use is associated with anaemia and is now rarely used.

— CNS dysfunction
Efavirenz has been associated with altered sleep patterns and vivid dreams. In some cases, more serious effects including psychosis, suicidal ideation, depression and mania have been reported, requiring efavirenz to be discontinued.

— Rash
Many antiretrovirals are associated with rash, including risk of Steven–Johnson syndrome (a potentially fatal skin disease resulting from an adverse drug reaction) with the NNRTIs or PIs such as darunavir. Some of the NRTIs may also be associated with nail discoloration or skin pigmentation problems.

— Bones
Osteonecrosis is reported as a possible side effect of most antiretrovirals. Tenofovir use is also possibly associated with an increased tendency to develop osteomalacia.

— Appropriate antiretrovirals in this case
The aim in primary HIV is to minimise the damage done during acute infection when the viral load is very high and the CD4+ count very low. The choice of first-line treatment should follow the recommendations in the BHIVA guidelines. Treatment needs to be started as soon as possible in Mr JR's case to reduce his symptoms of acute HIV. Some drugs require additional tests before safe treatment can be initiated so other drugs may be chosen in preference because they don't require

tenofovir

emtricitabine

atazanavir   ritonavir

further tests. Treatment should begin with two NRTIs and a boosted PI. Fixed dose combinations of NRTIs are available and help to simplify regimens

The choice of a boosted PI therapy as first-line therapy can be justified for the following reasons. In this case, ART needs to be started quickly. There is no time to wait for the results of a genotypic resistance test. In the USA and Europe it is reported that there is transmitted resistance to NNRTIs at a rate of between 8% and 14%. Either atazanavir or darunavir boosted with ritonavir would be suitable for Mr JR.

A variety of combinations of NRTIs is possible and the choice will be need to be evaluated on a case by case basis.

Kivexa is a combination product containing abacavir and lamivudine. Before use of Kivexa (or any other combination therapy that includes abacavir), a genetic test (HLA*B5701) needs to be undertaken to check if there is predisposition to a hypersensitivity reaction with abacavir. As HAART needs to be started quickly there is no time to wait for the results of this test. A positive HLA*B5701 test result would mean that abacavir cannot be used.

The fixed dose combination of zidovudine and lamivudine is very rarely used because zidovudine is associated with anaemia and lipoatrophy with long-term use.

Truvada, a combination product containing tenofovir and emtricitabine, is well tolerated as initial therapy and would be a suitable option for Mr JR.

On day 5 of admission, Mr JR's ceftriaxone was stopped and the i.v. aciclovir was changed to oral aciclovir at a dose 400 mg five times daily to treat his perianal herpes. He was started on co-trimoxazole to prevent *Pneumocystis jiroveci* pneumonia because his CD cell count was low, putting him at risk of developing this opportunist infection.

On day 6 of admission, Mr JR started his antiretroviral combination of Truvada along with atazanavir and ritonavir (both PIs). He was prescribed 10 mg domperidone to prevent nausea and vomiting. The ward pharmacist discussed the common side effects with Mr JR and explained how the drugs work against HIV.

EXTENDED LEARNING

- List common opportunistic infections associated with HIV
- Describe the morphology of viruses, including HIV and hepatitis
- What is the difference between a nucleoside analogue reverse transcriptase inhibitor (such as emtricitabine) and a nucleotide analogue reverse transcriptase inhibitor (such as tenofovir)?
- HIV is most prevalent in low-income countries. How are issues of access to medicines (especially ARTs) and rational use addressed in these settings?
- Describe the mechanisms of action, abuse potential and regulation of the recreational drugs mentioned in this case study
- Comment on the potential value and limitations of clinical trials to inform therapy decisions

References and further reading

British HIV Association (2008). *Guidelines for HIV Testing*. Available at: www.bhiva.org/HIVTesting2008.aspx (accessed 2 October 2013).

British HIV Association (2012). *Guidelines for the Treatment of HIV-1 Positive Adults with Antiretroviral Therapy*. Available at: www.bhiva.org/TreatmentofHIV1_2012.aspx (accessed 2 October 2013).

British National Formulary (current edition). London: BMA and RPSGB.

SPARTAC Trial Investigators (2013). Short course anti-retroviral therapy in primary HIV infection. *N Engl J Med* **368**:207–17.

Case 14
Immunisations against infectious diseases and malaria chemoprophylaxis

LARRY GOODYER

LEARNING OUTCOMES

At the end of this case, you will be able to:

- Outline the major health risks that may be encountered by travellers
- Describe the common travel immunisations that may be required by travellers
- Summarise how to minimise the risks of contracting malaria when travelling
- Explain the advantages and disadvantages of different agents that may be taken for malaria chemoprophylaxis
- Outline the World Health Organization's strategy for prevention and treatment of malaria

Case study

Miss HW is a single, 32-year-old accountant. She has only ever taken a few holidays overseas and never before outside of Europe. After saving up for a number of years, Miss HW is now looking forward to a 6-week trip to South America. To start off, she has chosen a tour with an established company and will be arriving in Lima, Peru, on 21 October, but she does not visit the nurse at her local GP run travel clinic until 25 September.

During her tour with the established company, she will be staying in good hotels and following a route well used by tourists. She will fly via Amsterdam to Lima, where she will spend a couple of nights. After that, she will visit various tourist sites along the Inca trail such as Machu Pichu (at 8000 feet/ 2400 m) and Lake Titicaca, travelling by road and train. She will travel to Brazil on day 14 of her holiday.

She then plans to spend a day or two in Rio de Janeiro before embarking on an excursion into the Amazon basin, in which she would like to include a rain forest trek and overnight camping. She has not actually booked this last trip yet but has the name of a local company recommended by a reputable specialist organisation. She is therefore unsure of the exact itinerary but has allowed about 3 weeks for this part of her travels.

She has had all of her childhood immunisations, but none specifically for travel overseas. She has no drug or other allergies, and her only prescribed medication is a salbutamol inhaler that she uses occasionally.

- What are the major health risks that might be encountered by Miss HW during her travels, and how can they be identified?
- What further questions should Miss HW be asked?
- What are the general principles of planning a travel immunisation schedule?
- What vaccines would you advise for Miss HW?
- What are the risks of Miss HW contracting malaria, and how can these be minimised?
- What are the advantages and disadvantages of different antimalarial agents?

Case discussion

— Potential health hazards when travelling overseas

This case has focused on immunisations against infectious diseases and malaria chemoprophylaxis. However, there are a large range of other potential health hazards for travellers, in many cases representing a greater risk than diseases for which vaccines are used, which need to be identified and mitigated against. The principles of travel medicine are therefore greatly concerned with risk assessment and management.

In this case, Miss HW is visiting an area where a range of immunisations would be necessary, and, when in Amazonia, there is a high risk of encountering chloroquine-resistant *Plasmodium falciparum* malaria. There is also a range of other potential health hazards including:

- Travellers' diarrhoea
- Other insect-borne diseases, particularly dengue fever
- Altitude sickness when in Peru
- Potential issues related to warm climates in the tropics
- Accidents and injury.

Information about the range of potential health hazards and recommendations for prophylaxis can be found through two important websites in the UK:

- TRAVAX or Fitfortravel – Health Protection Scotland
- National Travel Health Network and Centre (NaTHNaC) – Health Protection England.

— Current medication

Always enquire about current or repeat medicines and chronic medical conditions. In this case, you should make enquiries about Miss HW's control of her asthma and ensure adequate supplies of inhalers.

In relation to vaccines, it is important to identify any potential for immunosuppression that might limit their effectiveness, or in the case of live vaccines to contraindicate their use. This may be due to an impaired immune response resulting from illness or medication. Any allergies to vaccines or their excipients should be identified, as should any adverse drug reactions to antimalarial medication. Pregnancy contraindicates live vaccines and also some antimalarials; in general, travel to malaria-endemic areas is discouraged in pregnancy. Also specifically with respect to mefloquine, enquire after any history of mental illness, including family history. A history of epilepsy or certain cardiac conditions could also contraindicate some antimalarials.

— Travel immunisation schedules

Generally, it is advised to visit a travel clinic 6–8 weeks before departure to allow for optimal scheduling of all vaccines; in this case, Miss HW is presenting somewhat late. Some vaccines, such as

rabies, require a schedule of three injections at appropriate spacing, whereas others, such as typhoid, require a single injection. However, some schedules can be given more rapidly, and travellers should normally be encouraged to begin immunisations no matter how close to the time of departure. In general, inactivated vaccines will not interfere with each other or with live vaccines, so they can be administered at one appointment. Live vaccines can be given together but at different sites, or on separate occasions three weeks apart.

The cost of immunisation may be an issue for some travellers. Only typhoid, cholera, hepatitis A and tetanus/polio/diphtheria are currently available on the NHS.

The detailed regimens of the vaccines required by Miss HW are not given here and can be found on either the TRAVAX/NaTHNaC websites or in the Department of Health's *Green Book*. Brief notes are given below relating to the vaccines that may be required.

Recommended vaccines: consideration in this case

— Hepatitis A

Hepatitis A is transmitted by food and drink, and is common in countries where public health systems are poor. Immunisation is probably best given as a combined vaccine with typhoid in this case. Alternatively, a combined immunisation product with hepatitis B could be given. Miss HW will need a full course and can be reassured that it is highly effective.

— Hepatitis B

Hepatitis B is contracted from sexual activity and contaminated blood products or poorly sterilised equipment. It is worth considering this vaccine for Miss HW because she is away for more than 1 month and in the Amazon, at risk from accidents, and therefore has a chance of needing surgery/blood products. She may also be at risk from sexual activity. However, she is presenting just 4 weeks before travel so will require the accelerated course. Note that this has a high cost but is free on the NHS if given as Twinrix (hepatitis A inactivated and hepatitis B [recombinant] vaccine).

— Typhoid

Typhoid is a systemic infection transmitted via the faecal/oral route, most commonly through ingestion of contaminated food and water. The vaccine is not very effective and, in Miss HW's case, the risk of typhoid is moderate, but as she is

chloroquine

mefloquine

atovaquone

proguanil

travelling to remote areas and villages then it could be recommended.

— Tetanus

Tetanus is contracted from cuts and grazes. As Miss HW may be in situations far from medical help, with poor access to immunoglobulins and undertaking activities that could lead to possible injury, immunisation is recommended. Although Miss HW had the immunisation as a child, this would be more than 10 years ago, so a booster is required.

— Diphtheria

Diphtheria is most commonly contracted by droplet infection and from close contact with local populations. It seems that Miss HW will not be greatly exposed to such contact. However, as diphtheria is available only as a combined vaccine with tetanus, she will receive this anyway.

— Yellow fever

Yellow fever is spread by the mosquito *Aedes* sp. and is a potentially fatal condition. The vaccine is very effective and a certificate of immunisation should be issued, but is not actually a requirement for entry. Travellers must have this vaccine 10 days before departure as a minimum, otherwise the certificate will not be valid. Miss HW does need this for her trip to Brazil.

— Rabies

Rabies can result from the bite of any infected mammal and is 100% fatal if untreated. A rabies vaccine could be considered for Miss HW because she is likely to be in situations in the Amazon away from medical help and also where immunoglobulin is in poor supply. There is a further risk from infected vampire bats. Miss HW should be informed that medical help should be sought in the event of a bite, and to obtain further immunisation. Cost may be an issue.

— Tuberculosis

Tuberculosis is spread by droplet infection and close contact with the population. Miss HW is not at a great risk because she is unlikely to be in such close contact. Miss HW should be asked about her BCG (Bacillus Calmette–Guérin) status because she may have been be immunised in childhood.

Malaria: risks, prevention and antimalarials

The malaria parasite does not develop in the mosquito at high altitudes so this is not a risk for Miss HW in Peru. It is only a major risk when she is travelling in the Amazon. Both *Plasmodium vivax* and *Plasmodium falciparum* malaria are present, but falciparum malaria poses the greatest risk to the traveller. Appropriate chemoprophylaxis should be taken in Brazil as identified from the NaTHNaC/TRAVAX websites or the *BNF* for quick reference. Chloroquine should not be used, because falciparum malaria has developed resistance to this agent. Therefore, there are three potential agents for Miss HW: doxycycline, atovaquone with proguanil, and mefloquine.

In all areas where malaria is present, mosquito bite avoidance measures should be advised, because no prophylactic is 100% effective, and poor adherence is a common reason for contracting malaria. Such advice includes covering the skin with long sleeves or trousers, applying a 50% DEET (*N,N*-diethyl-*m*-toluamide) repellent to exposed skin, and sleeping in well-screened, air-conditioned rooms kept clear of mosquitoes by insecticide sprays or vaporisers. In some situations a treated bed net is required.

The three agents mentioned above are all equally effective in preventing malaria. Therefore a concordance approach should be taken in which discussion with the traveller could consider the adverse effect profile, regimen and cost.

A combined preparation of atovaquone with proguanil hydrochloride (Malarone) is the most expensive choice but it is taken only 1 day before exposure and then just 1 week after return, because it acts on the liver and blood stages. A slight disadvantage to starting when Miss HW is away is making sure that she can get alternatives if the preparation does not suit her due to adverse effects.

Doxycycline is the cheapest alternative and could also be started while Miss HW is away, a few days before travelling to the Amazon. There is a small risk of photosensitivity so Miss HW should be warned to use a sunscreen. Doxycycline can also cause vaginal candida (thrush) infection. It is important to swallow doxycycline in an upright position with plenty of water due to a risk of severe oesophagitis. It needs to be taken for 4 weeks after return.

Mefloquine has the advantage of once-a-week dosing but it also has potential CNS side effects (neuropsychiatric reactions: depressed mood, anxiety, unusual thoughts or behaviour, hallucinations). It is best to take test doses 3 weeks in advance of travel and it must be taken for 4 weeks after returning. The traveller should be questioned carefully about family and his or her own psychiatric history. It may not be a good choice in Miss HW's case because she may already be an 'anxious' individual.

— **International perspectives and malaria**
Malaria remains highly prevalent and a major cause of mortality in many parts of the world. The WHO estimates that there are still over 200 million cases per year (although this incidence has declined by around 25% in the last decade) and more than 600 000 deaths. Most cases and deaths are in children and in sub-Saharan Africa, where a child dies every minute from malaria.

Artemisinin combination therapies are recommended for the treatment of malaria in endemic areas. Use of artemisinin compounds in combination with other drugs is vital to prevent the spread of resistance. These recommendations for the treatment of malaria are part of a wider strategy that includes the provision of insecticide-treated nets free of charge to all people at risk, indoor residual spraying to eradicate parasites, intermittent preventive treatment in pregnancy (as pregnant women are at an increased risk) and more emphasis on diagnostic tests so that therapy can be targeted to confirmed cases of malaria, rather than given to all who experience fever (which may or may not be a result of malaria).

EXTENDED LEARNING

- What is the recommended treatment for travellers' diarrhoea?
- What should be prescribed for malaria prophylaxis for children?
- Outline the recommendations for malaria chemoprophylaxis for long-term travellers (>6 months)
- How are vaccines formulated, and why do they frequently include an adjuvant?
- How are biopharmaceutical products such as vaccines sterilised?
- What routes, other than by injection, are possible for vaccine delivery, e.g. nasal delivery?

ADDITIONAL PRACTICE POINT

- Consider approaches to achieving concordance in pharmacists' consultations

Reference/further reading

Department of Health (2006). *Immunisation against Infectious Disease (The Green Book)*. London: DH. Available at: https://www.gov.uk/government/uploads/system/uploads/attachment_data/file/239274/Green_Book_updated_110913.pdf (accessed 1 October 2013).

— **Resources**
Fit for Travel: www.fitfortravel.nhs.uk
National Travel Health Network and Centre: www.nathnac.org
TRAVAX: www.nathnac.org

6

Endocrinology cases

INTRODUCTION

This section contains 10 cases focused on patients with endocrine diseases, namely: diabetes (types 1 and 2), Cushing's disease, Addison's disease, hypothyroidism, osteoporosis (in a young and a postmenopausal patient) and hypercalcaemia in hyperparathyroidism.

Case 1
Insulin pump use in a child ▸ 228

This case is based on an 8-year-old girl with type 1 diabetes that is not being well controlled with a standard insulin injection regimen. The case starts with an outline of the basic structure and properties of the insulin molecule, its physicochemical properties and bioavailability, and then describes how an insulin pump works to deliver regular subcutaneous doses from an insulin reservoir, and its advantages over conventional therapy in providing tight blood sugar control. Some possible disadvantages of the pump therapy are also mentioned. The types of insulin that can be used in the pump are discussed, along with a usual dosage plan. The case also raises the important principle of carbohydrate counting by the patient's mother, to aid in the assessment of insulin requirements for her child, particularly as the girl wishes to participate in sports activity at school. Some general advice on how parents and carers can support young people with long-term medical conditions, such as type 1 diabetes, is also given.

Case 2
Hyoglycaemia during insulin therapy ▸ 232

This case continues the theme of type 1 diabetes, with a case study focusing on a young teenage student who is on standard biphasic insulin therapy, but finding it difficult to control his blood glucose level and experiencing disturbing episodes of hypoglycaemia. The case explains the main signs and symptoms of hypoglycaemia and their physiological causes, as well as the immediate treatment. The biphasic insulin regimen is explained, as well as the mechanism by which insulin exerts its biological effect of lowering blood glucose. Recommendations on how better to control blood glucose levels for this patient are also described, particularly avoiding excessive alcohol intake and strenuous physical activity, a change in dietary habits and a possible switch to a basal bolus insulin regimen. The learning programme DANFE and the 'insulin passport' are also described.

Case 3
Type 2 diabetes mellitus ▸ 235

This case describes a patient presenting to his GP after a pharmacy health check that detected an elevated blood glucose level in the diabetic range. The patient had exhibited some classic early symptoms of type 2 diabetes mellitus, namely increased tiredness and polyuria. The case describes the treatment options and health advice that a GP and pharmacist can provide for this condition and explains the causes of type 2 diabetes, along with the risk factors, long-term complications and goals of therapy with oral anti-diabetic drugs. Possible management with the newer GLP-1 receptor agonists, or a glucose transport inhibitor, is also considered.

Case 4
Serious lactic acidosis induced by metformin ▸ 239

This case describes an elderly patient with established type 2 diabetes taking metformin, who is admitted to hospital with a dangerously high blood level of lactic acid (metformin-associated lactic acidosis – MALA). Her condition progresses to severe and she is admitted to the intensive care unit (ICU) with renal failure. The chemical properties, pharmacology and problems associated with the use of metformin are described, in particular MALA and its causes plus other serious side effects. The treatment received by the patient in the ICU is outlined, together with a mention of the feasibility of using succinate for specific MALA therapy.

Case 5
An unusual case of Cushing's syndrome ▶ 242

This unusual case describes a female patient initially presenting to her GP with some classic symptoms of Cushing's syndrome (hypercortisolaemia) which eventually turns out to be derived from the release of excessive cortisol from the adrenal glands (secondary Cushing's syndrome), stimulated by an atypical 'ectopic' pulmonary (tumour) source of ACTH. The patient is referred to an endocrine clinic for further investigation. The case begins by going through the patient's symptoms and the standard laboratory tests that would normally be undertaken for such a patient and the outcomes. Imaging tests are also made to further establish the diagnosis including MRI (magnetic resonance imaging) of the head (looking for pituitary or hypothalamic tumours) as well as a radiograph, PET (positron emission tomography)/CT (computed tomography) and somatostatin receptor radioimaging scans of the chest to try to localise the ectopic ACTH-secreting tumour(s) in the lung. Basic descriptions of Cushing's syndrome and Cushing's disease are given, considering the pathophysiology, signs, symptoms, and expected diagnostic tests and outcomes in each case. How the patient was treated and her prognosis are discussed. The preparation of radiopharmaceuticals in a hospital environment is also considered.

Case 6
Addisonian crisis ▶ 248

This case deals with a young female patient who presents at a local hospital accident and emergency department (A&E) with severe weakness, nausea and abdominal pains that developed while she was out shopping on a particularly cold winter's day. After observing that the patient looked thin and dehydrated, the doctor

on duty admitted her to the ward for standard blood tests and rehydration/oxygen therapy. On the basis of the initial blood results and the patient's recent history, she is suspected of having adrenal insufficiency (Addison's disease). The case goes on to describe how, during the course of her hospital stay, she develops an 'addisonian crisis' with imminent cardiovascular collapse, which requires immediate emergency treatment to stabilise the condition. The nature and basis of subsequent blood tests done to confirm the diagnosis are discussed, together with life-long combined corticosteroid therapy on discharge from hospital and the advice normally given to such patients to avoid similar recurrence of symptoms.

Case 7
Hypthyroidism ▶ 254

This case concerns a mother with a young baby who is showing some recognised signs of hypothyroidism, including weight gain, cold intolerance and fatigue. The case begins with a basic description of thyroid gland function, the possible causes and classic signs of hypothyroidism, and the kind of tests that would normally be used to diagnose the condition. It continues by outlining the chemistry and mechanism of action of thyroid hormones, and then discusses the standard replacement thyroid hormone therapies, and the goals and counselling points that would be applicable for this patient. The strategies for paying for thyroid hormone treatment in the UK and other countries are also mentioned.

Case 8
Osteoporosis in a younger woman ▶ 258

This case is based on a postmenopausal patient who presents at her GP for a review of pain control after a wrist fracture, and is then referred to hospital for a DXA bone scan and advice on osteoporosis management. The case starts by describing what osteoporosis is and how it is diagnosed, and then outlines the most common sites that are susceptible to osteoporotic fracture and the risks of developing the condition. Prolonged glucocorticoid-induced osteoporosis is also highlighted. The case continues with a description of the most commonly recommended osteoporotic treatment options that could be used for her management and considers an individualised HRT risk–benefit evaluation.

Case 9
Osteoporosis in an elderly woman ▶ 262

This case continues the theme of osteoporosis with a case study of an elderly postmenopausal woman who is admitted to hospital after a fall, but does not sustain a fracture. The pathophysiology, signs and symptoms of osteoporosis and the risk factors playing a role in the pathogenesis of fractures are discussed, together with treatment options with bisphosphonates (including their chemistry, mechanism of action and absorption properties), calcium and vitamin supplements and some other available therapeutic possibilities. The FRAX algorithm tool for predicting the 10-year risk of a fracture is mentioned. Lifestyle change recommendations to reduce the general risk of osteoporosis in women are discussed.

Case 10
Treatment for hypercalcaemia ▶ 266

This case describes the treatment of an elderly patient who presents to a hospital A&E with a swollen leg (suspected DVT), but also complaining of decreased mobility, constipation and slurred speech. Blood tests revealed abnormally high blood levels of urea, creatinine, calcium (hypercalcaemia) and parathyroid hormone. The case starts with a general description of hypercalcaemia, its signs/symptoms and causes (including drug therapies), adverse effects and treatments, and then progresses to a diagnosis of primary hyperparathyroidism (confirmed by an ultrasound scan of the thyroid gland) which is complicated by acute hypercalcaemic kidney damage. Signs/symptoms and treatment options for primary hyperparathyroidism (including surgery) are discussed along with their risks. The chemical structures, properties and mechanisms of action of some common bisphosphonates used to reduce bone cell resorption in hypercalcaemia are also presented.

Endocrinology cases | Introduction

Case 1
Insulin pump use in a child
FATEMAH ALSALEH

Case study

Jenny is an 8-year-old girl who was diagnosed with type 1 diabetes when she was 5 weeks old. Her diabetes is difficult to manage and is not well controlled by her current insulin injections. In previous years, she has had numerous hospital admissions for the treatment of diabetic ketoacidosis (DKA). In spite of increasing insulin doses, she has continued to have high and fluctuating blood sugar values. The diabetes specialist physician has decided to start insulin pump therapy (continuous subcutaneous insulin injection – CSII) to manage her condition.

You are responsible for pharmacy services to the paediatric diabetes clinic. Jenny and her mother come to you for guidance on the use of the new insulin pump.

- ❷ Outline the structure of insulin and comment on its stability
- ❷ Why is insulin not orally bioavailable?
- ❷ Explain how an insulin pump works, and how it is used in the treatment of diabetes
- ❷ Why do you think that an insulin pump might be a better method of insulin delivery than the traditional insulin injections for Jenny?
- ❷ What advantages (and disadvantages) does insulin pump therapy offer over injection therapy?

You are asked to supply insulin for use with the pump.

- ❷ What type of insulin should be supplied, and how would you calculate the amount of insulin to be dispensed, based on the units that she would use?

Jenny's mother tells you that, because of her uncontrolled diabetes, she has recently been less able to participate in sport lessons at school, especially gymnastics and swimming.

- ❷ What will you advise them to do with the pump before participating in sporting activities?
- ❷ How can the pump offer better diabetes control, enabling physical activity?

Jenny's mother is concerned about how she will measure doses based on food intake.

- ❷ Outline the principles of carbohydrate (carb) counting and explain how insulin doses are modified based on glucose levels, physical activity and food ingested

Case discussion

— Insulin structure and properties

Insulin is a polypeptide hormone made up of two chains of amino acids (the amino acids are represented using their single letter codes in the structure on page 229). The primary structure comprises an 'A' chain of 21 amino acids and a 'B' chain of 30 amino acids. It contains one intra-chain and two inter-chain disulfide bridges. Insulin folds up into a globular conformation in which many of the hydrophobic amino acid side chains are positioned in the interior of the peptide, with the polar side chains exposed. This allows the peptide to be soluble in water. The secondary and tertiary structures are a consequence of the primary sequence alone.

Solutions of insulin should be stored in the refrigerator *but never frozen.* Modern preparations of insulin undergo very gradual chemical degradation when stored at 4°C. This degradation occurs more rapidly at room temperature and solutions stored out of the refrigerator for a period of a few months will lose most of their activity.

```
GIVEQCCTSICSLYQLENYCN

FVNEHLCGSHLVEALYLVCGQRGFFYTPKT
```

Alanine: A
Arginine: R
Asparagine: N
Aspartic acid: D
Cysteine: C
Glutamine: Q
Glutamic acid: E
Glycine: G
Histidine: H
Isoleucine: I
Leucine: L
Lysine: K
Methionine: M
Phenylalanine: F
Proline: P
Serine: S
Threonine: T
Tryptophan: W
Tyrosine: Y
Valine: V

— Bioavailability of insulin

Insulin is not orally bioavailable as a consequence of its physicochemical properties, which are, in turn, a consequence of its chemical structure. Human insulin has a high molecular mass (>5 kDa) and is a highly polar protein, containing many polar bonds, many hydrogen bond donors and acceptors, and several groups that are charged at physiological pH. These properties mean that insulin will be extremely poor at crossing the gastrointestinal epithelium because it is too polar to diffuse through the cell membrane (transcellular) and too large to be absorbed between cells (paracellular). Insulin is also chemically unstable, particularly in the low pH environment of the stomach. Such conditions rapidly lead to denaturation of the peptide's three-dimensional structure. Finally, and importantly, the abundance of proteolytic enzymes in the stomach and small intestine lead to extensive enzymatic degradation (in the same manner as dietary proteins) and hence abolition of activity.

— Routes and means of insulin administration

Insulin pumps: an insulin infusion pump is a small external device with an insulin reservoir, connected to the body via a soft plastic tube that ends with a fine, soft, flexible cannula which is inserted subcutaneously, usually in the abdomen area, although other sites are possible, such as the arm, thigh or lower back.

Insulin pumps are designed to mimic the function of the pancreas, delivering a programmed basal insulin dose continuously throughout the day and night. Bolus doses are also administered, usually before meals, based on blood sugar levels, food intake (amount of carbohydrates consumed) and physical activity. If blood glucose levels remain high after a meal, then a 'supplemental' or 'correction' bolus dose of insulin can be administered to achieve the target blood sugar level.

Insulin pumps or injections: insulin pump therapy has many advantages over conventional subcutaneous insulin injection therapy. Tight control of blood sugar can be achieved with conventional insulin injection therapy via multiple daily injections. This requires patients to have three or more injections. Similar control can be achieved by CSII using an insulin pump. This frees patients from painful injections, which can be a particular advantage for children and young people.

Using insulin pumps in the management of diabetes also allows better glycaemic control. This is because CSII uses only soluble insulin and enables continuous delivery via an injection site. The ability to set various basal profiles throughout the day reduces the risk of nocturnal hypoglycaemia and activity-induced hypoglycaemia.

Insulin pumps allow patients to adopt a flexible lifestyle without loss of diabetes control. Insulin pumps permit flexible timing of meals and snacks, because various programming options enable patients to adjust their doses according to need.

Some modern insulin pumps can deliver basal rates as low as 0.025 units/h, and they can be programmed for intermittent insulin administration if required. This is beneficial for infants and very young children with diabetes, who often require extremely small basal and bolus doses.

Patients may experience some disadvantages with pump therapy, e.g. pain at the cannula site, and there is a lot to learn when commencing therapy.

— Types of insulin and insulin dosing

Recently, several studies have shown that rapidly acting insulin analogues (insulin lispro, aspart and glulisine) achieve a more physiological profile than soluble insulin when used in CSII, providing bolus/basal insulin doses without increasing the risk of hypoglycaemia or DKA.

Conventional, soluble insulin tends to complex with zinc in the blood, forming hexamers. In this form, insulin will not bind to insulin receptors, though the hexamer slowly reverts back to the biologically active monomer. Consequently, subcutaneously administered soluble insulin is not readily available when needed in large doses, such as following a meal. By genetic engineering, the amino acid sequence of insulin can be manipulated to produce an insulin analogue with altered pharmacokinetic properties. Fast-acting analogues are absorbed more rapidly from the absorption site and thus act faster subcutaneously than soluble natural insulin, achieving appropriate therapeutic concentrations after a meal.

When starting pump therapy, the pre-pump total daily dose of insulin is usually reduced by 20–30%. Half of this reduced total daily dose is given as a total daily basal dose, which can also be calculated as 0.22 units/kg, and the remaining half as the total daily bolus dose. For young patients, pump therapy is usually started with 40% basal and 60% bolus doses. This is summarised in Figure 6.1.

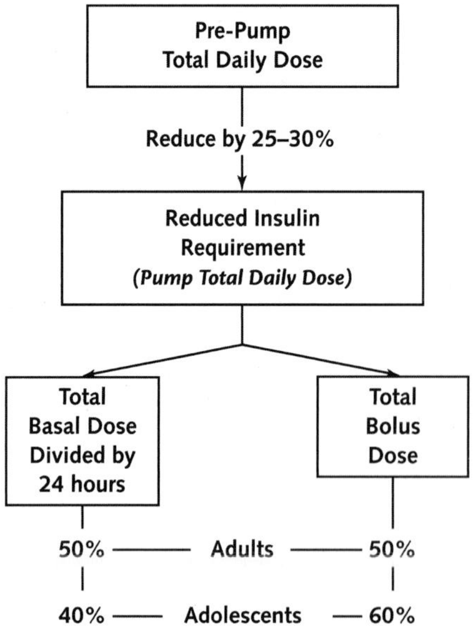

— Carbohydrate counting and adjustments of insulin doses for patients receiving pump therapy

Patients receiving CSII are required to calculate the amount of carbohydrates in their food ('carb counting') in order to calculate the size of insulin bolus to be injected. This requires them to use an insulin:carbohydrate ratio (to cover carbohydrates in the ingested food) and a blood glucose correction factor (to lower the blood glucose level to a target range after the ingestion of food). These are usually determined by the physician or dietician (Table 6.1).

For patients to carb count accurately, they are usually taught to read 'nutritional information' on food labels for total carbohydrates in grams. In addition, patients are normally provided with a

▼ TABLE 6.1

Example of how to calculate an insulin dose using insulin:carbohydrate ratio and blood glucose correction factor

Insulin:carb ratio = 1 unit rapid acting insulin/15 g carbohydrate[a] **Blood glucose correction** = 1 unit of rapid acting insulin per 50 mg/dL over 150 mg/dL blood glucose[a]	
Example school lunch	
6 baked chicken nuggets	15 g carbohydrate
½ cup mashed potatoes	15 g carbohydrate
½ cup green beans	5 g carbohydrate
½ cup canned fruit in natural juices	15 g carbohydrate
1 carton 2% white milk	12 g carbohydrate
Total	62 g carbohydrate

Pre-meal blood glucose = 250 mg/dL
Total carbohydrate = 62 g
Insulin needed for carbs = 62 ÷ 15 = 4 units
Blood glucose in excess of target level (150 mg/dL) = 250 − 150 = 100 mg/dL
Insulin needed to lower blood glucose to target level = 100 ÷ 50 = 2 units
Total dose = 4 + 2 = 6 units
[a]Insulin:carb ratios and blood glucose corrections are individualised for each child.
Note that this example should not be used as a recommendation for dosing.

```
            ┌─────────────────────┐
            │     Pre-Pump        │
            │  Total Daily Dose   │
            └─────────────────────┘
                      │
             Reduce by 25–30%
                      │
            ┌─────────────────────┐
            │  Reduced Insulin    │
            │   Requirement       │
            │ (Pump Total Daily   │
            │       Dose)         │
            └─────────────────────┘
               ╱            ╲
    ┌──────────────┐   ┌──────────────┐
    │    Total     │   │    Total     │
    │  Basal Dose  │   │  Bolus       │
    │ Divided by   │   │   Dose       │
    │  24 hours    │   │              │
    └──────────────┘   └──────────────┘
          │                   │
        50% ──── Adults ──── 50%
          │                   │
        40% ─── Adolescents ── 60%
```

▲ FIGURE 6.1

Establishing initial basal and bolus doses for insulin pump therapy.

book or reference list to which they can refer for unlabelled food.

Ongoing monitoring of blood glucose levels is extremely important, because basal and bolus doses have to be adjusted accordingly. Adjustment of basal doses (typically by 0.1 unit/h) is usually undertaken in the daytime, depending on factors such as skipped meals or physical activity; sometimes, when taking part in sporting activities, the pump can be removed. This helps to prevent any hypoglycaemic events. In contrast to the basal dose, bolus insulin doses are usually adjusted according to blood glucose values, measured 2 hours after meals.

— Supporting young people with long-term medical conditions

Children with long-term medical conditions such as type 1 diabetes need support to manage their condition and optimise their medical treatment. The National Service Framework for Children, Young People and Maternity Services – Diabetes Type 1 in Childhood (Department of Health, 2010) highlighted the importance of responding to the views of children and their parents, involving them in key decisions, providing early identification, diagnosis and intervention, and delivering flexible, child-centred, holistic care. Particular challenges can arise when the primary responsibility for medicines moves from parents to the young person. Care needs to be integrated between different settings, and to be sensitive to the individual's changing needs. Key areas identified for advice and support were:

- Monitoring blood glucose levels
- Taking medication and supporting changes to treatment regimens
- Treating emergency situations, e.g. hypoglycaemia or illness that has associated effects on diabetes
- Access to a healthy balanced diet
- Participation in extracurricular and social activities.

EXTENDED LEARNING

- How does the body regulate blood sugar?
- What is the cause of type 1 diabetes? How does it differ from type 2 diabetes?
- What is the function of the pancreas, and how is endogenous insulin synthesised and secreted?
- What is the mechanism of action of insulin at the biochemical and cellular level?
- How are synthetic 'human' insulins manufactured?
- What are the latest developments in insulin pumps, including pumps with continuous glucose monitoring, and implantable insulin pumps?

ADDITIONAL PRACTICE POINTS

- It is important for patients with diabetes to carry an ICE (in case of emergency) MedicAlert card at all times (or an ID bracelet, necklace or watch), showing important patient information for first responders in an emergency situation: type of diabetes and medication being taken, together with contact details of next of kin or people to be notified when the patient may not be able to speak for him- or herself.
- What extra support might be available for children or adolescents with diabetes?

References and further reading

Alsaleh F, Smith FJ, Taylor KMG (2010). Insulin pumps: past, present and future. *J Clin Pharmacy Therapeut* **35**:127–38.

Department of Health (2010). *National Service Framework for Children, Young People and Maternity Services – Diabetes type 1 in childhood.* London: DH.

Kawamura T (2007). The importance of carbohydrate counting in the treatment of children with diabetes. *Pediatr Diabetes* **8**(Suppl 6):57–62.

Spiegel G (2008). Carbohydrates counting for children with diabetes: why, what and how? *School Nurse News* **25**:36–8.

Case 2
Hypoglycaemia during insulin therapy
ELIZABETH HACKETT

LEARNING OUTCOMES

At the end of this case you will be able to:

- Describe the symptoms and causes of hypoglycaemia
- Advise on the most effective treatment of hypoglycaemia
- Decipher which dose of insulin or component of a biphasic (or pre-mixed) insulin relates to which blood glucose level associated with pre-meal and pre-bedtime testing
- Advise on methods to avoid hypoglycaemia

Case study

Mr JW is a 19-year-old university student with type 1 diabetes that was diagnosed 6 months ago. He was placed on a twice-daily biphasic insulin regimen (NovoMix 30, 12 units in the morning and 10 units in the evening), which he is finding difficult because his blood glucose readings are rather erratic. He finds this regimen very restrictive and is having hypoglycaemic episodes (at least three or four times a week), which frighten him.

He monitors his blood glucose levels at home four times a day and obtained the readings in Table 6.2 over the past week.

▼ TABLE 6.2
Blood glucose readings for Mr JW

	Before breakfast (mmol/L)	Before lunch (mmol/L)	Before dinner (mmol/L)	Before bed (mmol/L)
Sunday	7.8	5.7	6.4	7.7
Monday	8.7	3.2	13.3	10.8
Tuesday	5.6	6.8	8.2	12.5
Wednesday	7.0	3.1	10.8	16.9
Thursday	3.3	2.9	11.7	8.0
Friday	5.9	9.2	7.8	17.5
Saturday	3.8	5.6	6.3	8.1

Mr JW likes to have an alcoholic drink in the student bar with his mates, particularly on Wednesday and Friday nights; however, this is giving him high pre-bed readings and low next-morning readings. He is also having hypoglycaemic episodes before lunch, on the days that he visits the gym and undertakes a work-out.

- What is hypoglycaemia and what are the classic symptoms?
- What are the main factors that cause hypoglycaemia?
- How should hypoglycaemia be most effectively treated?
- NovoMix 30 is a biphasic insulin. What is a biphasic insulin?
- How do biphasic and other insulin regimens help achieve steady blood glucose levels throughout the day?
- Which components of his biphasic insulin are responsible for the readings that he obtains before breakfast, before lunch, before dinner and before bed?
- What is the mechanism of action of insulin at receptor level?

Mr JW likes to go to the gym three times a week, in the morning when he has a gap between his university lectures. As he has put on weight as a result of starting insulin, he does not want to reduce the amount of exercise that he does.

- What can be recommended to help Mr JW maintain steady blood glucose readings within the desired range (pre-meal and bedtime 4–7 mmol/L)?
- What is an 'insulin passport'?

Case discussion
— Hypoglycaemia
Hypoglycaemia is normally defined as a blood glucose level of ≤3.5 mmol/L. Some people may experience symptoms of low glucose at 3.5 mmol/L; others may not until glucose levels are lower. Hypoglycaemia may be rapidly corrected by the administration of glucose.

— Symptoms of hypoglycaemia

Most of the symptoms of hypoglycaemia can be divided into two categories: autonomic symptoms, which are caused by the release of adrenaline, and neuroglycopenic effects, which occur as the brain becomes affected and starved of glucose.

The autonomic (sympathetic) symptoms include sweating, trembling, tachycardia, palpitations and pallor. These symptoms often occur first and serve as a 'warning' to the individual that carbohydrates need to be consumed soon.

Neuroglycopenic symptoms include: light-headedness, loss of concentration, drowsiness, visual disturbances, abnormal behaviour (often even mild-mannered people can become quite aggressive), confusion and coma. Once the brain becomes involved, it is potentially a more dangerous situation, because confusion often means that the person affected is unable to act appropriately to overcome the hypoglycaemia, and is therefore reliant on someone else being able to recognise the problem and offer the right treatment. If hypoglycaemia is severe and prolonged, permanent brain damage may occur. Diabetic coma and death may even result if the condition is not treated in time.

Other classic symptoms of hypoglycaemia that are not autonomic or neuroglycopenic include hunger, headache and perioral numbness/tingling – these also serve as 'warning symptoms'.

A normal body response to hypoglycaemia is to produce counter-regulatory hormones (e.g. glucagon and adrenaline), which increase glucose levels through glycogenolysis and gluconeogenesis. However, for those who have taken insulin or oral hypoglycaemic agents, the effects of these drugs may outlast the effects of the counter-regulatory hormones, hence causing hypoglycaemia that must be corrected by consuming carbohydrates (or administering intravenous glucose or glucagon).

At blood glucose levels of 3.5 mmol/L some people will experience symptoms. For others, there may be no symptoms until blood glucose levels drop lower. Most people experience their own unique combination of symptoms of hypoglycaemia, so the warning symptoms experienced by one individual may be different from those experienced by another. However, the most important thing is for the person experiencing the hypoglycaemia to heed the warning symptoms and act as quickly as possible to reverse the hypoglycaemia by consuming carbohydrates to avoid the situation from becoming potentially dangerous.

— Causes of hypoglycaemia?

For people on insulin or insulin secretagogues (oral hypoglycaemic agents that cause the release of insulin), the most common cause of hypoglycaemia is a delay in eating, or missing a meal altogether. This delay or lack of carbohydrate intake (which is required for the insulin to act on) causes a decrease in glucose levels. In the same way, a reduction in the amount of carbohydrate normally consumed may also result in low glucose levels. An increase in the dose of insulin (or insulin secretagogue) may also cause hypoglycaemia, particularly if the amount of available carbohydrate is not sufficient, as may the addition of another oral anti-diabetes agent. Likewise, an increase in the amount of energy expended (increase in physical activity) may cause low blood sugar levels as the glucose is more readily taken up into the cells. Excessive alcohol consumption may cause hypoglycaemia (even in someone without diabetes) because it can impair the process of gluconeogenesis. In the same way, liver disease may predispose to hypoglycaemia due to impaired gluconeogenesis and glycogenolysis.

— Treatment of hypoglycaemia

Many guidelines suggest starting treatment for hypoglycaemia if the blood glucose level falls <4 mmol/L. This is to allow for a small margin of error if using capillary glucose testing equipment. Before treating hypoglycaemia, an assessment needs to be made as to whether or not the individual can swallow safely without the risk of aspiration. In most cases, if the hypoglycaemia is being treated in response to autonomic symptoms, the patient should be able to treat himself, or to follow instructions and swallow safely, in which case oral treatment is recommended. If unable to swallow, or if there is a risk that aspiration might occur, parenteral treatment should be given (either intravenous glucose or glucagon).

The most rapidly effective oral treatments are pure sources of glucose, e.g. glucose tablets, glucose powder, glucose drinks (e.g. Lucozade). Hot drinks should be avoided in an emergency situation because there is a risk that they could burn. Likewise, drinks containing milk are not advisable because the fat in milk slows down the absorption of the sugars.

After treating the hypoglycaemia, blood glucose levels should be measured about 10–15 min later. If still <4.0 mmol/L more glucose should be consumed and, if >4.0 mmol/L and the next meal is more than 1 hour away, then a long-acting carbohydrate is also required, e.g. a piece of bread or a couple of biscuits. It must be remembered that, if the person is taking an α-glucosidase inhibitor (e.g. acarbose) then monosaccharide carbohydrates must be given, because disaccharides and polysaccharides will not be absorbed due to inhibition of the necessary enzymes for cleaving the carbohydrate into absorbable monosaccharide units. If parenteral treatment is required, it is recommended to use intravenous glucose or glucagon (which may be administered intramuscularly, intravenously or subcutaneously). Glucagon takes approximately 15–20 min to work. However, if the person has liver disease (cirrhosis) or is malnourished, then glucagon may not work, in which case intravenous glucose should be given.

— **When do the components of a twice-daily biphasic insulin regimen exert their effects?**

NovoMix 30 comprises 30% insulin aspart (a rapid-acting insulin analogue) and 70% protamine-bound insulin aspart (giving a delayed or 'intermediate' release). In this twice-daily regimen, the morning dose of insulin relates to pre-lunch and pre-evening meal glucose levels – the rapid-acting insulin in the mix (peak of action at about 2–5 hours) will influence the pre-lunch level and the longer-acting insulin, the pre-evening meal level. The evening dose of insulin relates to the pre-bedtime reading (the rapid-acting component) and the intermediate (protamine-bound component) will influence the pre-breakfast (or fasting) reading.

The amino acid sequence of insulin (51 amino acids) can be altered by genetic engineering, to produce analogues with altered pharmacokinetic properties. Insulin aspart (rDNA origin) is a rapid-acting insulin analogue, which is a synthetic derivative of human insulin, prepared by substitution of a proline residue with an aspartic acid residue. This results in faster systemic absorption, with no change in receptor binding affinity. Injected immediately before a meal, rapid-acting analogues, such as insulin aspart, rapidly produce a large peak in insulin levels, comparable to that produced physiologically, though with a short duration of action.

When mixed with insulin, protamine, a protein extracted from the nucleus of fish sperm, slows down the onset, and increases the duration of insulin action.

— **Mechanism of action of insulin at receptor level**

The mechanism by which insulin produces its physiological effects, involving a stimulation of glucose uptake principally in muscle (myocyte) and fat (adipose) cells, has now been studied in great detail and involves a number of complex internal cellular signalling steps, ultimately leading to an increase in the number of high-affinity GLUT4 glucose transporter molecules in the plasma cell membrane. The receptor itself, after the extracellular binding of insulin, undergoes a conformational change that triggers a tyrosine kinase domain (adds phosphate groups to tyrosine residues) residing on the intracellular portion of the receptor protein; this then activates a multistep signalling cascade leading to an increase in glucose uptake. Termination of the signal mainly involves endocytosis and degradation of the insulin-bound receptor complex by the cell.

— **Stabilising blood glucose levels and preventing hypoglycaemia**

In this case, Mr JW needs to reduce his alcohol intake. If he binges on alcohol, his blood glucose levels will increase in the short term, causing hypoglycaemia afterwards.

In Mr JW's case, his bursts of increased physical activity mid-morning appear to be causing a problem. He is reluctant to stop exercising, but he could be encouraged to undertake a more gentle workout. Otherwise, he could eat a carbohydrate-rich snack before exercising, which would provide carbohydrates to replace those being used up by the activity. He could also reduce his insulin dose a little on the days that he exercises. However, this may then adversely affect his pre-evening meal readings. The other option to improve the situation is to switch regimens and change to a basal bolus regimen (pre-meal rapid-acting insulin plus an overnight intermediate-/longer-acting insulin). This allows more flexibility for people with an erratic lifestyle, although it involves more injections (four to five daily). If he were on a basal bolus regimen, he could undertake a learning programme such as DAFNE (dose adjustment for normal eating), which would teach him the skills required to adjust insulin doses depending on exercise taken and calories consumed.

— Insulin safety and the 'insulin passport'

Due to the reporting of patient safety incidents involving insulin which led to serious harm or death, the UK's National Patient Safety Agency (NPSA) has recommended that all adult patients on insulin therapy should receive a patient information booklet and an 'insulin passport'. The types of reported incidents involved:

- Wrong insulin dose, strength or frequency
- Omitted medicine
- Patients prescribed or dispensed the wrong insulin product.

The passport is a patient-held record aimed at empowering patients with diabetes to take a more active role in their treatment, avoid being given the wrong insulin and help improve accurate identification of the current insulin product. This will act as a safety check for the correct prescribing, dispensing and administration of insulin, supporting safer insulin treatment.

EXTENDED LEARNING

- What is nocturnal hypoglycaemia?
- What is hypoglycaemia unawareness?
- How can hypoglycaemia unawareness be modified?
- What are the formulation strategies for short- and long-acting insulins?

- Compare subcutaneous and other routes of parenteral administration of insulin

ADDITIONAL PRACTICE POINTS

- What are the risks of lipoatrophy (localised loss of adipose tissue under the skin) and lipohypertrophy (lump under the skin caused by accumulation of extra adipose tissue) due to repeated use of the same injection site?
- As a hospital pharmacist, what would be your advice with regard to missed insulin doses such as when inpatients are 'nil by mouth'?

References and further reading

Amiel SA, Dixon T, Mann R, Jameson K (2008). Hypoglycaemia in type 2 diabetes. *Diabet Med* 25:245–54.

Frier B, Fisher M (2007). *Hypoglycaemia in Clinical Diabetes*, 2nd edn. Oxford: Wiley-Blackwell.

Gualandi-Signorini AM, Giorgi G (2001). Insulin formulations – a review. *Eur Rev Med Pharmacol Sci* 5:73–83.

Hackett E, Jacques N, Gallagher A (2013). Type 1 diabetes: pathophysiology and diagnosis. *Clin Pharmacist* 5:69–72.

Jacques N, Hackett E (2013). Type 1 diabetes: insulin management. *Clin Pharmacist* 5:75–81.

Joint British Diabetes Society (2010). *The Hospital Management of Hypoglycaemia in Adults with Diabetes Mellitus*. Available at: www.diabetes.org.uk/About_us/What-we-say/Improving-diabetes-healthcare/The-hospital-management-of-Hypoglycaemia-in-adults-with-Diabetes-Mellitus (accessed 1 October 2013).

National Patient Safety Agency (2011). *The Adult Patient's Passport to Safer Use of Insulin*. Available at: www.nrls.npsa.nhs.uk/resources/type/alerts (accessed 3 June 2013).

Case 3
Type 2 diabetes mellitus

JOSEPHINE FALADE

LEARNING OUTCOMES

At the end of this case, you will be able to:

- Briefly describe the pathophysiology and outline the signs, symptoms and diagnosis of type 2 diabetes mellitus
- Describe the risk factors and the complications of type 2 diabetes
- Outline goals of therapy

- Describe the available treatment choices and their appropriateness in type 2 diabetes

Case study

Mr DP, a 46-year-old IT technician, has been referred to his GP following a health check at his local pharmacy.

Before the health check, he had informed his community pharmacist of feeling very tired over the last 2 months and increased frequency of passing urine. After the health check, he was informed by the pharmacist that his blood glucose result was in the diabetic range and that more tests were required for a proper diagnosis in order to initiate treatment as necessary. Meanwhile, Mr DP was given lifestyle advice (diet and exercise) by the pharmacist.

Test results confirm that Mr DP has type 2 diabetes mellitus.

- What is type 2 diabetes? What are its causes? How does it differ from type 1 diabetes?
- What are the common symptoms of diabetes mellitus?
- What are the risk factors for type 2 diabetes?
- How is it diagnosed?

Mr DP weighs 70 kg and his body mass index (BMI) is 30 kg/m^2; he has been prescribed pioglitazone 15 mg twice daily for his hyperglycaemia.

- What treatment options are available for type 2 diabetes?
- Is the above choice of treatment appropriate for Mr DP?
- Draw the structure of pioglitazone. Which structural features are important in its clinical use? What is its mechanism of action?
- What are the long-term complications of untreated or poorly controlled diabetes?
- What are the goals of therapy?

Case discussion

— Diabetes

Diabetes mellitus is a metabolic condition in which the amount of glucose in the blood is too high (hyperglycaemia) because the body cannot use it properly to supply normal energy requirements. After eating food, carbohydrates are broken down into glucose molecules in the gastrointestinal (GI) tract. Glucose is absorbed into the bloodstream, thereby raising blood glucose levels. To help the body use glucose properly, insulin (a hormone produced by islet β cells of the pancreas), acting via cellular insulin receptors, helps the glucose to enter the cells where it is used as a source of energy. Excess glucose is stored in the liver in the form of glycogen, serving as a reservoir for future use. Any glucose filtered into the urine is normally reabsorbed back into the circulation by the sodium/glucose co-transporter 2 (SGLT2), so that

none is excreted; however, when the renal glomerular absorption threshold of the transporter is exceeded (about 11 mmol/L $\equiv$ 200 mg/dL), as can occur in uncontrolled diabetes, glucose begins to appear in the urine (glycosuria) where it acts as an osmotic diuretic.

— Symptoms of diabetes

The three classic symptoms of diabetes are therefore increased frequency of urination (polyuria), excessive thirst (polydipsia) and dehydration, together with an increased appetite (polyphagia). The presence of excess glucose in the body also predisposes patients to infections, such as vaginal candidiasis in women or balanitis (inflammation of the end [glans] of the penis) in men. Polyphagia and lethargy (feeling tired) result from not being able to make effective use of the glucose available to the body.

— Type 1 and type 2 diabetes

There are two main types of diabetes: type 1 (previously called *juvenile-onset* diabetes – where the body is unable to produce any insulin due to autoimmune destruction of the pancreatic β cells) and type 2 (previously *maturity-onset* diabetes – where there is insufficient insulin secreted or when the insulin produced does not work properly in the body, i.e. insulin 'resistance'). Type 2 diabetes is more common, accounting for around 90% of people with diabetes. In most cases, it is linked with being overweight. It also usually appears in people aged >40 (although in south Asian and African–Caribbean people it can appear earlier, from age 25). Apart from age, ethnicity and obesity, other risk factors include family history, sedentary lifestyle and social deprivation.

— Diagnosis of type 2 diabetes

Type 2 diabetes is diagnosed by the presence of symptoms and blood tests. In symptomatic patients, diagnosis can be confirmed by either measuring fasting glucose ($\geq$7.0 mmol/L; normal about 5.5 mmol/L $\equiv$ 100 mg/dL) or 2-hour post-glucose load from an oral glucose tolerance test (OGTT $\geq$11.0 mmol/L)). For asymptomatic people, diagnosis is made with at least two blood glucose tests performed on different days. The results must both be in the diabetic range.

Recently, the World Health Organization (WHO) approved the use of the glycated haemoglobin (HbA1c) blood test to diagnose diabetes. A laboratory venous HbA1c 48 mmol/mol (6.5%: normal 20–40 mmol/mol $\equiv$ 4–5.9%) is the cut-off point for diagnosing diabetes. However, a value <48 mmol/mol (<6.5%) does not exclude diabetes diagnosed by blood glucose tests. In patients without symptoms of diabetes, the laboratory venous HbA1c should be repeated in 6 months or earlier if symptoms develop. Caution is advised with the use of HbA1c for diagnosis as it is unsuitable (false results) in certain groups of people, e.g. individuals with genetic or chemical alterations in haemoglobin.

— Treatment of type 2 diabetes

Diet and lifestyle modification are fundamental to managing diabetes either before, or at the same time as, initiation of drug therapy. It is common to start immediate drug therapy, especially in symptomatic patients with markedly raised test results without waiting for a response to diet and lifestyle modification (e.g. restricting carbohydrate intake, increasing physical activity, smoking cessation).

Metformin, a biguanide, is the first-choice oral anti-diabetic agent in overweight or obese patients and should also be considered in those who are not overweight. It acts by increasing peripheral utilisation of glucose (increased insulin sensitivity at receptor level and enhanced cellular glucose uptake) and decreasing liver gluconeogenesis through activation of adenosine monophosphate-activated protein kinase (AMPK). Metformin is usually started at a low dose and increased gradually in order to reduce GI side effects. In this case, as Mr DP is obese (BMI >30), metformin should be considered first if there are no contraindications to its use. Side effects include GI upsets (nausea/vomiting, diarrhoea, skin reactions, taste disturbances [dysgeusia], vitamin B_{12} malabsorption and, rarely, lactic acidosis. Metformin (and sulfonylurea) use is supported by long-term data from the UK Prospective Diabetes Study (UKPDS).

Gliclazide is a sulfonylurea that can be used (usually in those who are not overweight) if metformin is contraindicated or not tolerated, or as an add-on to metformin where dual therapy is required. It acts by binding to specific sulfonylurea receptors (SUR-1) on the surface of the pancreatic β cells to close ATP-sensitive K^+ channels (K_{ATP}) thereby depolarising the cells and increasing insulin release. Side effects include hypoglycaemia, GI disturbances, skin reactions, and (rarely) hepatic dysfunction and blood abnormalities.

Pioglitazone is currently the only marketed thiazolidinedione product in the UK that can be used for third-line treatments. Pioglitazone stimulates the nuclear receptor peroxisome proliferator-activated receptor γ (PPAR-γ) that functions as a transcription factor regulating expression of genes; this leads to a reduction in peripheral glucose resistance. It can be used alone or added to metformin and/or a sulfonylurea. For overweight and obese patients, the combination of metformin and pioglitazone is preferred to sulfonylurea and pioglitazone. A small increased risk of bladder cancer has been associated with the use of pioglitazone and therefore patients should be assessed for bladder cancer risk factors before treatment is initiated. The risk factors for bladder cancer include age, smoking status and previous radiation therapy to the pelvic region. Pioglitazone should also not be used in patients with heart failure or a history of heart failure because it promotes fluid retention and oedema. Other side effects include increased bone fracture risk and weight gain.

The thiazolidinedione ring in pioglitazone is highlighted in red on the structure in the diagram. This is the key structural feature of all the so-called 'glitazone' drugs, which have included troglitazone and rosiglitazone, withdrawn in most countries because of toxicity concerns (mainly cardiac and hepatic). The sp^3-hybridised carbon atom in the thiazolidinedione ring is a chiral centre and the drug is manufactured as a mixture of enantiomers. The S-enantiomer is responsible for pioglitazone's biological activity as an agonist at PPAR-γ receptors. The pyridine ring of pioglitazone contains a basic nitrogen atom and this allows the drug to be formulated as the hydrochloride salt, which demonstrates more rapid dissolution in the GI tract. Overall, the drug has low polarity and, similar to many low polarity drugs, it is cleared by metabolism in the liver. *Consequently pioglitazone should be avoided in patients with hepatic impairment.*

pioglitazone

GLP-1 agonists are a recent discovery in the management of type 2 diabetes and are centred on the 'incretin effect'. This describes the phenomenon by which oral glucose stimulates greater insulin release compared with intravenous glucose. Hormones responsible for this effect are called incretin hormones, and glucagon like peptide-1 (GLP-1) appears to be the most potent. GLP-1 is released from the small intestine in response to food, stimulating insulin release and suppressing appetite. GLP-1 levels are noted to be low in humans with type 2 diabetes.

This discovery has led to drug options such as injectable GLP-1 receptor analogues (e.g. exenatide and liraglutide) being introduced recently for the management of type 2 diabetes. They work by suppressing glucagon secretion, increasing insulin secretion by activating the GLP-1 receptors and also slowing gastric emptying, therefore reducing the rate at which glucose from food appears in the circulation. In addition, by its action in the brain, patients feel fuller for longer, thereby contributing to weight loss, which is beneficial in overweight patients. Another related group is the dipeptidyl peptidase 4 (DPP-4) inhibitors (gliptins). These inhibit the enzyme responsible for breaking down GLP-1. DPP-4 inhibitors are administered orally and include sitagliptin and vildagliptin. A common concern with drugs acting on the GLP-1 pathway is pancreatitis. Hypoglycaemia, GI upsets and headache are also common side effects.

A newer therapy based on prevention of glucose reabsorption, thereby forcing excretion in the urine, is dapagliflozin (sodium/glucose transport protein subtype 2 [SGLT-2] inhibitor). Common side effects are genital and urinary tract infections relating to increased urinary glucose excretion (glycosuria) and back pain.

Insulin is also used in managing type 2 diabetes where good control has not been achieved with oral or injectable non-insulin therapies. It may also be needed temporarily before or after surgery or when patients are severely ill and/or unable to receive oral medication.

— Long-term complications of poorly controlled diabetes

The long-term effects of diabetes include: microvascular complications, e.g. retinopathy (which can lead to blindness); nephropathy (which can lead to chronic kidney disease and renal replacement treatment); and neuropathy (e.g. gastroparesis [delayed gastric emptying], erectile dysfunction, and 'tingling' and loss of peripheral sensation in the hands and feet). People with diabetes are also at increased risk of macrovascular complications such as cardiac (e.g. myocardial infarction), peripheral arterial and cerebrovascular disease (e.g. stroke).

There are also acute metabolic complications associated with uncontrolled diabetes, e.g. DKA or with excessive management or an imbalance of exercise, food intake and drug therapy, e.g. hypoglycaemia.

— Goals of managing type 2 diabetes

The main goals are to manage diabetic symptoms, prevent acute and long-term (chronic) complications, improve quality of life and avoid premature diabetes-associated death. It must be noted that the approach to therapy must be individualised, and treating type 2 diabetes is not just about managing hyperglycaemia. Blood pressure and lipids must also be managed appropriately (where necessary) to reduce cardiovascular risks.

Unlike patients with type 1 diabetes mellitus, patients with type 2 are not absolutely dependent on insulin for life. However, most patients may need treatment with insulin at some point. It is important that Mr DP be informed that diabetes is a progressive disease and that there may be a future need for insulin therapy. All treatment decisions should involve the patient and should focus on their preferences, needs and values. There are a number of validated patient education programmes (e.g. DESMOND – Diabetes Education and Self Management in Ongoing and Newly Diagnosed) that have been shown to be effective in supporting people in managing their diabetes.

Lifestyle measures are also an important part of the management of type 2 diabetes to limit disease progression and future complications, in particular observing dietary advice. Patients with diabetes who plan to fast as part of their religious belief (e.g. Muslims during Ramadan) could be at risk of hypo- or hyperglycaemia, which could have serious implications for their health. They should therefore be advised to discuss this with their diabetes team as some medication changes may be recommended.

EXTENDED LEARNING

- What is the NHS health check?
- How is the OGTT performed?
- What are the targets for treating type 2 diabetes?
- How is treatment monitored?
- What is the side-effect profile of newer agents used for treatment of type 2 diabetes?
- How are the complications of diabetes (both acute and chronic) managed?
- What are the nutritional and therapeutic options for obesity?
- What is gestational diabetes? What are its risks and how may it be managed?

ADDITIONAL PRACTICE POINT

- Make sure that you are aware of the typical symptoms of hypoglycaemia in patients with diabetes and how they can be rapidly counteracted in an emergency

References and further reading

García-Pérez LE, Alvarez M, Dilla T, Gil-Guillén V, Orozco-Beltrán D (2013). Adherence to therapies in patients with type 2 diabetes. *Diabetes Therapy* 4:175–94.

Gerich JE (2010). Role of the kidney in normal glucose homeostasis and in the hyperglycaemia of diabetes mellitus: therapeutic implications. *Diabet Med* 27:136–42.

— Websites

www.healthcheck.nhs.uk
This website is a collaborative resource between the Department of Health, Public Health England, NHS Improving Quality, local government association, and local health- and social care teams.

www.nice.org.uk
NICE is a non-departmental public body (NDPB). It is accountable to its sponsor department, the Department of Health, but operationally it is of government. Its guidance and other recommendations are made by independent committees.

www.diabetes.org.uk
Diabetes UK is the leading charity that cares for, connects with and campaigns on behalf of every person affected by or at risk of diabetes.

www.idf.org
The International Diabetes Federation (IDF) is an umbrella organisation of over 230 national diabetes associations in 170 countries and territories.

www.who.int/diabetes
The World Health Organization is the directing and coordinating authority for health within the United Nations system.

Case 4
Serious lactic acidosis induced by metformin

ROB SHULMAN AND MERVYN SINGER

LEARNING OUTCOMES

At the end of this case, you will be able to:

- Describe the signs, pathophysiology, incidence and outcomes of MALA
- Outline the contraindications of metformin in relation to MALA and discuss whether these are overstated
- Identify features of the chemical structure of metformin that determine its absorption and excretion profile
- Outline the mechanism of action of metformin at a cellular level that leads to lactic acidosis
- Outline the management strategy for the treatment of MALA

Case study

Mrs MM is a 74-year-old obese woman with adult-onset (type 2) diabetes admitted to the ICU via A&E with an initial blood (plasma) pH of 6.7 (normal: 7.35–7.45), a plasma lactate level of 15 mmol/L (normal: 0.3–1.3 mmol/L) and a plasma creatinine of 946 μmol/L (this was normal [50–110 μmol/L] for adult woman when measured 6 months ago). She was established on metformin before admission and had a past history of myocardial infarction.

- ❷ Was metformin a suitable drug for Mrs MM?
- ❷ What do the initial results indicate and what is the diagnosis?
- ❷ What are the incidence and presenting symptoms of MALA?
- ❷ How does metformin cause MALA?

❓ What is the treatment for severe cases of MALA and what is the chance of survival?

❓ Is the outcome from MALA different if the patient takes an overdose compared with a non-intentional cause?

Mrs MM undergoes a long ICU stay with multiorgan failure that required mechanical ventilation, renal replacement therapy and vasopressor support of her circulation. Her stay was complicated by episodes of melaena (passage of dark or black faeces due to bleeding from the stomach or duodenum) and chest pain.

The consultant tells you that he is aware of some animal data that suggest succinate could be a treatment for MALA.

❓ He asks you to investigate whether this could be given to your patient

Mrs MM was discharged to the ward after 53 days in the ICU.

Case discussion

— Metformin use in diabetes

Metformin is widely used in obese patients with type 2 diabetes. This follows from publication of the UKPDS in overweight patients, which studied intensive glycaemic control from a metformin group, a sulfonylurea/insulin group and a conventionally treated group of patients. The results favoured the metformin group, because these patients had fewer diabetes-related endpoints, diabetes-related deaths, myocardial infarctions, stroke and microvascular disease.

The key contraindications to metformin are related to actual renal failure and acute conditions that can predispose to renal deterioration, such as dehydration, severe infection, shock and intravenous contrast media. Furthermore, in acute or chronic disease causing tissue hypoxia, it is contraindicated, e.g. cardiac or respiratory failure, recent myocardial infarction and shock. These contraindications are not widely followed; it has been estimated that approximately a half to three-quarters of patients established on metformin have at least one or more contraindications to its use.

— Incidence and presenting symptoms of MALA

Metformin is a member of the biguanide group of anti-diabetic drugs. The biguanide, phenformin, was first associated with lactic acidosis in the 1970s, with an associated incidence of 1 in 4000 patients and a mortality rate of 50%. It was

withdrawn from the market in 1977 and the whole drug group was tarred with this reputation; another biguanide, buformin, was available only in Hungary and Romania. The incidence of MALA in the USA is quoted as 2–9 cases per 100 000 patient years. There are some 330 cases of MALA in the literature but the historical link of biguanides and lactic acidosis may have heightened awareness of cases. A systematic review comparing metformin, non-metformin-treated diabetics and placebo did not find any difference in lactate levels, or any cases of lactic acidosis in over 30 000 patient-years in each group. They reported that the incidence of lactic acidosis in the other non-biguanide treatments was 9.9/100 000 years. Hence the case for MALA may be overstated.

The presenting symptoms of MALA are anorexia, somnolence, lethargy, nausea, vomiting and epigastric pain. Serious effects include hypotension, hypothermia, respiratory failure and dysrhythmia.

— Metformin structure and absorption

The chemical structure of metformin (Glucophage) is shown in the diagram. Metformin (*N,N*-dimethylimidodicarbonimidic diamide hydrochloride) is a highly polar, low-molecular-weight drug. As a basic drug, it is positively charged in the small intestine after oral administration and also at physiological pH, further increasing its polarity. Despite its charge and high polarity, it is fairly well absorbed from the GI tract. Absorption of metformin most probably occurs via the paracellular route (a common feature for polar, low-molecular-weight drugs), but active transport may also play a role.

metformin

Metformin is excreted via the urine largely unchanged; its high polarity allows filtration into the urine without the need for prior metabolism. The fact that the drug is cleared renally is the main reason that its use is contraindicated in patients with impaired renal function. Accumulation of metformin can predispose to adverse drug reactions (ADRs) including lactic acidosis.

— Pharmacology of metformin

Metformin exerts its anti-hyperglycaemic effects by decreasing liver glucose production (gluconeogenesis) through activation of adenosine monophosphate-activated protein kinase (AMPK), decreasing intestinal absorption of glucose, and improving the sensitivity of responsive tissues (e.g. muscle, adipose tissue) to insulin by increasing peripheral glucose uptake and utilisation, thus counteracting the 'insulin resistance' that typifies this condition. It may also antagonise the action of glucagon.

— Understanding the initial findings in this case

A normal patient's plasma pH is 7.35–7.45. Her finding of 6.7 is extremely acidic and is virtually incompatible with survival. The lactate level of 15 mmol/L indicates *hyperlactataemia* as the normal range is below 2 mmol/L. So, she has a severe lactic acidosis. Her plasma creatinine level is elevated at 946 μmol/L (normally 50–110 μmol/L), indicating severe renal failure.

— Causes of MALA

To understand this, one needs a grasp of how cellular energy production is generated by the production of adenosine triphosphate (ATP). This occurs firstly in the cytosol via glycolysis, i.e. the metabolism of glucose molecules. This is fairly inefficient, as one molecule of glucose will generate a net gain of just 2 molecules of ATP. The main site of energy production is in the mitochondria. The end-product of glycolysis is pyruvate which enters the mitochondrion, where it is metabolised to acetyl CoA (acetyl coenzyme A). This feeds into the tricarboxylate cycle, producing a further 2 ATP molecules. Electrons generated by the tricarboxylate cycle pass down the electron transport chain (ETC) to enable oxidative phosphorylation. The movement of electrons results in a shift of protons across the inner mitochondrial membrane, generating the energy for ATP synthase to produce 26–32 molecules of ATP.

Metformin is an inhibitor of Complex I, the first part of the ETC. This leads to a reduction of ETC efficiency and a decrease in energy production. The consequence of the 'log-jam' on the Krebs' cycle is that pyruvate is not taken up into the mitochondria and is thus converted to lactate. Due to a lack of adequate energy production, there is an increased hydrolysis of ATP leading to an increase in hydrogen ions.

Together, this leads to the observation of lactic acidosis.

The trigger for MALA is unknown, but in this case, it is speculated that an infection triggers an amplified response leading to sepsis, organ dysfunction and MALA.

— MALA treatment and survival rate

The mainstay of MALA treatment is elimination of the drug via renal replacement therapy, managing acidaemia and concurrent disease. The literature describes several reports where metformin is effectively removed by haemodialysis. It takes approximately 15 hours of haemodialysis to return to the normal upper range of metformin levels (<2 mg/L), although levels are not routinely measured in practice. In the ICU, haemodialysis is not widely used, especially in haemodynamically unstable patients. Haemofiltration is preferred because this is a continuous process with less significant fluid removal from the circulation. There are few published data on the removal of metformin with haemofiltration.

The outcomes of MALA were reported over a 5-year period during which 160 patients were treated who were established on metformin therapy and saw 30 cases of MALA (1% of all admissions); 21 of the MALA patients survived (11 of whom were dialysed) and 9 died (5 of whom were dialysed).

— Outcome from MALA: suicide versus accidental cases

A 10-year retrospective study of ICU patients reported 42 cases (0.1% of all ICU admissions), of whom 13 were suicide attempts and 29 accidental cases of MALA. The mortality rate was 33% overall but, interestingly, this broke down to 0% in the suicide group and 48% in the accidental group. Three-quarters of these patients received haemodialysis. The suicide patients were younger and had less deranged plasma pH values, and lower lactate and creatinine levels but much higher metformin plasma concentrations.

— Succinate: a treatment for MALA?

Animal studies indicate that metformin inhibits mitochondrial complex I activity by up to 44%. Succinate acts as a substrate for complex II and was used to reduce the inhibitory effects of metformin on mitochondria.

Succinate is present in a number of pharmaceuticals such as erythromycin ethyl succinate suspension, hydrocortisone and chloramphenicol injections, but in small quantities. Succinate on its own is not available in pharmaceutical grade and, as such, must be regarded at present as a promising experimental treatment which requires further investigation before it is used in humans for this indication.

EXTENDED LEARNING

- How does MALA occur at a cellular level?
- Describe how, theoretically, succinate may be a treatment for MALA.
- What other medical conditions are associated with the development of hyperlactataemia?
- How would renal disease affect drug pharmacokinetics?

- Differentiate between transcellular and paracellular transport mechanisms for drugs

References and further reading

Peters N, Jay N, Barraud D et al. (2008). Metformin-associated lactic acidosis in an intensive care unit. *Crit Care* **12**:R149.

Protti A, Russo R, Tagliabue P et al. (2010). Oxygen consumption is depressed in patients with lactic acidosis due to biguanide intoxication. *Crit Care* **14**:R22.

Salpeter S, Greyber E, Pasternak G, Salpeter E (2003). Risk of fatal and nonfatal lactic acidosis with metformin use in type 2 diabetes mellitus. *Arch Intern Med* **163**:2594–602.

UK Prospective Diabetes Study (UKPDS) Group (1998). Effect of intensive blood-glucose control with metformin on complications in overweight patients with type 2 diabetes (UKPDS 34). *Lancet* **352**:852–65.

Case 5
An unusual case of Cushing's syndrome
ANDREW CONSTANTI

LEARNING OUTCOMES

At the end of this case, you will be able to:

- Outline the causes, symptoms, signs and diagnosis of Cushing's syndrome
- Describe the various treatment options in Cushing's syndrome and the likely prognosis for the patient using such treatments
- Outline the use of radiopharmaceuticals as diagnostic agents, and precautions to be considered in their handling, use and disposal

Case study

Mrs ND, a 45-year-old woman, presented to her GP complaining of weight gain, lethargy, muscle weakness, back pain and fatigue which she had noticed developing slowly over the past few years. She also mentioned that her face felt swollen and that strange dark patches had appeared on her skin, particularly around her elbows and knees. She often felt very depressed, and found it increasingly difficult to concentrate and remember things. Her periods had also become irregular.

> **On examination**
> - Weight: 65 kg
> - Height: 1.55 m
> - HR: normal
> - Mildly hypertensive
> - No previous history of cancer
> - Not on any medication

The GP decided to refer her to her local hospital endocrine clinic for further examination.

On admission, the consultant noticed her to be centrally obese, with distinct purple abdominal skin striations, a reddish 'moon' face with some facial hair and acne, thinning head hair, some swelling at the back of the neck, and a dark thin skin, with some bruised-looking areas on her arms and legs. Laboratory tests revealed that her fasting blood glucose level was elevated (10 mmol/L; normal 3.6–5.5 mmol/L) but serum K^+ and other blood electrolytes were normal. Her plasma cortisol level measured at 8 am was 1680 nmol/L (normal: 180–800 nmol/L) and plasma ACTH (adrenocorticotrophic hormone) was 525 ng/L (normal <50 ng/L). Urinary free cortisol was also raised to 820 nmol/24 h (normal 30–300 nmol/24 h) and diurnal (8 am and 12 midnight) changes of plasma cortisol and ACTH were not present.

After undergoing an overnight 1 mg oral dexamethasone suppression test, her plasma cortisol failed to decrease; no inhibitory effect was seen after an 8 mg dexamethasone test (normal suppression <50 nmol/L). A CRH (corticotrophin-releasing hormone) stimulation test and bilateral inferior petrosal sinus test were not carried out in this case. Other tests revealed normal serum levels of TSH (thyroid-stimulating hormone) and T_3/T_4 (total).

MRI of the head showed a normal-looking pituitary gland, but a chest radiograph revealed a small opaque area (about 2 cm × 2 cm) at the top of her left lung. An ^{18}FDG ([^{18}F]fluorodeoxyglucose) PET/CT scan suggested no unusual tracer uptake in the lung nodule or surrounding chest areas. A whole body ^{111}In-labelled pentetreotide (Octreoscan) scintigraphy scan likewise showed no abnormal pentetreotide uptake in the lungs or elsewhere. Abdominal CT scans indicated, however, a bilateral adrenal hyperplasia. A diagnosis of Cushing's syndrome of ectopic origin (ectopic ACTH syndrome) was made, and appropriate treatment was started.

❷ What is Cushing's syndrome and how may it arise?

❷ What is Cushing's disease?

❷ Do all the patient's symptoms accord with the diagnosis?

❷ Explain how the various Cushing's symptoms may develop

❷ How do the laboratory test results enable a distinction to be made between a primary and a secondary cause of Cushing's syndrome?

❷ What do the results of the dexamethasone suppression tests suggest as a likely cause for this patient?

❷ What is the reasoning behind the tests?

❷ Why did the consultant ask for TSH and thyroid hormone levels to be measured?

❷ Why were the CRH stimulation test and inferior petrosal sinus test considered unnecessary in this case?

❷ What was the purpose of doing the radiograph and various other scans?

❷ How might the patient's disorder be treated, and what would be a likely prognosis after therapy?

❷ Octreoscan is a radiopharmaceutical; how is it dispensed in the hospital environment?

Case discussion

— Cushing's syndrome: causes and symptoms

Cushing's syndrome is due to chronic excess glucocorticoid secretion from adrenal, pituitary or external (therapeutic) origin. The weight gain (BMI [body mass index] = 27.1), depression, mental confusion, mild diabetes, puffy, rounded 'moon'-shaped face, 'buffalo hump' (raised supraclavicular fat pads), hirsutism and dysmenorrhoea (increased facial hair and irregular menstruation in women, suggesting increased virilisation by adrenal androgens) fits into a classic Cushing's syndrome presentation. This could be either of primary origin (non-ACTH-dependent), due to an adrenal tumour (benign adenoma or carcinoma), or secondary (ACTH-dependent) due to pituitary (microadenoma) or ectopic (usually lung carcinoid) tumour secretion of ACTH (ectopic ACTH syndrome). It may also arise symptomatically after excess long-term therapeutic glucocorticoid intake (iatrogenic) for treatment of chronic inflammatory conditions, such as rheumatoid arthritis, asthma and multiple sclerosis. Such cases of Cushing's syndrome are generally easily reversible. Excess cortisol arising from a benign tumour of the hypothalamus secreting excessive CRH or an isolated ectopic CRH-secreting tumour (carcinoma) is also possible, though very rare.

Mrs ND is also mildly hypertensive, which could be compatible with mineralocorticoid excess, but serum electrolytes (which would be expected to show a hypokalaemia and alkalosis in mineralocorticoid [aldosterone] excess) were normal. In this case, the likelihood is that the hypertension arose from a combination of several mechanisms, possibly involving a direct mineralocorticoid-like effect of excess cortisol acting on aldosterone receptors, an upregulation of the renin–angiotensin system, and a direct effect of cortisol on peripheral and systemic vasculature (decreased vasodilatation and increased vasoconstriction due to enhancement of circulating catecholamine effects). The truncal obesity, bruising, purple abdominal striae (stretch marks) and skin hyperpigmentation (due to excess ACTH interacting with melanocyte-stimulating hormone [α-MSH] melanocortin type-1 receptors on skin melanocytes, to produce the pigment melanin) are also characteristic of progressive ACTH-dependent Cushing's syndrome development.

— Explaining how the various Cushing's symptoms may develop

The expected symptoms in Cushing's syndrome are due to excessive circulating cortisol acting over a prolonged period of time and include:

- *Muscle weakness and wasting:* an increase in protein catabolism, results in protein loss in the muscles of the extremities (causing muscle atrophy: thin arms and legs); in bone (leading to osteoporosis and back pain); in skin (resulting in skin thinning and purple stretch marks on the thighs and abdomen); and in blood vessel walls (causing increased tendency to bruise easily).

- *Bone loss and pain:* osteoporosis is common in Cushing's syndrome, caused by decreased intestinal and renal calcium reabsorption, coupled with decreased bone formation and increased bone resorption due to direct effects of excess cortisol on osteoblasts and osteoclasts, respectively. Bone fractures may also occur, resulting in severe pain.

- *Fat redistribution:* an increase in fat deposition in the face, trunk and between the shoulders, causes a rounded 'moon-shaped' face, a 'buffalo hump' and prominent abdomen (truncal obesity). Regional stimulation of lipoprotein lipase (LPL) by cortisol may be responsible for this fat redistribution effect.

- *Virilisation of female patients:* the general increase in activity of the adrenal glands may also lead to a significant increase in serum androgen levels, which in women may cause excessive hair growth on the face and body, development of facial acne, voice changes and cessation of menstruation (amenorrhoea).

- *Hyperglycaemia*: cortisol is a diabetogenic hormone; by promoting liver gluconeogenesis from circulating amino acids and inhibiting insulin-induced glucose uptake by muscle and adipose tissue (insulin resistance), it increases blood glucose levels, leading to polyuria (excessive urination), polydipsia (excessive thirst) and a tendency towards diabetes mellitus.

- *Psychological disturbances:* due to the effects of excess cortisol on neuronal function, significant mood changes, e.g. euphoria, depression and hallucinations, can occur in patients with hypercortisolism.

- *Increased risk of infections:* high cortisol inhibits both immune and inflammatory responses, thereby creating an increased susceptibility to infections (particularly fungal infections and also pneumonia and TB) and impaired wound healing. Cortisol decreases T-lymphocyte proliferation and suppresses the synthesis of important inflammatory mediators, e.g. prostaglandins and leukotrienes.

— Laboratory tests

The abnormally high level of plasma cortisol and loss of normal circadian rhythm (high cortisol in the morning, low cortisol at night) is a principal characteristic of Cushing's syndrome. The fact that both plasma/urinary cortisol levels *and* plasma ACTH were elevated suggests, however, a *secondary* origin of the syndrome in this case, although whether this is due to excess pituitary ACTH output (benign pituitary *microadenoma* or *macroadenoma)* or an ectopic (possibly malignant) tumour source cannot be discerned from this result alone. A primary cause derived from the adrenal gland(s) themselves would be characterised by high cortisol levels and a *low* level of ACTH due to direct and indirect negative feedback exerted by elevated cortisol on the hypothalamus and anterior pituitary respectively.

— Diagnosing Cushing's disease

The dexamethasone suppression tests showed a failure of plasma cortisol suppression at *both* the low and high dexamethasone doses. This finding is characteristic of hypercortisolism due to an ACTH-producing tumour of ectopic origin, more commonly found in the lung. If the plasma cortisol had failed to be suppressed with the low-dose dexamethasone, but suppressed at the higher dose, this would have indicated a pituitary adenoma (Cushing's *disease*), based on the principle that pituitary tumours retain some negative feedback inhibition, although at a higher set-point than normal.

In the CRH stimulation test, human CRH is injected by intravenous bolus, and plasma cortisol and ACTH levels measured at regular intervals thereafter. In patients with pituitary-dependent Cushing's disease, a significant rise in ACTH and cortisol levels would be expected, whereas in patients with an ectopic source of ACTH production, such a response would not be seen. What can be confusing is that a small percentage of ectopic ACTH-secreting tumours can also be suppressed by high doses of dexamethasone, and stimulated by CRH, thereby making diagnosis difficult.

Inserting a petrosal sinus catheter (usually done under local anaesthesia, via a vein in the thigh or groin under radiological control) allows blood sampling directly from the veins that drain from the pituitary gland and would normally be used to confirm the source of ACTH as pituitary in the case of Cushing's disease (level showing a characteristic central-to-peripheral ACTH gradient), but would not detect an abnormal excess sinus ACTH level in the case of an ectopic ACTH tumour.

Depression and mental confusion with a puffy face can also be compatible with *hypothyroidism*, hence the tests for TSH and thyroid hormone levels, although hypothyroidism associated with a normal heart rate would be unusual.

— **Imaging tests**
In this case, Cushing's syndrome derived from an ectopic (lung) neuroendocrine tumour source of ACTH was suspected. Approximately 10% of cases of Cushing's syndromes can usually be ascribed to ectopic ACTH production. Ectopic ACTH tumours in the pancreas, thymus, thyroid gland and GI tract can also sometimes be found. In about 12% of cases, the tumours are not locatable. ACTH-producing lung tumours are apparently more common in men than in women, although females are more prone to pituitary-based or adrenal-based hypercortisolism. Accordingly, an MRI of the head did not reveal any pituitary abnormalities in this patient. If a pituitary microadenoma had been detected, it would have needed subsequent removal by trans-sphenoidal resection. A routine chest radiograph, however, revealed a suspicious nodule in the left lung as the likely source of the ectopic ACTH.

MRI and CT are routinely used to look at the pituitary and adrenal glands in an attempt to confirm a Cushing's syndrome diagnosis and, where appropriate, to guide surgical intervention. In this case, there was no pituitary tumour, but the abdominal CT (which utilises several X-ray beams and a computer to create an image) revealed that both adrenal glands were abnormally enlarged, as might be expected after continual overstimulation by ACTH. Interestingly, many healthy people have benign tumours in their pituitary and adrenal glands (non-secreting incidentalomas) that produce no symptoms; thus, the presence of a pituitary or adrenal tumour might in itself not always confirm a Cushing's syndrome diagnosis.

— **Combined [^{18}F]fluorodeoxyglucose (^{18}FDG) PET/CT scan**
The radiolabelled glucose analogue ^{18}FDG is commonly used as an intravenous tracer in PET (combined with superimposed CT scan) to identify malignant, rapidly dividing cancerous cells in the body that have a high metabolic activity (and therefore a high glucose uptake and nucleotide retention), and to plan and monitor subsequent treatment strategies. The emitted positron radiation from the tumour focus collides with nearby ambient electrons to emit γ-ray photons that are detected coincidently by the PET scanner and analysed into an image which, when combined with a CT scan, shows the location of the suspected tumour 'hot spot(s)'.

— **^{111}In-labelled pentetreotide (Octreoscan) scintigraphy**
Pentetreotide is DTPA (diethylenetriamine pentaacetate)-D-phenylalanine conjugate of octreotide, a synthetic cyclic peptide analogue of the hypothalamic (and pancreatic) peptide hormone somatostatin. The structure of [^{111}In] pentetreotide is shown on page 246. The metal ion-chelating agent DTPA is covalently bonded to the *N*-terminal D-phenylalanine residue of octreotide. The carboxyl and tertiary amino groups of the DTPA form a coordination complex with ^{111}In^{3+} ions, resulting in tight binding through at least seven non-covalent interactions. The octreotide portion of the molecule is able to recognise and bind to somatostatin receptors, localising the ^{111}In at the site of the receptors.

^{111}In-labelled pentetreotide (Octreoscan) scintigraphy is a relatively new scanning method aimed at identifying sites in the body where somatostatin type 2 (SST$_2$) peptide receptors are located. Patients injected with [^{111}In]pentetreotide as an intravenous infusion would normally show some physiological tracer uptake in the pituitary gland, thyroid, liver, kidneys, spleen, urinary bladder, gallbladder and bowel. Certain metastatic neuroendocrine tumours, such as ACTH-secreting ectopic tumours of the lung, express high levels of somatostatin receptors on their surface, and can

[^{111}In]-pentetreotide

therefore be detected by such a method using a γ-scintillation SPECT (single-photon emission computed tomography) camera.

In this case, both scans did not indicate any abnormal tracer uptake, suggesting that the lung nodule detected by the chest radiograph was the likely source of ectopic ACTH, may not have spread to other tissues and did not possess somatostatin receptors.

— **Radiopharmaceuticals and radiopharmacy**
Radiopharmaceuticals are radiolabelled substances used in nuclear medicine to diagnose, prevent or treat disease. Many utilise the radioisotope technetium-99m (^{99m}Tc) because it has a very short half-life (6 h), decaying to technetium-99 through rearrangement of the nucleus to a lower energy state and emission of a γ-ray. Radiopharmaceuticals are highly regulated, being controlled as both medicinal products and radioactive substances.

Octreoscan is a kit for preparing [^{111}In] pentetreotide 111 MBq/mL. The kit comprises two vials: vial A is a radiopharmaceutical precursor (in a glass vial shielded with lead) and vial B is a lyophilised powder for yielding a solution for injection, following reconstitution. Reconstitution is undertaken by closely following the instructions provided by the product manufacturer, using aseptic technique, and wearing protective waterproof gloves and an adequately shielded syringe, which is supplied in the kit. After reconstitution, the content of [^{111}In]pentetreotide is determined using an ionisation chamber. Adequate shielding of the product is required at all times until the product is given to the patient.

It must be disposed of in an approved manner, or allowed to decay to safe levels of radioactivity.

Radiopharmaceuticals are prescription-only medicines, and radiopharmacy services are essential for the delivery of nuclear medicine to patients. Compounded radiopharmaceuticals for parenteral use are usually prepared locally, under the supervision of a pharmacist, in a clean room following the principles of good manufacturing practice (GMP).

— **Treatment and prognosis**
As a result of the significant morbidity associated with Cushing's syndrome, it is important to establish a firm diagnosis and initiate therapy as soon as possible. Thus, in any case of ectopic ACTH syndrome, it is necessary to control the high levels of cortisol and ACTH, even when the source of the ACTH remains unclear. If an ectopic tumour is identifiable and operable, as in this case, immediate therapy with a steroid synthesis inhibitor such as metyrapone (Metopyrone) would be recommended, to control hormone levels and prepare the patient for surgery. Metyrapone competitively inhibits the 11β-hydroxylase enzyme in the adrenal cortex, involved in cortisol (and aldosterone) synthesis. The dosages used and period of treatment are tailored to suit the patient, with careful monitoring of cortisol levels to check for possible development of *hypo*cortisolism. Metyrapone may also aggravate masculinising effects in females (due to a rise in adrenal androgens).

Ketoconazole, an imidazole antifungal agent, can be used as an alternative inhibitor of adrenal steroid synthesis (unlicensed application) but requires monitoring of liver enzymes for hepatotoxicity, which in rare cases can be fatal. Other steroid synthesis inhibitors – aminoglutethimide and trilostane – are no longer available. Treatment with a somatostatin analogue, such as octreotide or lanreotide, reduces tumour volume before surgery, but would be effective only if the tumour has somatostatin receptors, which this tumour does not appear to have. If an ectopic tumour is inoperable or not easily locatable, then pre-treatment with metyrapone followed by laparoscopic total bilateral adrenalectomy (TBA) plus supplementary corticosteroids/mineralocorticoids for life may be an effective treatment option, although this would not cure the cutaneous hyperpigmentation (Nelson's syndrome).

The bronchopulmonary carcinoid tumour remains one of the most prevalent sources of ectopic ACTH secretion; small cell lung cancer (SCLC) is the most frequent cause, but is usually highly malignant with a poor prognosis. The outcome for patients with ectopic ACTH syndrome therefore depends very much on the nature of the tumour found and its extent of spread. In the case of this patient, it seems that the tumour was *atypical* in being not as aggressive as a typical carcinoid, and had not apparently spread. It therefore could eventually be removed surgically to effect a lasting cure. In some cases, surgical removal supplemented by local radiotherapy may be considered.

Subsequent histology carried out on the excised lung tumour might in this case be expected to show specific immunostaining for ACTH, and also chromogranin A (CgA), synaptophysin and CD56 (cluster of differentiation antigen 56), which are all commonly found markers in neuroendocrine tumours.

When the ACTH source is unknown ('occult'), survival rates are slightly better but still not very good. Here, as the patient did not have any obvious metastases, Cushing's syndrome would be expected to improve gradually after onset of drug therapy and then quite quickly after resection of the lung nodule, so the patient's major symptoms should decline, and blood pressure and periods would eventually return to normal. Removal of the lung nodule should also resolve the excess ACTH secretion and therefore the hyperpigmentation effect. Her long-term prognosis would then be expected to be good.

EXTENDED LEARNING

- What other tests could have been used in the diagnosis of Cushing's syndrome, and what is their basis? What other method would you suggest for assessing midnight cortisol levels in Cushing's patients?

- It is common for Cushing's syndrome patients to develop some degree of osteoporosis characterised by a decrease in bone mineral density (BMD). How might this be measured? How reversible is this change in BMD after normalisation of cortisol levels? What type of drug therapy might be recommended in more extreme cases?

- It has been suggested recently that temozolamide might be useful in the treatment of certain forms of Cushing's disease and ectopic ACTH syndrome. What is the evidence for this, and how effective is this drug?

- What is mitotane? Under what conditions might it be used in the treatment of Cushing's syndrome?

- What is BMI and how is it calculated? How reliable is it as a measure of obesity level?

- What is lyophilisation (freeze drying) and why might it be employed in the preparation of injections?

ADDITIONAL PRACTICE POINT

- Make sure that you are familiar with and understand the basis of the information provided on the front of a patient steroid-warning card.

References and further reading

Asnacios A, Courbon F, Rochaix P et al. (2008). Indium-111-pentetreotide scintigraphy and somatostatin receptor subtype 2 expression: new prognostic factors for malignant well-differentiated endocrine tumors. *J Clin Oncol* **26**:963–70.

de Matos LL, Trufelli DC, das Neves-Pereira JC, Danel C, Riquet M (2006). Cushing's syndrome secondary to bronchopulmonary carcinoid tumor: report of two cases and literature review. *Lung Cancer* **53**:381–6.

Deb SJ, Nichols FC, Allen MS, Deschamps C, Cassivi SD, Pairolero PC (2005). Pulmonary carcinoid tumors with Cushing's syndrome: an aggressive variant or not? *Ann Thorac Surg* **79**:1132–6.

Kenchaiah M, Hyer S (2012). Cushing's syndrome due to ectopic ACTH from bronchial carcinoid: A case report and review. *Case Reports Endocrinol* doi:10.1155/2012/215038.

UK Radiopharmacy Group (2012). *Guidelines for the provision of radiopharmacy services in the UK*. Available at: www.bnms.org.uk (accessed 1 October 2013).

Case 6
Addisonian crisis

ANDREW CONSTANTI

LEARNING OUTCOMES

At the end of this case, you will be able to:

- Outline the causes, symptoms, signs and diagnosis of Addison's disease and an Addisonian crisis
- Describe the various standard treatment options in Addison's disease and the emergency management of an Addisonian crisis and the likely prognosis for the patient in each case

Case study

A 25-year-old woman, Mrs SN, presented at a local hospital A&E accompanied by her husband, who told the attending doctor that, while out shopping, his wife was suddenly overcome by a feeling of extreme weakness, nausea, uncontrolled shivering (it was a particularly cold day) and a cramp-like pain in her abdomen. She also complained of feeling very dizzy and faint, particularly on standing. On further enquiry, the doctor was told that Mrs SN had recently suffered a severe bout of flu and since then had been feeling very depressed and over-tired, and on two occasions had even fainted while riding to work on the underground in the morning rush hour. Apparently, over the past few months, and particularly since falling ill, Mrs SN had shown little appetite, except for salty foods such as crisps and peanuts; consequently she always felt very thirsty, and was drinking and passing a lot of water during the day. She also had difficulty sleeping and had lost about 12 kg in weight.

On examination

- Weight: 55 kg
- Height: 1.60 m
- BP: 90/60 mmHg (normal about 120/80 mmHg)
- HR: 115 beats/min
- Respiration: 25/min (normal about 12–20/min
- Temperature: 38° C (slightly elevated)
- Undernourished, thin and dehydrated
- Dark skin around creases of palms, elbows and knees
- Loss of underarm hair
- Postural hypotension on standing
- No current medication
- Non-smoker
- No excessive use of alcohol

The doctor decided to admit her to the ward for immediate blood tests to be carried out. Mrs SN was particularly anxious about being admitted because she 'did not like hospitals or needles'. Her husband tried to comfort her and accompanied her to the ward for reassurance.

On the ward, the attending doctor, after trying to calm Mrs SN down as much as possible, took blood samples for urgent analysis and ordered her to be started immediately on an intravenous infusion of 5% dextrose in 0.9% saline, together with O_2 at 2 L/min by intranasal cannula. Her BP (systolic/diastolic), heart rate and mean arterial pressure (MAP) were monitored continuously with a double finger cuff. On the basis of these results, the doctor

▼ TABLE 6.3
Blood tests on admission

Blood test	Level	Normal range
Plasma Na+ (mmol/L)	100	135–145
Glucose (mg/dL) (mmol/L)	60 3.3	59–105 3.3–5.8
Plasma K+ (mmol/L)	6.6	3.5–5

suspected that Mrs SN was showing the symptoms of an adrenal insufficiency, or possible Addison's disease, and asked for further measurements of plasma cortisol, aldosterone, adrenocorticotrophic hormone (ACTH) and renin activity levels to be made in the morning.

During the course of the afternoon, Mrs SN felt increasingly agitated and, at around 6 pm, her MAP suddenly dropped to 65 mmHg, triggering a monitor alarm. Luckily, the doctor who was still on the ward recognised the symptoms of an acute Addisonian crisis, and immediately administered an intravenous dextrose/saline bolus together with an intravenous bolus dose of 200 mg hydrocortisone. Her dextrose/saline infusion was switched for a continuous intravenous administration of a vasopressor, noradrenaline, at 4.5 micrograms/kg per min, which restored her normal blood pressure over about 45 min, whereupon the infusion was discontinued. As the patient's condition appeared to stabilise, it was decided to keep her in the ward under observation overnight until further diagnostic tests could be done. A 7.5 mg tablet of zopiclone was also given to help her sleep through the night, and her husband was advised to go home.

In the morning (8.00 am), further blood test tests revealed:

- decreased levels of cortisol (1.4 micrograms/dL; normal 5–25 micrograms/dL)
- aldosterone (1.5 ng/dL; normal 6–30 ng/dL)
- an elevated level of ACTH (1040 pg/mL; normal 10–100 pg/mL)
- a high level of plasma renin activity (9.5 ng/mL per h; normal 0.3–3.7 ng/mL per h)

All of which confirmed the initial diagnosis of Addison's disease. The patient was initiated on standard chronic hormone replacement therapy (HRT) with hydrocortisone (15 mg hydrocortisone in the morning, 5 mg at midday and 5 mg in the evening – trying to follow the normal physiological circadian variation in cortisol levels) and fludrocortisone (a synthetic mineralocorticoid: Florinef) 0.1 mg daily taken in the morning, and discharged. She was advised that she needed to take this medication for life and instructed on how to increase her doses of hydrocortisone when under stressful situations such as infection, pregnancy, trauma or surgery, and provided with an identifying bracelet and patient emergency steroid warning card to carry around with her at all times,

stating the type of medication and the need for increased steroid dosage (with proper dose indicated) during extreme stress or injury.

❷ What is Addison's disease and how may it arise? Do all the patient's symptoms accord with the initial diagnosis and subsequent reversion to crisis? Explain how the various Addison's symptoms may develop. What is an Addisonian crisis? What possible trigger factors would a clinician need to consider for an Addison's patient?

❷ What are the main laboratory diagnostic criteria for the disorder? Are the observed physical symptoms and laboratory results what you would expect if the diagnosis were correct? Explain the basis for these observations. Do the laboratory test results of hormone levels allow a distinction to be made between a primary and a secondary cause of adrenal insufficiency? What other type of tests might the doctor have called for to confirm the diagnosis of primary Addison's disease? What is the reasoning behind the tests and the expected outcomes?

❷ Comment on the patient's treatment while in hospital. What do you think could have precipitated the crisis condition in this case?

❷ What would be a probable treatment and prognosis for the patient after discharge? Compare the structures of the two prescribed steroids and comment on the rationale for their combination

Case discussion

Symptoms of Addison's disease

The patient's initial physical symptoms of progressive weakness, fatigue, nausea, abdominal cramps and dizziness/faintness, with loss of appetite and weight loss, are indicative of Addison's disease (primary hypoadrenalism), which is a state of adrenal insufficiency usually resulting from an autoimmune destruction or unknown (idiopathic) impairment of function or atrophy (physical shrinkage) of the adrenal glands (primary cause), or from some hypothalamic–pituitary disease that causes a deficit of pituitary ACTH release (secondary cause). It is also possible for the symptoms of Addison's disease to appear after an acute infection such as tuberculosis (which can cause dense calcification of the adrenal tissue), HIV/AIDS (human immunodeficiency virus/acquired immune deficiency syndrome), surgical removal of the adrenal glands or an abrupt withdrawal of long-term adrenocortical HRT in an adrenalectomised patient.

More rarely, some fungal infections (histoplasmosis), malignant adrenal carcinoma or acute adrenal haemorrhage (e.g. following a major traumatic accident) can also cause acute adrenal failure. The condition is typically slow to develop (over months or years), such that overt clinical symptoms may become apparent only when a significant portion (about 90%) of the adrenal glands are involved, and is characterised by a combined loss of both glucocorticoid and mineralocorticoid adrenocortical function to levels that are inadequate to meet the patient's need for adrenal corticosteroids. Sometimes unexplained fatigue is the only symptom, so Addison's disease may not be immediately suspected by GPs. Patients may be told that their tiredness is due to depression or that 'it's all in your head'. Some patients may also exhibit other psychiatric symptoms such as agitation, poor concentration, confusion, irritability and poor quality of sleep. Normally, adrenal corticosteroids maintain the ability of the body to handle physiological and psychological 'stress' situations (glucocorticoids), and also to retain Na^+, and excrete K^+ ions via the kidney (mineralocorticoids). Deficient levels of these hormones would thus cause an increased renal loss of Na^+ (and water) and excessive reabsorption of K^+, resulting in a decreased blood volume, cardiac output and renal perfusion. This consequently leads to a decrease in BP and a compensatory rise in heart rate. Mrs SN's observed symptoms of diuresis, dehydration, excessive thirst (polydipsia), salt craving, postural hypotension and tachycardia would therefore also accord with the initial diagnosis of Addison's disease.

The expected symptoms in primary Addison's disease are due to a combined lack of both glucocorticoids and mineralocorticoids over a prolonged period of time and include:

- *Postural hypotension and dehydration:* the deficiency in aldosterone (mineralocorticoid) would lead to loss of body Na^+/water (hyponatraemia) and an increased absorption of renal K^+ (hyperkalaemia), accompanied by low BP, low blood volume and dehydration.
- *Muscle weakness, fatigue, tiredness and malaise, dizziness, nausea, vomiting, abdominal pain:* unexplained fatigue, weight loss, muscle cramps and dizziness result from the effect of a combined loss of cortisol and aldosterone on brain and muscle cells.
- *Anorexia, loss of appetite and decrease in body weight, depressed mood and increased irritability, rapid respiration (tachypnoea), tachycardia, hypoglycaemia:* such unspecific symptoms are difficult to ascribe to a specific glucocorticoid or mineralocorticoid deficiency because they can also occur in other disorders such as anorexia nervosa.
- *Loss of pubic and axillary hair:* this is due to lack of adrenal androgens which, in females, is the only source of the male hormone testosterone. This is not seen in male patients with Addison's disease, because, in men, androgens are principally produced by the testes.
- *Low levels of plasma cortisol, associated with high levels of ACTH:* this is due to a lack of negative feedback by cortisol on the hypothalamus and anterior pituitary (note: *low* plasma cortisol levels with *low* levels of ACTH would be expected in patients with secondary hypoadrenalism where either the hypothalamus or the anterior pituitary is dysfunctional).
- *Increased skin pigmentation:* lack of circulating cortisol leads to an *increase* in plasma ACTH which can interact with melanocortin type-1 receptors for melanocyte-stimulating hormone (α-MSH) on skin melanocytes, producing the pigment melanin; the pigmentation is particularly prominent around scars, skinfolds, elbows, knees, knuckles, buttocks and the gums (more difficult to discern in darker-skinned patients).

The detection of circulating, specific, destructive autoantibodies (21-hydroxylase antibodies) directed against the key enzyme involved in adrenal steroid synthesis (21-hydroxylase) is also a typical biochemical feature of autoimmune Addison's disease (AAD) and these antibodies usually appear well before a full clinical Addison's disease diagnosis is made (pre-clinical AAD) and could therefore be early markers of the condition. In some cases, adrenal cortex autoantibodies (ACAs) may also be detected in the serum. Other autoimmune conditions can sometimes accompany the disorder, e.g. thyroid disease (Hashimoto's thyroiditis), type 1 diabetes or pernicious anaemia.

A further characteristic of Addison's disease is a raised level of plasma renin activity. Renin is an enzyme released by renal juxtaglomerular cells when there is a fall in renal BP and an excessive reduction in circulating blood volume (e.g. during severe haemorrhage, or excessive salt or water loss). Renin promotes the production of angiotensin I from a circulating angiotensinogen precursor, which is then converted by angiotensin-converting enzyme (ACE) to the active octapeptide angiotensin II; the latter directly stimulates the synthesis and release of aldosterone from the outermost zona glomerulosa region of the adrenal glands (note that angiotensin II also has a direct vasoconstrictor action that helps to maintain the blood pressure of the arterial circulation under extreme conditions, and a further important central effect [via the subfornical organ] to control water intake [dipsogenic effect]).

— Addisonian crisis

Addisonian crisis, or acute adrenal insufficiency, is a clinical emergency that may develop suddenly when an ongoing adrenal insufficiency goes undetected and therefore untreated or an Addison's disease patient undergoes any type of physical stress situation such as a serious infection, surgery, cold exposure, severe burns, overexertion or severe psychic stress/over-anxiety, despite any previous corticosteroid/mineralocorticoid supplementation that the patient may be taking to ensure adequate stabilisation. In women, the stress of labour or hyperemesis gravidarum (severe 'morning' sickness), or the period during or immediately after childbirth (*puerperium* to 6 weeks post-birth) could also be a trigger. Such patients then run a serious risk of developing an acute hypovolaemic shock state (an emergency situation in which severe fluid [or blood] loss in a patient makes the heart unable to pump sufficient blood around the body), which can lead to possible circulatory collapse and death.

Laboratory tests

A preliminary diagnosis of Addison's disease would normally be established on the baseline laboratory findings of a low plasma cortisol level, increased plasma ACTH level (due to lack of negative feedback) and a low or undetectable plasma aldosterone with increased plasma renin activity (triggered by the drop in BP, blood volume and loss of Na^+). Her observed physical symptoms due to the combined lack of corticosteroids and

rise in ACTH (stimulating skin α-MSH receptors) would certainly accord with these laboratory results and the initial diagnosis of Addison's disease. To confirm an autoimmune origin, measurement of positive antibodies to the 21-hydroxylase and/or adrenal cortex (due to autoimmune attack of the adrenal glands) would need to be made.

— ACTH stimulation test

The ACTH stimulation test is also commonly used for diagnosing primary Addison's disease. In the low-dose (short or rapid) test, baseline morning ACTH and cortisol blood levels would be measured, followed by intravenous administration of a low dose (1 microgram) of Synacthen (a synthetic analogue, containing the first 24 amino acids of ACTH) to test the function of the adrenal glands. Post-Synacthen plasma cortisol levels would then be measured 30 and 60 min after injection. A cortisol level rising from about 25 μg/dL to $\geq$50 μg/dL, would be considered normal after this procedure. However, in primary Addison's disease, where both glands are dysfunctional (and therefore unable to respond correctly), the baseline cortisol level would be well below normal to start with ($<$10 μg/dL) and barely rise 1 hour after injection in response to the ACTH stimulation. Where the adrenal insufficiency arises from a secondary source (i.e. inadequate endogenous ACTH stimulation due to pituitary or hypothalamic disease), the short test would typically double or triple the cortisol level from its low baseline value, confirming that the adrenal glands are indeed functional. There is also a high-dose (long or prolonged stimulation) test that can be used when the short test is inconclusive. Here, 250 micrograms of Synacthen is injected either intravenously or intramuscularly to produce maximal adrenal activation, and cortisol levels measured at 30-min intervals over 48–72 h. Patients with a primary adrenal insufficiency would still fail to produce any cortisol during the test period, whereas those with a secondary adrenal insufficiency eventually respond to the test on the second or third day.

At this point, when the ACTH stimulation test produces a significant rise in cortisol level (adrenal glands are functional), further distinction between a pituitary or hypothalamic source for the secondary adrenal insufficiency could be made using two further tests: the insulin tolerance test and the corticotrophin-releasing hormone (CRH) stimulation test.

— Insulin tolerance test

In the insulin tolerance test (to confirm secondary cause of insufficiency), an intravenous dose of insulin (Actrapid, 0.1–0.15 units/kg) is injected to induce hypoglycaemic stress (plasma glucose level <40 mg/dL [<2.2 mmol/L]), which would normally be expected to trigger release of the counteractive hyperglycaemic hormones cortisol and growth hormone (GH) via stimulation of the hypothalamic–anterior pituitary axis (pituitary prolactin would also be released). In patients with secondary hypopituitarism, or hypothalamic dysfunction, an adequate cortisol (and GH/prolactin) response would not be obtained. This test can be potentially dangerous, so it needs to be carried out under careful medical supervision and monitoring. It would certainly not be advised in the case of this patient, whose baseline cortisol level was very low and was close to Addisonian crisis. Intravenous dextrose and hydrocortisone must always be made available during the test.

— CRH stimulation test

The CRH stimulation test can then be used to distinguish between hypothalamic and anterior pituitary failure. CRH is normally produced by the hypothalamus to stimulate the anterior pituitary gland to produce ACTH, which then stimulates the adrenal glands to produce cortisol. After injecting synthetic CRH 100 micrograms (or 1 microgram/kg) intravenously the normal response would be a rise of plasma ACTH and cortisol; individuals with primary Addison's disease (underactive or damaged adrenal glands) would respond by producing high levels of ACTH but little or no cortisol. Patients with secondary hypothalamic disease (pituitary intact) would also usually respond with a delayed rise in both ACTH and cortisol, but, in those with a pituitary dysfunction, there would be no change in the level of either hormone.

Consideration of the cause and Addisonian crisis in this case

In this case, it seems that the main symptoms of Addison's disease were developing slowly over a period of time, and the disease was not suspected until she was almost in an addisonian crisis, most likely precipitated by that fact that she was out shopping on a particularly cold day. Her general,

dark, sickly, undernourished and dehydrated appearance prompted the A&E doctor to admit her for immediate blood tests, which revealed a significant electrolyte imbalance suggestive of an adrenal insufficiency. While waiting for the initial blood test results, the ward doctor started her on standard dextrose/saline rehydration therapy with supplemental intranasal O_2 at 2 L/min. The further stress of being in a hospital environment and having blood samples taken undoubtedly triggered the crisis, characterised by the sudden dramatic drop in BP, which was fortunately diagnosed in time by the ward doctor, before more severe low BP, hypoglycaemia, fever and hypovolaemic shock could develop. The immediate goal in an Addisonian crisis is to restore the vascular volume and replace adrenal corticosteroids. Patients usually respond well to a large dose of glucocorticoid with dramatic improvement in BP, which can be further improved with a systemic vasoconstrictor until stabilisation has been achieved. Any delay in diagnosis could have had a fatal outcome. The doctor thus responded correctly with a rapid intravenous bolus of dextrose in physiological (0.9%) saline together with hydrocortisone and a slow infusion of noradrenaline (as tolerated) until Mrs SN's systolic blood pressure was restored. The intranasal O_2 was also continued until her symptoms subsided.

hydrocortisone

fludrocortisone acetate

Treatment and prognosis after discharge

Provided that the patient takes her hormone replacement steroids on a regular basis and avoids or compensates for stressful situations, her vital signs, electrolyte abnormalities and other associated symptoms should rapidly return to normal, and she should be able to lead a normal life, although, of course, the primary adrenal autoimmunity would remain.

— Hydrocortisone and fludrocortisone

Fludrocortisone is the 9α-fluoro-synthetic derivative of hydrocortisone. Fludrocortisone is administered as the acetate ester (at the primary hydroxyl group) derivative. The acetate ester (among others) of hydrocortisone is also used clinically, but these acetate esters are hydrolysed during first-pass metabolism to generate the parent steroid. Hydrocortisone possesses good glucocorticoid but weak mineralocorticoid activity. The use of hydrocortisone alone in Addison's disease is not usually sufficient for mineralocorticoid replacement so it is usually used in combination with a potent mineralocorticoid such as fludrocortisone. The simple introduction of the fluorine atom in fludrocortisone increases glucocorticoid activity around 10-fold, but increases mineralocorticoid activity by a factor of several hundred.

EXTENDED LEARNING

- Although not immediately relevant in the case of this patient, imaging tests could provide further supporting information to help diagnosis of primary or secondary adrenal insufficiency. What imaging tests would you suggest might be useful for clarifying the origin of Addison's disease? Would you rely on these tests alone for making a definite diagnosis?

- Would there be any contraindication in administering zopiclone to an Addison's disease patient?

- What would be the best strategy to follow for an Addison's disease patient who becomes pregnant: during the pregnancy, at time of birth and postpartum?

- What other esters of hydrocortisone are used clinically? How are their properties (particularly polarity) important in their formulation and administration?

ADDITIONAL PRACTICE POINT

- Adddison's disease is a fairly rare but serious, potentially life-threatening condition. To prevent unnecessary death from Addisonian crisis, it is important that patients with known adrenal insufficiency (as well as their immediate relatives and GPs) receive adequate verbal and written instructions on how to deal with any severe physical and psychological stress situations. Patients and their relatives need to be taught how to recognise symptoms and to use an emergency injection of hydrocortisone or increase their dose of oral hydrocortisone in times of stress, as necessary.

References and further reading

Allolio B, Lang K, Hahner S (2011). Addisonian crisis in a young man with atypical anorexia nervosa. *Nat Rev Endocrinol* 7:115–21.

D'Silva C, Watson D, Ngaage D (2012). A strategy for management of intraoperative Addisonian crisis during coronary artery bypass grafting. *Interact Cardiovasc Thorac Surg* 14:481–2.

Falorni A, Minarelli V, Morelli S (2012). Therapy of adrenal insufficiency: an update. *Endocrine* 43:514–28.

Frederick R, Brown C, Renusch J, Turner L (1991). Addisonian crisis: emergency presentation of primary adrenal insufficiency. *Ann Emerg M* 20:802–6.

Nieman LK, Chanco Turner ML (2006). Addison's disease. *Clinics Dermatol* 24:276–80.

O'Donnell M (1997). Emergency! Addisonian crisis. *Am J Nursing* 97:41.

Small M, MacCuish AC, Thomson JA (1987). Missed Addisonian crisis in surgical wards. *Postgrad Med J* 63: 367–9.

Case 7
Hypothyroidism
JOSEPHINE FALADE

LEARNING OUTCOMES

At the end of this case you will be able to:

- Outline the pathophysiology, signs, symptoms and diagnosis of hypothyroidism
- Outline goals of therapy in treating hypothyroidism
- Describe the chemistry of thyroid hormones
- Outline the role and methods of dissolution testing of solid dosage forms
- Describe the available treatment choices and their appropriateness in treating hypothyroidism
- Identify relevant counselling points and issues of relevance to a pharmacist

Case study

Ms LT is a 30-year-old mother of a 12-month-old baby. She complains that she has been unable to lose most of the weight gained during pregnancy, feels cold even when it is hot, has noticed a general feeling of fatigue in the last 3 months and now finds it very difficult to keep up with the demands of her growing son. In addition, she feels very low especially now that her hair is falling out. Her bowel habit has changed a lot and she is now constipated most of the time, despite having no changes to her diet.

> **On examination**
>
> - Palpable goitre (thyroid enlargement)
> - Puffy face and yellowish skin
> - HR: 60 beats/min (normal 60–100 beats/min)

The results of laboratory tests confirm that Ms LT has hypothyroidism.

- Describe the structure of the thyroid gland and thyroid hormones
- What is hypothyroidism and how is it caused? Identify signs and symptoms that suggest Ms LT has hypothyroidism
- What laboratory tests are normally used in the diagnosis of hypothyroidism?

Ms LT weighs 60 kg; she has been prescribed levothyroxine 100 micrograms once daily as replacement therapy.

- What treatment options are available for hypothyroidism and how long does levothyroxine need to be taken?
- List the goals for treating Ms LT and relevant counselling points for the new medication
- The synthetic drug levothyroxine is identical to thyroxine, naturally produced in the thyroid gland (also known as thyroid hormone T_4). Draw the structure of levothyroxine and describe its stereochemistry. Why is the levorotatory isomer active and the opposite (dextrorotatory) isomer inactive?
- Levothyroxine is prescribed generically. However, variation has at times been reported, believed to be based on differences in the dissolution behaviour of tablets from different manufacturers, resulting in changed therapeutic response. How is the dissolution behaviour of solid dosage forms, such as tablets, determined?

Case discussion

— Thyroid gland and thyroid hormones

The thyroid gland is a small butterfly-shaped structure overlying the trachea and is the largest endocrine organ, weighing about 20 g. It produces three hormones: triiodothyronine (T_3) and tetraiodothyronine (or thyroxine [T_4]) and calcitonin (released directly from the thyroid gland in response to changes in blood calcium levels). The thyroid hormone levels are regulated via a direct negative feedback mechanism mediated by the anterior pituitary gland. T_4 is the major circulating hormone secreted by the thyroid; it is approximately 99% protein bound. For activity, T_4 needs to be converted to T_3 (deiodination) in the target tissues.

— Hypothyroidism: causes, signs, symptoms and diagnosis

Hypothyroidism is hyposecretion or deficiency of thyroid hormone. It is a chronic disorder with a prevalence of 2–3% and is approximately 10% more common in women than in men. It can be caused by a malfunction of the thyroid gland itself (primary hypothyroidism) or the hypothalamus–anterior pituitary system (secondary hypothyroidism). Primary hypothyroidism is more common and often presents as an autoimmune disease (Hashimoto's thyroiditis), which is characterised by the destruction of thyroid cells by various cell- and antibody-mediated immune processes. Other causes of hypothyroidism include:

- Surgery (removal of the thyroid gland [thyroidectomy])
- Radioactive iodine therapy, used for the treatment of *hyper*thyroidism
- Iatrogenic hypothyroidism from use of drugs such as amiodarone, interferon or lithium
- Dietary iodine deficiency.

The thyroid hormones are essential for the function and maintenance of the body's metabolic processes and systems. They increase the body's metabolism (BMR or basal metabolic rate), resulting in increased oxygen consumption, intestinal motility, contraction of the heart and, among others, the breakdown of substances such as cholesterol, as well as carbohydrates and protein. Therefore, a general metabolic slowing down is expected where there is insufficient production of the hormones.

In this case, Ms LT has some of the typical features of hypothyroidism; these are weight gain and general fatigue (secondary to a low BMR); cold intolerance (impaired calorigenesis), constipation, yellowish skin (due to build-up of β-carotenes, normally converted to vitamin A), puffy face (myxoedema), hair loss and bradycardia (low heart rate). Hypothyroidism can also present with an enlargement of the thyroid gland (goitre) as in this case.

One of the differential diagnoses for a patient with suspected hypothyroidism is depression, because some of the presenting symptoms of hypothyroidism can be confused with depression. In primary hypothyroidism, the thyroid fails to produce enough thyroid hormone, leading to low T_3 and T_4 levels. As the hypothalamus and anterior pituitary are still intact, the levels of TSH from the pituitary rise. In the negative feedback regulation, TSH from the anterior pituitary is normally stimulated to secrete TSH in response to low T_3 and T_4 levels. The increase in TSH then results in the normalisation of T_4 levels.

A raised TSH level in the blood is therefore a sensitive indicator of primary hypothyroidism. Other laboratory findings that aid diagnosis are a low free thyroxine level (FT_4). However, in subclinical hypothyroidism, the FT_4 levels can be normal.

— Chemistry of thyroid hormones
Thyroxine is 3,5,3′,5′-tetraiodothyronine and contains four iodine atoms, which is why the hormone is also referred to as T_4. Triiodothyronine (T_3) is 3,5,3′-triiodothyronine. The T_4 molecule is an amino acid, and contains a single chiral centre indicated in the structure in the diagram with an asterisk (*). T_4 produced by the thyroid gland and the synthetic drug levothyroxine are identical. Each is produced as only the single stereoisomer shown below.

levothyroxine

There are several ways to describe stereoisomers. We can describe the three-dimensional arrangement of the groups bonded to the chiral centre – its *configuration*. Levothyroxine has S absolute configuration. We usually use *relative* configuration to describe amino acids, so we can also describe levothyroxine as having L-configuration (all of the amino acids found in proteins in the body have L relative configuration). In the thyroid gland, T_4 is produced from the simple amino acid tyrosine. As the body only uses amino acids of L-configuration, we expect thyroxine to also have an L-configuration. (Note: the thyroid also synthesises 'reverse T3' [3,3′,5′-T_3] which is inactive.)

We can also describe how stereoisomers interact with polarised light. Stereoisomers that rotate polarised light in a clockwise direction are called dextrorotatory and those that rotate polarised light in an anticlockwise direction are called levorotatory. This property of the molecule has, however, *nothing* to do with configuration (which describes structure). T_4 produced in the thyroid gland is levorotatory and so can also be called levothyroxine.

Levothyroxine, after intracellular transport and deiodination to T_3, binds to specific intracellular nuclear receptors present on specific sequences of the DNA of target tissue cells to alter gene expression (up- or downregulation), and therefore mRNA/protein synthesis directly (compare intracellular cytosolic/nuclear receptors for steroid hormones). As these nuclear receptors are DNA-binding proteins, they have very specific three-dimensional shapes. Only molecules with a matching (or *complementary*) shape are able to fit into the binding site, similar to a key fitting into a lock. The mirror image of levothyroxine has a very different three-dimensional shape (configuration) and so will not fit in to the binding site and will not be active, in the same way that your left foot does not fit into your right shoe.

— Treatment of hypothyroidism

Hypothyroidism is easily treated with replacement therapy, *but this needs to be taken for life.* The main goal of treatment is to achieve and maintain a *euthyroid* state such that clinical signs and symptoms of hypothyroidism are reversed. The preferred treatment option is synthetic T_4, levothyroxine; it has a long half-life and can be given once a day. Synthetic T_4, just like the natural hormone, is converted to active T_3 in target tissues. The usual starting dose is 1.6 micrograms/kg per day. However, older patients or those with a history of cardiac disease should be initiated on low doses, which are then titrated according to tolerance and response to treatment. Hypothyroidism can mask pre-existing cardiac disease, and excessive levothyroxine can lead to tachycardia and increased risk of cardiac mortality.

Monitoring of TSH and FT_4 levels are required to assess efficacy and/or toxicity. This is usually done 6–8 weeks after starting therapy, and doses adjusted where necessary. Once stable, annual TSH measurement is acceptable.

T_3 is approximately four times more potent than T_4, is less bound to plasma protein but has a shorter half-life. The synthetic preparation of T_3, liothyronine, is mainly used in hypothyroid emergencies where a rapid effect is desired. It can also be preferred in patients who have impaired conversion of T_4 to T_3. Due to its short half-life, liothyronine has to be given in multiple daily doses. It is more expensive than levothyroxine.

Desiccated thyroid preparations are claimed to be closer to the physiological production of thyroid hormones. However, they do not contain the same ratio $T_4 : T_3$ as secreted by the human thyroid and are unlicensed. They are not recommended for use in the UK because of the variation in manufacturing processes and therefore potency.

— Dissolution testing

The MHRA (Medicines and Healthcare products Regulatory Agency) has reported that levothyroxine tablets are difficult to manufacture and may be prone to instability once formulated. To ensure that different levothyroxine products may be used interchangeably, it is important that they exhibit equivalent dissolution behaviour demonstrated using a suitable and discriminative test method. Dissolution of a drug from a solid dosage form is often the rate-limiting step in drug absorption, when the drug has limited aqueous solubility. Drug dissolution can be correlated to oral bioavailability and dissolution testing is a key quality control test for solid dosage forms, such as tablets. The aim of dissolution testing is to measure the rate at which drug is released from the dosage form and dissolves in a particular dissolution medium. The test conditions are based on the properties of the drug, type of product and the reason for testing, i.e. to ensure compliance with product specifications (e.g. as specified in a pharmacopoeia), to evaluate the effect of formulation (e.g. a change of excipient) and process variables (e.g. compaction force) or to provide an indication of *in vivo* performance. Dissolution tests are usually performed under sink conditions and use simple buffer solutions, including a surfactant if appropriate, though more biologically relevant dissolution media are available. International pharmacopoeias include four types of dissolution apparatus, namely: basket apparatus, paddle apparatus, reciprocating cylinder and the flow-through cell. The former two methods are most frequently used for immediate-release tablets, such as levothyroxine, while the latter two methods are more frequently employed to determine the dissolution behaviour of modified-release preparations.

— Counselling points

Once a patient is on thyroid replacement therapy, he or she will probably be taking the medication

▼ TABLE 6.4
Normal blood levels of thyroid hormones

Test	Reference range[a]
TSH (mU/L)	0.4–4.5
Free T$_4$ (pmol/L)	9.0–25
Total T$_4$ (nmol/L)	60–160
Free T$_3$ (nmol/L)	3.5–7.8
Total T$_3$ (nmol/L)	1.2–2.6

[a]Reference values may vary across laboratories.

for life. Levothyroxine is available in strengths of 25, 50 and 100 micrograms (in the UK).

The prescribed dose is best taken on an empty stomach. Patients are advised not to eat for at least 30 min to an hour, and not to take iron supplements or antacids within 2–4 hours of the medication because these affect absorption. Calcium can also interfere with the absorption, so, if the patient is taking calcium supplements, he or she should take them at least 2–4 hours after the levothyroxine. (Remember that some fruit juices are calcium-fortified.)

Some other drugs that interfere with the metabolism of levothyroxine include rifampicin, carbamazepine and phenytoin (increase metabolism thereby increasing requirements). Oral contraceptives may also increase thyroxine requirements. An increase in dosage requirements of insulin or other anti-diabetic therapy may also occur with thyroid replacement therapy. (See www.bnf.org and manufacturers' product information on www.medicines.org.uk for further information.)

The normal blood levels of thyroid hormones are shown in Table 6.4.

— **Paying for thyroid treatment**
In England, there are charges associated with receiving prescription medicines. However, there are also a number of people and conditions that are exempt from prescription charges. If patients require thyroid hormone replacement, they are entitled to a Medical Exemption Certificate, allowing for free NHS prescriptions. The patient does not have to pay for any of their prescription medicines, whether or not related to the hypothyroidism.

In other countries around the world, the ways in which healthcare is structured and financed varies, and therefore charges associated with prescription medicines, vary. Health systems can be funded in different ways, e.g. by general taxation, social health insurance, voluntary or private health insurance, direct payment or donations to charities. Variations in health systems can lead to disparities in universal health coverage. Finance systems can influence the types of health services (promotion, prevention, treatment and rehabilitation) used by local populations. Direct payment systems, which require people to pay for health services at the time that they receive them, can be a barrier to people using health services. Prepayment systems, by which the resulting funds may be pooled, can increase access to services and spread the financial risks of ill health across the population. However, this does not remove the need for countries having to make hard choices about how best to use these limited funds.

EXTENDED LEARNING

- What are the autoantibodies normally found in the blood of patients with Hashimoto's thyroiditis directed against? How do they differ from the antibodies found in patients with Graves' disease (*hyper*thyroidism)?

- What are the risks of untreated maternal hypothyroidism during and after pregnancy? Is thyroid hormone replacement therapy safe to take while pregnant? Would any adjustment of dosage be necessary, and why?

- How does hypothyroidism affect fertility?

- What are the usual methods used in dissolution testing of pharmaceuticals?

- Differentiate between disintegration testing and dissolution testing of tablets

ADDITIONAL PRACTICE POINTS

- What information does the Drug Tariff present in order to assist in your practice as a pharmacist in England and Wales?

- Who is entitled to free prescriptions in England?

- For which conditions may people apply for Medical Exemption Certificates?

- What are the advantages and disadvantages of the different methods of funding health systems around the world?

References and further reading

Constanti A, Bartke A, Khardori R (1998). *Basic Endocrinology: For students of pharmacy and allied health sciences.* Amsterdam: Harwood Academic Publishers.

Freire AC, Basit AW (2013). Dissolution testing of solid dosage forms. In: Aulton ME, Taylor KMG (eds), *Aulton's Pharmaceutics: The design and manufacture of medicines,* 4th edn. London: Elsevier, 611–22.

Koda-Kimble MA, Young LY, Alldredge BA et al. (2009). *Applied Therapeutics: The Clinical Use of Drugs,* 9th edn. Baltimore, MD: Lippincott Williams & Wilkins.

Neal JM (2001). *How the Endocrine System Works.* London: Blackwell Science.

Roberts CG, Ladenson PW (2004). Hypothyroidism. *Lancet* **363**:793–803.

Case 8
Osteoporosis in a younger woman
NUTTAN TANNA

LEARNING OUTCOMES

At the end of this case, you will be able to:

- Discuss the risk factors for osteoporosis, including the possibility of disease secondary to drug therapy
- Understand how osteoporosis may be identified and diagnosed
- Describe the treatment options available for osteoporosis, in particular the place of HRT
- Help patients with a management plan that includes prescribed bone-sparing therapy and lifestyle interventions to maintain healthy bones

Case study

Mrs AM, a 49-year-old woman with stable asthma, who is a single mother with twin teenage girls, sustains a wrist fracture and sees her GP for review of pain control after being discharged from the hospital fracture clinic. Her GP prescribes anti-inflammatory painkillers, and refers her for physiotherapy, as she has some muscle wastage in the arm that had been in plaster for 6 weeks. The patient's GP refers her to the hospital specialist unit for a DXA (dual-energy X-ray absorptiometry) bone scan and requests advice on osteoporosis management.

CASE NOTES

Medical history
- The patient's body mass index (BMI) is 19
- She went through the menopause with last normal menstrual period 3 years ago aged 46
- She is a smoker and drinks alcohol

- She sustained a wrist fracture after slipping on a broken pavement. She had been on her way to drop her 13-year-olds to school, wearing high heels and put her hand out to break the fall

❷ What is osteoporosis and how is it diagnosed?
❷ What are the most common sites for osteoporotic fragility fractures?
❷ What are the risks for osteoporosis?
❷ What further medical and drug history will you need to elicit from this patient?

A full history is taken in the specialist unit, the patient is referred for a DXA scan and the pharmacist attached to the specialist unit is asked to discuss bone-sparing therapy options with the patient, including HRT, as the patient is aged only 49 years, to help decisions with her management plan.

Current medicines being taken include painkillers, and salbutamol and beclometasone inhalers used for the management of asthma. In the past, she has had various courses of corticosteroids, prescribed when she has had asthma exacerbations. She is trying to reduce the number of cigarettes that she smokes, and has got down to five a day. She is honest and tells you that, when she is stressed, she reverts back to 20 a day. At the moment, she is without a partner and feels lonely but her two children keep her busy.

❷ What treatment modalities are available and when should they be prescribed?

HRT is licensed for menopause symptom control and some regimens have an indication for osteoporosis.

? What types of HRT are available?

? In this case, what further medical history will you need to help determine the patient's individualised HRT risk–benefit evaluation?

? How does this guidance influence the decision of prescribing bone-sparing therapy?

Case discussion

— Osteoporosis

Osteoporosis is internationally defined as a progressive, systemic, skeletal disease characterised by low bone mass and microarchitectural deterioration of bone tissue, with a consequent increase in bone fragility and susceptibility to fracture. Although fractures of the spine, hip and wrist are most typical, fractures of other bones such as the ribs, humerus and pelvis are not uncommon.

Osteoporosis is a silent condition. Bone loss or failure to attain peak bone mass is not associated with any obvious signs or symptoms. In most patients, osteoporosis will be diagnosed on presentation of a low trauma fracture. Fractures of the wrist or spine are presenting signs of osteoporosis in younger menopausal women, whereas hip fractures are more common in elderly people. Generally, the lower the bone mass, the lower the trauma necessary to incur a fracture. Bone density and its closely related factor, bone strength, change considerably throughout life. Age-related bone loss is seen in both men and women, with loss of around 1% of bone mineral density from age 40 onwards. However, up to 20% of a woman's expected lifetime bone loss can occur in the years immediately after menopause.

— Diagnosis of osteoporosis

This is based on bone mineral density (BMD) measurement, which is based on a DXA scan report. A DXA report will provide BMD values for the spine, femoral neck and total hip for the patient scanned. The BMD of the tissue studied is presented as grams per centimetre squared and interpreted using *T* and *Z* scores:

- A *T* score is the number of standard deviations that separate the patient from the mean value of a healthy young population.

- A *Z* score is the number of standard deviations that separate the patient from an age-matched healthy population.

In general, the fracture risk doubles for each standard deviation fall in BMD, and a previous fracture is associated with an increased risk of a subsequent fracture. With daily quality control and appropriately trained technologists, the DXA equipment should deliver a precision of about 1% at the spine and 2% at the hip.

— Risk factors for osteoporosis

BMD is just one component of fracture risk. Assessment of fracture risk should also take into account other proven risk factors. Although the size and shape of each bone, and of the whole skeleton, are genetically predetermined, bone density and the risks of osteoporosis are influenced by many factors.

Osteoporosis has been shown in studies to have a large genetic component. A parental history of fracture (particularly hip fracture) confers an increased risk of fracture that is independent of BMD.

Physical inactivity and a sedentary lifestyle, as well as impaired neuromuscular function (e.g. reduced muscle strength, impaired gait and balance), are risk factors for developing fragility fractures. Conversely, low body weight and weight loss are associated with greater bone loss and increased risk of fracture. Some young women, particularly those training for elite athletic competition, exercise too much, eat too little and consequently experience amenorrhoea, which makes them at risk for low bone mass and fractures.

Smoking can also lead to lower bone density and higher risk of fracture, and this risk increases with age. A high intake of alcohol confers a further significant risk of future fracture (e.g. >4 units of alcohol/day can double the risk of hip fracture). The risk of vertebral and hip fractures in men increases greatly with heavy alcohol intake, particularly with long-term intake.

Proton pump inhibiting drugs can reduce the absorption of calcium from the stomach and long-term use of these drugs can significantly increase the risk of an osteoporosis-related fracture.

After an initial low-trauma fracture from a simple fall, both older men and women have an increased equivalent risk of all types of subsequent fractures, especially in the next 5–10 years.

Middle-aged and older men and women with annual height loss >0.5 cm are at increased risk of hip and any other fracture. Falls contribute to fractures, and around 90% of hip fractures result from falls. A third of people aged >65 fall annually, with approximately 10–15% of falls in elderly people resulting in fracture, and almost 60% of those who fell the previous year will fall again.

— **Glucocorticoid-induced osteoporosis**
Prolonged therapeutic use of glucocorticoids is the most common cause of secondary osteoporosis. It is estimated that 30–50% of patients on long-term corticosteroid therapy will experience fractures, with an increased risk of hip fracture 2.6-fold in men and twofold in women. This is of particular relevance in this case, because there is the possibility of steroid-induced osteoporosis as a consequence of the patient's chronic asthma therapy. Long-term use of corticosteroids leads to an increased risk of osteoporosis. This could include long-term use of a high-dose steroid inhaler, as well as oral therapy (e.g. prednisolone), especially if longer courses are required to control asthma or other inflammatory conditions (e.g. rheumatoid arthritis).

The molecular mechanisms involved in the significant bone loss seen during prolonged high-dose corticosteroid therapy are multiple and complex but, overall, both bone resorption by bone-cell osteoclasts and bone formation by osteoblasts are known to be affected (the latter more so), and it is likely that not all these changes are fully reversed after the corticosteroid therapy is stopped. Essentially, glucocorticoids decrease the number and function of osteoblasts (thereby *suppressing* new bone formation) whereas decreasing the apoptosis (programmed cell death) of mature osteoclasts and prolonging their lifespan *enhance* bone resorption. Corticosteroids are also known to decrease the absorption of calcium from the GI tract by opposing the actions of vitamin D, and to increase the amount of calcium lost in the urine by inhibiting renal tubular calcium reabsorption — both effects contributing to the defective bone mineralisation and increase in fracture risk.

— **Treatment options for primary and secondary osteoporotic fracture prevention**
Drugs used to treat bone density loss and reduce the risk of fracture include the following: oral and injectable bisphosphonates (alendronate, etidronate, risedronate, ibandronate and zoledronate), the selective oestrogen receptor modulator (raloxifene), strontium ranelate with its dual anti-resorptive and bone-forming modes of action, and teriparatide, a parathyroid hormone anabolic treatment given by injection, and reserved for high-risk patients intolerant to more traditionally used osteoporotic treatments. Denosumab, a human monoclonal antibody that inhibits osteoclast formation, function and survival, is a newer licensed bone-sparing therapy also reserved for high-risk patients and given as 6-monthly subcutaneous injections.

It is also important that all patients are calcium and vitamin D replete and, if there is a nutritional deficiency, that supplements are prescribed, before bone-sparing therapy is initiated. Compliance and persistence rates for bone-sparing therapy are poor, especially for the bisphosphonate drugs, where these range between 30% and 80%. These drugs are very sensitive and patients need to adhere to a strict routine for good bisphosphonate taking to ensure treatment efficacy.

— **Hormone replacement therapy and osteoporosis**
HRT is also being considered for this patient. Most women use HRT for the relief of menopausal symptoms that can affect quality of life and wellbeing. In these instances, HRT tends to be used for relatively short durations in the perimenopausal and early postmenopausal period. HRT is generally prescribed for women at an age when fracture risk is low.

At one time, HRT was widely used to prevent osteoporosis. However, findings reported, from 2002 onwards, on the potential *long-term* health risks of HRT have meant that it is now less commonly used for this purpose. This is because of the small increased risk of breast cancer and cardiovascular disease (venous thromboembolism and stroke) if HRT is taken on a long-term basis. HRT comprises medication that includes two components: an oestrogen and a progestogen. These combinations may be administered as tablets or transdermal patches, which deliver a constant, controlled dose of drugs that have systemic activity over a prolonged period of time. Combined products are prescribed unless the patient has undergone a hysterectomy, in which case an 'unopposed' oestrogen product is indicated. Progestogens are taken to reduce the risk of developing endometrial carcinoma in women with an intact uterus.

Direct effects of circulating oestrogens on osteoclast and osteoblast cells in premenopausal women lead to inhibition of bone remodelling, or a decrease in bone resorption and maintained bone formation, respectively, through a variety of mechanisms, thereby protecting the skeleton from bone loss and osteoporosis. The oestrogenic component of HRT is well known to be effective in preserving bone density and preventing osteoporosis in the spine and hip, as well as reducing the risk of osteoporosis-related fractures. The progestogenic component of combined HRT is not, however, believed to offer any significant protective action of its own or to subtract from the effectiveness of the oestrogens on the bones.

Although not considered a treatment option for older women with osteoporosis, HRT is viewed as having a role in the management of osteoporosis in women aged <60 years. For peri- and postmenopausal women aged <60 who do not have risk factors for breast cancer, stroke and venous thromboembolism, the risks associated with HRT are low, and when prescribed for these women, it is considered to have an overall favourable risk–benefit ratio. Thus, HRT can be considered a potential treatment option.

Effective prevention and management of osteoporosis, low bone density and fractures should be a priority for health services. A high-risk case-screening approach is used in some areas, but patients are often identified opportunistically or after a fracture. The health and social care costs of fractures in older people is high. Fractures also impact on the quality of life of individuals affected. Resultant poor mobility can lead to greater frailty and susceptibility to falls. Falls have also been linked with higher morbidity and mortality rates.

EXTENDED LEARNING

- Outline the various designs of transdermal drug delivery patches. What factors limit the sorts of drugs that can be administered by these systems?

References and further reading

Canalis E, Mazziotti G, Giustina A, Bilezikian JP (2007). Glucocorticoid-induced osteoporosis: pathophysiology and therapy. *Osteoporos Int* 18:1319–28.

Endocrine Society, The (2010). Postmenopausal hormone therapy: An Endocrine Society scientific statement. *J Clin Endocrinol Metab* 95(Suppl 1):S1–66.

Fancis R, Aspray T, Fraser W et al. (2013). *Vitamin D and Bone Health: A practical clinical guideline for patient management*. London: National Osteoporosis Society, 2013.

Khosla S, Oursler MJ, Monroe DG (2012). Estrogen and the skeleton. *Trends Endocrinol Metab* 23:576–81.

National Institute for Health and Clinical Excellence (2008). *Alendronate, Etidronate, Risedronate, Raloxifene, and Strontium Ranelate for the Primary Prevention of Osteoporotic Fragility Fractures in Postmenopausal Women*. NICE Health Technology Appraisal 160. London: NICE. Available at: www.nice.org.uk/Guidance/TA160 (accessed 7 August 2009).

National Institute for Health and Clinical Excellence (2008). *Alendronate, Etidronate, Risedronate, Raloxifene, Strontium Ranelate and Teriparatide for the Secondary Prevention of Osteoporotic Fragility Fractures in Postmenopausal Women*. NICE Health Technology Appraisal 161. London: NICE. Available at: www.nice.org.uk/Guidance/TA161 (accessed 7 August 2009).

National Institute for Health and Clinical Excellence (2010). *Denosumab for the Prevention of Osteoporotic Fractures in Postmenopausal Women*. NICE Health Technology Appraisal 204. London: NICE. Available at: http://guidance.nice.org.uk/TA204/Guidance/pdf/English [accessed 13 August, 2013).

Tanna N (2009). Osteoporosis and fragility fractures: identifying those at risk and raising public awareness. *Nursing Times* 105:28–31. Available at: www.nursingtimes.net/nursing-practice-clinical-research/primary-care/osteoporosis-and-fragility-fractures-identifying-those-at-risk-and-raising-public-awareness/5006668.article (accessed 1 July 2014).

Tang BM, Eslick GD, Nowson C, Smith C, Bensoussan A (2007). Use of calcium or calcium in combination with vitamin D supplementation to prevent fractures and bone loss in people aged 50 yrs and older: meta analysis. *Lancet* 370:657–66.

World Health Organization (2013). *FRAX® WHO Fracture Risk Assessment Tool*. WHO Collaborating Centre for Metabolic Bone Diseases, University of Sheffield, UK. Available at: www.shef.ac.uk/FRAX (accessed 27 June 2013).

Case 9
Osteoporosis in an elderly woman

LELLY OBOH

LEARNING OUTCOMES

At the end of this case, you will be able to:

- Outline the pathophysiology, signs and symptoms of osteoporosis

- Describe the role of osteoporosis, falls and other clinical risk factors in the pathogenesis of fragility fractures*

- Describe the therapeutic options for the treatment of osteoporosis and prevention of fractures in postmenopausal women

- Outline the chemistry, absorption and administration of bisphosphonates

- Outline the adverse effects and practical problems associated with bisphosphonate therapy in older people, and their solutions

*Fragility fractures are fractures that result from low-level trauma, which means mechanical forces that would not ordinarily cause fracture

Case study

Mrs ED is an 83-year-old white woman who lives alone and is housebound. She weighs 43 kg, has bilateral cataracts, chronic renal failure (CRF), and a history of depression with increasing confusion, aggression and agitation. She has ill-fitting dentures and can swallow only small tablets or liquids.

Her daughter, who is her carer, visits the pharmacy regularly and rings to inform you that Mrs ED has been admitted to hospital after a fall. Although Mrs ED did not sustain a fracture on this occasion, her daughter is quite concerned that, next time, she may not be so lucky.

Her repeat prescription is as follows:

Lansoprazole gastro tablets 30 mg o.d.
Citalopram tablets 20 mg o.m.
Lisinopril tablets 2.5 mg o.d.
Quetiapine tablets 50 mg o.m. 25 mg o.n.
Diazepam sugar free solution 5–10 mL b.d. p.r.n. (for agitation)
Ferrous sulphate tablets 200 mg t.d.s.
Aspirin-dispersible tablets 75 mg o.d.
Lactulose solution 10 mL b.d.
Fortisip 200 mL

❔ What is osteoporosis?

❔ What are the signs and symptoms of osteoporosis and how is it diagnosed?

❔ How does it increase the risk of fragility fractures?

❔ In this case, what other factors predisposed Mrs ED to having a fracture?

❔ What therapeutic interventions are available to treat osteoporosis in postmenopausal women?

Three days later the daughter presents a new prescription for:

Alendronate tablets 70 mg once weekly
Calcium and vitamin D 500 mg/400 units tablets one b.d.

❔ How do these drugs work to reduce the risk of fragility fractures?

❔ Draw the structure of alendronate sodium and relate its physicochemical properties to its clinical use, precautions and adverse effects

❔ In this case, what are the adverse drug effects and the practical problems associated with the use of these drugs?

❔ What recommendations and practical advice would you give Mrs ED's daughter to help reduce these problems?

❔ What lifestyle changes would you advise Mrs ED to make at this time?

Three months later, quetiapine and diazepam have been discontinued and Mrs ED's behaviour has improved. However, the swallowing difficulty is worse so she has been unable to take the alendronate and calcium and vitamin D tablets in the last 2 weeks. The daughter says that her auntie is taking an injection for osteoporosis which she wants the GP to prescribe and wants your advice.

❔ What other therapeutic options including parenteral preparations are available to treat osteoporosis in postmenopausal women, and when is it appropriate to prescribe each one?

Case discussion

— **Pathophysiology, signs and symptoms of osteoporosis**

Osteoporosis is a degenerative disease characterised by low bone mass and microarchitectural deterioration of bone tissue, which leads to increased bone fragility and susceptibility to fracture. Fractures are the main consequence of osteoporosis and they usually occur in the hip, spine or wrist. The WHO defines osteoporosis as having a T score ≤ 2.5 standard deviations (SDs) on DXA. However, a diagnosis may be assumed in women aged ≥ 75 years or older without the need for DXA confirmation (T score relates to the measurement of bone mineral density [BMD] using central [hip and/or spine] DXA scanning, and is expressed as the number of SDs from peak BMD).

Peak bone mass is achieved around the age of the mid-20s, followed by gradual bone loss and a more rapid loss around the menopause in women. Black people usually reach higher values of peak bone mass, which makes them less susceptible to osteoporosis compared with white people. This age-related bone loss is due to increased osteoclast (destroying bone) and decreased osteoblast (creating bone) cell activity, which leads to increased loss and resorption of old bone that surpasses the formation of new bone. The resulting reduction in bone mass makes the bone brittle and easily broken. Also, bone mass is positively related to oestrogen levels and the reduced oestrogen level associated with menopause makes postmenopausal women more susceptible to the disease.

Calcium is needed for bone formation, and reduced calcium intake or excessive loss from the kidneys will have a negative effect on bone mass. Consequently, vitamin D which supports calcium absorption has a positive effect on bone mass. Housebound elderly individuals and those in institutionalised care settings are at higher risk of calcium and vitamin D deficiency.

Osteoporosis is usually asymptomatic until a bone fracture occurs or symptoms become noticeable. Signs and symptoms include clinically evident fractures, height loss, spinal deformity and back pain. Generally, by the time a diagnosis is made, the condition has reached an advanced stage where even the slightest trauma can cause fractures.

— **Osteoporosis, falls and other risk factors that play a role in the pathogenesis of fractures**
Apart from increasing age and low BMD, other clinical risk factors are associated with increased fractures. Some of these factors are partly independent of BMD and include parental history of hip fracture, ≥ 4 units alcohol intake per day,

previous fracture, use of long-term corticosteroids and rheumatoid arthritis. Other risk factors relate to low BMD and include BMI <22 kg/m^2, medical conditions such as ankylosing spondylitis, Crohn's disease, conditions that result in prolonged immobility and untreated premature menopause.

Falling is a high predictor of fracture risk and most fractures in older people result from a fall from standing height. The risk of falling is higher in older people and a previous fall predisposes to further falls. Therefore, the factors associated with falling, such as poor lighting, uneven surfaces, poor eyesight, muscle weakness, postural instability, poor coordination, polypharmacy and the use of drugs, including opiates, sedatives and antipsychotics, must be addressed to prevent fractures.

— **Treatment of osteoporosis and the prevention of fragility fractures in postmenopausal women**
Treatment of osteoporosis aims to preserve bone mass and prevent fractures: this involves modification of risk factors, calcium and vitamin D supplementation, and use of drugs that improve bone health.

The decision to start drug therapy depends on whether there has been a fracture (secondary prevention) or not (primary prevention), the patient's age, BMD (confirmed by DXA, but not compulsory in over-75s if the clinician considers a DXA scan to be inappropriate or unfeasible), as well as the number of clinical risk factors and indicators of low BMD present. Primary prevention is about identifying those at a high risk of sustaining fractures before it occurs. The FRAX tool is an example of an algorithm developed by the WHO that utilises age, BMD and clinical risk factors to predict the 10-year risk of a fracture.

— **Bisphosphonates**
Once the decision has been made to treat, NICE recommends bisphosphonates as the choice of treatment for primary prevention of fragility fractures in postmenopausal women. Alendronate is the first choice, but etidronate and risedronate can be used if patients unable to comply with the special instructions for the administration of alendronate have a contraindication to, or cannot tolerate, alendronate.

Once bound to the bone matrix (hydroxyapatite sites), bisphosphonates, being similar in structure to pyrophosphate (a product of bone cell metabolism) are taken up by osteoclasts and prevent bone resorption, by inhibiting the activation of the pyrophosphate-using enzyme, farnesyl pyrophosphate synthase (FPP), which ultimately controls osteoclast activity and bone turnover. Depending on the individual drug used, they can reduce hip, vertebral and non-vertebral fractures. However, bisphosphonates can take 6–12 months to have an effect and will often be continued for a number of years.

GI adverse effects, such as abdominal pain, dyspepsia, diarrhoea and constipation, are common. If patients develop symptoms of oesophageal irritation, such as dysphagia, pain on swallowing or retrosternal pain, or new or worsening heartburn, they should stop taking the drug immediately and seek medical attention. Severe oesophageal reactions with oral preparations sometimes occur, and osteonecrosis of the jaw is rare, but can be checked for by the dentist. Good oral hygiene should be maintained and patients requiring dental procedures should inform their dentist about taking bisphosphonates. Atypical femoral (thigh) fractures and renal toxicity (IV formulations) are rare, but important, adverse effects associated with bisphosphonates that patients should look out for.

— Chemistry, properties, administration and absorption of alendronate

The structure of alendronate sodium is shown in the diagram.

alendronate sodium

Phosphonic acids have the structure R-PO$_3$H$_2$ and the negatively charged anions derived from them are called phosphonates. The presence of two phosphonic acid groups in alendronate sodium and similar drugs gives rise to the name 'bisphosphonates'. Each phosphonic acid group has two acidic protons and alendronate is highly negatively charged at physiological pH. Alendronate is a so-called nitrogen-containing, second-generation bisphosphonate.

After oral administration, absorption of alendronate from the GI tract is poor. Both phosphonate groups are negatively charged in the small intestine, contributing to the very high polarity of the drug. Consequently, its ability to diffuse across the GI tract epithelium is very limited. Absorption is further diminished in the presence of food, and alendronate must be administered on an empty stomach. Calcium preparations (including antacids) can reduce the absorption of alendronate (most likely through a combination of pH effects and complex formation with metal ions).

Bisphosphonates are excreted by the kidneys, so caution should be exercised in older people with already compromised renal function. The rapid clearance of alendronate by the kidneys is also a consequence of the drug's high polarity (and high water solubility).

Bisphosphonates are available as oral, intramuscular and i.v. preparations. Oral preparations have complex dosing and administration instructions to ensure effective drug delivery and prevent severe oesophageal reactions. Bisphosphonates are typically highly irritant and can cause direct damage of the oesophageal mucosa. They must be taken whole on an empty stomach with a full glass of water and the patient must remain upright for ≥30 min after taking the oral preparation. NICE advises that bisphosphonates should not be prescribed if patients cannot adhere to these instructions. It is important that patients are able to recognise and differentiate between their tablets in order to follow the instructions.

Adherence and persistence are poor with bisphosphonates, particularly within 3 months of initiation. Weekly, monthly, 3-monthly and yearly preparations (depot injections) have been developed to assist with these problems.

— Calcium and vitamin D

Vitamin D aids the absorption of calcium, which helps to strengthen the bone and prevent fractures. Oral preparations are usually available in combination with calcium as swallowable chewable, effervescent or soluble tablets, sachets or solutions. The chewable tablets (plain or flavoured) are usually large, which could be problematic in people with swallowing or chewing difficulties. Non-adherence is common and the patient's preference is an important consideration when choosing treatment options.

Drug treatment options for osteoporosis

Drug	Action	Comments
Strontium ranelate	↓ bone resorption and ↑ bone formation	Increased risk of venous thromboembolism
Raloxifene	Oestrogen agonist	
HRT	Oestrogen effect on bone	Increased risk of venous thromboembolism and breast cancer. Unlicensed use for <50s when others not tolerated
Calcitriol	↑ reabsorption of calcium	Hypocalcaemia
Parathyroid hormone	Stimulates bone formation	
Teriparatide	Stimulates bone formation	Last resort in severe cases and when other options have failed

— Other therapeutic options

Other drug options for treating osteoporosis are summarised in Table 6.5. However, strontium ranelate is the only drug recommended by NICE when bisphosphonates are not suitable in primary prevention. The choice of drug will depend on the safety profile and patient factors, such as co-morbidities, ability to comply with administration instructions and tolerance.

Raloxifene is an orally active selective oestrogen receptor modulator (SERM) that exerts an oestrogen-like protective action on the bone and can therefore also be used to treat osteoporosis, but only in postmenopausal women. Interestingly, it has *anti*-oestrogenic activity in breast tissue so it has been suggested as a possible treatment for certain types of oestrogen-dependent breast cancers; however it is not currently licensed for this purpose. It is contraindicated in patients with a history of thromboembolic events.

— Risk modification and lifestyle changes

Although osteoporosis is relatively common among older women, it should not be seen as a normal part of the ageing process. Many measures to reduce the risk of osteoporosis are similar to lifestyle modifications that are recommended to reduce the risks of other long-term conditions, i.e. regular exercise, healthy diet and not smoking.

Although an individual's genes will determine the potential size and strength of the skeleton, lifestyle factors can influence bone health. The following are of particular relevance to osteoporosis:

- Regular exercise, especially weight-bearing exercise, where the feet and legs support the weight of the body, such as walking, running, dancing (but not swimming and cycling)
- Maintaining the recommended daily calcium intake (700 mg daily), e.g. from milk, leafy green vegetables, yoghurt
- Vitamin D, which promotes the absorption of dietary calcium in foods including eggs, milk and oily fish. Some exposure to sunlight is important in promoting the production of vitamin D in the skin
- Not smoking: cigarette smoking is associated with increased risk of osteoporosis.

EXTENDED LEARNING

- How would corticosteroid-induced osteoporosis be treated?
- What is the role of medication review in the prevention of falls?
- How are depot injections formulated and manufactured?

ADDITIONAL PRACTICE POINT

- How would you calculate BMI?

References and further reading

McClung M, Harris ST, Miller PD et al. (2013). Bisphosphonate therapy for osteoporosis: benefits, risks, and drug holiday. *Am J Med* **126**:13–20.

National Institute for Health and Care Excellence (2013). *The Assessment and Prevention of Falls in Older People.* Clinical Guideline. London: NICE.

National Institute for Health and Clinical Excellence (2008). *Alendronate, Etidronate, Risedronate, Raloxifene, and Strontium Ranelate for the Primary Prevention of Osteoporotic Fragility Fractures in Postmenopausal Women.* NICE Health Technology Appraisal 160. London: NICE. Available at: www.nice.org.uk/Guidance/TA160 (accessed 7 August 2009).

National Institute for Health and Clinical Excellence (2008). *Alendronate, Etidronate, Risedronate, Raloxifene, Strontium Ranelate and Teriparatide for the Secondary Prevention of Osteoporotic Fragility Fractures in Postmenopausal Women.* NICE Health Technology Appraisal 161. London: NICE. Available at: www.nice.org.uk/Guidance/TA161 (accessed 7 August 2009).

Case 10
Treatment for hypercalcaemia
MEE-ONN CHAI

LEARNING OUTCOMES

At the end of this case, you will be able to:

- Outline the pathophysiology, signs, symptoms and diagnosis of hypercalcaemia
- Describe the common causes of hypercalcaemia
- Describe the treatment options in hypercalcaemia
- Outline the chemistry of bisphosphonates
- Outline the place of bisphosphonate therapy and describe the choice of bisphosphonates available
- Outline the place of hydration therapy and describe the choice of fluids available

Case study

Mrs JH is a 76-year-old African–Caribbean woman. She has a history of type 2 diabetes mellitus and has been on insulin therapy for 13 years. She has well-controlled asthma, hypertension and arthritis. She presented to A&E with a 1- to 2-week history of swollen right leg. According to her daughter, Mrs JH had recently completed a 7-day course of amoxicillin, obtained from her GP, for a

▼ TABLE 6.6

Mrs JH's blood results on day 1 of admission to A&E

Blood test	Result	Normal range
Urea (mmol/L)	12.0	3.3–6.7
Serum creatinine (μmol/L)	478	45–120
eGFR (mL/min)	8	>90
Sodium (mmol/L)	136	135–145
Potassium (mmol/L)	3.8	3.5–5.0
Calcium (mmol/L)	4.84	
Corrected calcium(mmol/L)	4.76	2.20–2.60
Albumin (g/L)	44	35–50
Phosphate (mmol/L)	1.22	0.80–1.40
Magnesium (mmol/L)	0.76	0.7–1.0

eGFR, estimated glomerular filtration rate.

urinary tract infection but no improvements were noted. She also reported a 1- to 2-week general deterioration in her mother's mobility and that her mother was constipated and experiencing slurred speech.

On examination

- No shortness of breath or haemoptysis
- Glasgow Coma Scale (GCS) score of 15 (a neurological scale used to assess the conscious state of a person; maximum score 15 = normal)
- HR: 92 beats/min
- Respiratory rate: 18/min
- Blood glucose: 7.8 mmol/L
- Temperature: 38.60°C
- No family history of renal disease or stones
- GP blood test showed previous serum creatinine in April 2011 was 120 μmol/L

Mrs JH was admitted from A&E with differential diagnoses of acute kidney failure, hypercalcaemia, probable right leg DVT (deep vein thrombosis) and altered bowel habit – with a need to rule out malignancy such as sarcoidosis or myeloma.

Table 6.6 describes Mrs JH's blood results on day 1 of admission.

OTHER RESULTS

- Arterial blood gases: normal
- ECG result: normal sinus rhythm
- D-dimer: >8000 ng/mL (normal: <500 ng/mL) (a specific screening test for suspected DVT – detects degradation fragments of fibrin blood clot in the circulation)
- Acute myeloma screen: normal

- What is hypercalcaemia?
- What are the most common causes of hypercalcaemia?
- What are the signs and symptoms of hypercalcaemia?

▼ TABLE 6.7
Relevant blood results for Mrs JH

Blood test	Result	Normal range
Hb (g/dL)	13.2	11.5–15.5
Platelets ($\times 10^9$/L)	117	150–450
ESR (mm/h)	7	1–10
TSH (mIU/L)	0.92	0.3–5.5
Free thyroxine (pmol/L)	15.4	9–25
iPTH (ng/L)	1644	10–70
Vitamin D (μg/L)	5.6	10–42
Calcitonin (ng/L)	16	<4.8
Serum ACE (IU/L)	27	8–25

ACE, angiotensin-converting enzyme; ESR, erythrocyte sedimentation rate; iPTH, intact parathyroid hormone (entire PTH molecule); TSH, thyroid-stimulating hormone.

❓ What are the adverse effects of hypercalcaemia?
❓ What drugs can cause hypercalcaemia?
❓ How is hypercalcaemia treated?

The following drugs were prescribed for Mrs JH on admission:

Heparin infusion at 1 mL/h
1 L NaCl 0.9% infusion and a stat dose of sodium pamidronate 30 mg i.v.
Other relevant blood results are given in Table 6.7.

RESULTS FROM IMAGING

- Ultrasonography results:
- Parathyroid gland: right inferior 14-mm parathyroid adenoma
- Thyroid gland: showed normal size thyroid gland, no cysts or masses detected
- Renal ultrasonography showed no hydronephrosis (kidney swelling due to back flow of urine)
- Renal artery Doppler sonography showed no evidence of renal vein thrombosis

---

All of Mrs JH's blood tests were within the normal range, except for the raised serum levels of urea, creatinine, calcium and intact PTH. These results support the diagnosis of severe hypercalcaemia secondary to primary hyperparathyroidism. Results from the ultrasound scan of the parathyroid gland provided confirmation of the diagnosis. Mrs JH also has acute kidney injury secondary to the severe

hypercalcaemia, as indicated by the elevated urea and creatinine levels.

Mrs JH was given i.v. pamidronate 30 mg 2 days later, because there was no change in her serum calcium levels after saline hydration.

On day 4, Mrs JH received urgent haemodialysis while waiting for an urgent parathyroidectomy.

Case discussion

The most effective management of hypercalcaemia is to recognise and treat the underlying disease.

— Hypercalcaemia and its pathophysiology

Calcium is an important cation in the body. Approximately 45% of it is bound to plasma protein (mainly albumin and globulins) and is therefore biologically inert. The unbound calcium (about 50%), or the free ionised calcium is the metabolically and physiologically active form responsible for cellular transport, membrane function and bone metabolism; the remainder (about 5%) is complexed with several anions, e.g. bicarbonate, citrate, phosphate and sulfate (also biologically inert). Calcium levels in the extracellular fluid fluctuate with protein-binding capacity, e.g. a patient with low serum albumin usually has low serum calcium levels. This means that the total plasma calcium levels must be corrected for the lowered albumin level. Calcium levels usually change by 0.02 mmol/L for every 1 g/L change in plasma albumin concentration below the usual mean of 40 g/L. The corrected calcium concentration is then given by:

$$Ca_{corr} = Ca_{meas} + [0.02 \times (40 - Alb)]$$

where Ca_{corr} is the corrected calcium concentration in mmol/L, Ca_{meas} is the measured calcium concentration in mmol/L and Alb is the albumin level in g/L.

See www.globalrph.com/calcium.htm

The protein binding of calcium is pH-dependent, such that acidosis decreases the amount of calcium bound to albumin, whereas alkalosis increases the bound fraction of calcium.

PTH, vitamin D and to a lesser extent calcitonin (secreted by the thyroid gland parafollicular C-cells), regulate the exchange of calcium in the extracellular fluid across the bones, gut and kidneys. Normal (total) plasma calcium levels are in the range 2.13–2.63 mmol/L and free ionised calcium is 1.15–1.28 mmol/L, with serum albumin level of 45 g/L.

— Causes of hypercalcaemia

The two most common causes of hypercalcaemia are hypercalcaemia secondary to malignancy and primary hyperparathyroidism (excess secretion of PTH). Other less frequent causes of hypercalcaemia are bone diseases, granulomatous conditions (e.g. sarcoidosis, a chronic skin disorder, where an enhanced synthesis of vitamin D_3 occurs in the skin after sun exposure), hyperthyroidism, diet (excessive calcium intake) and drugs (e.g. thiazides, lithium, vitamin D analogues, vitamin A). The incidence of primary hyperparathyroidism is $1:2000$ in older women, and about 85% of cases are due to a single benign adenoma of one of the four parathyroid glands (embedded posteriorly within the thyroid capsule), and the other 15% are a four-gland disease. A raised intact PTH level is not usually associated with severe hypercalcaemia, secondary to malignancy; the latter is believed to be due to the secretion of a PTH-related peptide (PTHrP) by the malignant tumour cells, which mimics the action of native PTH.

— Signs and symptoms of hypercalcaemia

The signs and symptoms of hypercalcaemia are usually non-specific. They are often related to the severity and the rate of change of the serum calcium level. Symptoms are more severe with acute changes than with a chronic rise in calcium level. A good history can aid in the identification of hypercalcaemia, e.g. history of renal stones. Other common signs and symptoms are complaints of tiredness, lethargy, easy fatigue, confusion, depression, irritability, constipation, polyuria and polydipsia. Chronic symptoms can relate to hyperparathyroidism, whereas a sudden onset of symptoms is more likely to suggest malignancy.

Untreated high calcium in blood serum will exceed capacity for calcium reabsorption in the kidneys, and lead to nephrolithiasis (renal stone disease) and precipitation of calcium in the kidney tubules, thereby causing damage to the kidneys.

— Drugs that can cause hypercalcaemia

Drugs such as thiazide diuretics can cause mild hypercalcaemia by reducing the renal tubular excretion of calcium, which is reversible when it is discontinued. High intake of calcium carbonate, usually from excessive intake of calcium-containing antacids, can also lead to hypercalcaemia, alkalosis and renal insufficiency.

Such excessive intake is rare, but results in an uncommon disorder termed 'milk-alkali syndrome'. Lithium carbonate (used in the treatment of bipolar disorder) can increase PTH secretion, which results in a rise in calcium levels. Vitamin D overdose is related to excessive intake of vitamin D supplements but is uncommon at doses <3000 IU/day. Large doses of vitamin A and its analogues can cause hypercalcaemia through increased bone resorption.

— Treatment of hypercalcaemia

Treatment is usually not needed for asymptomatic mild-to-moderate hypercalcaemia. However, severe hypercalcaemia is a medical emergency requiring an urgent response to prevent death. Excessive calcium is detrimental to the function of excitable membranes and leads to skeletal muscle and GI smooth muscle fatigue. Effects on cardiac muscles include shortening of the QT interval and increased risk of cardiac arrests.

Treatment of severe hypercalcaemia usually includes fluid resuscitation using 0.9% sodium chloride – at least 3–4 L/day, for up to 3 days is generally required. The aim is to achieve a urine output of at least 200 mL/h. Sodium chloride infusion is used instead of dextrose-containing infusion because the sodium salt is needed to replace the salt loss and increase renal calcium clearance. Fluid resuscitation can lower serum calcium by 0.25–0.75 mmol/L. It is crucial to tailor fluid volume and monitor central venous pressure in patients with concomitant cardiorenal failure. Administration of high fluid volumes in this patient group can exacerbate heart failure.

The volumes of fluid that can be administered intravenously range from <1 mL to several litres. Although small volumes can be administered as a bolus (i.e. all at once), larger volumes are infused at a controlled slow rate. Sodium chloride 0.9% infusion is 'isotonic' (as is 5% glucose/dextrose), which means that it has an osmolality approximating to that of blood plasma. This is necessary for a number of routes of administration to avoid damage to tissues, e.g. a large-volume infusion that is hypotonic (lower osmotic pressure than plasma) will cause swelling and bursting of red blood cells (erythrocytes), which are surrounded by a semipermeable membrane, leading to serious health consequences. Such solutions can be adjusted to isotonicity, by addition of excipients such as glucose or sodium chloride. Infusion of a hypertonic solution will result in shrinkage of the blood cells due to loss of water by osmosis. Such solutions would need to be diluted before administration.

Once intravascular volume has been restored, then a loop diuretic, such as furosemide, can be used. Usually the dose of furosemide is 10–20 mg. Loop diuretics can inhibit calcium reabsorption in the distal renal tubule. Monitoring of serum potassium is needed, because loop diuretics can cause hypokalaemia and/or dehydration if the patient is not well hydrated.

Treatment of primary hyperparathyroidism is usually by surgical removal of the overactive parathyroid tissue (parathyroidectomy), although, in some cases, the tumours may be difficult to locate. Postoperative persistence of the hyperparathyroid symptoms, or even development of permanent *hypo*parathyroidism (with consequent *hypo*calcaemia) is common. In very rare cases, parathyroid surgery may cause inadvertent damage to the recurrent laryngeal nerves. In patients with hypercalcaemia associated with malignancy, bisphosphonates are often used. Bisphosphonates reduce osteoclast bone cell activity, reducing bone turnover and hence calcium levels in plasma. Caution is needed when bisphosphonates are used in patients with hyperparathyroidism because they can cause an increase in calcium.

Oral bisphosphonates have a bioavailability range of 1–5% under ideal conditions, whereas the bioavailability of intravenous preparations is 100%. Concurrent administration with food or anything containing divalent cations inhibits their absorption and therefore intravenous administration is needed for treating severe hypercalcaemia. The onset of action of bisphosphonates is slow, such that peak action occurs 48–72 hours after administration. About 50–80% of the dose binds to bone surfaces, most avidly at sites of active remodelling. The rest of the unbounded bisphosphonate is excreted rapidly via the kidneys. Renal toxicity may occur with rapid intravenous administration of bisphosphonate and may cause further complications in a dehydrated patient.

— Properties of bisphosphonates

There are several bisphosphonates available on the market and each has a different potency of binding to bone to reduce osteoclastic bone cell resorption.

pamidronate disodium   zoledronic acid

pyrophosphate

Pamidronate disodium reduces hypercalcaemia after 4 days and has a mean duration of action of 28 days, whereas zoledronic acid is slightly more effective than pamidronate. Zoledronic acid is 100–850 times more potent than pamidronate and has the advantage of bolus administration rather than infusion.

The structures of these two bisphosphonates are shown in the diagram. They owe their mechanism of action to their ability to mimic native pyrophosphate, which is involved in normal bone turnover processes. All of the bisphosphonates are highly polar molecules with sufficient water solubility for formulation and administration as injections and infusions.

In the case of life-threatening hypercalcaemia, haemodialysis is warranted. Dialysis against a low-calcium dialysate is effective in lowering serum calcium levels.

EXTENDED LEARNING

- Describe calcimimetics as a new therapy for hyperparathyroidism
- Describe the action of bisphosphonates on the HMG-CoA (3-hydroxy-3-methylglutaryl-coenzyme A) reductase pathway
- What is osmolarity? How is the osmolarity/isotonicity of a solution for injection adjusted to render it isotonic?

References and further reading

Boovalingham P, Conroy S, Sahota O (2009) *Hypercalcaemia in Adults: A guide to diagnosis and management*. Available at: http://learning.bmj.com (accessed 1 October 2013).
Fraser WD (2009). Hyperparathyroidism. *Lancet* 374:145–58.

7

Malignant disease, immunosuppression and haematology cases

INTRODUCTION

This section contains eight cases that are based on patients with cancer, autoimmune disease or haematological disorders. Various types of cancer are discussed, including lung cancer, breast cancer, colorectal cancer and leukaemia, along with their management using chemotherapeutic drugs and the challenges that this may present. The treatment of multiple sclerosis and vaso-occlusive crises in sickle cell disease are also discussed.

Case 1
Lung cancer ▸ 274

This case concerns a patient recently diagnosed with lung cancer and initiated on systemic anticancer therapy with cisplatin and pemetrexed. The epidemiology and pathophysiology of lung cancer are outlined, along with its diagnosis and staging, and the bearing that the latter has on treatment options. The mechanisms of action of the chemotherapeutic drugs initially prescribed are described, along with the management of neutropenic sepsis – a serious adverse effect that can occur with systemic anticancer therapy. The use of erlotinib is also briefly outlined, together with its common associated adverse drug reactions, and alternative means of oral administration in patients who have difficulty swallowing tablets. Finally, the role of the pharmacist in the early detection of lung cancer is introduced.

Case 2
The use of antimetabolites in the treatment of breast cancer ▸ 278

This presents a case in which adjuvant chemotherapy with cyclophosphamide, methotrexate and 5FU is initiated in a patient with breast cancer after a partial mastectomy. This regimen is more suitable than a conventional anthracycline-containing regimen in the case discussed, due to the patient's history of cardiac impairment. Antimetabolites in general are introduced, before considering the mechanisms of action of methotrexate and 5FU in detail. A short summary of the grading system for chemotherapy adverse drug reactions developed by the National Cancer Institute is presented, followed by discussion of the roles of folic acid and folinic acid in the prevention and counteraction of methotrexate toxicity. In addition, this case considers the facilities and precautions required when handling cytotoxic drugs in the hospital pharmacy environment.

Case 3
Clinical verification of prescriptions for oral anticancer medicines ▸ 282

This case considers a patient with metastatic colorectal cancer receiving oral capecitabine, the chemistry and mechanism of action of which are discussed in detail. The case goes on to consider the use of oral anticancer medicines and their sites of action within the cell cycle, as well as the differences between traditional and targeted oral therapies. The safety concerns for oral anticancer medicines are then identified, along with the specific steps that pharmacists must undertake to verify clinically prescriptions for these agents.

Case 4
Thromboprophylaxis in a patient undergoing surgery for cancer ▶ 287

This case is centred on a patient about to undergo surgical intervention to remove a recently diagnosed adenocarcinoma of the colon. Cancer patients are at increased risk of venous thromboembolism, and the reasons for this, along with signs and symptoms of DVT and PE, are discussed. The different classes of drugs used for thromboprophylaxis (including low-molecular-weight heparins, dabigatran, rivaroxaban and fondaparinux) are identified and their suitability or otherwise for use together with cancer surgery is considered. The relationship between the physicochemical properties of heparins and their clinical use is also summarised.

Case 5
Febrile neutropenia in paediatric oncology ▶ 291

This case begins by outlining the pathophysiology and diagnosis of childhood leukaemia. It concerns a 5-year-old child with acute lymphoblastic leukaemia (ALL) who presents with pyrexia and a low neutrophil count, leading to a diagnosis of febrile neutropenia. The criteria for making such a diagnosis are presented, along with a consideration of the choice of initial antibiotic therapy. In addition to a general discussion of ALL chemotherapy, the mechanisms of action of the cytotoxic drugs specific to this case (methotrexate and mercaptopurine) are explained. The classes of antibiotics most commonly prescribed in febrile neutropenia are also identified and further considerations relating to ALL treatment, such as the use of analgesics and administration of chemotherapeutic drugs via a port, are briefly introduced. Freeze drying is often employed in the preparation of antibiotics for reconstitution before injection and the details of the freeze-drying process are presented. Finally, the design and features of clinical trials are summarised.

Case 6
Managing chemotherapy-induced nausea and vomiting in a patient with lung cancer ▶ 295

This case concerns a patient diagnosed with non-small cell lung cancer experiencing severe nausea and vomiting after her first cycle of chemotherapy. The emetogenic potential of chemotherapeutic drugs is discussed, along with the classification, mechanism and risk factors for chemotherapy-induced nausea and vomiting (CINV). The different antiemetic agents used in the management of CINV are examined, including metoclopramide, dexamethasone, aprepitant and the $5HT_3$ antagonists ondansetron and palonosetron. The chemical structures and properties of the last two agents are explored in detail. Genetic differences between patients can affect their ability to metabolise and inactivate ondansetron, so the scope for personalised medicine is also discussed.

Case 7
Drug therapy of multiple sclerosis ▶ 299

This case focuses on a patient newly diagnosed with multiple sclerosis (MS). The typical signs and symptoms associated with MS are outlined, along with the principal means by which a diagnosis is confirmed. The use of the Expanded Disability Status Scale to measure the severity of functional disability in MS is described, followed by a detailed discussion of the immediate and longer-term therapeutic options for MS patients. Drug therapies detailed include oral and intravenous methylprednisolone for acute episodes, interferon-β products, glatiramer acetate and natalizumab. The commonly encountered adverse effects associated with these treatments, particularly the risk of depressive illness with interferon-β, are also discussed.

Case 8
Management of vaso-occlusive crisis in sickle cell disease ▶ 304

This case presents a patient with sickle cell disease (SCD) who has been admitted to hospital with a severe vaso-occlusive crisis. The pathophysiology of SCD is described, along with the symptoms of a vaso-occlusive crisis and the common clinical complications associated with the disease. Vaso-occlusive crises are associated with significant pain. The measurement of pain and the use of analgesic strategies to manage pain are detailed. The structures, chemical properties and pharmacological mechanism of action of several opioid analgesics are discussed, along with the value of patient-controlled analgesia in the management of sickle cell crises. Additional approaches to manage vaso-occlusive crises are further outlined, including incentive spirometry and prevention using hydroxycarbamide therapy.

Case 1

Lung cancer

FIONA MACLEAN

LEARNING OUTCOMES

At the end of this case, you will be able to:

- Briefly describe the epidemiology of lung cancer in the UK and understand its impact on UK healthcare
- Outline the risk factors for lung cancer
- Understand the staging of lung cancer and its relevance to treatment options and decisions
- Describe how community pharmacy can support early diagnosis of lung cancer and contribute to UK public health initiatives

Case study

Mr JM is a 62-year-old white man, ex-smoker of 10 years. He presented to his GP with haemoptysis (coughing of blood) and right shoulder pain. On further questioning, he reported a persistent cough and some weight loss. He was referred for an urgent chest radiograph, which showed a 4-cm rounded opacity in the right lung upper zone. A CT scan followed which confirmed a 3.6 × 4 cm lesion in the right upper lobe, with multiple variable-sized nodules in both lungs. Bronchoscopy and biopsy confirmed a stage IV adenocarcinoma. Mr JM consented to combination systemic anticancer therapy (SACT) with cisplatin and pemetrexed. Four cycles were planned, given every 21 days.

- What is the incidence of lung cancer in the UK? What are the typical signs and symptoms of lung cancer?
- How is a diagnosis of lung cancer confirmed and how is the cancer staged?
- Draw the structures of cisplatin and pemetrexed and describe their modes of action
- What are the significant toxicities expected from SACT? Outline the counselling points you would discuss with this patient

Mr JM began to feel unwell and had a temperature of 38.9°C 7 days after his second cycle of SACT. He attended the accident and emergency department (A&E) as instructed and was found to be neutropenic (abnormally low neutrophil count: 0.5

× 10⁹/L; normal 2.5–7.5 × 10⁹/L). He was admitted to hospital for treatment with intravenous antibiotics and discharged 5 days later. He completed a course of antibiotics and received his final two cycles of chemotherapy as planned.

- What is neutropenic sepsis and how is it managed?

When Mr JM attended the cancer follow-up clinic 6 months later he complained of back pain, difficulty swallowing and increasing shortness of breath. A CT scan showed a new mass in the left lung and a mass in the neck, and MRI confirmed bone metastases. Mr JM was offered second-line treatment with erlotinib.

- What is the therapeutic goal of second-line SACT?
- Draw the structure of erlotinib and outline its mode of action
- What counselling points would you discuss with the patient?
- What are the challenges of oral SACT compared with parenteral SACT?

Mr JM presents to his community pharmacist after 10 days of erlotinib therapy. He has a widespread, itchy, acne-like rash. Some pustules look infected and he is having difficulty swallowing the erlotinib tablets. He wants to stop taking the erlotinib and asks you for advice.

- What adverse effects is he experiencing?
- What recommendations would you make for rash management?
- What advice would you offer with regard to crushing the tablets?

Case discussion

— Lung cancer: epidemiology and pathophysiology

Lung cancer is the second most common cancer in the UK. Each year in the UK there are >39 000 new cases of lung cancer and >35 000 people die from it. In women, lung cancer is the leading cause of cancer death. The mean age at presentation is 70 years and about 90% of lung cancers are caused by smoking. Other causative agents include ionising radiation, asbestos and air pollution.

The male:female death rate ratio has changed in line with a change in smoking patterns. Fewer men smoke and this has been reflected in a reduction in male lung cancer deaths. Conversely, the number of female smokers has increased, resulting in an increase in female deaths from lung cancer. The 5-year survival rate is poor and only about 5.5% of lung cancers are currently cured. Early detection is vital because advanced disease is inoperable and hence incurable. Lung cancer is diagnosed by PET/CT, bronchoscopy and biopsy. PET (positron emission tomography) is a technique that uses a positron-emitting tracer (commonly ^{18}F-FDG [^{18}F-labelled fluorodeoxyglucose]) to produce a three-dimensional image with the aid of a CT scan, which is performed at the same time.

— Symptoms, signs and diagnosis of lung cancer

Presenting symptoms depend on the size and location of the primary tumour. Patients with lung cancer might experience symptoms of shortness of breath, persistent cough or a change in cough, weight loss, finger clubbing, weakness, fatigue, haemoptysis or pain. Lung cancer most commonly metastasises to the brain, liver, adrenal glands and bones. A patient who has brain metastases might complain of headache, being unsteady or falls.

Diagnosis of lung cancer will include all or most of the following: clinical examination, chest radiograph, CT (with or without biopsy), bronchoscopy, biopsy and CT/PET. Lung function tests will be carried out if the tumour is operable and an MR or bone scan may be requested to confirm the presence or absence of bone metastases. Generally, haematology and biochemistry tests are all within reference ranges.

— Staging and treatment

There are two major subdivisions of lung cancer: small cell lung cancer (SCLC), which accounts for about 20% of cases, and non-small cell lung cancer (NSCLC), which accounts for the remaining 80% of cases.

Lung cancer is staged using the TNM classification system. T refers to tumour size, N to the presence or absence or lymph node metastases and M to the presence or absence of distant metastases. In its early stages (stages I, II and IIIa), the primary treatment of NSCLC is surgery. Most patients, however, present with advanced disease that is stage IIIb or IV. Stages IIIb and IV are incurable and are treated with palliative intent using SACT with or without adjuvant radiotherapy.

The primary treatment of SCLC is SACT with or without radiotherapy. There is increasing importance placed on histology of NSCLC because the cell type (adenocarcinoma, squamous cell carcinoma or large cell carcinoma), molecular markers and presence of activating mutations may determine the choice of drug therapy.

— Systemic anticancer therapy (SACT)

The choice of drugs is guided by current evidence-based protocols, which are based on the type of lung cancer, histology, patient background including patient performance status (a measure of how well a person is able to undertake ordinary daily activities while living with cancer), organ function and, to a certain degree, patient choice. In stage IV disease all treatments are palliative, the goals of therapy aimed at symptom control and improving quality of life.

— Structure and mode of action of pemetrexed and cisplatin

Mr JM has an adenocarcinoma and the recommended first-line SACT is cisplatin and pemetrexed. Pemetrexed is a folate antimetabolite that is structurally related to methotrexate. In addition to its inhibition of dihydrofolate reductase (DHFR), it also acts as an inhibitor of thymidylate synthase and glycinamide ribonucleotide formyltransferase (GARFT) – two enzymes also involved in purine and pyrimidine biosynthesis. These multiple mechanisms of action interfere with the ability of cells to synthesise RNA and

pemetrexed

cisplatin

DNA. Cisplatin contains an electron-deficient platinum atom that can bond separately to two electron-rich DNA bases, resulting in (mainly) intrastrand cross-linking and eventual cell death. The most common toxicities from this combination are myelosuppression, nausea and vomiting, neurotoxicity and renal toxicity. Early clinical trials with the antifolate pemetrexed identified a correlation between poor folate status and increased pemetrexed toxicity. This led to the requirement for folic acid and vitamin B_{12} supplementation during pemetrexed therapy to reduce the risk of bone marrow suppression.

Early recognition of sepsis is vital – fever, rigors and feeling generally unwell should be investigated urgently. Neutropenic sepsis is an oncological emergency and requires prompt administration of parenteral antibiotics. The recommended antibiotics vary across the UK and local protocols should be available. Platelets should also be checked and intramuscular injections avoided if they are low. Drugs associated with bleeding are best avoided and the ongoing use of heparin when platelets are $<50 \times 10^9/L$ should be discussed with the cancer care team.

— Prescribing of SACT
In most cases, and unless there is an agreed shared-care protocol, all SACT for lung cancer will be prescribed by an oncologist. With the exception of some oral therapies where a local arrangement is in place, all SACTs are dispensed from a hospital pharmacy. There are national standards for SACT quality and safety and each SACT prescription is verified by a suitably trained pharmacist before dispensing. It is important therefore that the patient is given clear instructions on where and how they will receive treatment and what to do when a problem arises out of hours.

Chemistry and mode of action of erlotinib
Erlotinib is an oral therapy for locally advanced or metastatic NSCLC. It is an inhibitor of the epidermal growth factor receptor tyrosine kinase (EGFR-TK). By blocking signalling pathways in cell proliferation, it slows down the growth of the tumour. It is one of only a few drugs to contain an alkyne ($C\equiv C$) functional group.

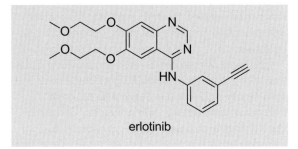

erlotinib

Rashes are one of the most commonly reported adverse drug reactions. These often develop in the first 2–3 weeks of treatment and resolve when treatment ends. Steps such as avoiding certain skin products, caution in sunlight and moisturising the skin after bathing may help to relieve symptoms. Otherwise, cancer networks have protocols for management of SACT-induced toxicity and the cancer care team should be contacted for advice. A standard approach is to use topical or systemic antibiotics such as clindamycin 1% lotion or oxytetracycline, or topical or oral corticosteroids. The patient may be given written information, or maintain a diary or patient-held card to aid communication with and between healthcare professionals.

— Erlotinib tablets: patient considerations
Crushing erlotinib tablets is outside its product licence and the manufacturer does not recommend this. The use of a licensed medicine in a way that is not recommended by the manufacturer (outside its marketing authorisation or Summary of Product Characteristics [SPC]) is referred to as 'off-label' or 'off-licence' use. In such a case, the prescriber should be made fully aware because the prescriber and pharmacist then assume greater responsibility for any associated risks, e.g. adverse effects or potential treatment failure. The erlotinib tablets may be dissolved in 100 mL water. The resulting solution is bitter tasting and may be masked with fruit juice (except grapefruit juice). There are no stability data and so the tablets should be dissolved immediately before administration. After administration, the container in which the solution was prepared should be rinsed twice with about 40 mL water and this also administered to ensure that the full dose has been taken.

— Early disease detection and the role of the community pharmacist
As stated previously, patients with lung cancer often present with advanced disease. This narrows

the treatment options and prognosis is poor. So what can be done to change this? Prevention and early detection are key to improving the survival rates. The vast majority of lung cancer cases are linked to smoking and passive smokers are also at risk. Smoking is also an important determinant of other chronic and life-threatening conditions. Thus, smoking cessation (see Case 12, Section 4) is a public health priority and all health professionals, including community and hospital pharmacists, need to recognise that they can have an impact. There have been many public awareness campaigns to raise awareness of the signs of lung cancer. November has been designated as the UK Lung Cancer Awareness month. Three key triggers for referral to the GP are:

- Persistent cough
- Breathlessness
- Haemoptysis.

If patients seek advice about a troublesome cough, ask them the right questions. How long have they had it? Has it changed recently? A cough of >3 weeks' duration and/or haemoptysis with clear sputum should be referred to the GP. Ask about smoking and occupational exposure to, for example, asbestos. Are they breathless? Don't forget that never smokers and ex-smokers can develop lung cancer too. What about weight loss, pain, hoarseness? Without causing undue alarm, be specific with the patient and if you refer to the GP be clear that this should be done as soon as possible.

EXTENDED LEARNING

- How do non-small cell lung cancer and small cell lung differ in their response to SACT?

- What are the latest developments in histology and tests for activating mutations in lung cancer?

ADDITIONAL PRACTICE POINTS

- How is the *performance status* of cancer patients normally assessed?

- Interactions have been identified between various drugs and grapefruit/grapefruit juice. What are the principal drugs and drug classes that are affected? What is believed to be the mechanism of these interactions?

- Discuss the place and operation of healthy living programmes in the prevention of chronic disease.

References and further reading

National Institute for Health and Clinical Excellence (2011). *The Diagnosis and Treatment of Lung Cancer.* NICE Clinical Guideline 121. London: NICE. Available at: http://guidance.nice.org.uk/CG121 (accessed 30 September 2013).

National Institute for Health and Clinical Excellence (2012). Erlotinib for the first-line treatment of locally advanced or metastatic EGFR-TK mutation-positive non-small cell lung cancer – NICE Technology Appraisal 258. [online]. Available at: http://guidance.nice.org.uk/ta258 (accessed 30 September 2013).

— **Resources**

British Lung Foundation: www.britishlungfoundation.org/lung-cancer

Cancer Backup: www.cancerbackup.org.uk/Cancertype/Lung

Cancer Research UK: www.cancerhelp.org.uk/help/default.asp?page=2787

It's time to focus on lung cancer: www.lungcancer.org

The Roy Castle Lung Cancer Foundation: www.roycastle.org

Case 2
The use of antimetabolites in the treatment of breast cancer

ADAM TODD AND ANDY HUSBAND

LEARNING OUTCOMES

At the end of this case, you will be able to:

- State the chemotherapeutic agents commonly used in the treatment of breast cancer
- Explain the differences between metabolites and antimetabolites
- Outline the criteria used to grade adverse drug reactions associated with chemotherapy
- Describe the chemical and clinical differences between folic acid and folinic acid
- Describe the facilities and safety precautions necessary when handling cytotoxic drugs in hospital pharmacy

Case study

Mrs AF is a 54-year-old woman who has recently been diagnosed with breast cancer. She underwent a quadrantectomy (partial mastectomy to remove a tumour in one breast tissue quadrant) around 6 weeks ago and is now being considered for adjuvant chemotherapy. Mrs AF has had cardiac problems in the past and is therefore not suitable for any anthracycline-containing chemotherapy regimens. As a result, the consultant oncologist has decided to prescribe six cycles of classical CMF combination therapy treatment.

Administration is as follows:

Day 1

Cyclophosphamide 600 mg/m² i.v. bolus (C)
Methotrexate 40 mg/m² i.v. bolus (M)
5-Fluorouracil (5FU) 600 mg/m² i.v. bolus (F)

Day 8

Cyclophosphamide 600 mg/m² i.v. bolus
Methotrexate 40 mg/m² i.v. bolus
5FU 600 mg/m² i.v. bolus

- —What other regimens can be used in the treatment of breast cancer?

- Why do cardiac problems contraindicate the use of anthracycline-containing regimens?
- What is the rationale for prescribing cyclophosphamide, methotrexate and 5-fluorouracil in combination?
- What facilities and safety precautions are necessary when handling these cytotoxic drugs in the hospital pharmacy?

After the first cycle of chemotherapy, Mrs AF complains of a sore mouth; she also has several mouth ulcers (mucositis), which are making it painful to eat solid food, although she can still drink fluids.

- What side effects are commonly observed with this regimen of chemotherapy?
- How do we grade the severity of side effects associated with chemotherapy?

You recommend adding oral folinic acid to be taken 24 hours after chemotherapy, to minimise the mucositis; you also supply Mrs AF with an antiseptic mouthwash to use twice a day.

- What is the rationale for using folinic acid to manage the mucositis?
- What chemotherapeutic agents are associated with commonly causing mucositis?

Mrs AF returns 3 weeks later and explains that her mouth is much better; she is now able to eat food without any problems. However, she is unsure about taking the folinic acid again, because she does not like taking tablets. Her sister has recommended that she take folic acid, which sounds very similar to folinic acid, as it is a natural supplement.

- What is the difference between folic acid and folinic acid?
- Will folic acid have the same effect as folinic acid?

Case discussion
— Treatment of breast cancer
Breast cancer is the most common form of cancer in the UK; it is most prevalent in women, although it can, on rare occasions, occur in men. There are many forms of chemotherapy that can be used to

folic acid

methotrexate

uracil

5-fluorouracil

treat breast cancer. When used after surgery, it is called adjuvant chemotherapy.

The decision of what chemotherapy regimen to use is based on many factors, including if the cancer is node negative (has not spread to the lymph nodes) or node positive (has spread to the lymph nodes).

Generally, for node-negative patients, an anthracycline-containing regimen is used, e.g. epirubicin (an anthracycline) can be used in combination with cyclophosphamide (an alkylating agent).

As outlined in this case, anthracyclines can cause cardiotoxicity and heart failure and are therefore contraindicated in patients who have current or previous history of cardiac impairment (e.g. myocardiopathy). The cellular mechanisms underlying this anthracycline cardiotoxicity (which can apparently still manifest many years after initial exposure) are multifactorial and not entirely understood, but are believed to involve a combination of injury processes leading to apoptosis and cell necrosis. Although cardioprotection using the iron chelator dexrazoxane was once considered useful as a prophylactic treatment during anthracycline chemotherapy, it is now licensed for use only in patients with advanced or metastatic breast cancer who have received cumulative doxorubicin or epirubicin treatment and require further anthracycline therapy. In cases where anthracyclines are contraindicated, a regimen consisting of cyclophosphamide, methotrexate and 5-fluorouracil (collectively known as classical CMF) can be used.

For node-positive patients, a taxane-containing regimen is often recommended, e.g. docetaxel (a

taxane) can be used in combination with 5-fluorouracil, epirubicin and cyclophosphamide – a regimen collectively known as 'FEC-T'.

— Antimetabolites

'Metabolite' is a general term for a compound that is required for normal biochemical reactions in cells. An antimetabolite is therefore, structurally similar to a metabolite, but cannot directly take its place; they often interfere with the normal cellular function, including cell division, which make them useful agents for the treatment of cancer. In the regimen prescribed for Mrs AF, both methotrexate and 5-fluorouracil are examples of antimetabolites.

Antimetabolites are often designed by taking a metabolite and performing a bioisosteric change, i.e. substituting an atom or group on a metabolite with another atom or functional group with similar chemical properties (e.g. substituting a hydrogen atom with a fluorine atom). If we examine the structures of the antimetabolites methotrexate and 5-fluorouracil and compare them to the corresponding metabolites, folic acid and uracil, we can see that they are very similar (differences are shown in red in the diagram).

— Methotrexate

Due to the structural similarities between folic acid and methotrexate, it should be no surprise to learn that methotrexate works by interfering with the folic acid cycle in cells. More specifically, methotrexate inhibits an enzyme called dihydrofolate reductase: an enzyme that is responsible for reducing dihydrofolic acid to tetrahydrofolic acid.

In the absence of methotrexate, folic acid is reduced to dihydrofolic acid and then tetrahydrofolic acid, which eventually forms N^5,N^{10}-methylenetetrahydrofolate and N^{10}-formyltetrahydrofolate (or, more simply, 'one-carbon donors'); these compounds act as building blocks for DNA synthesis.

When methotrexate is present, dihydrofolate reductase is inhibited; this prevents the formation of tetrahydrofolic acid (which, in turn, stops the formation of the one-carbon donors), and, ultimately, results in the inhibition of DNA synthesis.

There are other clinically used drugs that also inhibit the enzyme dihydrofolate reductase; these are trimethoprim (an antibacterial) and pyrimethamine (an antimalarial). Thankfully, however, trimethoprim and pyrimethamine have far greater selectivity for bacterial and protozoal dihydrofolate reductase, respectively, compared with human dihydrofolate reductase.

— 5-Fluorouracil

5FU is very similar in structure to uracil (the only difference is a fluorine atom). 5FU, once in the body, is converted by a series of cellular enzymes to 5-fluorodeoxyuridine monophosphate (5FdMUP), which irreversibly inhibits an enzyme called thymidylate synthase (TS). This enzyme is responsible for the synthesis of deoxythymidine monophosphate (an essential building block of DNA), which results in the inhibition of DNA synthesis.

— Facilities and safety precautions for handling these cytotoxic drugs in the hospital pharmacy

Cytotoxic drugs include anticancer drugs, monoclonal antibodies and immunosuppressive drugs. Direct exposure to these agents can result from skin contact, inhalation or ingestion, and consequently protective precautions are necessary for both patients and healthcare staff, including those in the hospital pharmacy reconstituting and dispensing such products.

Within the hospital pharmacy, ideally all preparation, reconstitution and dilution of cytotoxic injections should take place in a dedicated clean room with an environment controlled for particulate and microbial contamination levels, and with restricted access, used solely for that task. Preparation of the product takes place in a suitable safety cabinet or in an isolator. After preparation, the product should be labelled to indicate that it is cytotoxic and packaged to prevent spillages. Clear written standard operating procedures (SOPs) are necessary for all activities, including dealing with spillages and safe disposal of waste.

— Grading of adverse drug reactions associated with chemotherapy

Adverse drug reactions caused by cancer chemotherapy are graded according to the common toxicity criteria (CTC) – a system developed by the National Cancer Institute to promote consistency in the reporting of side effects associated with chemotherapy. The criteria, which include toxicities, such as nausea, vomiting and neutropenia (abnormally low level of neutrophils), are based on a set of predefined standards, whereby the toxicity is graded on a scale of 0–4. Typically, a grade of 0 means that there is no toxicity, whereas a grade of 3 or 4 means that the toxicity is severe or, in some cases, life threatening.

Mucositis (often associated with antimetabolite chemotherapy) is graded as:

- **Grade 1**: erythema (reddening) of the mucosa
- **Grade 2**: patchy ulceration, symptomatic but can eat and swallow
- **Grade 3**: confluent ulcerations, unable to adequately eat and drink normally
- **Grade 4**: symptoms associated with life-threatening consequences.

From the symptoms described in this case, Mrs AF would be classed as experiencing grade 2 mucositis.

— Folic acid and folinic acid in methotrexate toxicity

As shown in the diagram on page 281, the structures of folic acid and folinic acid are very similar (the only differences, shown in red, are the presence of a formyl group and, importantly, a reduced pyrazine ring in folinic acid). Folinic acid is used clinically to counteract methotrexate toxicity (including methotrexate overdose), whereas folic acid is used in patients who are taking oral methotrexate to reduce the possibility of developing toxicity. So, to summarise, folinic acid is used to *counteract* methotrexate toxicity, whereas folic acid is be used to *prevent* methotrexate toxicity.

folic acid

folinic acid

The differences in clinical use can be explained by examining what happens to these compounds once they enter the body. In the case of folinic acid, it can be converted to tetrahydrofolic acid without the need for the enzyme dihydrofolate reductase; thus, it can help replenish the one-carbon donors required for DNA synthesis – even in the presence of methotrexate.

Folic acid, on the other hand, requires the enzyme dihydrofolate reductase to be converted to tetrahydrofolic acid; thus, in the presence of methotrexate, folic acid cannot be converted into tetrahydrofolic acid and, ultimately, DNA cannot be made.

What does all of that mean for the patient? Folinic acid should always be used to manage methotrexate toxicity – especially in the case of overdose – because it can be converted into tetrahydrofolic acid without the enzyme dihydrofolate reductase, whereas folic acid should never be used to manage acute methotrexate toxicity.

In the case of Mrs AF, she should be advised to continue with the folinic acid because, even though it has a similar name (and structure) to folic acid, its biochemical effects in the body are quite different.

EXTENDED LEARNING

- Give examples of other antimetabolites used in oncology
- Compare and contrast 5-bromouracil and 5-fluorouracil
- When a patient takes methotrexate in combination with folic acid for the treatment of a non-malignant condition (such as rheumatoid arthritis), why is it taken on a different day to the folic acid?
- What are the sources of contamination in a pharmaceutical clean room?
- How are clean room facilities for preparation and reconstitution of sterile products designed, so as to exclude particulate, microbial and chemical contamination?

ADDITIONAL PRACTICE POINTS

- What are the common side effects of chemotherapy for cancer? How can patients be advised to minimise or manage these?

References and further reading

Chen B, Peng X, Pentassuglia L, Lim CC, Sawyer DB (2007). Molecular and cellular mechanisms of anthracycline cardiotoxicity. *Cardiovasc Toxicol* 7:114–21.

Health and Safety Executive (2003). Handling of cytotoxic drugs in isolators in NHS pharmacies. Available at: www.hse.gov.uk/pubns/cytotoxic-drugs.pdf (accessed 1 October 2013).

Health and Safety Executive (2003). Safe handling of cytotoxic drugs. Available at: www.hse.gov.uk/pubns/misc615.pdf (accessed 1 October 2013).

International Society of Oncology Pharmacy Practitioners (2007). Section 6 – Facilities for sterile cytotoxic reconstitution and personal protective equipment. *J Oncol Pharmacy Pract* 13(Suppl):17–26.

Lima LM, Barreiro EJ (2005). Bioisosterism: a useful strategy for molecular modification and drug design. *Curr Med Chem* 12:23–49.

National Cancer Institute (2013). *Common Terminology Criteria for Adverse Events (CTCAE) and Common Toxicity Criteria (CTC)*. Available at: http://ctep.cancer.gov/protocolDevelopment/electronic_applications/ctc.htm (accessed 1 October 2013).

National Institute for Health and Clinical Excellence (2009). *Advanced Breast Cancer: Diagnosis and treatment*. NICE Clinical Guideline 81. London: NICE. Available at: www.nice.org.uk/guidance/CG81 (accessed 1 October 2013).

Case 3

Clinical verification of prescriptions for oral anticancer medicines

KUMUD KANTILAL

LEARNING OUTCOMES

At the end of this case, you will be able to:

- Outline the sites of action of anticancer medicines
- Outline the risks associated with oral anticancer medicines
- Outline the chemistry and mode of action of capecitabine
- Describe the checks undertaken by a pharmacist when clinically verifying a prescription containing oral anticancer medicines
- Outline current resources available to aid pharmacists to verify prescriptions containing oral anticancer medicines clinically

Case study

Mr AS is a 73-year-old white man who has been diagnosed with metastatic colorectal cancer. His oncologist started him on capecitabine, an oral anticancer medicine licensed for his disease. Mr AS was seen by the cancer nurse and pharmacist, who reviewed the medication with him, including the side effects that he may experience and how to manage them, who to call in the event of an emergency, and the procedure for further clinic visits and capecitabine supply.

❷ What are the sites of action of oral anticancer medicines?

❷ What are the risks associated with oral anticancer medicines?

❷ What information will the pharmacist need in order to verify the prescription clinically?

❷ What information should pharmacists provide to patients taking oral anticancer medicine(s)?

❷ Draw the structure of capecitabine and outline how this prodrug is converted to its active metabolite preferentially in tumours (with respect to normal tissue)

Case discussion

— Oral anticancer medicines

Previously, most patients receiving anticancer medicines would have received their treatment via the parenteral route. In recent years, however, many new oral anticancer medicines have been developed, as a result of increased knowledge and understanding of the biological pathways involved in cancers. Advancing technologies ensure better bioavailability and predictable pharmacokinetics, and these drugs are now in routine clinical use. The usage of oral anticancer medicines is increasing in hospitals and the community. During 2006–2007, almost 18 million doses were used in hospitals and 6 million doses in the community in England.

— Sites of action of oral anticancer medicines

Traditional oral anticancer medicines cause damage to cancer cells by interfering with cell growth or cell division. The agents are grouped according to the phase of the cell cycle on which they act. Figure 7.1 shows the major classes of traditional anticancer medicines and their sites of action within the cell cycle.

Many traditional anticancer medicines target DNA synthesis or replication directly or indirectly (e.g. through intercalation of DNA, by blocking constituents such as antifolates or purine antagonists, or through inhibition of topoisomerase enzymes needed for DNA repair), or by inhibition of microtubules needed for mitosis and cell division. The side effects of these agents are the result of their non-specific effects on healthy cells as well as cancer cells.

Over the last few decades, new targets that play a role in cancer cell development and growth have been identified. As a result, new anticancer medicines that affect these targets have emerged in clinical practice. These targets include various tyrosine kinases from receptors that regulate cellular differentiation, growth and survival. These receptors are often over-expressed or mutated in cancers. The mechanism of action and side-effect profiles of these targeted oral anticancer medicines differ from those of the traditional anticancer medicines.

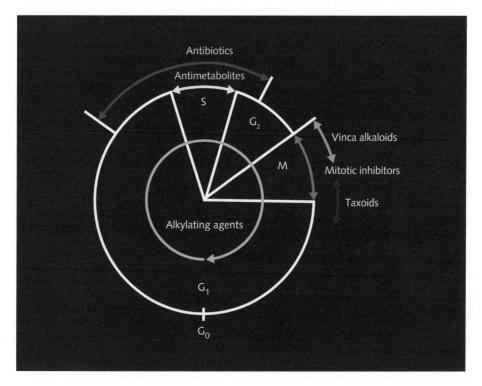

▲ FIGURE 7.1

Sites of action of traditional anticancer medicines within the cell cycle. Stages in the cell cycle are designated G_0, G_1, G_2, S and M phases.

Many of the current, targeted, oral, anticancer medicines are given continuously, so the cancer cells are continually exposed. This requires daily oral administration. The daily low-dose schedules often do not have the same dose-limiting side effects as high-dose intermittent schedules that have been used for parenteral administration. The traditional anticancer medicines are used for a limited number of cycles, then stopped. By contrast, many of the newer oral anticancer medicines used in current practice require prolonged treatment.

The term 'targeted' suggests that toxicity will be less than that encountered using the traditional parenteral anticancer medicines. In practice, however, it has been observed that side effects of the newer agents may be quite significant. Table 7.1 gives some examples of anticancer medicines.

— **Chemistry and mode of action of capecitabine: a traditional oral anticancer medicine**

Capecitabine contains an unusual carbamate (-NH-CO-OR) side chain, highlighted in the diagram in red. After oral administration, the ester (-CO-OR) bond is hydrolysed in the liver to give an unstable intermediate that decomposes to give the free amino (-NH$_2$) group. Further metabolism (catalysed by the enzymes cytidine deaminase, then thymidine phosphorylase) gives the well-known anticancer agent 5FU. As thymidine phosphorylase is much more active in tumour tissues than normal tissues, a degree of selective toxicity is possible, with fewer side effects compared with the use of 5FU itself. Once produced in the tumour, the antimetabolite 5FU ultimately inhibits the biosynthesis of pyrimidines or is incorporated as a 'false' nucleotide into DNA or RNA, resulting in cell death.

▼ TABLE 7.1

Examples of anticancer medicines

Traditional oral anticancer medicines (direct antitumour activity)			
Bexarotene	Busulphan	Capecitabine	Chloram-bucil
Cyclo-phosphamide	Estramustine	Etoposide	Fludarabine
Hydroxy-carbamide	Idarubicin	Lomustine	Melphalan
Mercapto-purine	Methotrexate	Mitotane	Procarbazine
Tegafur/uracil	Temozola-mide	Tioguanine	Topotecan
Treosulphan	Tretinoin (ATRA)	Vinorelbine	
Immunomodulatory drugs (IMiDs)			
Lenolidamide	Thalidomide		
Targeted therapies			
Axitinib	Crizotinib	Dasatinib	Erlotinib
Everolimus	Gefitinib	Imatinib	Lapatinib
Nilotinib	Pazopanib	Ruxolitinib	Sorafenib
Sunitinib	Vandetanib	Vemurafenib	

Table 7.2 lists key differences between traditional and targeted oral anticancer medicines. Many parameters are drug specific, so individual drug product literature must be referred to for detailed information. Table 7.2 attempts to give a broad general overview of the major differences between the traditional and newer targeted anticancer medicines currently available in the UK.

Please refer to individual drug product literature for detailed information.

— Safety concerns for oral anticancer medicines

Although oral treatment offers advantages to patients and health professionals, it nevertheless carries the same risks as parenteral anticancer treatment in terms of toxicity and potential for harm from medication errors. This is due to the narrow therapeutic index of these drugs. Between November 2003 and July 2007, the National Patient Safety Agency (NPSA) received reports of three deaths and 400 patient safety incidents concerning oral anticancer medicines.

The risks are increased if non-specialist practitioners prescribe, dispense or administer

▼ TABLE 7.2

Summary of major differences between traditional and targeted anticancer medicines

	Traditional anticancer medicines	Targeted anticancer therapies
Mode of action	Direct antitumour activity; affects different phases of the cell cycle	Act on specific targets known to be involved in cancer cell development
Adminis-tration	Mainly parenteral, some oral Pulsed therapy Short-term treatment, e.g. six cycles Mainly administered in secondary care setting	Mainly oral, some parenteral Continuous therapy (drug dependent) Prolonged treatment, e.g. until disease progression May be administered in primary or secondary care setting
Dosing	High doses given to maximise cell kill Individualised: based on weight or body surface area, e.g. capecitabine	Lower doses given to inhibit/suppress cell growth Flat dosing for many agents, e.g. erlotinib
Side effects	Common Generalised Predictable	Rare Specific Unpredictable
Nurse role	Pre-chemotherapy consultation, administration, monitoring	Pre-chemotherapy consultation, monitoring, e.g. assessment of toxicity by telephone
Pharmacy role	Aseptic preparation of parenteral doses, verification of clinical appropriateness of doses, patient information and support	Verification of clinical appropriateness of doses, patient information and support
Patient/carer role	Inform healthcare professionals of any adverse events related to anticancer medicine	Administration and monitoring of adverse events related to anticancer medicine

these medicines and bypass the normal safeguards used for parenteral anticancer medicines.

Parenteral anticancer medicines are prepared under strict environmental controls, in a suitable safety cabinet or an isolator, by trained pharmacy personnel and administered by specialist chemotherapy nurses, mainly in the hospital setting. The recent introduction of oral anticancer medicines allows the supply to take place in the community setting and administration in the homes of patients.

This transfer to the community setting could increase the risk of dosing errors, side effects, drug interactions and non-adherence to treatment plans. Patients will be expected to assume greater responsibility for taking their oral anticancer medicines at home. Consequently, appropriate counselling will be important to ensure that the proper dose is taken in the correct manner at the appropriate time.

The increasing use of oral anticancer medicines poses various other challenges, such as drug interactions with other medicines and complementary therapies, e.g. herbal products. Administration in relation to food can also be a specific issue for these agents; some (e.g. sorafenib) should not be taken with food because of reduced drug absorption and bioavailability, whereas other agents (e.g. imatinib) should be taken with food to reduce gastrointestinal irritation.

Dysphagia (difficulty in swallowing or inability to swallow), odynophagia (painful swallowing), nausea and vomiting can present barriers to oral administration and can cause missed doses or reduced drug absorption in patients who vomit within a short time of taking a dose.

Patient non-adherence to the prescribed treatment (as a result of confusion, misunderstanding or failure to remember to take doses) is another potential problem with the use of oral anticancer medicines. Patient counselling on the use of their oral anticancer medicines is vital to minimise potential non-adherence issues.

Patients with cancer are believed to be particularly motivated to adhere to their anticancer treatments. Over-adherence can, therefore, also pose risks.

Regimens used to treat cancer may include the traditional anticancer medicines and/or targeted therapies and may comprise a single agent or multiple agents, making the dosing regimens extremely complex. The need to monitor side effects and titrate doses accordingly further increases the complexity of oral anticancer medicines.

— **Steps undertaken by pharmacists to verify prescriptions containing oral anticancer medicines clinically**

The National Cancer Action Team report, *Chemotherapy Services in England: Ensuring Quality and Safety*, published in August 2009,

states that 'All chemotherapy prescriptions should be checked by an oncology pharmacist, who has undergone specialist training, demonstrated his or her appropriate competence and is locally authorised/accredited for the task.' The British Oncology Pharmacy Association (BOPA) standards for clinical pharmacy verification of prescriptions for cancer medicines (updated in April 2013) describe the steps that a pharmacist must take when checking prescriptions for anticancer medicines, and are described in detail below. The term verification has been used to describe this checking process.

— **Anticancer prescription verification checks**

Prescriber details: prescribing of anticancer medicines should be undertaken only by appropriately trained staff (medical staff and non-medical independent and supplementary nurse and pharmacist prescribers) working within the oncology/haematology services. There should be local policies in place describing which staff groups (e.g. consultant, registrar) may prescribe anticancer medicines and who can prescribe the first and subsequent cycles of chemotherapy. A list of designated prescribers should be available and this list should be maintained and updated at least annually.

The pharmacist should have access to the list of designated prescribers to confirm that they are authorised to prescribe anticancer medicines.

Regimen details: anticancer medicines should be prescribed in the context of written protocols, which should be approved for local use.

The pharmacist should check that the regimen has been through a local approval process, e.g. clinical governance and financial approval and/or is included in a list of locally approved regimens. For the first cycle, where access to clinical notes, treatment plans or electronic records is available, the pharmacist should ensure that the regimen prescribed is the intended treatment and is appropriate for the patient's diagnosis, medical history, performance status and chemotherapy history.

Administration details: the pharmacist should check that the timing of administration (i.e. interval since last treatment) and method of administration (e.g. can the patient swallow the oral dose units?) is appropriate for the patient.

Patient details: the pharmacist should check that the patient's weight and height have been correctly recorded and the body surface area correctly calculated, as appropriate for the regimen being used. The pharmacist should also note any drug allergies.

Dosing information: the pharmacist should check that the doses are correctly calculated as per the protocol and adhere to any local dosing guidelines, e.g. dose rounding/banding. The pharmacist should also check for maximum cumulative doses as appropriate. If doses have been adjusted, the pharmacist should check that the reason is documented and the dose adjustment appropriate, and that local guidelines and protocols are adhered to.

Relevant laboratory tests: the pharmacist should check the full blood count, biochemistry results, renal function, liver function and results of any other relevant tests as stipulated in the protocol.

Supportive and other medicines: the pharmacist should check that the appropriate supportive therapy has been prescribed, e.g. antiemetics, antibiotics, as per the protocol. The pharmacist should also check what other medicines the patient is currently taking to check for any drug interactions. Note that some patients may be on complementary therapies that could interact with the anticancer medicine prescribed.

— Patient counselling points

All healthcare professionals have a role to play in providing patients with information with respect to treatment. The NPSA emphasises the need to ensure that patients are fully informed about their oral anticancer medicines and should be provided with verbal and up-to-date written information. The information should include contact details for specialist advice, intended treatment regimen, treatment plan and monitoring arrangements.

BOPA and the United Kingdom Oncology Nursing Society (UKONS) have made recommendations for information and education that must be provided to patients to ensure patient safety, adherence and treatment success.

Information that should be provided to patients is listed in the box.

Intended regimen and treatment plan

- Name of the oral anticancer medicine(s)
- The number of different tablets/capsules to be taken

- When/how often to take them, e.g. morning, evening
- When they need to start
- When they need to stop
- Any treatment gaps

Need to swallow tablets/capsules whole

- Do not open capsules, or crush/chew tablets, unless specific local information is available
- Contact doctor/nurse if cannot swallow tablets/capsules

When and how to take oral anticancer medicines in relation to food

- With food
- Before food

What to do if one or more doses are missed
What to do if the patient vomits after taking a dose
What side effects to expect and how to manage them

- Explain when and how to start taking any supportive medicines being supplied at the same time
- Explain when they need to contact the hospital

Possible interactions with other drugs, food, supplements and herbal remedies

- Remind patient to inform healthcare professionals about all their current treatments, including copies of medicines list, diaries, etc.

Need for, and how to obtain, further supplies

- Role of the GP/community nurse in their treatment

Principles of safe handling, storage and disposal

- Store oral anticancer medicine(s) in a secure manner, away from children
- Refrigeration requirements, if applicable
- Wash hands well with soap and water before and after handling oral anticancer medicine(s), and/or use disposable gloves depending on local practice

- Avoid/minimise the handling of tablets/capsules by patient/carers
- The need to return any unused tablets/capsules to the hospital, depending on local practice

Patients must be provided with a 24-hour contact number so that they have access to specialist staff to whom they can direct queries. NHS cancer centre and cancer charities' websites should be used to access patient information. Patient alert cards, treatment plans and diaries may also be useful for helping patients manage their own treatment.

All the information above should be provided at the pre-treatment consultation and reinforced on subsequent visits.

EXTENDED LEARNING

- Describe DNA synthesis and replication
- What is meant by parenteral administration? What are the advantages and disadvantages of parenteral routes of administration?
- Describe the mechanisms of action of the newer oral anticancer medicines

- Identify medications that may interact with oral anticancer medicines
- Discuss the requirements for a safe oral anticancer medicines service
- What factors need to be considered for the supply of oral anticancer medicines in primary care/or via a homecare service?

References and further reading

British Oncology Pharmacists Association (2004). Position statement on the care of patients receiving oral chemotherapy. *Pharmaceut J* 272:422–3.

British Oncology Pharmacy Association (2010). *Guidance to Support BOPA Standards for Clinical Pharmacy Verification of Prescriptions for Cancer Medicines.* London: BOPA.

British Oncology Pharmacy Association (2013). *Standards for the Clinical Pharmacy Verification of Prescriptions for Cancer Medicines.* London: BOPA.

National Chemotherapy Advisory Group (2009). *Chemotherapy Services in England: Ensuring quality and safety.* London: Department of Health.

Williamson S (2011). *A Report on the Dispensing and Supply of Oral Chemotherapy and Systemic Anticancer Medicines in Primary Care.* London: BOPA, RPS, NPA.

Williamson S, Polwart C (2008). *The Oral Anticancer Medicines Handbook: A reference guide to oral chemotherapy and oral anticancer medicines including advice on safe prescribing, handling and administration,* 3rd edn. Gateshead: North of England Cancer Network (NHS).

Case 4
Thromboprophylaxis in a patient undergoing surgery for cancer
BARBARA CLARK

LEARNING OUTCOMES

At the end of this case, you will be able to:

- Describe the signs and symptoms of deep vein thrombosis (DVT) and pulmonary embolism (PE)
- Explain why cancer patients are at increased risk of VTE
- Explain the importance of carrying out a VTE risk assessment for all patients admitted to hospital
- Recommend a suitable thromboprophylaxis regimen for a cancer patient undergoing surgery

- Appreciate the properties of the different low-molecular-weight heparins

Case study

Mr MH is a 68-year-old investment banker who is still very active at his office and church and enjoys sailing on summer weekends. He had an acute myocardial infarction in 2005, for which he had a stent inserted. Since then, his cardiovascular health has been good and until recently he rarely saw his doctor. Mr MH has no other past medical history.

Four weeks ago, Mr MH started having persistent stomach cramps and a full or bloated feeling. He had also found blood in his stool. As his brother died from colorectal cancer 3 years previously, Mr

MH decided to see his GP. Due to his family history, Mr MH's GP sent him for a colonoscopy and CT scan. A 2-cm mass was detected in his descending colon and pathology revealed tumour cells indicating colon adenocarcinoma. Mr MH was referred to a colorectal surgeon and an oncologist.

Two weeks later, Mr MH was scheduled for surgery to remove the tumour. Before his scheduled surgery, he attended the pre-admission clinic where he underwent a number of investigations to prepare him for his surgery. At this appointment, the nurse was concerned about Mr MH's risk of venous thromboembolism (VTE).

❷ What is VTE?
❷ What are the signs and symptoms of VTE?
❷ Why are patients undergoing surgery for cancer at high risk of VTE?

The nurse ordered a full blood count (FBC). To address her concerns, she also completed a VTE risk assessment.

❷ What is a VTE risk assessment?
❷ Why is it important for all hospitalised patients to undergo a VTE risk assessment?
❷ What are Mr MH's risk factors for VTE?

Two weeks later Mr MH was admitted for his procedure. The junior doctor wants to prescribe an appropriate thromboprophylactic agent and asks for your advice.

❷ What classes of drugs are most commonly used for VTE prophylaxis?
❷ Before starting thromboprophylaxis, what blood parameters should be checked?

The relevant blood results were within the normal ranges and Mr MH was prescribed an appropriate thromboprophylactic agent.

❷ According to the BNF, which of the following is/are recommended for thromboprophylaxis in patients undergoing cancer surgery?
1. Enoxaparin 40 mg subcutaneously once daily
2. Dalteparin 15 000 units subcutaneously once daily
3. Rivaroxaban 10 mg once daily
4. Tinzaparin 3500 units once daily
5. Dabigatran 150 mg twice daily
6. Fondaparinux 2.5 mg once daily

Mr MH's surgery went well. However, after surgery his renal function deteriorated and, as a result, his current thromboprophylaxis regimen was no longer suitable. His current treatment was stopped.

❷ Which of the following options should Mr MH be prescribed to replace his previous therapy?
1. Enoxaparin 40 mg subcutaneously once daily
2. Dalteparin 15 000 units subcutaneously once daily
3. Unfractionated heparin 5000 units two or three times daily.
4. Tinzaparin 3500 units once daily
5. Dabigatran 150 mg twice daily
6. Fondaparinux 2.5 mg once daily

Mr MH has recovered well. His kidney function has recovered and he is now ready for discharge. You are the ward pharmacist. The junior doctor is writing Mr MH's discharge prescription and asks your advice about his thromboprophylaxis regimen.

❷ Which of the following is the most appropriate action?
1. Stop thromboprophylactic therapy
2. Continue thromboprophylactic therapy for one more week
3. Continue thromboprophylactic therapy for 28 days
4. Reduce the dose of the thromboprophylactic therapy and continue for 1 week
5. Reduce the dose of the thromboprophylactic therapy and continue for 28 days

Case discussion

— Venous thromboembolism

Venous thromboembolism is the general term to describe the blocking of a blood vessel by a blood clot. This term includes both DVT and PE. DVT occurs when a blood clot blocks a deep vein, usually in the leg. PE is a potentially life-threatening complication and occurs when the blood clot escapes into the circulation and becomes lodged in the lungs. VTE is the most common preventable cause of death in hospitalised patients and pregnant women.

— Signs and symptoms of VTE

VTE is generally a silent disease associated with a low frequency of clinical symptoms; most DVT cases are asymptomatic. If there are symptoms, they usually occur in just one leg and may include pain, tenderness and swelling of the leg and/or skin discoloration that is pale, blue or a reddish-purple colour. Symptoms of PE, if they present before severe complications, include shortness of breath, rapid pulse, sweating, chest pain and sudden collapse.

— VTE in cancer patients

Cancer patients are hypercoagulable, primarily because of tumour-related alterations in the coagulation cascade. Tumours contain cell-surface proteins (e.g. tissue factor and cancer procoagulant) that lead to activation of the clotting cascade via interactions with factors IX and/or X. In addition, tumour-released cytokines cause prothrombotic changes in the vascular endothelium. This hypercoagulability is exacerbated by cancer-associated treatment events, including immobility, central venous catheters, and packed red blood cell and platelet transfusions.

Cancer-related therapy further confounds VTE management. Drug interactions, chemotherapy-induced thrombocytopenia, malnutrition, bleeding risk from surgery, or tumour location and liver dysfunction make safe management of cancer-associated VTE a challenge.

Overall, cancer patients are at a sixfold increased risk of developing VTE compared with the general population, and these patients represent approximately 20% of all VTE cases. VTE is a leading cause of mortality among hospitalised cancer patients; evidence of VTE exists in up to 50% of cancer patients *post mortem*.

— VTE risk assessment

VTE is the most common preventable cause of death in hospitalised patients. Approximately 30 000 patients die every year from VTE. As a result, the Department of Health has stated that all patients admitted to hospital should have a documented VTE risk assessment, and a risk assessment tool has been designed. VTE risk assessment is now mandatory practice and failure to comply results in a financial penalty for the NHS trust.

Based on the Department of Health VTE risk assessment tool, Mr MH (in this case) has the following VTE risk factors:

- Age >60 years
- Active cancer
- Heart disease
- Surgery with total anaesthetic time >90 min.

As a result, Mr MH can be considered to be at high risk of VTE after his surgical procedure and will require thromboprophylaxis.

— Classes of drugs used for VTE prophylaxis

Low-molecular-weight heparins (LMWHs) are the most commonly used class of medicine for VTE prophylaxis.

Heparin is a polysaccharide, comprising a variable sequence of alternating N-acetyl-D-glucosamine and uronic (either D-glucuronic or L-iduronic) acid residues, linked by 1→4 glycosidic bonds. The constituent units are highly and variably sulphated, giving heparin a significant negative charge at physiological pH. Endogenous heparin consists of a mixture of polysaccharides of variable length, from around 3 kDa to 30 kDa in molecular mass. The LMWHs typically consist of shorter polysaccharides in the 3- to 8-kDa range, isolated by fractionation of heparin by gel filtration. The different LMWHs differ in their size ranges and distributions, their physical, chemical and biological properties, and their methods of production.

Enoxaparin is an LMWH licensed for numerous indications: prevention of DVT in medical and surgical patients, treatment of VTE, treatment of acute ST-segment elevation myocardial infarction (STEMI), treatment of unstable angina and non-ST-segment elevation

part of a heparin polymer

myocardial infarction (NSTEMI). Enoxaparin is not licensed for VTE prevention in patients undergoing surgery for cancer.

Tinzaparin is an LMWH licensed for the prevention of VTE in patients undergoing general and orthopaedic surgery. It is also licensed for the treatment of DVT and PE. Tinzaparin is not licensed for VTE prevention in patients undergoing surgery for cancer.

Dabigatran is a direct thrombin inhibitor that is given orally for the prophylaxis of VTE in adults undergoing elective total hip or knee replacements. It is not licensed for VTE prevention in patients undergoing surgery for cancer.

Rivaroxaban is a direct inhibitor of factor Xa, which is given orally for the prophylaxis of VTE in adults undergoing elective total hip or knee replacement, and for the treatment of VTE. It is not licensed for VTE prevention in patients undergoing surgery for cancer.

Fondaparinux is a synthetic pentasaccharide that inhibits activated factor X. It is licensed for the prevention of VTE in medical and surgical patients. It is also licensed for the treatment of VTE, unstable angina and STEMI. Fondaparinux is not licensed for the prevention of VTE in patients undergoing surgery for cancer.

Dalteparin is a LMWH licensed for numerous indications: prevention of VTE in surgical patients, treatment of VTE and treatment of unstable angina and non-Q-wave myocardial infarction when used concurrently with aspirin. Dalteparin is also licensed for extended treatment of VTE and prevention of its occurrence in patients with solid tumours.

LMWHs are renally cleared and most agents are contraindicated at a creatinine clearance <30 mL/min. LMWHs are also contraindicated at a low platelet count (75–100 $\times$ 10^9/L: normal 150–400 $\times$ 10^9/L) due to potential risk of bleeding.

Therefore, before initiation of therapy it is essential that Mr MH's renal function and platelet count are determined to ensure that he is not put at risk of bleeding.

— **Thromboprophylaxis in renal impairment**
The half-lives of unfractionated heparin and LMWH differ. This is because unfractionated heparin is cleared by two mechanisms: a saturable mechanism in which clearance is by the reticuloendothelial system and endothelial cells, to which heparin binds with a high affinity, and a non-saturable process of renal excretion. Which of these two mechanisms dominates depends on the dose administered (at high doses the non-saturable process predominates) and the molecular weight. By contrast, LMWHs are mainly removed by non-saturable renal excretion. The half-life of unfractionated heparin is typically approximately half that of LMWH. Due to its decreased half-life, the risk of accumulation with unfractionated heparin is much lower. The recommended dose of unfractionated heparin for VTE prophylaxis is 5000 units two or three times daily.

— **Duration of therapy in cancer patients undergoing surgery**
According to the NICE guidance published in 2010, VTE prophylaxis in cancer patients undergoing surgery should be continued after discharge and for a total of 28 days after the surgical procedure.

EXTENDED LEARNING
- Describe the clotting cascade
- What advice would you offer to a patient who was soon to embark on a long-haul flight and was concerned about the risk of DVT?
- Describe the process whereby a new drug product is licensed for a particular clinical indication.

References and further reading

Department of Health (2010). *Risk Assessment for Venous Thromboembolism (VTE)*. London: DH.

National Institute for Health and Clinical Excellence (2010). *Reducing the Risk of Venous Thromboembolism (Deep Vein Thrombosis and Pulmonary Embolism) in Patients Admitted to Hospital*. NICE Clinical Guideline 92. London: NICE. Available at: www.nice.org.uk/CG092 (accessed 18 August 2013).

Weaver AC, Barsuk JH (2010). What is the appropriate treatment of cancer-associated venous thromboembolic disease? *The Hospitalist*. Available at: www.the-hospitalist.org/details/article/689495/What_Is_the_Appropriate_Treatment_of_Cancer-Associated_Venous_Thromboembolic_Dis.html (accessed 18 August 2013).

Case 5
Febrile neutropenia in paediatric oncology
SHANI CORB

LEARNING OUTCOMES

At the end of this case, you will be able to:

- Outline the pathophysiology and diagnosis of childhood leukaemia
- State the criteria for a diagnosis of febrile neutropenia
- Explain the rationale for the initial antibiotic regimen
- Describe the therapeutic drug monitoring required
- Identify the principal features of a randomised controlled trial

Case study

IB is a 5-year-old child who weighs 18 kg and has a surface area (SA) of 0.74 m². She was diagnosed with acute lymphoblastic leukaemia (ALL) about 18 months ago. She has been enrolled on a clinical trial to compare different treatment regimens for ALL. IB is in the 'intensive treatment' arm because she was low risk at presentation (i.e. she has a favourable outcome).

❷ What is ALL?

Mum checks IB's temperature daily using an ear thermometer and this morning it was 38.1°C. Mum phoned the ward for advice and they told her to check IB's temperature in 4 hours' time. If it was still >38°C then she was to take her straight to the ward.

❷ What are the trigger criteria given to parents with regard to temperature?
❷ Why are parents advised not to give their child paracetamol or ibuprofen if they are on chemotherapy?

Mum takes IB to the hospital as her temperature doesn't settle. She is seen immediately on arrival at the ward and a nurse accesses her port while the doctor prescribes antibiotics and takes blood cultures.

The doctor prescribes the following antibiotics:

Antibiotic	Unit dose	Prescribed dose	Route	Frequency
Tazobactam/ piperacillin	90 mg/kg	1.62 g	i.v. bolus	q.d.s.
Gentamicin	7 mg/kg	126 mg	i.v. infusion over 30 min	o.d.

❷ What is a 'port' and how may it be accessed?
❷ In this case, what classes of antibiotics have been prescribed and what are their mechanisms of action?
❷ What organisms is the doctor covering by using this regimen?
❷ What therapeutic drug monitoring (TDM) needs to be performed?
❷ Tazobactam/piperacillin injection is available as a sterile freeze-dried powder for reconstitution. What is freeze drying (lyophilisation) and why is this product likely to be supplied in a powder form, rather than as a liquid?

IB's current oral chemotherapy/analgesic medication is:

Mercaptopurine suspension 100 mg/5 mL: 2.75 mL once daily
Methotrexate 2.5 mg tablets: 6 tablets once a week on Wednesday
Co-trimoxazole 240 mg/5 mL: 5 mL twice a day on Saturday and Sunday
Codeine phosphate 25 mg/5 mL: 3 mL every 4–6 hours, when needed

Her FBC comes back as shown below:

Parameter	Result	Usual range
Hb (g/dL)	11	11.3–14.1
Platelets ($\times\ 10^9$/L)	252	150–450
WCC ($\times\ 10^9$/L)	2.9	5–17
Neutrophils ($\times\ 10^9$/L)	0.1	1.5–8.5

As IB has a neutrophil count $<1 \times 10^9$/L and is pyrexial, a diagnosis of febrile neutropenia is made and she is to continue on her antibiotics for 7 days.

❷ Draw the structures of the two oral ALL chemotherapy medications currently prescribed

◯ What are their mechanisms of action with respect to the treatment of ALL?

◯ Should IB continue her current oral chemotherapy medication? Explain your answer

Case discussion

— Acute lymphoblastic leukaemia: pathophysiology and diagnosis

ALL is a cancer of the white blood cells. Normally, white blood cells grow and divide in an orderly and controlled way. In leukaemia, this process gets out of control because the normal signals that stop the body making too many cells are ignored, so the cells go on dividing and do not mature.

In ALL, there is an overproduction of immature lymphocytes, called lymphoblasts (sometimes referred to as blast cells). These immature cells fill up the bone marrow and stop it from making blood cells properly. As the lymphoblasts do not mature, they cannot do the work of normal white blood cells (fight infection). Also, as the bone marrow is overcrowded with immature white cells, it cannot make enough healthy red cells and platelets.

ALL occurs most frequently in children aged under 15 years old; in adolescents/adults it is more common between the ages of 15 and 25 years and in older people. It is slightly more common in males than in females.

— ALL treatment

Chemotherapy drugs circulate throughout the body in the bloodstream. However, the chemotherapy drugs cannot get into the fluid around the brain and spinal cord (cerebrospinal fluid, CSF), so they need to be injected directly into the fluid through a lumbar puncture. This is done even if leukaemia cells are not detectable in the CSF, because research has shown that there will almost always be some leukaemia cells in the CSF that need to be destroyed. For people who have just been diagnosed with ALL, it is important to start treatment quickly. Treatment is divided into three different phases: induction, intensification (consolidation) and continuing therapy (maintenance).

Induction: this is the initial intensive phase of treatment, aimed at destroying as many leukaemia cells as possible. It usually achieves a remission of the disease. Common chemotherapy drugs that may be used in this phase include: vincristine, daunorubicin or doxorubicin, methotrexate, asparaginase, mercaptopurine and cyclophosphamide.

Corticosteroids, usually dexamethasone, can also be given as part of the treatment. In addition, allopurinol, which helps to protect the kidneys against damage caused by the increase in uric acid (a waste product produced when the leukaemia cells are destroyed), may be used. The induction phase of treatment normally lasts 3–8 weeks and, as this is a very intense phase, patients need to stay in hospital for about 4 weeks.

Intensification (consolidation): after the induction phase, more chemotherapy is given to increase the chance of destroying any remaining leukaemia cells that cannot be seen in the blood or bone marrow. Drugs used during consolidation may include cytarabine, etoposide and mercaptopurine, as well as some of the same drugs used during induction. The consolidation phase of the treatment usually lasts for several months.

Continuing therapy (maintenance): continuing therapy reduces the risk of the leukaemia coming back at a later stage after treatment has finished. It is a less intensive course of chemotherapy. Common drugs used are mercaptopurine and methotrexate, given by mouth, and vincristine, which is given by injection. The steroid dexamethasone is given by mouth as a 5-day pulse every 4 weeks and patients also receive an intrathecal injection of methotrexate once every 3 months. This phase may last for a couple of years and is usually given as an outpatient procedure. Patients don't usually need to be admitted to hospital unless they develop problems such as infections.

Throughout these three phases of treatment, patients have regular blood tests and lumbar punctures to check for leukaemia cells. The doctor will check the results of the tests and will make changes to treatment accordingly.

— The role of a port/portacath

A port (or portacath) is a small device that is implanted under the skin to allow easy access to the bloodstream. Insertion of a port is usually a surgical procedure requiring a local anaesthetic. It can be used to draw blood, or administer drugs or other blood products if necessary. Cancer patients will often require repeated administrations of cytotoxic drugs, as well as blood tests to check recovery between successive chemotherapy administrations. Sometimes it can be difficult to access veins, and repeated attempts can be painful. A port means that separate i.v. injections are not required each time. To access the port, a needle is inserted into a resealing rubber centre. As the port is completely under the skin, patients can bathe and swim without risking infection.

— Structures and mechanisms of cytotoxic action of methotrexate and mercaptopurine

IB's current oral chemotherapy regimen includes methotrexate and mercaptopurine (6-mercaptopurine). Both these agents are antimetabolites (see Case 2 in this chapter) that interfere with the assembly of new DNA through inhibition of the synthesis of the component nucleotides. Both drugs act via more than one mechanism. Methotrexate is an inhibitor of the dihydrofolate reductase (DHFR) enzyme. Inhibition of DHFR results in increased levels of the usual substrate for this enzyme, 7,8-dihydrofolate, which in turn inhibits the biosynthesis of pyrimidine nucleotides (catalysed by thymidylate synthase). Methotrexate also inhibits another enzyme that is involved in the biosynthesis of purine nucleotides.

6-Mercaptopurine is a prodrug that first requires metabolic activation by conversion to its corresponding ribonucleotide. This ribonucleotide, after methylation, is a potent inhibitor of the key step that initiates purine biosynthesis (catalysed by amidophosphoribosyl transferase). A second mechanism also operates in which 'false' mercaptopurine ribonucleotides are incorporated into DNA and RNA, preventing strand elongation and resulting in cell death by apoptosis.

— Definition of febrile neutropenia

- Neutrophils $<0.75 \times 10^9$/L
- *and* fever* $>38.0°$C for >4 h or on two occasions at least 4 h apart
- *or* fever* $>38.5°$C on one occasion

- *or* clinical suspicion of sepsis in the absence of fever, e.g. unexplained abdominal pain or generally unwell.
  (*Fever should be unrelated to the transfusion of blood products.)

Blood counts can change quickly and therefore parents do not always know when their child becomes neutropenic (low neutrophil count). It is very important that parents monitor temperature if they suspect that their child is unwell and follow the prompts of $>38.0°$C for >4 h or on two occasions at least 4 h apart, $>38.5°$C on one occasion or any suspicion that the child is unwell. IB's low neutrophil count (0.1 $\times$ 10^9/L) and elevated temperature ($>38.0°$C on two occasions at least 4 h apart) are indicative of febrile neutropenia.

— Use of analgesia

If analgesia is required at home, patients are usually given codeine. Parents are advised not to give paracetamol as it may mask the signs of fever. Paracetamol can be given in hospital once the criteria for initiating antibiotics have been fulfilled.

Ibuprofen and other non-steroidal anti-inflammatory drugs (NSAIDs) are avoided in children on chemotherapy as blood counts can fall quickly, leading to bleeding risk with low platelets. NSAIDs are also antipyretics and can mask the signs of fever in the same way as paracetamol.

Under no circumstances are oncology children to be given any medicines by the rectal route, including enemas. This is due to the infection risk.

— Empirical antimicrobial regimen: consideration of this case

- Piperacillin/tazobactam (Tazocin) 90 mg/kg four times daily **and**
- Gentamicin 7 mg/kg once daily (*check level before second dose) **plus**
- Teicoplanin or vancomycin if child has a pain/inflammation round an endoprosthesis (port) or a tunnel infection.

methotrexate

6-mercaptopurine

Piperacillin/tazobactam is a combination product containing a broad-spectrum penicillin with good activity against *Pseudomonas aeruginosa* and a β-lactamase inhibitor. This combination works in synergy with gentamicin, which gives good Gram-negative cover.

Gentamicin is an aminoglycoside antibiotic drug that requires therapeutic drug monitoring (TDM) and trough levels should be taken 20 h after the previous dose with a target of <1 mg/L.

Teicoplanin and vancomycin principally cover infections caused by *Staphylococcus aureus*, a common inhabitant of the skin's natural flora that can cause opportunistic infections.

— Antibiotic injection: freeze drying to improve stability

Tazobactam/piperacillin injection is available as a sterile freeze-dried powder for reconstitution because the combined injection will not have long-term stability as a solution and the materials will degrade if a traditional drying process is employed.

Freeze drying (lyophilisation) is employed to dry very-heat-sensitive materials, including antibiotics. In the process, liquid (most commonly an aqueous solution) is frozen, the pressure above the frozen liquid is reduced and then the water removed by sublimation.

Freeze drying comprises three principal stages:

1 Freezing the solution.
2 Applying a vacuum above the ice to reduce the pressure to below that of the triple point of the product. The triple point is the unique point on the pressure–temperature phase diagram of water, where the three phases – gas, liquid, solid (ice) – coexist.
3 Applying heat to the system sufficiently to cause sublimation of water vapour. Drying occurs in two phases. *Primary drying*: the ice sublimes, leaving a porous solid with about 0.5% residual moisture after primary drying. *Secondary drying*: raising the temperature to remove the residual moisture left after primary drying.

The final dried product is a porous network of solid (cake) occupying the same volume as the original solution. The solid readily dissolves during reconstitution with solvent.

— Continuation of regular medication

It is generally thought to be safer for children to stop their oral chemotherapy medication on admission to hospital, rather than to continue it. If the child is neutropenic, as is the case with IB, they should stop medication regardless.

If patients are febrile but non-neutropenic, their blood counts could be about to fall and so it would be prudent to omit the doses for that evening and wait for the oncology team to review them the following morning.

While on intravenous antibiotics, prophylactic co-trimoxazole and required analgesia should continue.

— Clinical trials: design and features

Randomised controlled trials (RCTs) are employed to test hypotheses about the relative benefits of different treatment options. This may be to compare different drug therapies or treatment regimens, such as dose, timing or duration of therapy. Sometimes they will be employed to compare a new treatment with 'care as usual' or an active drug with a placebo. Thus, they are experimental studies. Eligible patients are randomised into one or more 'arms'. This structure is referred to as the design of the study. Randomisation helps ensure that there are no systematic differences between individuals in each arm. Some important features of RCTs are:

- Precise specification of study population (eligibility criteria)
- Adequate sample size to detect potential differences in outcomes between the groups
- Randomisation of the sample between arms (e.g. intervention and control groups, or different treatment arms)
- Ensuring that the experience of the two arms is similar (except with regard to the intervention)
- Blinding of participants, professionals and researchers as far as possible to the allocation of participants to intervention or control groups
- Selection of appropriate outcomes measures and methods for collecting relevant data.

When well conducted, RCTs are often seen as a 'gold standard' in research, producing findings that should not be influenced by possible confounding factors and biases. However, in practice they are not always feasible and have some limitations, e.g. restrictive eligibility criteria can confine the study to a non-representative population, blinding may not be achievable because the nature of the intervention may mean that participants will be aware of which group they are in. Sometimes randomisation is not possible; in these cases 'quasi-experimental' designs, which involve 'matching' of intervention and control groups instead of randomisation, may be employed.

References and further reading

Aulton ME (2013). Drying. In: Aulton ME, Taylor KMG (eds), *Aulton's Pharmaceutics: The design and manufacture of medicines*, 4th edn. London: Elsevier, 487–503.

Great Ormond Street Hospital for Children NHS Trust, Royal Marsden NHS Trust, University College London Hospital NHS Trust (2009). *Supportive Care Protocols: Paediatric Haematology & Oncology*. A collaborative publication from Great Ormond Street Hospital for Children NHS Trust, The Royal Marsden NHS Trust, The University College London Hospital NHS Trust.

Case 6
Managing chemotherapy-induced nausea and vomiting in a patient with lung cancer

ADAM TODD AND ANDY HUSBAND

LEARNING OUTCOMES

At the end of this case, you will be able to:

- Outline the emetogenic potential of commonly prescribed chemotherapy drugs
- List the different risk factors for developing chemotherapy-induced nausea and vomiting (CINV)
- Outline the different types of CINV
- Examine the different agents used in the management of CINV
- Outline the chemistry and mechanism of action of ondansetron and palonosetron

Case study

Mrs DM is a 47-year-old woman who has recently been diagnosed with non-small cell lung cancer (NSCLC) of non-squamous histology. Staging of the cancer revealed a tumour in her right lung, approximately 6 cm in diameter; there is local lymph node involvement, but no distant metastasis.

After discussion with the oncologist, Mrs DM was prescribed four cycles of carboplatin and pemetrexed. The administration schedule was as follows:

Dexamethasone 8 mg i.v. bolus
Ondansetron 8 mg i.v. bolus
Pemetrexed 500 mg/m² i.v. infusion
Carboplatin: target AUC = 5 mg min mL⁻¹ i.v. infusion

The Calvert formula for carboplatin dosing takes into consideration the patient's renal function:

$$\text{Total carboplatin dose (mg)} = \text{Target AUC} \times (\text{GFR} + 25)$$

where AUC is the target area under the carboplatin plasma clearance pharmacokinetic time–concentration curve and GFR the glomerular filtration rate (in mL min⁻¹).

— **Discharge medication**

Metoclopramide 10–20 mg four times daily, when required
Ondansetron 8 mg twice a day for 2–3 days
Dexamethasone 4 mg twice a day for 1 day

- What is the difference between nausea and vomiting?
- Explain how CINV is classified
- What is the rationale for prescribing ondansetron, dexamethasone and metoclopramide?

Around 36 hours after her first cycle, Mrs DM has severe nausea and vomits uncontrollably despite having taken her discharge medication as prescribed. The nausea and vomiting eventually subside over a number of days.

- How is the emetic potential of chemotherapy classified?
- What is the emetic potential of the chemotherapy regimen prescribed for Mrs DM?
- What are the risk factors for developing CINV?

For the next cycle, Mrs DM is very anxious about receiving her chemotherapy because 'she hated being sick the last time'. In fact, she is so fearful of being sick again, she is considering stopping her chemotherapy altogether. As she was walking to the oncology day unit (ODU) for her monthly clinic appointment with the oncologist, the smell of the hospital made her nauseous.

❷ What are the options for CINV prophylaxis for Mrs DM's second cycle of chemotherapy?

❷ Why has the hospital environment made Mrs DM nauseous?

As Mrs DM experienced severe CINV after her first cycle of carboplatin and pemetrexed, a decision is made to replace the ondansetron with palonosetron and add aprepitant to her therapy.

❷ What advantages does palonosetron offer over ondansetron?

❷ What is the rationale for using aprepitant?

Case discussion

— Nausea and vomiting

Vomiting (or emesis) is the physical event that results in the forceful evacuation of stomach contents through the mouth, whereas nausea is the sensation of wanting to vomit; it may be accompanied by retching, but without the discharge of the stomach contents. CINV is a major problem with cancer chemotherapy and can have a significant impact on the quality of life of patients, their families and caregivers. Some patients are so fearful of the sickness associated with chemotherapy that potentially curative treatment is either delayed or refused, all of which has negative outcomes for patients.

— Classification of CINV

Broadly speaking, there are three classes of CINV:

1 Acute CINV occurs within 24 hours of receiving chemotherapy

2 Delayed CINV occurs >24 hours after receiving chemotherapy

3 Anticipatory CINV occurs before chemotherapy and is a conditioned response; previous stimuli (such as sights or smells associated with previous chemotherapy cycles) can stimulate it as in the case of Mrs DM.

— Mechanism of CINV

The mechanism of CINV is complex and is thought to involve multiple neurotransmitter systems including: 5-hydroxytriptamine (5HT – also known as serotonin), substance P and dopamine. Briefly, it is thought that administration of chemotherapy (both i.v. and oral formulations) causes, through free radical generation, 5HT release from enterochromaffin cells located in the small intestine. This, in turn, stimulates sensory receptors on vagal afferent nerves in the small intestine to produce a signal that travels to a group of associated cells, known collectively as the nucleus tractus solitarius (NTS), and the chemoreceptor trigger zone (CTZ) in the brain. The NTS and CTZ then activate the vomiting centre (sometimes referred to as the central pattern generator), which results in the initiation of the vomiting reflex.

— Emetic potential of chemotherapy

Not all chemotherapy has the same emetogenic risk; it tends to be categorised by four levels:

- Level 1 (minimal risk: <10%)
- Level 2 (low risk: 10–30%)
- Level 3 (moderate risk: 31–90%)
- Level 4 (high risk: >90%).

The percentage figures indicate the risk of vomiting in the absence of antiemetic prophylaxis. Antiemetic therapy is therefore directed according to the emetic risk of the prescribed chemotherapeutic regimen.

In terms of the chemotherapy prescribed for Mrs DM, carboplatin is level 3 (moderate risk) and pemetrexed level 2 (low risk).

— Antiemetics

There are many agents used for the treatment of CINV, all with differing pharmacology, including ondansetron and palonosetron (selective $5HT_3$ receptor antagonists), dexamethasone (a corticosteroid), metoclopramide (a dopamine D_2-receptor antagonist) and aprepitant (a neurokinin-1 [NK_1]-receptor antagonist). These agents all target signals that contribute to the vomiting reflex.

In the UK, *ondansetron* is the most commonly used $5HT_3$ receptor antagonist; it is one of the most effective antiemetics in the prevention of acute CINV, but is less effective for prevention of delayed CINV, possibly because delayed CINV is thought to be mediated by neurotransmitters other than 5HT. This is why $5HT_3$ antagonists are only used for 2–3 days after chemotherapy.

Palonosetron is a newer $5HT_3$ antagonist and has a significantly longer half-life when compared with other agents in the class (such as ondansetron). It also has a higher binding affinity at $5HT_3$ receptors and, as you would expect, is more effective at preventing CINV – and is significantly more expensive – than ondansetron.

— Chemical properties of ondansetron and palonosetron

Both ondansetron and (more recently) palonosetron are available in oral and parenteral formulations. Both drugs are basic, each containing a single basic nitrogen atom, highlighted in red in the diagram. Ondansetron contains a five-membered imidazole ring. The highlighted nitrogen atom shares one electron with each of the two bonded carbon atoms to form two σ-bonds and contributes one electron to the aromatic π system; it consequently has a free lone pair of electrons (within an sp^2 orbital). The highlighted nitrogen in palonosetron is part of a tertiary amino group; three electrons are shared to form the three σ-bonds, leaving a lone pair of electrons in the remaining sp^3 orbital. None of the remaining nitrogen atoms in either drug are basic centres as none has available lone pairs of electrons. Both drugs are formulated as their hydrochloride salts, which are sufficiently water soluble to allow administration as injections.

ondansetron   palonosetron

Metoclopramide works directly to block dopamine D_2-receptors in the periphery and central nervous system and, at high doses (typically >40 mg/day), also has weak antagonist activity at $5HT_3$ receptors. This explains why high-dose metoclopramide (in this case 10–20 mg four times daily, when required) is used to manage CINV. The higher doses do, however, increase the risk of developing extrapyramidal symptoms such as tardive dyskinesia. Metoclopramide, used in combination with a corticosteroid (e.g. dexamethasone), is useful for preventing delayed CINV.

Dexamethasone is a glucocorticoid, thought to have an effect on both acute and delayed CINV; it is an integral component of almost all antiemetic regimens. The mechanism of action is not entirely clear, but it is thought that inhibition of prostaglandin synthesis plays a part. Dexamethasone has been shown to work better when given in combination with other antiemetics. *Aprepitant* is a NK_1-receptor antagonist and blocks substance P from exerting an effect both peripherally and centrally. The development of the NK_1-receptor antagonists was based on the finding that substance P, when injected intravenously, induced vomiting. When used in addition to standard antiemetic therapy (such as ondansetron and dexamethasone), it significantly improves antiemetic control – particularly with delayed CINV. Aprepitant is an inhibitor of the cytochrome P450 (CYP) enzyme CYP3A4 and an inducer of CYP2C9, so it has the potential to interact with other drugs that are substrates for these important CYP isoforms involved in drug metabolism and clearance.

— Risk factors for CINV

Not all patients have the same risk of CINV – some will experience it, whereas others will not. There are several patient-based factors that can increase the risk of CINV:

- Being female
- Previous nausea and vomiting during pregnancy
- Previous history of motion sickness
- Younger age (typically <50 years)
- Previous uncontrolled CINV
- A history of low alcohol intake.

The evidence for these patient-based risk factors is poor and tends to be based on small-scale studies examining a single regimen of chemotherapy. However, despite this limited evidence, patient-based risk factors do influence prescribing decisions associated with antiemetic treatment.

— Personalised medicine

As we have seen, ondansetron, alongside other antiemetics, is commonly used to prevent CINV due to the antagonistic effects on $5HT_3$ receptors. Ondansetron is metabolised through hydroxylation at positions 7 and 8 by the liver enzymes CYP2D6 and CYP3A4 (Figure 7.2). Once this occurs, the hydroxylated metabolites do not have any antiemetic activity, thus rendering the ondansetron inactive.

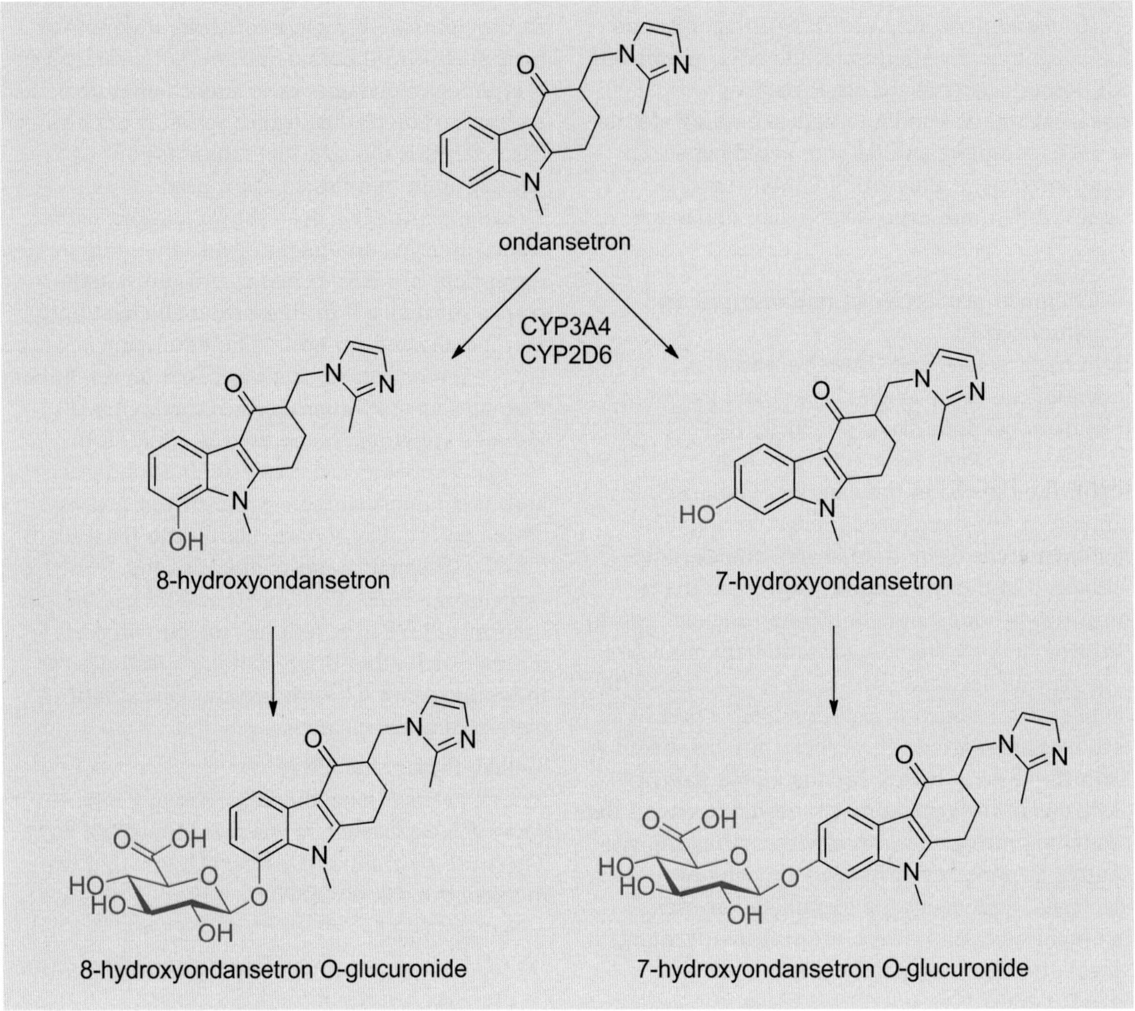

▲ FIGURE 7.2
The metabolism of ondansetron.

Interestingly, the enzyme CYP2D6 has variable activity depending on the patient's genotype. Research suggests that patients who have high CYP2D6 activity (known as ultra-rapid metabolisers) are more likely to have a less than optimal response to ondansetron compared with patients with low CYP2D6 activity (known as poor metabolisers). Screening patients to establish genotype in relation to ondansetron metabolism may therefore help predict which patients will be at risk of antiemetic failure. Such patients may then be prescribed optimised therapy, such as palonosetron and/or aprepitant to reduce the risk of developing CINV. Personalising antiemetic therapy for patients undergoing chemotherapy is therefore a distinct possibility for the future.

EXTENDED LEARNING

- Describe the pharmacological signalling associated with CINV

- What is anticipatory nausea? How can it be managed?

- What drug interactions are associated with aprepitant?

- What is the role of cannabinoid derivatives in the treatment of CINV?

References and further reading

Calvert AH, Newell DR, Gumbrell LA et al. (1989). Carboplatin dosage: prospective evaluation of a simple formula based on renal function. *J Clin Oncol* 7:1748–56.

Grunberg SM, Deuson RR, Mavros P et al. (2004). Incidence of chemotherapy-induced nausea and emesis after modern antiemetics. *Cancer* **100**:2261–28.

Jordan K, Sippel C, Schmoll HJ (2007). Guidelines for antiemetic treatment of chemotherapy-induced nausea and vomiting: past, present, and future recommendations *Oncologist* **12**:1143–50.

Kaiser R, Sezer O, Papies A et al. (2002). Patient-tailored antiemetic treatment with 5-hydroxytryptamine type 3 receptor antagonists according to cytochrome P-450 2D6 genotypes. *J Clin Oncol* **20**:2805–11.

Likun Z Xiang J, Yi B, Xin D, Tao ZL (2011). A systematic review and meta-analysis of intravenous palonosetron in the prevention of chemotherapy-induced nausea and vomiting in adults. *Oncologist* **16**:207–16.

Multinational Association of Supportive Care in Cancer (MASCC) (2013). MASCC/ESMO antiemetic guidelines 2013. Available at: www.mascc.org/antiemetic-guidelines (accessed 1 October 2013).

Sharma R, Tobin P, Clarke SJ (2005). Management of chemotherapy-induced nausea, vomiting, oral mucositis, and diarrhoea. *Lancet Oncol* **6**:93–102.

Case 7
Drug therapy of multiple sclerosis

CHARLES TUGWELL

LEARNING OUTCOMES

At the end of this case, you will be able to:

- Describe the signs and symptoms most commonly associated with MS

- Outline the main means of arriving at a diagnosis of MS

- Describe the disability scale that is used to measure severity of the disease

- Discuss the immediate and longer-term drug treatment options for patients with MS, including their adverse effects

Case study

Mr RW is 29 years old and has been admitted onto your ward for investigations under the care of the neurologists. He has been suffering for more than 2 weeks with pain in his left eye and increasing difficulty in walking due to his legs feeling very heavy and fatigued. He had a similar episode 8 months ago, which resolved without treatment over a period of 3 weeks. Mr RW states that the symptoms are more severe this time and understandably they are making him very anxious. He has been told on this occasion that there is a possibility that he has multiple sclerosis (MS). The neurologist has assessed Mr RW using the Expanded Disability Status Scale; the result was 6.0.

- Comment on Mr RW's presenting symptoms. Are they typical for a patient with MS?
- On the assumption that he does have MS, what is the likely cause of his eye pain?

- List the other common signs/symptoms that can be associated with MS
- What investigations or tests do you think would be appropriate to carry out?
- Briefly outline the relevance of the result using the Expanded Disability Status Scale

The results of Mr RW's scan are available and confirm the provisional diagnosis of MS. Treatment with methylprednisolone was commenced yesterday and he is told that a diagnosis of MS is confirmed. He is informed by his neurologist that various forms of ongoing drug therapy can help with the condition, and he is given a very brief outline of these. During your regular clinical ward round, he wants to discuss potential drug therapies with you and asks that you explain in more detail the drugs that can be used; he was told by the neurologist that these are known as 'disease-modifying drugs'.

- Why has methylprednisolone been prescribed? Outline the route, dosage and duration of this form of treatment that would be appropriate for Mr RW
- List the 'disease-modifying drugs' available for treating MS at this stage of Mr RW's disease. What benefits do they produce in clinical outcome terms?

Mr RW has now been in hospital for 9 days. He feels much better; the pain in his eye has resolved and he finds walking much easier (at times it is more or less normal). Having had several discussions with you and the neurologists, he has decided to proceed with a 'disease-modifying drug' and feels that Avonex would be the most convenient. He has come to this conclusion after discussing with you the advantages and disadvantages of the products available.

❓ What is Avonex? What is the probable reason for him to choose this product over the others available?

❓ What are the side effects that can occur with this drug? Which common side effect should you warn him about, for which you might advise him to take a drug that is very frequently used as an analgesic?

❓ Which drugs in this class would you recommend?

You see Mr RW in your regular clinic session 3 months later. He is pleased with the treatment because he has had no further relapses. Results of his blood tests are within the normal range. Although delighted about being free of relapses, you notice that Mr RW does not seem overly happy. You make a further appointment to see him in 2 months time. At this appointment it is clear that Mr RW is quite depressed, a fact that he readily acknowledges. You discuss this development with his neurologist who agrees with your proposed course of action to change his 'disease-modifying drug'.

❓ Comment on the development of depression in this patient

❓ Which other 'disease-modifying drug' would you recommend and why?

❓ What are the possible side effects associated with this drug?

The change in therapy that you have recommended is tolerated with no apparent side effects and works well for 3 years. However, Mr RW has had a number of relapses in recent months, and recovery after each episode no longer seems to be complete. The neurologist examines and reassesses him and arranges for repeat MRI. When the scan is available, the neurologist concludes that Mr RW's condition is now 'rapidly evolving'. He discusses a form of licensed drug therapy that is more specific for this severity of MS. Mr RW is then referred to you so that you can provide him with further details. You explain that this form of therapy consists of a regular intravenous infusion every 4 weeks.

❓ Which drug, given as an intravenous infusion, is available and approved by NICE for use in specific patients with rapidly evolving MS?

❓ Briefly outline the pharmacology of this drug and give details of the dose and administration for the drug

❓ Which potentially fatal adverse effect can occur with this form of therapy that the patient must be warned of, even though it occurs rarely?

Case discussion

— Symptoms, signs and diagnosis of multiple sclerosis

Multiple sclerosis is a chronic incurable autoimmune disease that is characterised by neuroinflammation, axonal demyelination and axonal damage. Mr RW's presentation is characteristic of relapsing–remitting MS (RRMS), a condition that develops about once or twice a year, usually with good remission in between, but with a disposition towards recurrence and worsening of attacks with time. The eye pain is probably due to optic neuritis (inflammation of the optic nerve). This is a presenting symptom in approximately a quarter of patients; the pain is often made worse by eye movement and is accompanied by tenderness of the eyeball. Sometimes, patients have double or blurred vision. The other symptoms that Mr RW experiences are typical. The limbs often feel stiff and heavy, making walking difficult; sometimes the foot will tend to drag. Muscle fatigue is a common symptom associated with MS.

Other symptoms and signs that can be associated with MS include:

- Numbness or tingling feeling – typically in the limbs or face
- Impaired coordination and balance
- Bladder problems
- Memory impairment
- Difficulty in concentrating
- General tiredness and fatigue
- Pain
- Hyposmia (reduced ability to smell).

The history given by Mr RW is in line with a diagnosis of MS. He should have an MRI scan and blood tests to rule out other conditions, which may present in a similar way to MS. Sometimes, other tests may be carried out including lumbar puncture, evoked potentials and electrical tests of nerve function.

— Expanded Disability Status Scale

The Expanded Disability Status Scale (EDSS) is used to measure the severity of functional

▼ TABLE 7.3
The Expanded Disability Status Scale

Score	Severity of function
0.0	Normal neurological examination
1.0–2.0	No disability; minimal signs
2.0–3.0	Minimal disability, but fully ambulatory
3.0–4.0	Moderate disability, but fully ambulatory
4.0–5.0	Relatively severe disability, e.g. able to walk without aid for 500 m
5.0–6.0	Disability impairs full daily activities; ambulatory without aid for about 200 m
6.0–7.0	Assistance required to walk
7.0–8.0	Restricted to a wheelchair
8.0–9.0	Restricted to bed or chair
9.0–10.0	Confined to bed
10.0	Death

Adapted from MSdecisions.org.uk (an independent source of assistance and advice funded by the Department of Health).

disability in MS. This rates a patient's functionality from 0 (normal neurological function) to 10 (death due to MS). A score of 6.0 reflects Mr RW's problems with walking. An abridged version of the assessment scale is given in Table 7.3.

The EDSS steps 1.0–4.5 refer to people with MS who are fully ambulatory. EDSS steps 5.0–9.5 are defined by the impairment of ambulation.

It has been shown that the EDSS correlates with measures of health-related quality of life in MS, but the relationship is weak and therefore additional measures of quality of life may reveal less obvious aspects of life that are affected by the disease, such as everyday tasks, independence and decision-making, relationships and long-term goals.

Scales to rate health status and health-related quality of life are commonly used to measure the impact of long-term conditions. These scales are often classified as either 'generic measures', which are those that can be used in many population groups to provide a measure of overall health-related quality of life (e.g. SF-36), or 'disease-specific measures', which focus on the impact of a condition on particular aspects of health status. The EDSS is a measure of disability in MS, and is therefore a disease-specific measure.

— Treatment of patients who have MS
Treatment of acute attacks: High-dose corticosteroids (typically methylprednisolone, a synthetic glucocorticoid) are used to treat acute attacks of MS. Methylprednisolone can speed up the recovery from an acute attack. Mr RW was prescribed a 5-day course of intravenous methylprednisolone at a dose of 1 g daily. It should be noted that a course of steroids has no long-term effect on the disease. The dosage is usually 500 mg or 1 g intravenously for 3–5 days. Oral methylprednisolone can also be given in high doses. This is more convenient for patients who have an acute attack, but do not require admission to hospital. It is not considered necessary to gradually taper the dose when stopping the drug after a course such as this.

— Chemistry and properties of methylprednisolone
The form of methylprednisolone used for intravenous administration differs from that used for oral administration. Like most steroids, methylprednisolone is a highly lipophilic drug with poor water solubility. The drug lacks sufficient water solubility for formulation as an injection and is converted to the sodium salt of the succinate ester for intravenous use. Methylprednisolone sodium succinate is much more polar and water soluble than methylprednisolone itself. The succinate ester is hydrolysed by plasma and hepatic esterases.

— Disease-modifying drugs for treatment of MS
Specific disease-modifying drugs for treating MS have been available for more than 15 years and are well established. Interferon-β and glatiramer acetate are suitable drugs for treating Mr RW's condition. These drugs reduce the frequency and severity of relapses. They may also decrease the disability occurring from progressive relapses as the disease advances. Table 7.4 summarises the interferon-β and glatiramer acetate products available in the UK.

— Use of Avonex (interferon-β1a)
Avonex contains interferon-β1a (a glycoprotein of 166 amino acids, with a molecular mass of approximately 22.5 kDa, produced by recombinant DNA technology) and is injected once weekly at a dose of 30 micrograms (6 million units). It is the only product that is suitable for once-weekly injection and therefore patients who prefer not to have the worry or inconvenience of a higher

methylprednisolone

methylprednisolone sodium succinate

frequency of injection may choose this option. However, unlike the other products, Avonex needs to be given by intramuscular injection (the others are subcutaneous). Avonex is available as a prefilled syringe or pen device, or as a sterile lyophilised powder, for injection after reconstitution with Water for Injections.

The side effects and efficacy of the interferon-β1a and interferon-β1b products are considered to be similar. The most commonly encountered side effects are:

- Injection site reaction
- Flu-like symptoms
- Depression and mood changes
- Short-term increase in spasticity
- Increased blood levels of liver enzymes
- Leukopenia, thrombocytopenia, anaemia.

The flu-like side effects (fever, chills, aching muscles) tend to diminish as treatment continues over the first few months. However, at the start of treatment, these symptoms can be quite severe. Many patients find that paracetamol 1 g taken 30 min before the injection, then every 4–6 hours, is helpful (only two to four doses are usually necessary). Alternatively, ibuprofen can be taken if preferred.

— Using an alternative to interferon-β1

A significant number of patients with MS develop depression as a co-morbidity. This can be severe and can warrant discontinuing interferon-β. One of the contraindications to using interferon-β is a history of severe depressive illness. In such a situation, the use of glatiramer acetate is more appropriate. Glatiramer (Copaxone) is a 6.4-kDa polymer consisting of four amino acids – glutamic acid, lysine, alanine and tyrosine (present in myelin basic protein) – available as a 20 mg/mL solution in a pre-filled syringe for injection given subcutaneously once a day.

Although glatiramer acetate itself is not without potential side effects, most patients tolerate the drug well. The side effects that can be associated with glatiramer acetate include:

- Injection site reactions
- Flushing of chest or face
- Palpitations
- Tightness in the chest
- Shortness of breath

▼ TABLE 7.4

The interferon-β and glatiramer acetate products available in the UK

Proprietary name	Drug	Route	Maintenance dose	Frequency
Avonex	Interferon-β1a	Intramuscular injection	30 micrograms (6 million units)	One injection each week
Betaferon	Interferon-β1b	Subcutaneous injection	250 micrograms (8 million units)	One injection on alternate days
Copaxone	Glatiramer acetate	Subcutaneous injection	20 mg	One injection each day
Extavia	Interferon-β1b	Subcutaneous injection	250 micrograms (8 million units)	One injection on alternate days
Rebif	Interferon-β1a	Subcutaneous injection	22 micrograms (6 million units) or 44 micrograms (12 million units)	One injection three times a week

- Nausea
- Headache.

Similar to interferon-β, glatiramer acetate can cause depression and flu-like symptoms, but these are less common.

It is suggested that interferon-β may exert its anti-inflammatory and immunomodulatory effects by inhibiting the activation and proliferation of T cells involved in the autoimmune response, and release of proinflammatory cytokines in the peripheral and central nervous systems. Glatiramer is also believed to act as an immunomodulator by altering the properties of proinflammatory T cells, involved in the pathogenesis of MS.

— Rapidly evolving MS

Natalizumab (Tysabri) is licensed for use in the UK for the management of patients who have a rapidly evolving form of relapsing–remitting MS (REMS). It was approved by NICE in 2007 for use in the NHS in patients meeting certain criteria, i.e. patients with REMS that is severe and rapidly evolving. NICE defined this as having two or more disabling relapses within 1 year, and one or more gadolinium-enhancing lesions showing on a MRI scan or a significant increase in T2 lesion load compared with that shown on a previous MRI scan.

Natalizumab is a humanised monoclonal antibody that binds to the cellular adhesion molecule $\alpha_4\beta_1$-integrin. It works by reducing the passage of inflammatory immune cells into the brain, which lead to the MS lesions in the CNS.

The dose of natalizumab is 300 mg every 4 weeks given by intravenous infusion over 1 hour. Patients should be monitored during the infusion and for 1 hour afterwards for any signs of adverse reactions. Cases of anaphylaxis have occurred. If a severe hypersensitivity reaction does occur, treatment with this drug should be discontinued.

Cases of progressive multifocal leukoencephalopathy (PML – a viral disease causing progressive damage of central white matter in immunosuppressed patients) have been reported after the use of natalizumab. This is a very serious adverse effect that can prove fatal. It is therefore important that patients on natalizumab are regularly monitored for symptoms that may indicate the development of PML. This can be difficult because the first neurological signs may be indistinguishable from those of the patient's MS.

EXTENDED LEARNING

- MS can produce a range of symptoms. List these symptoms, together with a summary of drug therapies that are used to provide symptomatic treatment
- What new therapies are in the pipeline for the management of MS?
- Describe developments in the use of recombinant DNA technology for the production of biopharmaceuticals
- What are the funding arrangements for disease-modifying therapies? How do these relate to: risk-sharing schemes, NICE recommendations, payment by results (PBR), exclusions and commissioning arrangements?
- There are marked inequalities in levels of disability due to long-term health conditions between populations across the world. How can these be explained?

ADDITIONAL PRACTICE POINT

- The EDSS is one example of a disease-specific measure of functioning, which measures the limitations in functioning experienced by people with MS. The choice of a measure may be influenced by its psychometric properties. What is meant by this?

References and further reading

Dhib-Jalbut S, Marks S (2010). Interferon-beta mechanisms of action in multiple sclerosis. *Neurology* **74**(Suppl 1):S17–24.

Kurtzke JF (1983). Rating neurologic impairment in multiple sclerosis: an expanded disability status scale (EDSS). *Neurology* **33**:1444–52.

Mitchell AJ, Benito-León J, Morales González J-M, Rivera-Navarro J (2005). Quality of life and its assessment in multiple sclerosis: integrating physical and psychological components of wellbeing. *Lancet Neurol* **4**:556–66.

National Institute for Health and Clinical Excellence (2003). *Management of Multiple Sclerosis in Primary and Secondary Care.* Clinical Guideline 8. London: NICE. Available at: http://guidance.nice.org.uk/CG8 (accessed 1 October 2013).

Rolet A, Magnin E, Millot JL et al. (2013). Olfactory dysfunction in multiple sclerosis: evidence of a decrease in different aspects of olfactory function. *Eur Neurol* **69**: 166–70.

Tugwell C, Giovannoni G (2010). The treatment of multiple sclerosis: update on oral therapies. *Hosp Pharmacy Europe* **51**:42–5.

Case 8
Management of vaso-occlusive crisis in sickle cell disease

STEPHANIE KIRSCHKE

LEARNING OUTCOMES

At the end of the case, you will be able to:

- Outline the pathophysiology of sickle cell disease (SCD) and common clinical complications
- Understand the rationale of pharmacological prevention measures in SCD
- Outline the structure and metabolism of opioids
- Describe the mechanisms by which opioids produce pain relief
- Describe the management of a vaso-occlusive crisis

Case study

Mr JD is a 21-year-old African–Caribbean man who has a diagnosis of sickle cell disease (Hb SS). His disease was generally mild in nature with very few complications. However, over the last 2 years, Mr JD experienced five episodes of severe vaso-occlusive crises (VOCs) requiring hospitalisation.

At his most recent hospital admission, Mr JD was complaining of flu-like symptoms over the previous 3 days, sharp pain in both legs and abdomen for 1 day, productive cough, lethargy and loss of appetite.

His drug therapy on admission was:

Phenoxymethylpenicillin 250 mg b.d.
Folic acid 5 mg o.d.
Paracetamol 1 g q.d.s.
Codeine phosphate 30 mg q.d.s. p.r.n.

❷ What is sickle cell disease (SCD)?
❷ What are the common complications of SCD?
❷ How is VOC managed?

Initially Mr JD received 2.5 mg diamorphine subcutaneously every 2 hours when needed. On day 2 of admission, Mr JD has been started on a diamorphine PCA (patient-controlled analgesia).

❷ What are the advantages of PCA?

❷ Compare the structures of codeine and diamorphine and explain how both are related to the active metabolite, morphine
❷ How do opioids exert their pharmacological pain-relieving effects in the body?
❷ What is a pain measurement scale?

Mr JD is on 2-hourly incentive spirometry.

❷ What is incentive spirometry and what is the rationale for its use in SCD?

On day 4, Mr JD was complaining of worsening abdominal pain. He had an enlarged, palpable spleen, the Hb count was 4.9 g/dL (8.5 g/dL on admission). Mr JD was transfused with 3 units blood to correct his Hb count.

❷ What was the likely cause of Mr JD's abdominal pain, spleen enlargement and the drop in Hb?

At his follow-up appointment, Mr JD has been started on hydroxycarbamide.

❷ What is the rationale for treatment with hydroxycarbamide?
❷ What are the monitoring requirements?

Case discussion

— Causes and pathophysiology of SCD

Sickle cell disease – or sickle cell anaemia – is an inherited blood disorder that affects red blood cells (RBCs). The protein part of normal adult haemoglobin (HbA), the oxygen-carrying component of RBCs, consists of four peptide chains – two α chains and two β chains. Point mutation of the β-globin gene leads to the substitution of valine for glutamic acid in the β-globin chain, resulting in sickle haemoglobin (HbS). Individuals who carry two sickle cell genes (HbSS) have sickle cell disease. Homozygous SCD (HbSS) is the most common sickle genotype and most severe form of SCD. HbSC (sickle cell haemoglobin C disease) and HbS/thalassaemia are sickle genotypes with a less severe clinical picture. The presence of one normal haemoglobin gene (HbA) and one sickle cell gene (HbS) constitutes sickle cell trait (HbAS) but the individual has no disease.

The sickle haemoglobin is poorly soluble and crystallises in the deoxygenated state, causing RBCs to be sickle-shaped and making them rigid. The sickling process is reversible on reoxygenation. Repeated sickling, however, damages the membrane of the RBCs, leading eventually to irreversibly sickled cells and premature red cell destruction (chronic haemolytic anaemia). Sickled RBCs have lost their membrane flexibility and form aggregates that obstruct smaller blood vessels and reduce blood flow to organs, resulting in ischaemia, pain, tissue necrosis and often organ damage.

Common complications of SCD

— Infection

Life-threatening bacterial infections are a major cause of morbidity and mortality in patients with SCD. Recurrent occlusions of the splenic vasculature induce splenic infarction, which leads to functional hyposplenism or autosplenectomy, predisposing to severe infections with encapsulated organisms, e.g. *Streptococcus pneumoniae* or *Haemophilus influenzae*. *Salmonella* sp. is the common organism to cause osteomyelitis in infarcted bone. People with SCD need to keep their immunisation up to date, including *Haemophilus influenzae*, pneumococcal, meningococcal, hepatitis B (recommended for all patients with HbSS; mandatory for patients receiving blood transfusions) and influenza immunisations. Currently, infants with SCD should receive the conjugated pneumococcal vaccine (Prevenar 13), followed by the standard 23-valent vaccine (Pneumovax II), which is given at the age of 2 years and repeated at 5-yearly intervals. Pneumococcal prophylaxis with oral phenoxymethylpenicillin should start at the age of 3 months.

— Vaso-occlusive crisis

Acute painful crisis is a common sequela that can cause significant morbidity and negatively impact on the patient's quality of life. Although the exact cause of an acute sickle cell crisis cannot always be determined, there are a number of factors known to precipitate acute crises: dehydration, infection, sudden changes in temperature, low oxygen tension, strenuous exercise and psychological stress.

Patients need to be aware of these factors and should be counselled to keep hydrated during hot weather, wear warm clothes in cold weather and avoid exercising to exhaustion.

— Haemolytic crisis

The term 'haemolytic crisis' refers to an acute reduction in Hb levels; this is particularly common in SCD patients who lack the enzyme glucose-6-phosphate dehydrogenase (G6PD deficiency). Due to the high RBC turnover in SCD, folate stores are often depleted. Folic acid supplementation should therefore be taken for healthy regeneration of new RBCs.

— Splenic sequestration

Sickling with pooling of blood in the spleen leads to rapid spleen enlargement and a decrease in Hb levels. This can result in life-threatening circulatory collapse due to the loss of circulating blood volume. In these cases, urgent simple (top-up) transfusions are indicated.

— Acute chest syndrome

A life-threatening vaso-occlusive crisis involving the lungs may develop after an acute chest infection or painful crisis affecting the back or ribs. Acute chest syndrome is the most common cause of death and one of the most common causes of hospital admission for patients with SCD.

— Stroke

Vaso-occlusion of the cerebral vessels leads to infarction. Children usually present with ischaemic stroke, but haemorrhagic stroke is more common in adults. Urgent exchange transfusion is warranted in cerebrovascular events, followed by a transfusion programme for secondary stroke prevention.

— Eye problems

Sequestration of RBCs in the conjunctival vessels leads to retinopathy and sight impairment.

— Bone and joint problems

Inadequate circulation of the blood in bone tissue causes bone infarction and osteonecrosis. Bones of the thighs, legs and arms are most commonly affected, with permanent damage or deformation of the hips, shoulders or knees. Total joint replacement may be needed to restore function.

— Leg ulcers

Vaso-occlusive injury to the skin of the legs or ankles can promote skin damage and ulceration. Leg ulcers most commonly occur in adults and usually form over the ankles and sides of the lower legs. Due to impaired wound healing, the ulcers can become severe and are prone to infection.

— Use of analgesia to manage VOC

Painful crises typically affect the back, legs, knees, arms and abdomen. The severity of pain varies widely between patients. Patients with a mild crisis may manage at home with simple analgesia (paracetamol, NSAIDs or weak opioids), bed rest and increased fluid intake. Some patients may experience excruciating pain, necessitating hospital admission and the use of strong opioids for pain control.

Pain management should follow the WHO three-step 'ladder'. Pain scales are a useful tool for quantifying the intensity of pain and assessing the degree of pain relief while on analgesia. Patients with severe pain should receive parenteral opioids in appropriate therapeutic doses at fixed intervals combined with regular paracetamol and an NSAID (if no contraindications). The usual starting dose of subcutaneous diamorphine is 2.5–5 mg, which can be repeated at 15 to 20-min intervals until pain has been controlled. If pain persists, subcutaneous diamorphine is administered 2-hourly when needed at a dosage required to achieve good pain control, or patient-controlled analgesia (PCA, see below) is initiated. Careful monitoring of the respiratory rate, oxygen saturation and sedation score is necessary during opioid therapy. To manage potential opioid side effects, antiemetics (e.g. cyclizine), laxatives (e.g. senna, lactulose), anti-pruritus medicines (e.g.

hydroxyzine) and naloxone (opiate receptor antagonist for reversal of opioid-induced respiratory depression) should be prescribed. Once the pain diminishes, the opioid doses are tapered and the patient switched to oral analgesic therapy.

— Opioid structure and metabolism: morphine, codeine and diamorphine

Codeine is the 3-O-methylated derivative of morphine. It has very little analgesic activity itself but a small proportion of it (around 10%) undergoes O-demethylation in the liver (catalysed by the cytochrome P450 enzyme CYP2D6) to morphine, which is mostly responsible for its analgesic activity. The analgesic activity of morphine is due to activation of μ opioid receptors. Up to 10% of individuals lack the CYP2D6 isoform and therefore experience very little or no pain relief with codeine. Other drugs that inhibit CYP2D6 also have the potential to reduce the analgesic effect of codeine through inhibition of conversion to morphine.

Diamorphine (diacetylmorphine; heroin) is similarly inactive. When administered subcutaneously, hydrolysis of both ester groups by plasma and tissue esterases produces morphine as an active metabolite. Hydrolysis of the 3-O-acetyl group alone gives 6-acetylmorphine, which is a more potent μ-receptor agonist than morphine itself. Diamorphine is more lipophilic than morphine and readily penetrates the blood–brain barrier to exert central effects. Ester hydrolysis in CNS tissues releases both active metabolites resulting in intense euphoria, making diamorphine highly addictive and thus prone to abuse.

Opiate drugs, similar to morphine and codeine are derived from the opium poppy *Papaver somniferum* and, unlike general anaesthetics, produce their central analgesic effects without loss of consciousness or vital functions. They do this by modulating the sensory pain information normally relayed from primary ascending pain fibres (Aδ and C fibres) through the spinal cord to central brain stem (and higher) processing sites by interacting with G-protein-coupled opioid receptors – μ, δ and κ – which are widely distributed in the CNS. These receptors are also the targets for endogenously produced opiate analgesic peptides, such as the endorphins and enkephalins.

— Patient-controlled analgesia

A PCA system allows the patient to self-administer analgesia by using a computerised pump. Before initiating PCA, it has to be established that the patient understands the principles of PCA and is willing to assume the responsibility of managing the pain. During an acute sickle cell crisis, most patients require a continuous background infusion of the analgesic plus demand doses for breakthrough pain. To minimise the risk of overdose, the size of the bolus dose and the minimum time interval between doses (lockout time) is pre-set (e.g. diamorphine PCA, bolus dose = 3 mg [range 2–10 mg], lockout time = 30 min [range 20–30 min], continuous infusion dose = 2.5 mg/h [range 0–10 mg/h]).

The patient can be weaned off PCA if the pain has fully settled or the patient has only mild pain with low opioid requirements and is able to tolerate oral medication. The patient should be maintained on oral analgesia for 12–24 hours with regular pain assessment before discharge.

— Advantages of PCA

- Reduces the time between perception of pain and the administration of the analgesic; no need to wait for nursing staff to administer dose
- No need for repeated injections, which can cause pain and discomfort at the injection site
- Reduced workload for nursing staff (no preparation of single doses)
- Provides a measurement of the severity of pain
- Patients have control over their pain and are involved in their own care.

— Measurement of pain: pain scales

Pain may be measured by using daily pain diaries, which can be used to record the presence or absence of pain, the intensity of pain, pain location, pain descriptors and precipitants of pain. Alternatively, pain measurement scales may be employed. These are questionnaire-based instruments that have been developed specifically to assist in the assessment of pain. Many types are available and the choice of instrument will depend on the characteristics of both the patient (e.g. age, cognitive ability) and the instrument (e.g. number of questions, reliability and validity). Single-item measures of pain such as a visual analogue scale (VAS) are frequently used for acute pain and are popular due to their simplicity and speed of administration. However, they measure only one aspect of pain (e.g. intensity) and do not indicate the quality of the pain. Multidimensional measures such as the McGill Pain Questionnaire (Melzack and Katz, 2001) allow for different aspects of pain to be measured such as the perception of pain, emotional response to pain and intensity of pain.

Publication of scales will include information about the instrument's properties such as reliability and validity, which will help to determine the appropriateness of the instrument for the purpose for which it is intended. Reliability is an indication of the random error associated with the measurement of pain. Validity is the extent to which the instrument measures the concept of pain and may be determined by considering the relationship between the pain measure and related variables such as disability and mood. The availability of the instrument in multiple languages may be a further consideration.

— Other approaches in the management of VOC

Fluids: dehydration occurs readily in patients with SCD due to an impaired ability to concentrate urine. Hyperhydration should be started on admission with daily reviews of fluid requirements. A fluid chart with careful recording of fluid input and output is used to monitor the hydration therapy. Hydration is usually administered parenterally, but can also be given orally in the less-ill patient who is able to drink the required amount.

Oxygen: this should be administered if the patient is hypoxic and has an underlying pulmonary problem. If the patient has only limb pain and normal oxygen saturation, oxygen may be given if the patient requests it. Oxygen saturation should be monitored by pulse oximetry with regular readings of room air.

Antibiotics: infection is a common precipitating factor of a painful sickle cell crisis. Antibiotics are given for the treatment of suspected or confirmed infections. Cephalosporins (e.g. i.v. cefuroxime), macrolides (e.g. oral clarithromycin) or amoxicillin–clavulanic acid are common first-line antibiotics.

Incentive spirometry

The incentive spirometer measures the inspiratory capacity of the lungs and encourages deep inspiratory effort. It is used to prevent or reverse pulmonary complications (e.g. acute chest syndrome) during a VOC. The patient breathes in as slowly and deeply as possible through the spirometer mouthpiece, with the aim of reaching a set inspiration volume. The exercise should be repeated 5–10 times every 2 hours.

Hydroxycarbamide (hydroxyurea) is an anti-neoplastic drug that can be used to reduce the frequency of painful sickle cell crises, acute chest syndrome, and the transfusion requirements in adults and children with severe SCD. The drug acts by increasing the amount of fetal haemoglobin (HbF) in the blood, most likely by increasing endogenous levels of nitric oxide (NO) messenger and stimulating production of intracellular cyclic guanosine monophosphate (cGMP). HbF then interacts with HbS, preventing the tendency of RBCs to sickle.

The starting dose of hydroxycarbamide is 15 mg/kg per day and can be increased by increments of 5 mg/kg per day every 4 weeks to a maximum of 30 mg/kg per day to achieve a response. Discontinuation of treatment should be considered if there is no clinical improvement after 9–12 months. Renal function, liver function, percentage of HbF (HbF%) and FBCs have to be monitored on a regular basis.

Hydroxycarbamide can be toxic to the bone marrow. Low blood counts require cessation of treatment until blood counts recover, at which point treatment can be resumed at a reduced dose. Patients should be counselled to contact their doctor immediately if they experience nose bleeds, increased bruising, develop fever or suffer from shortness of breath and fatigue while taking hydroxycarbamide.

EXTENDED LEARNING

- Differentiate between the terms 'opiate' and 'opioid'
- Outline the medical uses of opioid analgesics
- What are the various routes by which injections may be administered parenterally?
- How are injections formulated, manufactured, sterilised and packaged?

References and further reading

Ataga KI (2009). Novel therapies in sickle cell disease. *Hematology* 54–61.

Ball S (2004). Congenital disorders of haemoglobin and blood cells. *Medicine* **32**:520–7.

Ballas SK (2007). Current issues in sickle cell pain and its management. *Hematology* 97–105.

Bellet PS, Kalinyak KA, Shukla R, Gelfand MJ, Rucknagel DL (1995). Incentive spirometry to prevent acute pulmonary complications in sickle cell disease. *N Engl J Med* **333**:699–703.

Jensen MP, Karoly P (2001). Self-report scales and procedures for assessing pain in adults. In: Turk DC, Melzack R (eds), *Handbook of Pain Assessment*, 2nd edn. New York: Guilford Press, 15–34.

Melzack R, Katz J (2001). The McGill Pain Questionnaire: Appraisal and current status. In: Turk DC, Melzack R (eds), *Handbook of Pain Assessment*, 2nd edn. New York: Guilford Press, 35–52.

National Institute for Health and Care Excellence (2013). *Sickle Cell Acute Painful Episode: Management of an acute painful sickle cell episode in hospital.* NICE Clinical Guideline 143. London: NICE.

Rees DC, Olujohungbe AD, Parker NE, Stephens AD, Telfer P, Wright J (2003). Management of acute painful crisis in sickle cell disease. *Br J Haematol* **120**:744–52.

Sickle Cell Society (2008). *Standards for the Clinical Care of Adults with Sickle Cell Disease in the UK.* London: Sickle Cell Society.

Ware RE, Aygun B (2009). Advances in the use of hydroxyurea. *Hematology* 62–9.

8

Musculoskeletal and joint disease cases

INTRODUCTION

This section comprises six varied examples of musculoskeletal disease. These are potentially long-term conditions, for which medication is commonly the mainstay of treatment. The cases focus on gout, low-back pain, DMARDs for rheumatoid arthritis, glucosamine for osteoarthritis, juvenile idiopathic arthritis and systemic lupus erythematosus.

Case 1
Gout ► 311

A patient asks a pharmacist about pain in his toe and the pharmacist suspects that this may be gout. This case outlines the pathophysiology, signs and symptoms of gout. It discusses the rationale for the management of an acute attack, including relief from symptoms and lifestyle actions to reduce the likelihood of recurrence. The case also considers long-term prophylactic treatment options.

Case 2
Approaches to the effective treatment of non-specific, low back pain ► 314

This case is a common presentation in a community pharmacy. It considers the place of medication (especially analgesia) in the management of low back pain, alongside possible non-pharmacological interventions. 'Red flag' signs that would warrant a referral are raised. A treatment ladder can provide a strategy for selection of appropriate analgesics. This case focuses particularly on actions and potential complications of non-steroidal anti-inflammatory drugs (NSAIDs), which, although widely used, present significant risks that must be weighed carefully against potential benefits.

Case 3
DMARDs and treatment for rheumatoid arthritis ► 317

This case outlines the pathogenesis, classic symptoms and diagnosis of rheumatoid arthritis. A class of drugs referred to as 'disease-modifying anti-rheumatic drugs' is prominent in its treatment. The place of DMARDs and biological agents is outlined. The case focuses particularly on methotrexate and sulfasalazine, discussing the chemistry, modes of action, counselling points and monitoring for these drugs.

Case 4
Glucosamine supplements for osteoarthritis and joint stiffness ► 324

This case concerns a patient who has been recommended glucosamine for joint stiffness by a friend. It examines the chemistry and physiological properties of glucosamine and its place in the treatment of joint problems. It highlights the uncertainty surrounding the strength of the evidence base to support its use.

Case 5
Treating juvenile idiopathic arthritis in young people ► 327

This case focuses on a 15-year-old boy, and so highlights special considerations in providing care for young people. It looks at important differences in arthritic disease and its management in adolescents and adults. Adherence to medicine regimens is known to be poor among young people with long-term conditions. Providing support requires service provision that is sensitive to their needs, priorities and perspectives.

Case 6
Systemic lupus erythematosus ► 331

This case outlines the pathophysiology, known triggers and presentation of systemic lupus erythematosus (SLE). It summarises the use of different DMARDs, when there is no major organ involvement, as well as considerations when there are renal complications. The newer monoclonal antibody treatments are also discussed.

Case 1
Gout

GEMMA QUINN

LEARNING OUTCOMES

At the end of this case, you will be able to:

- Outline the pathophysiology and signs and symptoms of gout
- Identify the risk factors for gout, including drug-related causes
- Construct an appropriate short- and long-term treatment plan for gout

Case study

Mr JG is a 59-year-old white man who is a solicitor for a local company. He brought in his usual prescription for bendroflumethiazide 2.5 mg daily and asked for something to help control the pain in his left toe, which he said was red and felt hot. After asking some questions about Mr JG's lifestyle, including his diet and alcohol intake, the pharmacist told him that she thought that he had gout and referred him to his GP.

- ❓ What are the signs and symptoms of gout?
- ❓ What are the risk factors for developing gout?
- ❓ What are the alternative diagnoses when suspecting gout?

Mr JG returned to the pharmacy later that day with a prescription for indometacin capsules 50 mg three times a day and losartan 25 mg daily. The pharmacist issued the prescription and counselled him on his new medication. Mr JG explained that his blood pressure medication had been changed and asked whether there was anything else he could do to prevent another attack of gout.

- ❓ How should an attack of gout be treated?
- ❓ What are the lifestyle changes that can be made to reduce the risk of another gout attack?

Mr JG returned to the pharmacy 6 months later with another attack of gout. This time he brought a prescription for:

Indometacin capsules 50 mg three times a day
Allopurinol 300 mg daily
Colchicine 500 micrograms twice daily

The pharmacist dispensed the drugs and counselled him on his medication.

- ❓ When should long-term treatment be initiated for gout patients?
- ❓ What are the regimens of choice?

The next time Mr JG came into the pharmacy he said that he'd been asked to get some blood tests done and asked the pharmacist how often this was likely to happen because it was difficult for him to get away from work.

- ❓ How should treatment be monitored?

Case discussion

— The pathophysiology, signs and symptoms of gout

Gout is a common disease in both primary and secondary care, and is characterised by painful, red, hot and swollen joints, with shiny overlaying skin that may flake. It usually affects the first metatarsophalangeal joint (big toe), but can also affect other joints, including the ankles, knees, elbows, wrists and fingers.

Gout is caused by hyperuricaemia (high levels of uric acid in the blood), which eventually results in the deposition of monosodium urate crystals within the joints. It is important to note that hyperuricaemia does not necessarily result in gout, and that gout can also occur at relatively low blood urate levels.

— Risk factors for developing gout

Men are more often affected than women (ratio of 3.6 : 1) and incidence increases with age, with a prevalence of 7% and 4% in men and women aged >75 years, respectively.

Hyperuricaemia can occur as a result of under-excretion and/or over-production of urate. Urate is mainly (>70%) excreted by the proximal tubule of the kidney as the final oxidation product of purine metabolism in the body; therefore renal impairment is a common cause. Other causes of under-excretion include hypertension and hypothyroidism, as well as several drugs, e.g. low-dose aspirin, loop and thiazide diuretics, ciclosporin and alcohol. Over-production can be as a result of excessive dietary intake of purines (e.g. in herring, mackerel, sardines, kidney, liver, venison, mussels, oysters, yeast), severe psoriasis, and drugs such as cytotoxics, alcohol and vitamin B_{12}.

Other risk factors for gout include genetics and metabolic syndrome (glucose intolerance), insulin resistance, central obesity, hypertriglyceridaemia, low serum high-density lipoprotein (HDL) and high serum low-density lipoprotein (LDL) levels.

— **Alternative diagnoses when suspecting gout**
It is important to rule out a potentially serious diagnosis of septic arthritis, so all but the most minor of cases should be referred to a GP.

— **Treatment of an acute attack of gout**
An acute attack of gout is usually self-limiting and will resolve over 1–2 weeks. The options for the initial treatment of an attack include NSAIDs, colchicine and corticosteroids.

NSAIDs are usually prescribed first line unless contraindicated. There is no evidence to support the use of one NSAID over any others, so guidelines recommend the prescribing of any fast-acting NSAID with a short half-life with which the patient is familiar, at the full licensed dosage. They should be avoided in patients with a past medical history of heart failure, poor renal function, GI ulcers, gastric bleeds or perforations. Great caution should also be used when prescribing for frail elderly people, or those with multiple pathologies. Co-prescribing of a proton pump inhibitor (PPI, e.g. omeprazole) can be considered for patients at risk of GI side effects.

When NSAIDs are contraindicated, colchicine is usually prescribed, although a response is not often rapid. It has a high risk of toxicity, with the usual side effects being diarrhoea, abdominal cramps, nausea and vomiting. These are all more common in patients with impaired renal function, and the drug should be stopped immediately if diarrhoea and/or vomiting occurs. The recommended dosage regimen is now 500 micrograms two to four times daily, because of the high risk of toxicity if given more frequently. Colchicine can also cause constriction of blood vessels and so should be used with caution in patients with heart failure.

Corticosteroids may also be used in patients in whom NSAIDs and colchicine are contraindicated. They can be given orally or by intravenous (i.v.), intramuscular or intra-articular injection. The route is usually dependent on the number of joints affected; if just one joint, an intra-articular injection will often terminate an attack, but if more than one joint is affected systemic administration is likely to be more beneficial.

For patients for whom standard treatments for gout, including NSAIDs, colchicine and corticosteroids, have been optimised and whose condition has not responded adequately, or for those who are intolerant of them, subcutaneous canakinumab may be considered. Canakinumab is a recombinant monoclonal antibody that selectively inhibits interleukin-1β receptor binding.

As loop and thiazide diuretics are a potential cause of gout, their continued use should be reviewed according to the indication. Diuretics (e.g. bendroflumethiazide as Mr JG was taking) are no longer first-line therapy in hypertension and therefore should be changed to an alternative, whereas those being used for heart failure should be continued. The angiotensin II type 1 receptor (AT_1) antagonist losartan has been shown to have uricosuric properties (increased excretion of uric acid in the urine) and therefore may be useful in patients who suffer from gout.

— **Lifestyle changes that can be made to reduce the risk of recurrence**
There are several evidence-based measures that patients who have had an attack of gout can take to reduce their risk of a further attack:

- Aim for an ideal body weight
- Avoid 'crash' dieting
- Avoid high-protein/low-carbohydrate type diets (e.g. Atkins and Dukan diets)
- Include regular skimmed milk and/or low-fat yoghurt
- Favour soy bean and vegetable sources of protein
- Favour fresh or preserved cherries as fruit
- Restrict intake or avoid high purine-containing foods (<200 mg/day), e.g. oily fish, sea food, offal, game, meat and yeast extracts
- Restrict overall protein intake
- Reduce intake of red meat
- Drink at least 2 L water daily and avoid dehydration
- Restrict alcohol content to <21 units/week for men and <14 units/week for women
- Have at least three alcohol-free days per week
- Try to avoid beer, stout, port and other fortified wines

- Undertake moderate physical exercise but avoid intense muscular exercise.

— Long-term treatment for prophylaxis

Long-term treatment for the prophylaxis of gout should usually be initiated if the patient experiences a second attack within a year of the first. Patients who should receive prophylaxis after their first attack include those with gouty tophi (where crystals of uric acid have built up, resulting in small visible lumps known as tophi to form underneath the skin), an estimated glomerular filtration rate (eGFR) or creatinine clearance <80 mL/min, uric acid stones and gout, and those who need to continue to take diuretics.

Allopurinol is the drug of choice for gout prophylaxis. It is an inhibitor of the enzyme xanthine oxidase to which it competitively binds to inhibit the metabolism of adenine and guanine to uric acid. Allopurinol is structurally very similar (an isomer) to the normal substrate for xanthine oxidase, hypoxanthine, which explains its ability to interact with the same active site on the enzyme target.

allopurinol   hypoxanthine

Allopurinol should be started at a dose of 50–100 mg daily and gradually increased at intervals of 50–100 mg until a blood urate concentration of <300 μmol/L is reached. The maximum dose of allopurinol is 900 mg/day, although this is significantly lower in patients with renal failure. Allopurinol causes a rash in 2% of patients, which can usually be treated by reducing the dose. It can also cause more serious allergic reactions involving a fever, exfoliative dermatitis (widespread peeling of the skin) and mucositis (inflammation of the oral/GI tract mucosal lining), as well as damage to the liver and kidneys; if this is suspected, the drug must be stopped immediately and the patient referred to the GP.

Initiation of a uricostatic agent such as allopurinol can often *precipitate* a gout attack, so it is recommended that they are not started within 1–2 weeks of an episode. Colchicine is usually given at a low dose (500 micrograms twice daily)

for up to 6 months, or for 1 month after the uric acid level has dropped, to reduce the risk of a further attack.

Colchicine is a natural product derived from the ethanolic extracts of the bulbs (corms) and seeds of various colchicum plants, mainly *Colchicum autumnale*. Although total chemical synthesis is possible, it does not yet offer a viable alternative to extraction from the natural source. Colchicine provides relief from gout by modulation of the inflammatory response as well as via an indirect (but related) effect on synovial fluid pH, which decreases uric acid deposition.

colchicine

In some cases (usually those resistant to or intolerant of allopurinol), uricosurics such as benzbromarone, probenecid and sulfinpyrazone may be used. Newer agents for the long-term treatment of gout include febuxostat, rasburicase, pegloticase and canakinumab. However, the unfavourable cost–benefit ratio of these drugs means that allopurinol is expected to remain the drug of choice for the foreseeable future.

— Monitoring of treatment

The British Society of Rheumatology recommends checking renal function and plasma urate levels every 3 months for the first year, reduced to annually thereafter.

EXTENDED LEARNING

- Why do some diuretics increase the risk of developing gout? What is the mechanism?
- What is the link between excessive alcohol intake and hyperuricaemia?
- What is the relationship between units of alcohol and alcohol content (milligrams per litre)?
- What are the recommended limits of alcohol intake for men and women?

References and further reading

British Society for Rheumatology and British Health Professionals in Rheumatology (2007). Guidelines for the Management of Gout. *Rheumatology* **46**:1372–4.

Duffy M, Hughes S (2012). Gout: Clinical features and diagnosis. *Clin Pharmacist* **4**:73–5.

Gibson T (2011). Recommended management of acute gout and hyperuricaemia. *Prescriber* **22**(13–14):31–6.

Hughes S, Vincent M (2012). Gout: Managing gout and hyperuricaemia. *Clin Pharmacist* **4**:79–83.

Lipkowitz MS (2012). Regulation of uric acid excretion by the kidney. *Curr Rheumatol Rep* **14**:179–88.

National Institute for Health and Care Excellence (2013). *Gouty Arthritis: Canakinumab. Key points from the evidence ESNM 23* Available at: http://publications.nice.org.uk/gouty-arthritis-canakinumab-esnm23 (accessed 9 January 2014).

Singh JA (2012). Emerging therapies for gout. *Expert Opin Emerg Drugs* **17**:511–18.

Suresh E, Das P (2012). Recent advances in management of gout. *Q J Med* **105**:407–17.

— **Resources**

UK Gout Society website: www.ukgoutsociety.org

Case 2
Approaches to the effective treatment of non-specific, low back pain

CARL MARTIN

LEARNING OUTCOMES

At the end of this case, you will be able to:

- Demonstrate an awareness of the evidence base for treatment options for lower back pain
- Discuss the safe and effective use of all formulations of NSAIDs
- Use a treatment ladder
- Demonstrate an awareness of alternative treatments for lower back pain

Case study

Mrs BM is 55 years old and presents with a back pain query. As part of your normal practice – you run a very successful MUR (medicines use review)/ NMS (New Medicine Service) – you invite her into the quiet area next to your dedicated consultation room for further discussion.

You take note of her slightly stooped posture and pinched expression. After putting her at ease she seems to relax a little. You sense that a story is to be told and you ask her to talk about her recent health experiences. She explains that she has recently been made redundant after the closure of the secondary school where she had worked for many years as a kitchen dinner lady. She admits that she misses the physical exertion of the job and feels that it kept her healthy. She explains that her daughter, who usually helps with her medicines, is away at university so she had to come to see you.

She describes a pain in her lower back 'in the arch just above my bottom'; she has not had the symptoms before and asks whether her recent reduction in activity could be the cause of the pain.

❷ Considering both pharmacological and non-pharmacological options, what approach do you take in treating Mrs BM's pain?

Mrs BM returns in 7 days and you talk with her in your consultation room. She explains that she has been on the phone to her daughter who said that she should be careful taking pain tablets. She thanks you for the treatment, which in her opinion hasn't worked; Mrs BM wonders whether it's something serious and she should go to her GP.

❷ What elements of Mrs BM's history are important?
❷ What more serious conditions are possible?
❷ What signs would you look for?

Mrs BM has become quite chatty and tells you about her daughter who wants to become a pharmacist like you. In her last phone call she was telling her mother about a recent lecture she had attended on the side effects of medicines. Mrs BM admits that this worried her about taking tablets. She asks about other, safer, treatments that you could recommend.

❷ Is Mrs BM showing signs of intentional non-adherence?
❷ What other treatment options are available?
❷ What constitutes good advice with regard to preventing/limiting future problems?

Case discussion

— Clinical definition of back pain

Low back pain is characterised by a range of symptoms, which include pain, muscle tension or stiffness, or soreness, and is localised between the shoulder blades, bottom of the rib cage and the buttock creases, with or without spread to the legs (sciatica).

— What are the effective treatment options for back pain?

Acute back pain has the potential to develop into chronic back pain if not treated promptly and effectively. In summary, the current NICE (National Institute for Health and Care Excellence) guidance (NICE, 2009) to GPs is as follows:

- Promote self-management and advise people with lower back pain to exercise, be physically active and carry on with normal activities as far as possible.
- Offer drug treatments as appropriate to manage pain and to help people keep active. Follow treatment ladders as below.
- Consider offering one of the following: an exercise programme, a course of manual therapy or a course (controversially) of acupuncture.
- Keep diagnosis under review at all times.

NICE also provides comprehensive advice (note the NICE emphasis on patient participation in health decisions) aimed at people with low back pain for >6 weeks but <1 year.

— Treatment ladder for lower back pain

Start with paracetamol and if insufficient (taking into account individual risk factors) offer NSAIDs and/or weak opioids. NICE recommends adding in tricyclic antidepressants at the smallest possible therapeutic dose to relieve associated anxiety and depression, and then short-term use of strong opioids in severe pain.

NICE (2009) identifies a number of treatments that **should not be offered**, including:

- Selective serotonin reuptake inhibitors (SSRIs) for treating pain
- Injections into the back
- Therapeutic ultrasonography
- Transcutaneous electrical nerve stimulation (TENS)
- Lumbar supports
- Traction.

— Prevention of future problems

Reduce straining the back through weight loss (certainly avoid weight gain), maintaining a good posture, and develop good practice with respect to lifting. Advise to strengthen the back muscles through regular exercise such as walking, swimming, pilates or yoga. Relaxation strategies can reduce muscle tension.

— Possible serious conditions and red flag signs

The following red flag signs (serious warning signs) would require immediate referral:

- Chronic pain while aged <20 or >55
- Feeling generally unwell, with systemic symptoms, e.g. weight loss
- Chest pain
- A history of cancer, steroid use, drug abuse, HIV or other significant disease
- Widespread neurological signs, e.g. pain in both legs
- Structural deformity
- Numbness in crotch area; bladder function impairment.

Serious conditions include malignancy, a fracture, an infection or inflammatory disease (such as ankylosing spondylitis).

— Adverse drug reactions of NSAIDs

NSAIDs are associated with a number of adverse effects, including effects on the kidney, and exacerbating asthma in some people, but the most important adverse effect of NSAIDs, including aspirin, is that on the GI tract. They cause gastric erosions, which can become ulcers. They can cause symptoms of an ulcer in some people, the ulcers may bleed, and indeed some people may die of a bleeding ulcer caused by NSAIDs. The potential benefits of NSAIDs must be weighed against the risks. NSAIDs are **contraindicated** in patients with known active peptic ulceration and should be **used with caution** in elderly people and those with renal impairment or asthma.

The molecular targets of the NSAIDs are the cyclooxygenase (COX) enzymes. The two isoforms of the COX enzymes are called COX-1 and COX-2. COX-1 is produced constitutively in many tissues, and is a key enzyme involved in prostaglandin biosynthesis. Inhibition of COX-1 (among other things) results in inhibition of both platelet aggregation and alkaline mucus secretion, which protects the GI epithelium, both of which are mediated by prostaglandins. COX-2 production is induced in inflammation. The specificity of COX-2-specific NSAIDs for inhibition of inflammatory prostaglandins, rather than the constitutive COX-1 should mean that they have an improved side-effect profile. In principle, COX-2-selective drugs are associated with reduced risks of GI side effects, but their use is limited because they have been linked with other adverse effects such as cardiotoxicity. (However, it should be noted that cardiotoxicity may also be a consideration for non-COX-selective NSAIDs.)

— **Efficacy of alternative treatment options**
Topical NSAIDs: the use of topical NSAIDs is one of the more controversial subjects in analgesic practice. A recent Cochrane review confirmed that topical NSAIDs are more effective than placebo, so, in people where systemic side effects limit the use of oral NSAIDs, a trial of a topical preparation may be helpful. Topical NSAID products (e.g. gel formulations of ibuprofen and diclofenac) are formulated to ensure rapid and extensive penetration of drug through the skin to underlying soft tissues and joints. They produce relatively low plasma concentrations, resulting in a low incidence of adverse effects.

Efficacy of TENS: this involves passing an electric current through the body via electrodes taped to the skin – considered by some to be the electrical equivalent of acupuncture. The design is based on the gate control theory of pain, which claims that selective stimulation of certain nerve fibres can effectively block some or all of the nociceptive (pain) impulses and hence may reduce the sensation of pain. TENS can be used in either intermittent pulse mode or continuous impulse. A Cochrane review concluded that there is no evidence (i.e. a lack appropriate quality trials) that TENS provides effective pain relief. Thus, for TENS, as for many complementary and alternative approaches, there is limited scientific research evidence on which to base treatment recommendations. This 'absence of evidence' does not automatically equate to 'evidence of absence', i.e. a lack of evidence that a therapy is effective does not necessarily mean that it is ineffective.

EXTENDED LEARNING

- Pain is a subjective experience, influenced by many factors, and assessment can be challenging. It can be difficult for people to articulate and describe the pain that they are experiencing. There are a number of descriptive/pictorial validated pain scales available. The British Pain Society (www.britishpainsociety.org) is a good source
- How are pharmaceutical gels formulated and prepared?
- How is the rate of drug release from a topical product measured?
- What is intentional non-adherence?

ADDITIONAL PRACTICE POINTS

- Adjuvant therapies include tricyclic antidepressants. Have you encountered this? It could be potentially confusing for our patients who wonder how medications can have more than one clinical use
- If, on further questioning, Mrs BM had revealed that she does not feel as fit as she did before stopping work, has lost weight recently and also confessed that she was anxious about her deteriorating posture, how might you respond?

Reference and further reading

National Institute for Health and Clinical Excellence (2009). *Low Back Pain* (Early management of persistent non-specific low back pain). NICE Clinical Guideline 88. London: NICE.

— **Resources**

An *Effective Health Care* bulletin on the effectiveness of therapies for acute and chronic low back pain (Vol.6, No 5, November 2000) can be downloaded at www.york.ac.uk/inst/crd.

For a review of research into **adherence** see *Medicines Adherence*. NICE Clinical Guideline 76 (2009). Downloadable at www.nice.org.uk.

Case 3

Disease-modifying anti-rheumatic drugs and treatment for rheumatoid arthritis

SIMONE BRACKENBOROUGH

LEARNING OUTCOMES

At the end of this case you will be able to:

- Outline the pathophysiology, signs, symptoms and diagnosis of rheumatoid arthritis (RA)
- Describe the use of DMARDs for the treatment of RA
- Describe in detail how to initiate, titrate and monitor methotrexate and sulfasalazine
- Describe the main counselling points on methotrexate and sulfasalazine
- Outline the mode of action of methotrexate in RA
- Outline the chemistry and mode of action of sulfasalazine in RA
- Outline the formulation approaches to producing gastroresistant (enteric-coated) solid dosage forms
- Describe how the progression of RA is monitored
- Describe when patients should move to biologic treatments

Case study

Mrs PN, a 43-year-old administrator, presents to her GP with painful wrists and hands over a period of 6 months. Her symptoms are early morning stiffness lasting for 4–5 hours of the day, which is causing her problems in performing daily tasks such as dressing, and general fatigue. On examination, both wrists and the metacarpophalangeal joints (MCPJs) and proximal interphalangeal joints (PIPJs) of both hands are swollen and tender. She has no other significant past medical history.

Her GP prescribes naproxen 500 mg twice a day and advises her to return if there is no improvement. After 1 month, although there was some improvement, her knees are now beginning to become tender, swollen and stiff, with a reduced

range of movement in these joints. The GP refers Mrs PN to the rheumatology consultant at the local hospital.

Mrs PN's results were as shown in the box.

> CRP (C-reactive protein): 35 µg/L (normal 0–1 µg/L)
> ESR (erythrocyte sedimentation rate): 38 mm/h (normal 0–20 mm/h)
> Seropositive rheumatoid factor (sheep cell agglutination test for IgM antibody): >1/1049 (normal: <1/32)
> U&Es (urea and electrolytes) and FBC (full blood count) were normal

Her radiographs showed erosions on the second and third MCPJs and PIPJs of both hands. She is diagnosed with RA. It was decided that Mrs PN should be started on methotrexate. She was initiated on 7.5 mg methotrexate weekly and also prescribed folic acid 5 mg to be taken the day after the methotrexate. A short course of prednisolone was also prescribed.

- What is RA, its pathogenesis and the classic symptoms?
- How is a diagnosis confirmed?
- What are the aims of treating RA?
- What are DMARDs and when should they be initiated?
- What DMARDs are available?
- In this case, is methotrexate (MTX) a suitable first choice of DMARD for Mrs PN?
- What should be checked before initiating MTX?
- How is methotrexate initiated, titrated and monitored?
- What is the mechanism of action of methotrexate in treating RA?
- Why was folic acid prescribed?
- What would be your key counselling points for Mrs PN?
- What would you give to Mrs PN to aid your counselling?

❷ What type of side effects would you warn the patient about while on low-dose methotrexate therapy?

❷ How is the progression of RA monitored?

❷ What non-drug therapy can be offered?

Mrs PN was followed up in clinic regularly over the next few months. At 3 months she still has swollen, tender wrists and knees, and also stiffness. Her DAS (disease activity score) is 5.2. The consultant adds sulfasalazine E/C to her prescription along with methotrexate.

❷ How should sulfasalazine be initiated?

❷ Sulfasalazine has been prescribed as an enteric-coated (gastroresistant) product. Why is such a formulation desirable for sulfasalazine? What formulation approaches may be employed to produce gastroresistant solid dosage forms?

❷ How are tablets enteric coated?

❷ How would you counsel Mrs PN about the sulfasalazine?

❷ What monitoring is required with sulfasalazine?

❷ Sulfasalazine is a prodrug. What is a prodrug? Draw the chemical structure of sulfasalazine and explain how it undergoes conversion to its active metabolite(s). What is its mechanism of action?

❷ What drug therapy can be recommended if Mrs PN does not respond to methotrexate and sulfasalazine?

Case discussion

Rheumatoid Arthritis (RA)

RA is a chronic and progressive inflammatory condition of the joints. It is a polyarthritis that is symmetrical, deforming and affects both small and large joints. If left untreated it is disabling and approximately a third of people with the condition have to give up work because of it. It affects between 0.5% and 1% of the population and three times as many women as men. It has a peak age of onset of 40–70 years. Life expectancy is also decreased.

— Pathogenesis

The exact cause is unknown, but it is thought to be autoimmune and there is a genetic tendency. Environmental factors may also play a role. The earliest change is swelling and inflammation of the synovial membrane and adjoining connective tissues. This causes infiltration of lymphocytes (especially CD4 T cells), plasma cells and macrophages and eventually damage to the synovial membrane. Pannus (similar to scar tissue) forms over the synovium, which causes erosion of the cartilage, which in turn causes erosion of the bone (Figure 8.1).

— Classic symptoms

The classic symptoms of RA are tenderness and stiffness of joints, and morning stiffness with a symmetrical presentation. It can affect small or large joints and commonly affects the small joints of the hands, wrists and feet first. As RA is an autoimmune condition, it can also affect other areas of the body. Fatigue is common, as well as symptoms, such as anaemia, weight loss and dry eyes.

— Diagnosis

In 2010, the American College of Rheumatology, jointly with the European League against Rheumatism, released classification criteria for RA. These were devised to enable the identification of patients at high risk of persistent and/or erosive disease when presenting early with inflammatory synovitis. The criteria are:

- Confirmed presence of synovitis in at least one joint
- Absence of an alternative diagnosis that better explains the synovitis (e.g. gout or reactive arthritis triggered by an infection) and
- Achievement of a total score of ≥6 (out of a possible 10) from:
  - Number and site of involved joints (score range 0–5)
  - Serological abnormality (score range 0–3), e.g. autoantibodies
  - Elevated acute-phase response (score range 0–1), e.g. CRP or ESR
  - Symptom duration (2 levels; range 0–1).

— The aims of treating RA

The treatment of RA should relieve the acute symptoms and pain but also slow the disease progression, which will prevent joint damage, loss of function and disability.

— Disease modifying anti-rheumatic drugs (DMARDs)

DMARDs are a group of drugs that affect the immune response in RA and subsequently suppress the disease progression. DMARDs should be initiated soon after diagnosis, ideally within 3 months of the onset of persistent symptoms. They

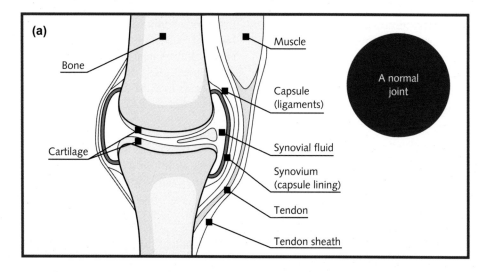

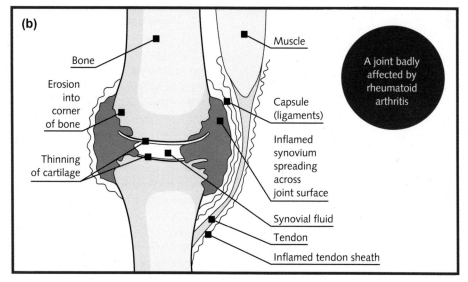

▲ FIGURE 8.1

(a) A normal joint; (b) a joint badly affected by rheumatoid arthritis. (Redrawn from Arthritis Research UK website.)

are usually given with short-term glucocorticoids initially to relieve symptoms until the DMARDs start to have an effect. NICE guidance (2009) recommends using two DMARDs together, unless the patient has contraindications.

There are a number of DMARDs available. Some are used more commonly than others:

- Auranofin (oral gold)
- Azathioprine
- Ciclosporin
- D-Penicillamine

- Hydroxychloroquine
- Leflunomide
- Methotrexate
- Sulfasalazine
- Mycophenolate mofetil
- Sodium aurothiomalate.

— **Methotrexate (MTX)**

Methotrexate (MTX) is often used first line because it is one of the quickest acting DMARDs. Before starting MTX, patients must have baseline tests performed. These include FBC, U&Es, LFTs and chest radiograph (unless done within the last 6 months). Pulmonary function tests should be considered in selected patients to assess pre-existing lung disease.

Mrs PN has no contraindications for MTX.

— Initiation, titration and monitoring of methotrexate

MTX should be started at a low dose (5–10 mg weekly) and titrated up by 2.5 mg or 5 mg dose increases every 2–6 weeks until the RA has been stabilised. The maximum licensed dose is 25 mg weekly, although doses up to 30 mg weekly are occasionally used. For elderly patients with poor renal function, initial doses should be smaller. Intramuscular or subcutaneous MTX could be considered if there are side effects or poor absorption with oral MTX. The same dose is used.

MTX is monitored by checking FBC, U&Es and LFTs every 2 weeks, until the dose of MTX and monitoring are stable for 6 weeks, and thereafter monthly until the dose and disease are stable for 1 year. After this, the monitoring may be reduced in frequency, based on clinical judgement with consideration of risk factors including age, co-morbidities or renal impairment when monthly monitoring is to continue.

Clinically serious liver disease is rarely seen in RA patients receiving low-dose MTX and routine liver biopsies are therefore not recommended.

MTX is also used in the management of other conditions, e.g. severe psoriasis. In these cases, both dosing regimens and monitoring will differ.

— Mechanism of action of methotrexate in treating RA

Methotrexate is a reversible dihydrofolate reductase (DHFR) inhibitor used primarily in the treatment of cancer (in high doses) and certain autoimmune diseases such as RA, severe psoriasis and Crohn's disease (in low doses). Interference with the function of the DHFR enzyme ultimately leads to an inhibition of RNA/DNA and protein synthesis (particularly in malignant, rapidly dividing cancer cells), therefore producing powerful cytotoxic effects. In treating RA, inhibition of purine (adenosine) metabolism, T-cell function/proliferation and synthesis/secretion of various proinflammatory cytokines may be the main mechanisms of anti-inflammatory action.

— Use of folic acid with methotrexate

As MTX is an anti-folate drug, folate supplementation, in the form of folic acid, is usually co-administered with MTX to minimise some of its adverse side effects, e.g. mouth ulcers and GI intolerance, which, in low-dose MTX patients with RA, essentially mimic folate deficiency. Folic acid is usually given once a week, the day after the MTX.

— Counselling points methotrexate

MTX is a complicated medicine to explain to patients. The National Patient Safety Agency (NPSA) made recommendations in 2004 that all patients are given an MTX booklet, which has patient information about MTX as well as their blood results. The key counselling points for MTX are as follows:

- MTX is used in other conditions as well as RA (specifically, cancer).
- It helps prevent the RA getting worse.
- MTX takes 4–6 weeks to work, so pain relief may still be needed until then.
- MTX is taken once a week, not every day: stick to the same day each week.
- Only take the 2.5 mg strength of MTX.
- Take the folic acid on the day after the MTX to prevent side effects.
- Both are yellow tablets so care should be taken not to mix them up.
- Always attend blood test appointments. They tell the doctors how well the MTX is working and any side effects can be spotted early.
- Blood tests are usually every 2–12 weeks, and may be more often at the start of treatment.
- Remember to bring the MTX book to clinic appointments, when collecting medicines from the pharmacy and if admitted to hospital.
- Side effects to watch out for include: nausea, dizziness/drowsiness, headache, sore mouth or mouth ulcers, stomach upset, skin rash and fever.
- Tell your doctor immediately if you have an infection, including fever, sore throat or chills, unexplained skin rash, swollen, tender or bleeding gums, black tarry stools or unexplained bruising, chest pain, difficulty in breathing, a dry persistent cough, severe and continuing diarrhoea or vomiting.
- MTX can make you more prone to picking up infections, so avoid people with chickenpox.
- Aspirin: avoid over-the-counter aspirin, but low-dose aspirin prescribed by a doctor is fine.
- Limit alcohol intake.

- Immunisations: live vaccines must be avoided, but the influenza vaccine is safe and is recommended. Check that any holiday vaccines are not live.
- When buying medicines over the counter remember to tell the pharmacist that you are taking MTX.
- Other medicines: some medicines can affect the way MTX works, e.g. aspirin at high dose (low dose is fine). Trimethoprim and co-trimoxazole should all be avoided with MTX.
- Pregnancy (if applicable to the patient): all patients, male and female, should be advised against conception and pregnancy during treatment with MTX because it is an abortificient as well as being a teratogenic drug.
- Patients should be advised to continue contraception for at least 3 months after stopping MTX.
- Breastfeeding is not recommended because the drug may be excreted into breast milk.

— **Monitoring of RA progression**

The Disease Activity Score (DAS) is a questionnaire-based instrument used to measure disease activity in patients with RA and is the most common monitoring system used in the UK. It has been extensively validated for use in clinical trials. There are two versions of the DAS available: the DAS measures 44 joints, whereas a validated simple version is the DAS28 in which 28 joints are measured.

In the DAS, the number of swollen and tender joints is assessed and the erythrocyte sedimentation rate (ESR) measured. Using this information, the DAS will provide you with a number between 0 and 10, indicating how active the RA is at that moment in time. It is calculated using a formula that includes four variables. The first two are the counts for tender and swollen joints (53 and 44 joints, respectively). The third variable is a measure of general health or global disease activity. Patients are asked to rate how active their arthritis was in the past week by marking a line on a 100-mm visual analogue scale (ranging from 'not active at all' to 'extremely active'). The final variable is a measure of circulating inflammatory markers.

DAS28 is similar to DAS, but uses only 28 joints for assessment. A DAS28 score >5.1 is considered to be indicative of high disease activity, between 5.1 and 3.2 of moderate disease activity,

and <3.2 of low disease activity. A patient scoring <2.6 is defined as being in remission. By comparing the DAS28 score for one patient at two different time points, it is possible to define improvement or response. It is easy to use and may be applied in everyday clinical practice.

A decrease in DAS28 score of ≤0.6 is considered to show a poor response to treatment, whereas decreases >1.2 points indicate a moderate or good response, dependent on whether an individual's DAS28 score at the endpoint is above or below 3.2, respectively. Inflammatory markers such as CRP (C-reactive protein) should also be measured. Both the DAS28 score and CRP should initially be measured monthly until the disease has been controlled. Thereafter, these should be measured periodically.

— **Non-drug therapies for RA**

These include:

- Improving general fitness and regular exercise
- Physiotherapy: to learn exercises for enhancing joint flexibility and muscle strength
- Occupational therapy: advice on splints, adapting the way things are done at home and offering specialist equipment
- Relief of short-term pain with wax baths or TENS
- Psychological support: to help with stress management, relaxation techniques
- Podiatry services: to help with general foot problems and to offer functional insoles and therapeutic footwear if necessary
- Surgery: for severe longstanding disease to improve pain and improve mobility in the joints.

— **Initiation of sulfasalazine**

Sulfasalazine should be initiated at 500 mg daily for 7 days, then increasing to 500 mg twice a day for 7 days, 1 g in the morning and 500 mg in the evening for 7 days, and then 1 g twice a day to continue.

— **Enteric-coated (gastroresistant) oral solid dosage forms**

To obviate the GI side effects of sulfasalazine, including diarrhoea, vomiting and abdominal pain, enteric-coated (gastroresistant) tablets are available. These are designed such that drug is released when a certain environmental pH is met, so in this instance drug is not released in the acid of the stomach, but in the higher pH of the small intestine or colon. Tablets are coated with a material that disintegrates or dissolves at a predetermined pH. Gastroresistant coatings are polymer coatings that are insoluble at low pH, but are soluble at higher pH (e.g. somewhere between pH 4 and 7 depending on the polymer). A gastroresistant coating may be employed for two possible reasons: (1) protecting the stomach from the drug or (2) protecting acid-sensitive drugs from the stomach environment.

— Tablet coating

Film coating is the most commonly used process for coating tablet cores. In the past, organic solvents were employed to dissolve the film-forming polymers, which are applied in a single-step process via a pan-coating technique. These are now largely replaced with aqueous coating formulations. Methacrylic acid copolymers and phthalate ester polymers, such as hydroxypropylmethylcellulose phthalate and polyvinyl acetate phthalate, can be applied as enteric coatings to tablets and microparticulates (filled into gelatine capsules), because they have low aqueous solubility at low pH, but solubility is increased at higher pH, such that they are soluble in the pH range encountered in the small intestine or colon, allowing subsequent dissolution of the tablet core.

— Counselling points for sulfasalazine

The main points to stress when counselling Mrs PN are:

- Sulfasalazine is used in other conditions as well as RA (ulcerative colitis, Crohn's disease)
- It helps prevent the RA getting worse
- It takes about 12 weeks to work, so pain relief may still be needed until then
- Always take the enteric-coated version
- Swallow whole with a full glass of water
- Always attend blood test appointments. They tell the doctors how well the sulfasalazine is working, and any side effects can be spotted early
- Blood tests are usually every month for the first 3 months and 3-monthly thereafter. After the first year these may reduce to every 6 months
- Side effects to watch out for include rashes and nausea or stomach upset
- Sulfasalazine will also cause your urine to be stained yellow
- Sulfasalazine may stain soft contact lenses yellow (rare)

- The ability of sulfasalazine to colour the urine and stain soft contact lenses is a direct consequence of its structure; sulfasalazine is highly coloured because it contains an extended system of conjugated π bonds and even low concentrations of drug can impart colour to fluids in which it is dissolved
- Do not take if allergic to sulfonamides, aspirin or co-trimoxazole
- Tell your doctor immediately if you have unexplained fever, sore throat or chills, unexplained bruising or bleeding or tiredness.
- Immunisations: check that any holiday vaccines are safe with your doctor. The flu vaccine is recommended if you are taking sulfasalazine
- Other medicines: some medicines can affect the way sulfasalazine works. Remember to remind your doctor and pharmacist that you are taking this if prescribed any new medicines
- Pregnancy (if applicable to the patient): patients should discuss with their doctor the benefits and risks of continuing treatment while pregnant
- Male patients: sulfasalazine may cause reversible temporary infertility
- Sulfasalazine is excreted into breast milk, but is not thought to be a risk to the baby.

— Monitoring with sulfasalazine

The following recommendations follow the British Rheumatology Society guidelines from 2008:

- Pre-treatment: check FBC, U&Es including creatinine and LFTs
- First 3 months: monitor FBC and LFTs (including AST/ALT) monthly
- Three months onwards: monitor FBC and LFTs (including AST/ALT) every 3 months
- Year 2: if, after the first year, dose and blood results have been stable, the frequency of blood tests can be reduced to every 6 months for the second year of treatment. Thereafter, monitoring of blood for toxicity may be disregarded
- After dose changes: repeat FBC and LFTs 1 month after dose increases.

Patients should be asked about the presence of rash or oral ulceration at each visit.

— Sulfasalazine as a prodrug

A prodrug is a substance that is administered in a chemical form other than that in which it will exert its pharmacological action. Prodrugs are often inactive themselves but undergo metabolism

sulfasalazine → sulfapyridine + 5-aminosalicylic acid

in the body to produce one or more active metabolites. Enteric-coated sulfasalazine passes through the small intestine and is released in the higher pH environment of the colon. On reaching the colon the azo group undergoes metabolic reduction by gut bacteria to generate 5-aminosalicylic acid (5-ASA: mesalazine), an active anti-inflammatory agent, and sulfapyridine. Sulfapyridine is an immunomodulator and may also contribute to the anti-arthritic activity of sulfasalazine.

— **Mechanism of action of sulfasalazine**

Although the precise mode of action of sulfasalazine and its metabolites in the treatment of RA are still not entirely clear, several complex mechanisms have been proposed including: reduced secretion of inflammatory cytokines, increased production of anti-inflammatory adenosine (see above for MTX) and inhibition of the activation of the transcription factor nuclear factor κB (NF-κB) – normally involved in the production of immune response mediators.

— **Alternatives to DMARDs**

Tumour necrosis factor α (TNF-α) inhibitors, e.g. adalimumab, etanercept and infliximab, are recommended if patients do not respond to DMARDs. NICE has set criteria for patient eligibility as:

- Patients must have active disease with a DAS28 score >5.1 confirmed on at least two occasions, 1 month apart.
- Patients must have undergone trials of two DMARDs, including MTX (unless contraindicated). A trial of a DMARD is defined as being normally of 6 months, with 2 months at standard dose, unless significant toxicity has limited the dose or duration of treatment.

Rituximab in combination with methotrexate is recommended as an option where TNF-α inhibitors have failed or the patient has developed adverse effects.

EXTENDED LEARNING

- What are the options for the management of pain in RA patients? What are the advantages and disadvantages of different classes of pain relief?
- Discuss the role of joint (intra-articular) injections and which drugs are commonly prescribed
- What are the adverse effects of oral corticosteroids and how can these be minimised?
- Outline the mechanism of action of anti-TNF-α drugs and their place in RA therapy
- How does rituximab work? What is its place in RA therapy?
- Describe the methods employed in tablet manufacture and coating
- What excipients are used in film-coating of tablets?

ADDITIONAL PRACTICE POINT

- How can health-related quality of life in RA be measured?

References and further reading

Callaghan C, Copeland R (2010). Rheumatoid arthritis: Features, causes and diagnosis. *Clin Pharmacist* 2:154–60.

Callaghan C, Copeland R (2010). Rheumatoid arthritis: Management. *Clin Pharmacist* 2:161–7.

McConnell EL, Basit AW (2013). Modified-release oral drug delivery. In: Aulton ME, Taylor KMG (eds), *Aulton's Pharmaceutics: The design and manufacture of medicines*, 4th edn. London: Elsevier, 550–65.

National Institute for Health and Clinical Excellence (2007). *Rheumatoid Arthritis – Adalimumab, etanercept and infliximab*. NICE Technology Appraisal Guideline 130. London: NICE. Available at: www.nice.org.uk/TA130 (accessed 9 April 2014).

National Institute for Health and Clinical Excellence (2009). *Rheumatoid Arthritis: The management of rheumatoid arthritis in adults*. NICE Clinical Guideline 79. London: NICE. Available at: www.nice.org.uk/cg79 (accessed 9 April 2014).

National Institute for Health and Clinical Excellence (2010). *Adalimumab, Etanercept, Infliximab, Rituximab and Abatacept for the Treatment of Rheumatoid Arthritis after the Failure of a TNF Inhibitor.* NICE Technology Appraisal Guideline 195. London: NICE. Available at: www.nice.org.uk/TA195 (accessed 9 April 2014).

Porter SC (2013). Coating of tablets and multiparticulates. In: Aulton ME, Taylor KMG (eds), *Aulton's Pharmaceutics: The design and manufacture of medicines*, 4th edn. London: Elsevier, 566–83.

Radboud University Medical Centre Nijmegen (2013). *DAS-score.* Available at: www.das-score.nl/das28/en/(accessed 9 April 2014).

— Resources

Arthritis Research UK: www.arthritisresearchuk.org

Case 4
Glucosamine supplements for osteoarthritis and joint stiffness

ELIZABETH M WILLIAMSON

LEARNING OUTCOMES

At the end of this case, you will be able to:

* Explain what glucosamine supplements are, and why they are sometimes used in arthritis-related conditions
* Describe the evidence for the use of glucosamine and its combination with chondroitin in arthritis and joint stiffness
* Recommend a course of action for the patient, taking into account any other medication and supplements that he may be taking

Case study

Mr FF is a 65-year-old man with joint stiffness in his knees, who is prescribed ibuprofen tablets (400 mg three times daily) by his doctor. You dispense these for him in your community pharmacy but he has told you that he does not take them very regularly because they give him indigestion. A friend has suggested that Mr FF should try a supplement of glucosamine, which he says is a natural substance found in the body. Mr FF has picked up a product containing both glucosamine and chondroitin from the shelf, and asks whether this might be even better.

❓ What is glucosamine and how is it thought to work?
❓ Does the addition of chondroitin increase efficacy?
❓ Is there any evidence to support the use of these supplements for treating arthritis?
❓ Why does the *BNF* give 'shellfish allergy' as a contraindication?
❓ Are these food supplements or medicines?

Mr FF tells you that he already takes a fish oil supplement (1000 mg) to help alleviate the condition.

❓ Is fish oil a common supplement for people with arthritis?
❓ Is there any evidence that it works?
❓ Would it be safe to add glucosamine and/or chondroitin to his drug regimen?
❓ What would you recommend that Mr FF does?

Case discussion

— Glucosamine

Glucosamine is a hexosamine sugar, and a natural constituent of glycosaminoglycans found in articular cartilage. It is a derivative of glucose, in which the secondary hydroxyl group at C2 is replaced by an amino group. Similar to all sugars found in mammalian systems, it has the D-relative configuration. Glucosamine is important for maintaining the elasticity and strength of cartilage in joints. The mode of action is not fully understood, although it is, of course, a component of connective tissue. *In vitro* studies have shown that glucosamine can increase collagen and mucopolysaccharide synthesis in fibroblasts, and that it also activates protein synthesis in chondrocytes.

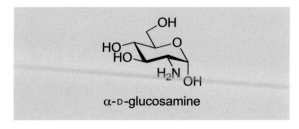

α-D-glucosamine

— Chondroitin

Chondroitin is a mixture of high-molecular-weight glycosaminoglycans and disaccharide polymers, which are usually variably sulfated. The chains are usually composed of alternating D-glucuronic acid and N-acetyl-D-galactosamine sugar residues, the latter being sulphated at either the C6 or C4 hydroxyl. It forms part of the cartilage matrix in which collagen is embedded. A major function of chondroitin is to absorb water, thicken cartilage and thus absorb pressure in the joints. It inhibits elastase and hyaluronidase enzymes which break down cartilage.

— Sources of glucosamine and chondroitin

Glucosamine is often extracted from the exoskeletons of shellfish, although it can be prepared from plant material or produced synthetically. If the source is not known, and if a patient is allergic to shellfish, they may be at risk of a reaction to particular brands of glucosamine. Chondroitin is extracted from both marine and bovine sources. These sources may be a concern for vegetarian patients.

— Evidence for efficacy of glucosamine for treating arthritis and joint stiffness

Glucosamine has been approved for the symptomatic treatment of mild osteoarthritis on prescription in the UK (see *BNF*) and is widely sold as a dietary supplement in the UK and the USA. The evidence for its use is mixed and, although clinical studies have shown positive effects (mainly in osteoarthritis of the knee), some of these are either of short duration or the studies have design flaws. But it is thought to be safe, and therefore it may be viewed as a low-risk alternative to NSAIDs, which can have marked adverse effects, indigestion and possible stomach ulcers being of principal concern. There is some evidence that chondroitin can provide pain relief in osteoarthritis but clinical studies have been small and of short duration. It is usually formulated in combinations with glucosamine.

The Arthritis Foundation statement on the Glucosamine/chondroitin Arthritis Intervention Trial (GAIT) concludes that a combination of both glucosamine and chondroitin is superior to either agent used alone. In fact, they also conclude that the evidence for the use of the individual supplements is limited.

— Food supplements or medicines

Products such as these can be sold as food supplements because they are indeed found in common foods. Food supplements do not have to comply with the same stringent regulatory requirements as medicines, although they are regulated by the EU Food Supplements Directive 2002/46. They are not allowed to make medicinal claims (such as 'for treating arthritis'), and do not have to contain a PIL (patient information leaflet), although they can make claims of health benefits (e.g. 'to help maintain healthy joints'). This means that the patient may not always receive suitable information about drug interactions, side effects or contraindications.

— Fish oil as a supplement for people with arthritis

Fish oil supplements are taken for many different real and perceived health benefits, of which the most important are probably their cardiovascular and anti-inflammatory effects. There is a substantial body of evidence in support of a role for fish oils in alleviating some of the symptoms of RA, such as tenderness of the joints and stiffness, and they can help decrease the need for NSAIDs.

— Clinical issues and evidence of effectiveness

Many people take a combination of fish oils and glucosamine/chondroitin with apparent benefit and no ill effects. Glucosamine can cause GI disturbances, headache and rash, and it has been suggested that it may alter glucose regulation, although a study on people with type 2 diabetes found no changes in serum insulin, glucose or glycated haemoglobin after 12 weeks of glucosamine administration. There are no reported

part of a chondroitin sulfate chain

drug interactions between ibuprofen and any of the other products.

— Possible recommendations for this case

Glucosamine is usually taken for a period of 3–6 months before deciding whether it is providing any benefit, so this would be a reasonable course of action for Mr FF to take. The evidence for a mixture of glucosamine with chondroitin seems to be stronger than for glucosamine alone, so a combination product would be a logical choice. The dose recommended by the manufacturer should be followed. You should check whether the patient has any allergies to shellfish and, if so, it is probably safer to advise the patient not to use this supplement. Remind the patient to tell his GP of his course of action at their next consultation, because this will help to identify any possible adverse reactions should they arise. If the product is effective, documentation also strengthens the evidence base for it.

EXTENDED LEARNING

- Discuss the importance of knowing the source of a supplement
- Comment on the strengths and weaknesses of the evidence base for the use of herbal remedies and nutraceuticals for long-term conditions
- Explain how dietary changes may help relieve some of the symptoms of arthritis

ADDITIONAL PRACTICE POINT

- What other lifestyle advice could you give to a patient with arthritis?

References and further reading

Aghazadeh-Habashi A, Jamali F (2011). The glucosamine controversy; a pharmacokinetic issue. *J Pharmacy Pharm Sci* **14**:264–73.

Henrotin Y, Mobasheri A, Marty M (2012). Is there any scientific evidence for the use of glucosamine in the management of human osteoarthritis? *Arthrit Res Ther* **14**:201.

Lockwood B (2007). *Nutraceuticals. A guide for healthcare professionals*. 2nd edn. London: Pharmaceutical Press.

Mason P (2011). *Dietary Supplements*, 4th edn. London: Pharmaceutical Press,

Reginster JY, Neuprez A, Lecart MP, Sarlet N, Bruyere O (2012). Role of glucosamine in the treatment for osteoarthritis. *Rheumatol Int* **32**:2959–67.

Sawitzke AD, Shi H, Finco MS et al. (2010). Clinical efficacy and safety over two years use of glucosamine, chondroitin sulfate, their combination, celecoxib or placebo taken to treat osteoarthritis of the knee: a GAIT report *Ann Rheum Dis* **69**:1459–64.

Wandel S, Jüni P, Tendal B et al. (2010). Effects of glucosamine, chondroitin, or placebo in patients with osteoarthritis of hip or knee: network meta-analysis. *BMJ* **341**:34.

Williamson EM, Driver S, Baxter K, eds (2013). *Stockley's Herbal Medicines Interactions. A guide to the interactions of herbal medicines*, 2nd edn. London: Pharmaceutical Press.

— Resources

Arthritis Foundation Statement on the Glucosamine/ Chondroitin: Arthritis Intervention Trial (GAIT): www. arthritis.org/files/images/newsroom/statements/ GAIT_Statement_FINAL_2_21_06.pdf

Arthritis Research UK (for dietary advice): www. arthritisresearchuk.org/arthritis-information/arthritis-and-daily-life/diet-and-arthritis.aspx? gclid=CJ2FnJab17kCFcfJtAodzkUAaw

British National Formulary: see www.bnf.org for latest edition and recommendations.

Food supplement legislation: www.dh.gov.uk/prod_consum_dh/ groups/dh_digitalassets/@dh/@en/documents/digitalasset/ dh_132124.pdf

Case 5
Treating juvenile idiopathic arthritis in young people

JANET E MCDONAGH AND NICOLA GRAY

Case 5 | Treating juvenile idiopathic arthritis in young people

LEARNING OUTCOMES

At the end of this case, you will be able to:

- Describe key differences in the drug management of arthritis in young people compared with adults
- Outline the chemistry and mechanism of action of piroxicam
- Evaluate adherence in young people with a long-term condition such as juvenile idiopathic arthritis (JIA)
- Describe the role of the community pharmacist in supporting the development of self-management skills in young people with JIA

Case study

You are a community pharmacist. One afternoon, MG a 15-year-old boy comes into your pharmacy with his mother – having had their first appointment at the paediatric rheumatology clinic – and presents you with a prescription for three-quarters (15 mg) of a Feldene Melt once daily. The mother tells you that the paediatric rheumatology team are suspecting juvenile idiopathic arthritis.

- What are the common side effects of Feldene Melt (piroxicam)?
- How frequent are they in this age group?
- Why is piroxicam a common choice of NSAID by paediatric rheumatologists for JIA in school-aged children?
- What other NSAIDs are licensed for use in this age group?
- What is your advice with regard to administration?

A few weeks later, the mother returns with a prescription for methotrexate tablets 15 mg once weekly orally. They have confirmed the diagnosis of JIA and it is the rheumatoid factor-negative polyarthritis subtype. The mother says that her son is unable to swallow tablets. She is also concerned that she has read on the internet that methotrexate is a chemotherapy agent used in cancer.

- What are the key differences between JIA and adult rheumatoid arthritis?

- What are the differences in DMARD use in childhood and adult arthritis management?
- What do you say regarding her concerns about methotrexate and cancer?
- What methotrexate tablet strength will you provide, and why?
- What strategies can you provide for the mother, to help the young person learn to swallow tablets?

A few weeks later, the mother comes in to ask about treatment for nausea as her son is troubled by this with the methotrexate.

- Describe the different patterns of nausea associated with methotrexate use in young people. What strategies can be used to manage each type of nausea?

A few weeks later MG comes into the pharmacy on his own to collect his prescription and asks if he could ask you a few questions. He then proceeds to ask you what would happen if he had a drink of alcohol while taking methotrexate.

- What advice do you give him?
- Do you inform his doctor?

A couple of months later MG comes in with a prescription from his GP for trimethoprim for a urinary tract infection.

- What advice do you give?
- What else do you do?

Case discussion
— Chemistry of piroxicam

Piroxicam is a common choice of NSAID by paediatric rheumatologists for young people with JIA.

It is structurally unusual compared with most other NSAIDs, particularly in that it lacks a carboxylic acid group. The hydroxyl group in the structure is still acidic, however, with a pK_a of approximately 5.1, as the negative charge formed by dissociation can be delocalised over several atoms by resonance. Piroxicam is thus negatively charged at physiological pH and is highly bound to plasma proteins. It has the potential to interact with other highly bound drugs because it can competitively displace them from their binding sites.

piroxicam

— Piroxicam for young people: side effects and dosing regimens

Piroxicam is not associated with as many side effects in children and young people compared with adults, where its use is limited to osteoarthritis, RA and ankylosing spondylitis. When they are seen, the main side effects in young people are GI symptoms. This is typical of most NSAIDs, due to their inhibition of COX-1, which is a key enzyme involved in the biosynthesis of the prostaglandins that regulate the secretion of protective alkaline mucus in the upper GI tract. When mild, these side effects are usually managed by the introduction of a gastroprotective agent such as ranitidine (histamine H_2-receptor antagonist) or omeprazole (proton pump inhibitor). Less common side effects are skin reactions including pseudoporphyria (a blistering skin condition triggered by excessive UV light exposure) in fair-skinned individuals.

The once-daily dosage of piroxicam is ideal for the school age group and helps promote adherence to this medication. Once-daily dosing is a consequence of the long half-life of piroxicam, which is in part due to the fact that it undergoes *enterohepatic cycling*. This is a process in which an absorbed drug is excreted into the bile by the liver. When the bile is secreted into the small intestine as part of the normal digestive process, the drug then becomes available again for reabsorption into systemic circulation. The Melt formulation (fast-dissolving freeze-dried tablet that is dissolved in the mouth) and other orodispersible formulations are also useful for young people who may have difficulty swallowing tablets.

— Other NSAIDs licensed for use in this age group

Unlike the wide range of NSAIDs licensed for use in adults, there is a more limited range for children and young people, and they include ibuprofen, piroxicam, diclofenac, indometacin and naproxen. Additional NSAIDs are also licensed for use in mid- to late-adolescence, e.g. meloxicam, which is another once-daily medication and hence particularly useful for the adolescent age group.

— Advice on administration of Feldene Melt

In this case, the young person and family should be advised to cut the Feldene Melt (20 mg strength is currently commercially available) into half, and then to cut one half in half again, and then to discard one of the quarters. He should then take the remaining three quarters, i.e. 15 mg. The freeze-dried tablets are more fragile than conventional tablets, and therefore they must be handled with care, including during removal from their packaging.

— Key differences between JIA and adult rheumatoid arthritis

Young people aged <16 years never get RA. JIA is the most common chronic inflammatory joint disease in this age group, and affects approximately 1 in 1000 children and young people. The causes are unknown. JIA is defined as an inflammatory arthritis lasting for >6 weeks in a young person aged <16 years. JIA is different from adult RA and there are, in fact, seven different recognised types of JIA (Table 8.1).

Unlike adult RA, there is a chance of remission in adulthood – although this varies from only a 30% to 70% chance, depending on the subtype. The other important differentiation is that JIA occurs in growing and developing young people, unlike adult RA, which occurs primarily in ageing adults. The reciprocal influences of the disease on the physical, psychological, social and vocational development of the young people must therefore be borne in mind by professionals to ensure that developmentally appropriate healthcare is provided.

— Use of methotrexate for JIA

There is essentially only one DMARD used in JIA, namely methotrexate, although it has never yet been licensed for this age group. Sulfasalazine may be useful, particularly in the enthesitis-related subtype of JIA, but the new biologics are now the next drug of choice for persistent inflammatory arthritis when methotrexate fails and/or young people become intolerant to it.

Being honest is important in a consultation and therefore, in this case, you should acknowledge that the mother is correct in thinking that methotrexate IS used to treat cancer BUT at different (lower)

ILAR classification of juvenile idiopathic arthritis (JIA) (Petty et al., 1998)

Type of JIA	Comments
Systemic arthritis	Systemic features (fever, rash, anaemia, etc.) with arthritis
Oligoarthritis persistent	Most common form of JIA affecting fewer than five joints
Oligoarthritis extended	Affecting fewer than five joints for the first 6 months, but extends to involve five or more joints afterwards. May be severe and persist into adulthood
Polyarthritis RhF negative	Often severe but may remit in later childhood
Polyarthritis RhF positive	Typically older girls with destructive arthropathy
Psoriatic arthritis	Oligo- or polyarticular, often asymmetrical
Enthesitis-related arthritis	Enthesitis (inflammation at insertion of tendons to bone) and synovitis
Undifferentiated arthritis	Features fit no category, or more than one

ILAR, International League Against Rheumatism (renamed International League of Associations for Rheumatology); RhF, rheumatoid factor.

doses from those used for arthritis. Evidence to date shows that current therapies for JIA are NOT associated with an increased rate of malignancy (Beukelman et al., 2012).

Although methotrexate is available in 2.5 mg and 10 mg strength tablets, the availability of these forms largely depends on local policy due to the potential for errors if patients get confused by the different strengths (NPSA, 2004). However, this can cause problems when young people find it difficult to swallow multiple tablets. A degree of flexibility with the appropriate safeguards is therefore often welcomed by both the clinician and the young person alike, particularly if it will mean improved adherence to therapy.

— Addressing swallowing difficulties

Learning to swallow tablets should be encouraged from a young age, particularly in long-term conditions that will require long-term medication with increasing dosage as the child grows. Crushing tablets is, however, an alternative for some medications – although it should be done with care in the case of methotrexate, particularly if there is any chance that the person crushing the tablet is pregnant. A useful strategy to help with the development of swallowing is to practise with small sweets such as TicTacs.

— Nausea associated with methotrexate use in young people and its management

Methotrexate-related nausea is mediated by central brain mechanisms and occurs within a few hours of administration, and can last for 24–48 hours after the dose. Also well recognised with methotrexate is nausea before (anticipatory) – or when thinking about (associative) – taking methotrexate, either of which can develop into significant phobic behaviours not seen with any other anti-rheumatic drug (Bulatović et al., 2011). In a recent study, 44.5% of young people with JIA reported intolerance to oral methotrexate and 67.5% to parenteral methotrexate (Bulatović et al., 2011).

Methotrexate nausea is best anticipated, and the young person provided with antiemetics to take before dosing, e.g. ondansetron 4 mg (serotonin $5HT_3$ receptor antagonist) 1 hour before methotrexate and, if necessary, 6- to 8-hourly afterwards. In addition, a weekly dose of folic acid, e.g. 5 mg taken on a *different* day from the methotrexate, can also help. Other strategies include omitting the NSAID dose on the day of methotrexate administration, because it may be compounding the nausea. Another simple measure is to take the methotrexate on Friday or Saturday evenings, so that the young person might sleep through the worst of it and will also limit any loss of schooling. OTC antiemetic medicines (e.g. domperidone: a peripheral dopamine D_2-receptor antagonist) will *not* be helpful because they act predominantly on the GI tract directly, and do not significantly influence central brain mechanisms (although there is some evidence that domperidone can also block dopamine receptors in the chemoreceptor trigger zone). Anticipatory and/or phobic behaviours are more challenging to treat and often require input from adolescent play therapists and/or clinical psychologists, who can teach young people skills such as guided imagery, which can help in such situations. In all cases, the young person and family should be encouraged to discuss such issues further with their rheumatology team.

— Advising a young person in the pharmacy

Engaging adolescents in their own treatment is an important aspect of successful management of long-term conditions. In this case, it would be important to acknowledge MG's expertise in coming in on his own, collecting his prescription, and asking a very sensible question that many other young people are also interested to know more about. It is important to assess the extent of his understanding of the use of alcohol and methotrexate first. It is essential to be honest and state that, ideally, alcohol should not be taken with methotrexate, due to the increased risk of toxicity. However, if a young person does drink, it is important to provide him or her with advice as to how to drink safely while on methotrexate – such as avoiding binge drinking (particularly around the day when methotrexate is taken), having alcohol-free days and limiting his weekly alcohol intake to a maximum of between 5 and 10 units (depending on his physical development, and with lower numbers of units for girls). Such advice is best given in the context that it is the same advice as you would give any young person. If giving advice about units, it is also important to assess the person's understanding of a unit of alcohol, i.e. 1 unit = half a pint of beer or cider, single measure of spirit, small bottle of alcopop.

You may also wish to consider what you would do if a young person presented a prescription for methotrexate to you. Would you insist on having a parent collect it? What message would it give to this young man – taking responsibility for his own medicines management – if you refuse to engage with him directly? In this case, being able to spend time on his own with the pharmacist has enabled him to receive accurate advice about a sensitive issue. Hopefully a trusting and supportive relationship will develop.

— Importance of confidentiality

In any discussion with a young person, the person's understanding of confidentiality should be assessed, particularly with respect to the circumstances when it may need to be broken, i.e. when a young person is at risk of serious harm by himself, by someone else, or that he is likely to harm someone else. But if confidentiality has to be broken, the young person should be told how, when and with whom this will happen. Confidentiality is a major issue for young people utilising healthcare and, if it isn't assured, young people may forego care or asking for advice (Lehrer et al., 2007). However, it is important to encourage the young person to discuss this further with the rheumatology team.

With respect to this case, trimethoprim, a commonly used antibiotic for the treatment of urinary tract infections, is contraindicated with methotrexate due to the risk of haematological toxicity and the patient should be advised not to take it. Contact the GP and ask for an alternative antibiotic for MG (a 3-day course of nitrofurantoin, amoxicillin or a cephalosporin may be suitable).

— Further considerations in advising adolescents on medicines use

The environmental setting of any consultation with a young person is an important consideration, particularly with respect to confidentiality. Ensuring compliance of pharmacy services to the 'You're welcome' quality criteria for a youth-friendly service (Department of Health, 2011) is of key importance to health policy and provision in the UK.

For regular customers to a community pharmacy, it is useful to establish communication with the paediatric or adult rheumatology team and to identify a key link person to whom queries can be directed. This is often the role of the rheumatology specialist nurses, who can work closely with the hospital pharmacists and, in the case of paediatric rheumatology nurses, are extremely knowledgeable about drug therapy for rheumatic disease in childhood and adolescence.

Community pharmacists may wish to consider opportunities for offering medicines use reviews to young people in England and Wales. In Scotland, there is a facility within the chronic medication service to carry out a focused high-risk medicine review for methotrexate. This service could be offered to young people with arthritis.

EXTENDED LEARNING

- Research resources available through patient charities and other agencies; these provide an insight to the experiences of long-term illness from the perspective of young people. An appreciation of these perspectives by health professionals will help to provide services that are responsive to the needs of young people:

- Arthritis Care: www.arthritiscare.org.uk Includes:

  - *The Source*: for young people with arthritis aged <25 years

- *Breakout*: a book written by young people with JIA for young people with JIA
- Arthritis Research UK: www. arthritisresearchuk.org Includes:
  - *Arthritis in Teenagers* booklet
  - Information leaflets about many drugs, although mainly written for adults
- Youth Health Talk Online: www. youthhealthtalk.org – Their 'Long-term conditions' module includes several young people talking about their experiences with methotrexate

References and further reading

Beresford MW (2011). Juvenile idiopathic arthritis: new insights into classification, measures of outcome, and pharmacotherapy. *Pediatr Drugs* 13:161–73.

Beukelman T, Haynes K, Curtis JR et al. (2012). Rates of malignancy associated with juvenile idiopathic arthritis and its treatment. *Arthrit Rheum* 64:1263–71.

Bulatović M, Heijstek MW, Verkaaik M et al. (2011). High prevalence of methotrexate intolerance in juvenile idiopathic arthritis: Development and validation of a methotrexate intolerance severity score. *Arthrit Rheum* 63:2007–13.

Department of Health (2011). *'You're welcome' quality criteria. Making health services young people friendly.* London: DH.

Lehrer JA, Pantell R, Tebb K, Shafer MA. (2007). Forgone health care among US adolescents: associations between risk characteristics and confidentiality concern. *J Adolesc Health* 40:218–26.

National Patient Safety Agency (2004). *Towards the Safer Use of Oral Methotrexate.* London: NPSA. Available at: http://publications.nice.org.uk/urinary-tract-infection-in-children-cg54/key-priorities-for-implementation (accessed 17 September 2013).

Petty RE, Southwood TR, Baum J et al. (1998). Revision of the proposed classification criteria for juvenile idiopathic arthritis: Durban, 1997. *J Rheumatol* 25:1991–4.

Wahezi DM, Ilowite NT (2013). Juvenile idiopathic arthritis: an update on current pharmacotherapy and future perspectives. *Expert Opin Pharmacother* 14:975–89.

Case 6
Systemic lupus erythematosus

STEPHEN HUGHES

LEARNING OUTCOMES

At the end of this case, you will be able to:

- Explain the pathophysiology and describe the signs and symptoms of systemic lupus erythematosus (SLE)
- Summarise the treatment options available for SLE with non-major organ involvement
- Describe the use of induction therapy of patients with severe SLE, e.g. lupus nephritis
- Discuss the different monoclonal antibody treatments available for patients with SLE

Case study

Mrs RM is a 24-year-old white woman who has been newly diagnosed with SLE based on her initial presentation of arthralgia (joint pain), recurrent mouth ulcers and fatigue. Her local rheumatologist has initiated therapy with prednisolone and hydroxychloroquine for the SLE.

- Explain the pathophysiology of SLE and its typical presentation
- What diagnostic tests can be used to confirm this diagnosis of SLE?
- What are the triggers of SLE?
- What advice would you offer Mrs RM with regard to starting hydroxychloroquine therapy?
- With the aid of the structure of hydroxychloroquine, explain the rationale for the need not to take it at the same time as antacids

At her 6-month review, it is clear that the patient's disease is relapsing each time the prednisolone dose is reduced <20 mg/day. The newly married Mrs RM is very anxious and is unhappy with her weight gain and irritability with the steroid treatment. She claims that the treatment is 'ruining her life' and 'affecting her marriage'. The consultant is concerned also with her worsening serology, with a decline seen in her complement (C3 and C4) as well as a trend of increasing anti-double-stranded DNA (anti-dsDNA) in the blood. It is decided to trial a steroid-sparing agent and Mrs RM is prescribed azathioprine 2 mg/kg daily, with the plan to reduce the steroids down to 10 mg daily.

- ❓ What serological monitoring can be used to guide therapy in patients with SLE?
- ❓ What is the significance of finding elevated levels of anti-dsDNA in the blood?
- ❓ What are the long-term complications of high-dose steroid treatment?

Two years later at a clinic review, Mrs RM complains of feeling short of breath and constantly tired.

> **On examination**
> - Fluid overloaded
> - Blood results appear normal with the exception of a markedly low albumin result (13 g/dL – reference range 35–50 g/dL)
> - Urine sample is tested and shows gross proteinuria (UPCR [urine protein : creatinine ratio] 10 mg/μmol: reference <20 mg/μmol)

After confirmation with a kidney biopsy, the doctor explains to the patient that she has nephrotic syndrome.

- ❓ What is nephrotic syndrome?
- ❓ What are the expected complications of this condition?
- ❓ What are the first-line induction treatments of lupus nephritis?

Upon diagnosis of class V (membranous) lupus nephritis with associated nephrotic syndrome, the nephrologist discusses the treatment options available.

On balance, Mrs RM decides against cyclophosphamide therapy because she plans to start a family in the near future. Although mycophenolate therapy is trialled, treatment has to stop due to severe diarrhoea.

The nephrologist and rheumatologist suggest starting monoclonal antibody therapy, which Mrs RM is keen to consider.

- ❓ What are rituximab and belimumab?
- ❓ What are their respective mechanisms of action?
- ❓ What complications are associated with the administration of monoclonal antibodies?
- ❓ How can these be minimised?

Case discussion

— Pathophysiology of SLE and its typical presentation

Systemic lupus erythematous is a chronic inflammatory disease involving many organs and systems, with prevalence in the UK of 25–28 cases per 100 000 population. SLE is classed as an autoimmune disease, where the immune system mistakes healthy body tissue for antigens and therefore develops destructive antibodies against them. There are many types of autoimmune diseases and the aetiology is unclear; however, there are also a number of drugs that can *cause* SLE (drug-induced lupus erythematous – DILE, e.g. hydralazine, procainamide, isoniazid, carbamazepine).

The most common symptoms of SLE include joint pain and swelling, particularly of the fingers, hands wrists and knees. Other symptoms include chronic fatigue and malaise, muscle pain, fever, swollen lymph nodes, skin rashes ('butterfly rash' on nose and cheeks, exacerbated by sunlight exposure), lung and heart inflammation (pleuritis, endocarditis), hair loss and possible headaches and personality changes.

Women of child-bearing age are predominantly affected; typically patients present from the age of 15 to 45 years. The clinical spectrum ranges from mild disease, with mainly mucocutaneous and musculoskeletal manifestations, to a severe life-threatening disease with major organ involvement, including kidneys, lungs or cardiac involvement. SLE is a relapsing–remitting disease, involving frequent flare-ups with severe symptoms followed by periods of disease remission.

— Tests used to diagnose SLE

A first step in the diagnosis of SLE is often the presence of antinuclear antibodies (ANAs). However, because a positive ANA result can be a consequence of an alternative diagnosis, more specific antibody tests will follow to confirm the diagnosis. These include tests for anti-dsDNA and anti-Smith (anti-Sm) antibodies. The appearance of extracellular DNA in the blood (and consequent antibodies against it) is believed to arise from a generally higher apoptosis (programmed cell death) in patients with SLE, although the precise mechanism involved is still unclear. Anti-Sm antibodies, which develop against so-called small nuclear ribonucleoproteins (snRNPs), are present in only about 20% of SLE patients. In patients with these ANAs present, titres may be used to monitor disease activity. The initiating factor in SLE is thought to be abnormal clearance of cells after apoptosis. Abnormal nuclear particles remain, which bind to specific antibodies and then deposit in tissues around the body. Here, the antibodies activate the complement immune response and damage local tissue. The complement proteins C3 and C4 are involved in this process, and therefore levels of these serological markers can be used to monitor disease activity, with low levels indicative of active disease. SLE can therefore affect any organ of the body and often mimics or is mistaken for other illnesses.

— **Triggers of SLE**

Sunlight and UV exposure are known triggers for SLE, particularly the cutaneous manifestations of the disease. This may be due to a direct alteration of DNA structure, through abnormal immune responses to UV-damaged cells or potentially to the body's complex relationship with vitamin D.

Hormones, particularly oestrogen, are thought to play a significant role in SLE disease. Women are nine times more likely to be affected than men and pregnancy is a known risk factor for SLE flares.

— **Treatment of SLE**

Triggers of SLE, if identifiable, such as stress, smoking and UV light should be avoided if possible. Regular use of simple analgesia, NSAIDs and antimalarials can help to manage mild symptoms. The antimalarials, such as hydroxychloroquine and chloroquine, possess anti-inflammatory activity and are used to treat and prevent SLE flares; they are particularly useful for cutaneous symptoms and arthralgias poorly controlled with NSAIDs. Drug-induced retinopathy may however occur with long-term antimalarial use, and annual review by an optometrist is generally advised. Other adverse effects include GI upsets (abdominal cramps), diarrhoea, nausea, vomiting, skin changes and cardiac toxicity.

chloroquine   hydroxychloroquine

The structures of the anti-malarial DMARDs are shown in the diagram; the presence of the additional primary hydroxyl group in hydroxychloroquine is clearly evident. Each drug contains a single chiral centre and is manufactured as a mixture of enantiomers. All three nitrogen atoms in hydroxychloroquine (and chloroquine) are basic. The tertiary amino nitrogen atom (highlighted in red) is most basic (lone pair of electrons most available), followed by the quinoline ring nitrogen. Both of these groups are protonated and positively charged for formulation of the drug as the water-soluble sulfate (SO_4^{2-}) salt. The remaining substituted aromatic amine is least basic. The side chain of hydroxychloroquine is able to form very poorly soluble coordination complexes (chelation) with some metal ions, such as found in most antacids, resulting in reduced absorption. Consequently, hydroxychloroquine should not be taken at the same time (within 4 h) as antacids.

Corticosteroids are a useful immunosuppressive treatment for all degrees of SLE disease. Pulse therapy with high-dose steroid (methylprednisolone 1 g/day for 3 days) can be used for life-threatening disease and low-dose prednisolone (up to 10 mg/day) is useful for treating mild flares and maintaining disease remission. Long-term therapy is usually limited by glucocorticoid steroid complications. Osteoporosis, gastritis, abdominal striae, psychosis and metabolic complications (weight gain, diabetes and hyperlipidaemia) can occur and must therefore be vigilantly monitored. Much like in rheumatoid arthritis, DMARDs are routinely used, particularly in a steroid-sparing role.

— **Lupus nephritis and its treatment**

Renal involvement is thought to affect at least 50% of all patients with lupus. Renal complications usually present with proteinuria (leaking of large amounts of protein from the blood into the urine) and/or kidney impairment. Nephrotic syndrome is defined as gross proteinuria (>4 g/day of protein loss) and is characterised by hypoalbuminaemia (albumin accounts for 60% of the body's protein), oedema (secondary to loss of albumin and reduced oncotic pressure [colloid osmotic pressure]) and hyperlipidaemia (loss of lipid enzyme lipoprotein lipase). Loss of clotting factors predisposes nephrotic patients to thrombotic complications, such as venous thromboembolisms and pulmonary embolisms.

The alkylating agent, cyclophosphamide, is sometimes used in severe cases of SLE especially where there is major organ involvement, such as lupus nephritis. This is a cytotoxic (alkylating) agent used to treat a number of malignancies; however, it also has immunosuppressant properties through the disruption of immune cells (lymphocytes). As a cytotoxic, complications of this therapy include hair loss, infections and irreversible infertility. The latter complication limits its use in patients hoping to start a family at a later date. The use of cyclophosphamide requires careful assessment of each patient with regard to the potential benefits and risks. Mycophenolate, an immunosuppressant commonly used post-transplantation, also has good success in severe SLE. Immune-related infections and diarrhoea are commonly seen adverse reactions that may however limit its use.

— **Use of monoclonal antibodies in SLE**

Advances in understanding the role of lymphocyte B cells in SLE have led to the successful development and use of anti-B-cell therapies such as rituximab and belimumab. Rituximab is a genetically engineered glycosylated mouse/human monoclonal antibody, produced using mammalian (Chinese hamster ovary) cell suspension culture which is subsequently highly purified. It is an antibody against the protein CD20, which is primarily found on the surface of B cells, and leads to the destruction of the target B cell.

Predominantly used in the treatment of RA and leukaemia, rituximab has shown some benefit in SLE with high antibody activity. It is currently unlicensed for SLE treatment but is commonly used by nephrologists and rheumatologists within the UK, in particular as second-line therapy to those intolerant or who have failed with first-line cyclophosphamide or mycophenolate treatment in SLE with major organ involvement.

Belimumab inhibits the activity of human B-lymphocyte stimulator protein (BLyS) by blocking it from binding to B cells and reduces cell survival. BLyS is over-expressed in SLE and is expected to

play a role in SLE. Belimumab is a human, IgG1λ monoclonal antibody, produced in a mammalian cell line by recombinant DNA technology. Despite being the only drug licensed for SLE in over 40 years, belimumab is not recommended by NICE for treatment of SLE at the time of print. Belimumab has shown moderate improvement in non-renal SLE and has been shown not to be cost-effective in comparison to other DMARDs available.

— **Complications associated with the administration of monoclonal antibodies**

Administration of monoclonal antibody therapy is complicated by infusion reactions. These range from slight chills and drops in blood pressure to serious anaphylactic reactions. This immune response is due to the introduction of foreign antibodies, often murine (mouse) derived, which stimulate systemic inflammatory responses. Prophylactic antihistamines and steroids before monoclonal antibody administration may reduce the initial immune response.

EXTENDED LEARNING

- Which other drugs might be implicated in drug-induced lupus erythematous?
- What are autoimmune diseases?
- Investigate some of the newer agents employed in the management of autoimmune diseases
- How are monoclonal antibodies manufactured? What are their therapeutic applications and limitations to their use?

References and further reading

Brown N, Hughes S, Venning M (2012). SLE: clinical features and diagnosis. *Clin Pharmacist* 4:195–9.

Frieri M (2013). Mechanisms of disease for the clinician: systemic lupus erythematosus. *Ann Allergy Asthma Immunol* 110:228–32.

Hughes S, Brown N, Vincent M (2012). SLE management. *Clin Pharmacist* 4:200–5.

Liu CC, Kao AH, Manzi S, Ahearn JM (2013). Biomarkers in systemic lupus erythematosus: challenges and prospects for the future. *Ther Adv Musculoskelet Dis* 5:210–33.

9

Eye, nose and throat cases

INTRODUCTION

This section comprises five cases centred on patients with conditions affecting the eye, nose or throat, namely conjunctivitis, glaucoma, age-related macular degeneration, sore throat and hay fever.

Case 1
Conjunctivitis in pregnancy ▶ 337

This case focuses on a woman who is 37 weeks' pregnant and presents at the pharmacy for advice about a sticky eye. First, the pathophysiology and diagnosis of conjunctivitis are outlined. The different presentations of conjunctivitis and the associated diagnoses are discussed, including the relevant issues that need to be considered for referral to a medical practitioner. Treatment options and important counselling points follow. The chemistry and mechanism of action of antimicrobial drugs used to treat conjunctivitis are explained. The properties of ophthalmic preparations, including isotonicity, pH, viscosity and preservatives, are outlined. Finally, the case concludes with particular considerations that need to be made when prescribing topical preparations for this patient.

Case 2
Chronic open-angle glaucoma ▶ 341

This is the second ocular case and focuses on a patient who has been newly diagnosed with chronic open-angle glaucoma. First, the pathophysiology, diagnosis and monitoring of chronic open-angle glaucoma are outlined, followed by a description of particular groups of patients that are at risk of developing glaucoma. Strategies for ensuring optimum use of, and the rationale for, topical ocular products are reported. This case chooses to focus on latanoprost and

reviews its chemistry and mechanism of action. A discussion of methods for reducing or preventing side effects from ocular products concludes the case.

Case 3
Wet age-related macular degeneration ▶ 345

This is the final ocular case and focuses on the immediate referral of a female patient to the hospital ophthalmologist for diagnosis of this sight-threatening condition. The case begins with a description of the pathophysiology, signs and presentation of wet age-related macular degeneration (wet ARMD). The role of vascular endothelial growth factor (VEGF) inhibitors in the treatment of wet ARMD, their mechanism of action and potential adverse effects are outlined. The advantages of intravitreal injections for the treatment of wet ARMD compared with other drug delivery routes are explained. The case closes with a discussion of the pharmaceutical considerations when designing intraocular preparations.

Case 4
Sore throat ▶ 348

This case involves a mother of two children who presents at the pharmacy with a sore throat. The pathophysiology, signs, symptoms and diagnosis of a sore throat are outlined and treatment options discussed. Solid dosage forms such as lozenges and pastilles are described. The chemistry and mechanism of action of local anaesthetics are outlined. Important information for a differential diagnosis or referral to another healthcare professional is highlighted.

Case 5
Hay fever ► 352

This case describes a student who visits the pharmacy for advice about his hay fever. The pathophysiology, signs, symptoms and diagnosis of hay fever are outlined and the criteria for referral to another healthcare professional discussed. The various treatment options available to relieve the different symptoms are detailed. The chemistry of chlorphenamine and cetirizine are outlined, and related to the sedating effects of some antihistamines. Information pertaining to lifestyle changes that may help with the management of hay fever is summarised.

Case 1
Conjunctivitis in pregnancy

NATALIE LEWIS

LEARNING OUTCOMES

At the end of this case, you will be able to:

- Outline the pathophysiology, signs and symptoms, and diagnosis of bacterial conjunctivitis
- Describe the treatment options available for bacterial conjunctivitis
- Outline the chemistry and mechanism of action of antimicrobial drugs used to treat conjunctivitis
- Describe the factors to be considered when formulating eyedrops
- Outline the factors to consider when prescribing topical products for pregnant patients

Case study

Mrs NC is 29 years old and currently 37 weeks' pregnant. She is concerned about her left eye, which has been producing a yellow discharge that has stuck her eyelids together. She has been experiencing some discomfort in the affected eye but her vision is normal once the discharge has been blinked away. On observation, the entire conjunctival surface, including the tarsal plates (dense, fibrous tissues that give shape and support to the eyelids), appears red. Apart from the generalised redness there are no other abnormalities of the tarsal plates.

- What is conjunctivitis and what are the main causes?
- How can a bacterial cause of conjunctivitis be identified?
- Which patients or symptoms will necessitate referral to a GP?

Seven days later, Mrs NC returns to your pharmacy. She has a prescription for fusidic acid eyedrops, one drop twice daily, having phoned the GP to ask for some eyedrops because her condition persisted during the week.

- What are the treatment options available for conjunctivitis?

- What are the formulation considerations for eyedrops?
- What additional factors have to be considered when treating pregnant women?
- Would chloramphenicol be safe to use in this patient?

Case discussion

— Pathophysiology of conjunctivitis

Conjunctivitis is inflammation of the conjunctiva, the semi-transparent, highly vascularised mucous membrane that covers the globe of the eye, starting from the edge of the cornea (limbus), flowing back behind the eye, looping forward to form the inner surface of the eyelids (tarsal plates). The purpose of the conjunctiva is to decrease friction when blinking and to protect the sclera. Due to the continuity of the conjunctiva, it also prevents objects such as eyelashes or contact lenses sliding back behind the eye. As the conjunctiva is the final ocular layer, it is regularly exposed to the environment and hence subject to trauma, infection and allergic reactions, which can induce inflammation.

— Establishing the cause of conjunctivitis

In cases of conjunctivitis, the whole of the conjunctiva will be involved (the globe and the tarsal plates) and so all surfaces should show redness. Where the redness is localised to just the limbus, another structure is affected and requires investigation. There will be generalised mild discomfort and ocular irritation; the presence of pain indicates involvement of the cornea and forms part of the differential diagnosis.

Discharge or increased lacrimation is generally the key to diagnosis for the most common causes of conjunctivitis. A thick yellow purulent discharge that can stick eyelids together in the morning indicates a bacterial origin. This cause is more common in infants and children than in adults. A more watery discharge is associated with viral conjunctivitis. Cases of viral conjunctivitis may also be distinguished by a recent flu-like illness, conjunctival follicles (small semi-translucent lymphatic swellings), lid oedema and excessive lacrimation. This type of conjunctivitis is more common in adults than in children. The most common causative agent is adenovirus; the others implicated to a much lesser extent are the Coxsackievirus and picornavirus. Viral conjunctivitis is very contagious and other people in close contact are likely to be affected. There can also be serious consequences with some patients developing keratoconjunctivitis, which affects vision.

Allergic conjunctivitis is not associated with any discharge, but will be associated with increased bilateral lacrimation. Itching will predominate with eyes appearing more pink than red. There may also be some degree of conjunctival swelling or ballooning (chemosis). Most patients presenting with allergic conjunctivitis at the pharmacy will do so with acute presentations and will have a history of contact with an allergen towards which the response is mounted, e.g. pollen, mite allergens. During the hay fever season it is termed 'seasonal allergic conjunctivitis'. Chronic allergic conjunctivitis may be present all year long. It commonly affects boys with a history of atopy (genetic disposition towards allergic disease). Due to the chronic nature, there may be more changes in the eye: follicles or white spots in the limbal region, papillary (raised, 'bumpy') lesions on the upper tarsal plate or punctate lesions (tiny white spots) on the corneal epithelium.

Chlamydial conjunctivitis caused by the obligate intracellular organism *Chlamydia trachomatis* is the least common type of conjunctivitis. Discharge can vary between watery and mucopurulent (containing mucus and pus), but the redness of the conjunctiva is deeper than seen with other causes. Raised follicles will be seen on the lower tarsal conjunctiva as well as symptoms of systemic infection. Patients are screened for chlamydial antigens to confirm diagnosis.

— **Bacterial cases requiring referral**
Although most cases of bacterial conjunctivitis are easily diagnosable in the community pharmacy, not all patients will be candidates for over-the-counter (OTC) treatment. The following patients will need referral to a doctor:

- Patients who are producing copious amounts of purulent discharge that reaccumulates quickly when wiped away, or infection that is not localised to the eye, because this indicates severe infection.
- Patients experiencing pain within the eye, which indicates corneal involvement needing investigation.
- Patients with loss of vision, indicating severe infection or other structures affected.
- Patients who have had surgery or laser treatment in the last 6 months because they will require examination of the surgical site before treatment.
- Contact lens wearers who are more prone to eye infections and more likely to become infected with *Pseudomonas aeruginosa*, which can go on to cause corneal ulceration, endophthalmitis (inflammation of the interior of the eye) and even permanent blindness.
- Patients who have failed to respond to initial topical antibiotic treatment, indicating that the antibiotic was not active against the causative organism.
- If the patient is pregnant or breastfeeding because exposure of the child to medication must be considered.

— **Treatment options for conjunctivitis**
Often, in bacterial conjunctivitis, no pharmacological treatment is necessary because the condition is usually self-limiting and will resolve within 7–10 days. Good hygiene is important to reduce transfer to the unaffected eye; this includes replacing any possible contaminated eye makeup. The use of eye bathing or sterile wipes to refresh the eye and remove discharge can help to reduce some symptoms. Often, patients will want some treatment in the form of a topical antibiotic. In the case of children, treatment may be requested by the nursery or school in order for the child to return to interaction with other children and prevent spread.

As well as bacterial conjunctivitis being more common in infants and children than adults, there is a difference seen in the probable causative organism. In adults the causative organisms are *Staphylococcus aureus* (55%), *Streptococcus pneumoniae* (20%), *Moraxella* sp. (10%), *Haemophilus influenzae* (5%) and *Pseudomonas aeruginosa* (5%), whereas in infants and children the most common bacteria are *S. pneumoniae, M. catarrhalis* and *H. influenzae*. Despite the differences in organisms, both groups have Gram-positive and Gram-negative bacteria implicated, so, when treating bacterial conjunctivitis, agents with a broad spectrum of activity are used.

Chloramphenicol 0.5% eyedrops are considered to be first-line treatment for bacterial conjunctivitis because it is broad spectrum with activity against both Gram-positive and -negative bacteria. It exerts its bacteriostatic effect by selectively inhibiting protein synthesis in ribosomes. Although considered the gold standard and effective for almost all cases of bacterial conjunctivitis, it is not active against *Pseudomonas aeruginosa* or *Chlamydia trachomatis,* so those patients who have not responded to treatment require immediate referral. Despite its effectiveness, OTC supply is prohibited to those who are aged <2 years or already using products for glaucoma or dry eye syndrome, have a personal or family history of bone marrow problems (due to link to aplastic anaemia) or take medication that may interact with chloramphenicol eyedrops.

chloramphenicol

In these patients, however, propamidine isetionate (isethionate) 0.1% eyedrops (Brolene eyedrops*)* could be supplied OTC. Propamidine is an aromatic diamidine (R-C[NH]NH$_2$) antibacterial disinfectant that is active against Gram-positive bacteria, but less active against Gram-negative bacteria; it also has limited antifungal properties. It blocks the permease transport system that is responsible for the uptake of purine nucleotides. Bacteria are therefore unable to synthesise the precursors for DNA, RNA or protein metabolism. Other less well-known interactions add together to give its bacteriostatic effect.

propamidine isethionate

Failure of OTC products necessitates referral to a doctor. Further investigation to determine the cause of the infection may be required and cultures taken. Before culture results are obtained, other broad-spectrum antibiotics would be prescribed such as ofloxacin (a fluoroquinolone), which can interfere with bacterial DNA replication, or fusidic acid (derived from the fungus *Fusidium coccineum*), a complex steroid-like molecule (no steroid activity), which acts by inhibiting bacterial protein synthesis.

— Formulation of eyedrops

To ensure that topical ophthalmic preparations are non-irritant, they are formulated to have properties approximating to those of lacrimal fluids (tears), have the appropriate viscosity and include an antimicrobial preservative if a multi-dose presentation is required (to prevent growth of microorganisms accidently introduced into the product during use).

Isotonicity: hypotonic and hypertonic solutions are irritant to the eye and thus hypotonic ophthalmic solutions (similar to many injections) are made isotonic by the addition of tonicity agents, such as sodium chloride, dextrose and buffer salts.

pH: the pH of tears is approximately neutral. Tears have some buffering capacity, and weak acids and bases, pH range 3.5–9 can be tolerated in the eye. Buffers may be included, such as borate and phosphate buffers.

ofloxacin

fusidic acid

Viscosity: water-soluble, viscosity-enhancing polymers, such as methyl cellulose and hydroxypropyl methylcellulose, may be included in formulations to increase their viscosity, prolonging retention of the drug in the eye and thereby increasing drug absorption.

Antimicrobial preservatives: antimicrobial agents with a broad spectrum of activity against Gram-positive and -negative bacteria, yeasts and moulds, and with low toxicity to humans, are required for multiple-use eyedrops, which may be accidently contaminated during use. The number of antimicrobial agents suitable for ophthalmic use is very limited, with benzalkonium chloride being the most commonly employed.

Fusidic acid is formulated as viscous eyedrops (Fucithalmic) in a preserved aqueous system containing the polymer Carbomer. The viscous formulation is easy to administer, and the polymer-containing formulation, which liquefies and becomes transparent on contact with the tear fluid, gives an increased precorneal residence time and sustained levels of the drug, compared with a conventional eyedrop formulation.

The decision to include any excipient within the formulation must take into account compatibility with the drug and the container.

— **Ocular treatment in pregnancy**

As with other minor ailments in patients who are pregnant, treatment initially will always tend towards conservative management with non-pharmacological therapies; this is to reduce the risk of exposing the unborn child to medicines and their metabolites. Despite the therapy in this case being topical, there is some systemic absorption of ocular products, hence their ability to cause systemic side effects. Medicines in ocular products penetrate the cornea, entering the aqueous fluid, which drains from the eye via the canal of Schlemm (circular canal at the sclerocorneal junction of the eye, draining aqueous humour from the anterior chamber into the conjunctival veins). In addition, some product will end up in the gastrointestinal (GI) tract, because it may drain via the nasolacrimal duct into the nasopharynx. Pharmacokinetic data on the amount of systemic absorption from ocular products are lacking. This, coupled with the lack of human data on the exposure of fetuses to topical ocular products, means that there are few published data on the potential for fetotoxic events of topical ophthalmic medications.

Many ocular medications have also been used systemically to treat conditions in pregnant women and have not produced evidence of birth defects above the normal background rate. Therefore, if a medication is not known to produce defects systemically, then it is not likely to do so topically due to the smaller amounts administered. Careful consideration is needed when prescribing medication and each patient must still be considered on a case-by-case basis. Even topical therapies will be subject to the same considerations: what is the severity of the infection? What are the potential consequences of not treating the mother? What is the potential toxicity to the fetus of the drugs under consideration?

— **Choice of treatment in this case**

In this case, conservative treatment has failed, and not treating the mother may lead to further ocular involvement and invasive infection. We are then left with the final consideration of which agent to use. A broad-spectrum agent would be required, so, on this first point, chloramphenicol would be a good choice. However, despite there being no published data on any associated risk of congenital malformation, there have been concerns that use near term is associated with grey baby syndrome. Due to this concern, the UK teratology information service advises that chloramphenicol use in pregnancy should be avoided where possible. In selecting a therapy that is believed to be the safest, fusidic acid is a potential alternative, for which the manufacturers state that it can be used in pregnancy.

EXTENDED LEARNING

- How can the systemic absorption of ocular products be reduced?
- Outline how eyedrops are packaged and sterilised
- What is ophthalmia neonatorum?
- How should allergic conjunctivitis be treated?
- What considerations should be taken when advising on topical dermatological preparations for pregnant patients?
- What is grey baby syndrome?

ADDITIONAL PRACTICE POINT

- How would you counsel the patient to administer the eyedrop product?

References and further reading

Chung CY Kwok AKH, Chung KL (2004). Use of ophthalmic medications during pregnancy. *Hong Kong Med J* **10**:191–5.

Elton M (2005). Conjunctivitis and chloramphenicol. *Pharmaceut J* **274**:725–8.

Fadda H, Khalili A, Khaw PT, Brocchini S (2013). Ocular drug delivery. In: Aulton ME, Taylor KMG (eds), *Aulton's Pharmaceutics: The design and manufacture of medicines*, 4th edn. London: Elsevier, 710–31.

Ghate D, Edelhauser H (2006). Ocular drug delivery. *Expert Opin Drug Delivery* **3**:275–87.

UK Teratology information service (2011). Use of eye drops in pregnancy, Version 1. Available at: www.bmec.swbh.nhs.uk/wp-content/uploads/2013/03/EYE-DROPS-IN-PREGNANCY.pdf (accessed 1 September 2013).

Case 2
Chronic open-angle glaucoma

NATALIE LEWIS

LEARNING OUTCOMES

At the end of this case, you will be able to:

- Outline the pathophysiology, diagnosis and monitoring of chronic open-angle glaucoma
- Describe the populations of patients who are at risk of developing glaucoma
- Describe the optimum use of topical preparations and the rationale for topical therapy in the case of ocular conditions
- Outline the chemistry and mechanism of action of latanoprost
- Outline methods for reducing or preventing side effects from ocular products

Case study

Miss NG is 34 years old and African–Caribbean. She regularly comes to your community pharmacy to collect medication for her father, Mr HG, who is 56 years old. During today's visit, she seems anxious and asks to speak to the pharmacist. She is concerned that her father has developed glaucoma and may go blind. The glaucoma was suspected by her father's optometrist who performed air puff tonometry as part of routine screening when he went to buy a new pair of glasses. He was then followed up and given latanoprost eyedrops, which she is collecting today.

- ❷ What is chronic open-angle glaucoma?
- ❷ How is it diagnosed?

- ❷ Which people are most likely to develop glaucoma?
- ❷ Is the patient likely to go blind?
- ❷ What class of drug is latanoprost and what is its mechanism of action? How is it related structurally to the naturally occurring biomolecule that it mimics?

Miss NG comes back the next day, because her father is having difficulty in using the eyedrops as his eyes seem to run with tears when he administers the drops. She asks if her father could have a tablet instead.

- ❷ What are the common formulations used for eyedrops?
- ❷ How should eyedrops be correctly administered to the eye?
- ❷ Why are topical medications used rather than oral therapy for ocular conditions?

At the end of the week, Miss NG has persuaded her father to come into the pharmacy because she is concerned that he is having a reaction to the latanoprost eyedrops as his eyes look pink.

- ❷ What is the side effect that Mr HG is experiencing?
- ❷ What can patients do to minimise side effects from ocular products?

Case discussion

— Chronic open-angle glaucoma and its pathophysiology

Glaucoma occurs when the drainage tubules (trabecular meshwork) in the eye are unable to drain the eye effectively of liquid aqueous humour, produced by the ciliary processes. As a result, intraocular pressure builds up, which, if left untreated, can permanently damage the optic nerve and nerve fibres in the retina, leading to visual field loss and eventual blindness. Intraocular pressure is the level of aqueous fluid pressure inside the eye. Normal intraocular pressure usually ranges from 12 mmHg to 21 mmHg and can be measured by means of a tonometer, nowadays using a non-contact air-puff method to detect small deflections of the cornea. Glaucoma is normally associated with a raised intraocular pressure >21 mmHg; however, some individuals with 'ocular hypertension' have an abnormally raised intraocular pressure without developing optic nerve damage.

Glaucoma encompasses a group of ocular conditions, typically, but not always, characterised by increased intraocular pressure, optic disc 'cupping' (due to thinning of the optic nerve head and enlargement of the optic cup observable at the back of the retina) and visual (peripheral) field loss. Chronic open-angle glaucoma is the most common type and develops slowly. In open-angle glaucoma, the drainage angle (Schlemm's canal) is open so that there is no structural obstruction to the drainage network. There is no visible abnormality of the trabecular meshwork. It is thought that something is wrong with the ability of the cells in the trabecular meshwork to carry out their normal function, or there may be fewer cells present, as a natural result of getting older. Some think that it is due to a structural defect of the eye's drainage system, others that it is caused by an enzymatic problem (e.g. microsomal CYP1B1 mutations or deletions in the galactosylceramidase gene [*GALC*]).

Primary angle-closure glaucoma is comparatively rare. Although onset may be insidious or rapid, a sudden painful increase in intraocular pressure occurs as a consequence of blockage to the drainage canals. Immediate medical attention is required.

Glaucoma is one of the leading causes of preventable blindness in the UK, accounting for around 15% of registered cases of blindness.

— **People most at risk of developing glaucoma**
There are several risk factors for the development of glaucoma. Age is a major factor, because the condition becomes much more common as people get older: in the white population, aged <40 years the prevalence is 1 in 50; in those >75 years, prevalence is 1 in 10. Glaucoma is also more likely in people of African or African–Caribbean origin and if there is a family history: people with relatives with the condition may have a four- to ninefold increased risk of its development. These risk factors may be relevant when targeting screening programmes to those most at risk.

— **Visual field loss**
Vision loss begins with peripheral or side vision. Patients compensate for this unconsciously by turning their head to the side, and may not be aware of a problem until significant vision is lost. If undiagnosed or untreated, the damage will progress and ultimately the whole visual field will be lost. Treatment can halt or slow down the progress of visual field loss, but it cannot regain any of the visual field that has already been lost. Thus, screening (especially in individuals most at risk) to identify disease early on is routinely undertaken by community optometrists.

— **Rationale for topical treatment of ocular conditions**
Glaucoma is most often treated using eyedrops. Systemically (often orally) administered ocular drugs are prevented from reaching therapeutic concentrations within the eye by a variety of physiological mechanisms as well as the characteristics of the drug itself. The blood–aqueous barrier (ciliary epithelium and capillary of the iris) and the blood–retinal barrier (non-fenestrated capillaries of the retinal circulation and tight junctions of retinal epithelium) are responsible for the regulation of drug/molecule transport from the systemic circulation to the anterior and posterior ocular tissues, respectively. In some cases, the vitreal drug level can be <10% of the serum concentration. Although increasing the systemic level would create a corresponding rise in vitreal concentration, this would be at the cost of increasing systemic side effects, and any issues that would normally be associated with the drug metabolism and excretion. It is therefore more clinically effective, cost-effective and safer to use a topical product.

— **Treatment options**
Classes of drug most commonly used are: prostaglandin analogues (e.g. latanoprost) which increase the flow of aqueous humour out of the

eye or β-adrenoreceptor blockers (e.g. timolol), thought to reduce intraocular pressure by slowing down production of aqueous humour. Other drugs that may be used are carbonic anhydrase inhibitors (e.g. dorzolamide or brinzolamide), sympathomimetics (α$_2$-adrenoreceptor agonists, e.g. brimonidine or apraclonidine) or miotics (parasympathomimetics, e.g. pilocarpine or anticholinesterases: physostigmine or echothiophate – although these are now less frequently prescribed in practice).

— Chemical properties of latanoprost
Latanoprost is a structural analogue of the naturally occurring prostaglandin F$_{2\alpha}$. As expected, the two molecules are very similar to each other. Latanoprost contains an isopropyl ester in place of the free carboxyl group in prostaglandin F$_{2\alpha}$. This ester must be hydrolysed by plasma esterases to generate the free carboxyl-containing metabolite, which is biologically active (latanoprost is a prodrug). In addition, on the other side chain, latanoprost lacks the additional alkene group and has an aromatic ring at the end of the alkyl chain. There are five chiral centres and an alkene capable of geometric isomerism in latanoprost. Of the 64 possible stereoisomers of this molecule, only latanoprost has the correct shape for effective interaction (after ester hydrolysis) with its prostanoid F$_{2\alpha}$ receptor target. The alkene in latanoprost has a *cis* (or *Z*) configuration.

— Formulations for the treatment of eye conditions
Eyedrop preparations may be solutions, suspensions or emulsions. Solution preparations are most common: latanoprost and timolol eyedrops are solution formulations. Solutions are homogeneous, allowing high dose uniformity and rapid onset of action. Poorly water-soluble drugs, such as corticosteroids, may be formulated as suspension eyedrops, e.g. prednisolone eyedrops. Homogeneity and dose uniformity, as with other suspension formulations, may be problematic and require the inclusion of suspending and thickening agents, such that the particles are readily dispersible on shaking, before administration. Much less frequently, drugs may be formulated in an oil-in-water submicrometre emulsion. An example of such a product is Restasis, an eyedrop formulation of ciclosporin dissolved in an oil phase, stabilised as an emulsion with the non-ionic surfactant Polysorbate 80.

latanoprost

prostaglandin F$_{2\alpha}$

In some cases, such as surgery, trauma and infection, it will be necessary to treat the structures surrounding the eye as well as the eye itself. Oral antibiotics, antivirals and anti-inflammatory agents are therefore given alongside topical treatment. During inflammatory states, the blood–ocular barriers are broken down, allowing for greater penetration. These barriers are usually restored once the inflammation has resolved. To increase ocular penetration of systemic therapy, the drugs chosen should have: a small molecular size, high lipid solubility and low protein-binding affinity.

— Administration of eyedrops
Regular application of eyedrops is vital to prevent disease progression, even if the patient is not experiencing any symptoms. The need for, and how to use, eyedrops should be carefully explained to the patient.

The use of topical ocular products, as for many other medicines, is associated with problems of adherence. A common problem is that patients may not know exactly where the product should be administered. Patients should avoid administering drops on, or close to, the cornea, which, as the most sensitive tissue in the body, is densely populated with nerves. Therefore, any contact with the cornea will produce an involuntary reflex to rapidly close the eyelid to protect it (blinking). Blinking may cause the bulk of the eyedrop to be removed from the ocular surface. An explanation of how to administer the drops should therefore be provided:

- Use your finger to gently pull down your lower eyelid
- Hold the bottle over your eye and allow a single drop to fall into the pocket you have created in your lower lid, so that the drop touches the sclera and *not* the cornea
- The pocket can then be gently released, allowing the drop to disperse across the ocular surface, closing your eye and keeping it closed for several minutes

If patients are using two different eyedrops, they should allow at least 5–10 minutes between using the different drops.

Sometimes, dexterity issues are a problem. If so, compliance aids can be helpful, as can different types of packaging, e.g. bottles that are easier to squeeze.

Latanoprost eyedrops are no longer required to be kept in a refrigerator before and after opening, but must not be stored >25°C. In general, eyedrops for domiciliary (home) use should not be used more than 4 weeks after opening the bottle.

— Side effects from ocular products for glaucoma

The ingredients in ocular products can produce side effects just like other dosage forms. These may be limited to the local area of administration or systemic effects after passage of the drug into the systemic circulation. Table 9.1 gives some examples of side effects that may occur locally and systemically after ocular use of glaucoma treatments.

The local effects of topical ocular products are hard to avoid, but for most patients are not troublesome, and in the case of conjunctival hyperaemia can be short-lived. The systemic effects can, however, be minimised by employing the technique known as punctual occlusion. The purpose of this technique is to place a finger close to the corner of the eye for a short period after administration of the product. This will prevent the product escaping through the punctum, which leads to the canaliculus, on to the lacrimal sac, which in turn leads to the nasolacrimal duct and the nasopharyngeal cavity. Drugs that enter this system are more likely to be absorbed, so blocking

this route is important for those patients who are likely to find the systemic effects problematic.

▼ TABLE 9.1

Examples of local and systemic side effects from ocular products

Product	Topical side effects	Systemic side effects
β-Adreno-receptor blockers	Redness of the eye, burning, loss of corneal sensation, reduced ocular blood flow	Exacerbation of asthma and COPD, hypotension, bradycardia, nightmares
Prostaglandin analogues	Conjunctival hyperaemia, darkening and lengthening of eyelashes, increased pigmentation of iris and periocular skin, macular oedema, uveitis	Reactivation of herpes, bitter taste
Parasympatho-mimetics (miotics)	Visual blurring (children), darkening of visual field (pupillary constriction), stinging	Headache (initially due to ciliary spasm), sweating
α_2-Adreno-receptor agonists	Redness of the eye, eyelid retraction, tearing, discomfort	Fatigue, drowsiness, hypotension, dry mouth, headache, drowsiness
Carbonic anhydrase inhibitors	Stinging	Headache, unpleasant taste

EXTENDED LEARNING

- Outline the stepwise treatment of open-angle glaucoma
- What is closed-angle glaucoma? What are its symptoms and why is it a medical emergency?
- What are the treatment options for closed-angle glaucoma?
- What surgical options are available for glaucoma?
- What is steroid-induced glaucoma?
- How are eyedrops formulated, manufactured, packaged and sterilised?

ADDITIONAL PRACTICE POINTS

- Who are optometrists? What is their role in eye health? How are their services accessed?

- What compliance aids are available for the administration of eyedrops?

References and further reading

Fadda H, Khalili A, Khaw PT, Brocchini S (2013). Ocular drug delivery In: Aulton ME, Taylor KMG (eds), *Aulton's*

Pharmaceutics: The design and manufacture of medicines, 4th edn. London: Elsevier, 710–31.

Ghate D, Edelhause H (2006). Ocular drug delivery. *Expert Opin Drug Delivery* 3:275–87.

Liu Y, Gibson J, Wheeler J et al. (2011). GALC deletions increase the risk of primary open-angle glaucoma: the role of Mendelian variants in complex disease. *PLoS One* 6:e27134.

Mookherjee S, Acharya M, Banerjee D, Bhattacharjee A, Ray K (2012). Molecular basis for involvement of CYP1B1 in MYOC upregulation and its potential implication in glaucoma pathogenesis. *PLoS One* 7:e45077.

Case 3
Wet age-related macular degeneration

HALA M FADDA

LEARNING OUTCOMES

At the end of this case, you will be able to:

- Describe the pathophysiology, signs and presentation of wet age-related macular degeneration (wet AMD)

- Outline the role of vascular endothelial growth factor (VEGF) inhibitors in the treatment of wet AMD, their mechanism of action and potential adverse effects

- Describe why intravitreal injections are the most suitable drug delivery route for the treatment of wet AMD and outline the limitations of the other drug delivery routes

- Outline the pharmaceutical considerations in the design of intraocular preparations

Case study

Mrs RT is 68 years old and has been noticing a change in her vision over the past couple of months. She can no longer read small print, even with her usual reading glasses. There is always a slight smudge in her sight and lines always appear wavy rather than straight. She visited her optometrist and explained these changes. On listening to these symptoms and performing some visual acuity tests, the optometrist suspected wet AMD and wrote a letter to her GP requesting immediate referral to an ophthalmologist at the hospital.

❷ What is wet AMD?

❷ Why did the optometrist suspect wet AMD and request immediate referral to an ophthalmologist?

The ophthalmologist at the hospital conducted several tests, one of which was a fluorescein angiogram of the eyes, which confirmed that Mrs RT suffered from wet AMD in her right eye. Prompt treatment with a VEGF inhibitor (anti-VEGF drug) was scheduled.

❷ What are VEGF inhibitors?

❷ How do they work?

❷ Which VEGF inhibitors are currently used for the treatment of wet AMD?

The ophthalmologist decides to treat Mrs RT with a once-monthly intravitreal injection of the anti-VEGF drug ranibizumab (Lucentis).

❷ Why is the intravitreal route of drug delivery most suitable here?

❷ Other common routes for drug delivery to the eye include oral, topical (eyedrops) and systemic. Discuss the limitations of these different routes for delivering ranibizumab to the retina

A single dose of Lucentis intravitreal injection comprises 0.05 mL of a 10 mg/mL solution. It contains the following pharmaceutical excipients: histidine hydrochloride, α,α-trehalose dihydrate, Polysorbate 20 and water for injection. It is formulated at a pH of 5.5.

❷ What are the important pharmaceutical considerations in the design of intraocular injections?

❷ What are the pharmaceutical functions of the different excipients present in Lucentis?

Case discussion

— AMD and its pathophysiology

Age-related macular degeneration (AMD) is the leading cause of blindness in adults aged >65 years in the developed world. It is a progressive degenerative disease attacking the macula, the region of the retina of highest visual acuity. AMD has two subtypes: the non-exudative (or dry) form and the exudative (wet or neovascular) form. Although the dry form is the most common, the wet form of AMD causes the worst visual impairment and accounts for 90% of blindness from AMD.

Vascular endothelial growth factor (VEGF) plays a pivotal role in physiological angiogenesis, including that of the eye. The retina is made up of a complex network of neurones and is the most metabolically active tissue within our body. Its nutrient and oxygen supply are maintained by the high blood flow and vasculature of the choroid layer that surrounds it. Over-expression of VEGF results, however, in pathological angiogenesis, which in wet AMD manifests as abnormal growth of choroidal blood vessels (choroidal neovascularisation, CNV). These choroidal neovascular vessels are leaky, leading to oedema and haemorrhage beneath the macula. Lesions are formed which turn into scars, resulting in destruction of the macula and loss of central vision. Ocular tissue hypoxia and inflammatory conditions are implicated in the upregulation of VEGF synthesis.

— Symptoms and need for immediate referral

In this case, Mrs RT displays typical symptoms of AMD. CNV progresses quickly, around 10 μm of choroidal blood vessel growth per day. Treatment of AMD must therefore be initiated promptly, ideally within 2 weeks of diagnosis. A delay in treatment of >1 month increases the risk of vision loss. Early detection and treatment can substantially improve clinical outcomes. If not treated, the patient can develop irreversible blindness.

— VEGF inhibitors and their mechanism of action

Four VEGF inhibitors have received regulatory approval for clinical use: Pegaptanib (Macugen), ranibizumab (Lucentis) and aflibercept (VEGF Trap-eye) have been approved for treatment of wet AMD, whereas bevacizumab (Avastin) is used off-label for wet AMD. All four are large molecules, which bind in different ways to certain isoforms of VEGF, thus preventing VEGF interaction with its receptors. They have all been shown to suppress CNV and improve visual acuity.

— Routes of drug delivery to the eye

The goals of drug delivery are to achieve effective concentrations of the therapeutic agent at the target site for sufficient lengths of time with minimum side effects. Several considerations need to be made when deciding on the best drug delivery route for a therapeutic agent including its physicochemical properties, mechanism and site of action, as well as its adverse effect profile. Ranibizumab is a biotechnology-derived therapeutic protein, specifically a humanised monoclonal antibody. It is the Fab fragment of immunoglobulin G1 (IgG1) and has a molecular mass of 48 kDa. It achieves its efficacy by local action in the posterior segment of the eye.

The oral route is an unsuitable route for ranibizumab. It is a protein and will therefore be subjected to enzymatic and/or non-enzymatic (chemical) degradation. Its large size will also prohibit it from traversing the membranes of the GI mucosa. The administration of eyedrops or semi-solids to the cornea (topical route) offer more patient convenience and far fewer risks than intravitreal injections, but it is ineffective at producing therapeutic concentrations of drug in the posterior segment tissue (back of the eye). Drugs administered topically to the eye need to overcome a multitude of barriers to reach the posterior segment. These include the long diffusional distance, rapid drug clearance from tear fluids by blinking and nasolacrimal drainage, absorption across the corneal and conjunctival epithelia, metabolism and efflux by the corneal and conjunctival epithelia, clearance from the different ocular compartments and absorption into the systemic circulation.

To target the posterior segment of the eye by the systemic route, high doses of drug need to be administered because only a small fraction of the blood flow circulates through the posterior segment of the eye. The VEGF pathway is critical to numerous cellular functions and physiological processes, including tissue vascularisation and angiogenesis. High systemic levels of ranibizumab can lead to inhibition of the VEGF pathway, giving rise to diverse adverse events, including hypertension, arterial thromboembolic events (cardiac ischaemia, stroke, peripheral arterial thrombosis), nephrotic syndrome and bowel perforations. Although the US Federal Drug Administration (FDA) has approved VEGF inhibitors for cancer therapy and inflammatory bowel diseases by the systemic route, risk–benefit assessment is always conducted before putting patients on these therapies. If administered systemically, some ranibizumab will also need to cross the blood–retinal barrier (BRB), which separates the retina from the circulating blood. The BRB is made up of a tight monolayer of cells with complex tight junctions that restrict the non-specific transport between the neural retina and circulating blood. Generally, therefore, drug permeability across the BRB is poor.

— Intravitreal route for treatment of AMD with ranibizumab

The intravitreal route is the most suitable route of administration for the treatment of wet AMD with ranibizumab. The vitreous is close to the target site and there are fewer biological barriers for the drug to overcome to reach the site of action. Moreover, only low doses of the therapeutic agent need to be administered locally, which reduces the incidence of systemic side effects. Systemic absorption of ranibizumab still occurs, however, from intravitreal injections, and side effects associated with VEGF suppression have been reported that pose a concern in patients receiving intravitreal anti-VEGF therapy. Nevertheless, the adverse effects are far fewer than those caused by systemic administration of the drug. A limitation of intravitreal injections is the associated risks including retinal detachment, endophthalmitis (severe inflammation of the intraocular vitreous space) and increases in intraocular pressure. Careful injection and the minimum needle gauge possible are used to reduce these risks.

— Important pharmaceutical considerations in the design of intraocular injections

Ocular preparations should be designed so that they are non-irritant to the eye and at the same time maintain drug stability. Stability is challenging, particularly in the case of proteins, which are at a high risk of degradation and aggregation. Lucentis has been formulated at a pH of 5.5; although this deviates from the pH of the

vitreous humour (about 7.3), it is the pH at which ranibizumab was found to be most stable in solution.

The pH plays a pivotal role in the maintenance of a protein's higher-order three-dimensional structure. Many amino acids contain ionisable (acidic and basic) groups as part of their side chains, and whether these groups are predominantly protonated or deprotonated (and hence whether they are charged) is highly dependent on the pH of the medium in which they are dissolved. Large changes in pH can have a marked effect on electrostatic forces of attraction between ionised groups and can disrupt the tertiary structure leading to denaturation, partial unfolding and aggregation. Proteins can also be subject to acid- and/or base-catalysed hydrolysis and therefore control of pH is even more important to ensure stability. Deviation of the pH of the injected solution from physiological pH of the vitreous humour increases the risk of ocular irritation. In this case, 0.05 mL Lucentis solution is injected, which is relatively small compared with the vitreous volume (approximately 3 mL), so the solution will be neutralised by the vitreous humour which is composed of >99% water. There is also a turnover of fluid in the vitreous humour, albeit at a very slow rate.

Histidine hydrochloride serves as a buffer in this formulation to control the pH of the injection. The pK_a value for the side-chain imidazole group of histidine is about 6, which makes it a suitable choice for ranibizumab solution. In ocular preparations, it is advisable to use buffers at as low a concentration as possible so that the injected solution is quickly restored to the pH of the ocular environment.

Another important feature is tonicity; ocular preparations should be as close as possible to the osmolality of ocular fluids to avoid irritation. α,α-Trehalose dihydrate is included in Lucentis injection as a tonicity agent. Polysorbate 20 is a surfactant that reduces the interfacial and surface tension, thereby lowering the risk of agitation-induced aggregation of ranibizumab. Lucentis is available in single use vials, which obviates the need for a preservative. This is desirable because preservatives have an inherent toxicity.

The product is sterile filtered under aseptic conditions. Sterile filtration is a non-terminal sterilisation process. Pharmaceutical products are terminally sterilised (sterilised in their final container) wherever possible, most frequently by moist heat sterilisation in an autoclave. This provides a high level of assurance that the product will be sterile. However, some pharmaceutical products, including biopharmaceuticals, such as ranibizumab, are not stable to the temperatures used for sterilisation, and hence are sterilised by passing through a sterile, sterilising filter using aseptic processing, before filling into containers under carefully controlled environmental conditions.

EXTENDED LEARNING

- What are monoclonal antibodies? For what conditions, and under what circumstances, might they be a treatment option?
- What are the differences between the VEGF inhibitors used in the treatment of wet AMD?
- How are VEGF inhibitors manufactured?
- What is the role of Visudyne (verteporfin) photodynamic therapy in the treatment of certain subtypes of wet AMD?
- Discuss suprachoroidal and intrascleral injections as investigative drug delivery

approaches in preclinical studies for treating the posterior segment of the eye

- Discuss the formulation, manufacture and sterilisation of products for ophthalmic use
- What are the advantages and disadvantages of the pharmacopoeial methods for sterilising pharmaceutical products?
- What are osmolality, isotonicity and colligative properties of solutions?

References and further reading

Fadda HM, Khalili A, Khaw PT, Brocchini S (2013). Ocular drug delivery. In: Aulton ME, Taylor KMG (eds), *Aulton's Pharmaceutics: The design and manufacture of medicines*, 4th edn. London: Elsevier, 710–31.

Kompella UB, Edelhauser HF, eds (2011). *Drug Product Development for the Back of the Eye*. Berlin: Springer.

National Institute for Health and Clinical Excellence (2008). *Ranibizumab and Pegaptanib for the Treatment of Age-related Macular Degeneration*. London: NICE. Available at: http://guidance.nice.org.uk/ta155 (accessed 29 September 2013).

Stewart M (2012). The expanding role of vascular endothelial growth factor inhibitors in ophthalmology. *Mayo Clinic Proc* 87:77–88.

Case 4
Sore throat

KATIE GREENWOOD

LEARNING OUTCOMES

At the end of this case, you will be able to:

- Outline the pathophysiology, signs, symptoms and diagnosis of a sore throat
- Discuss treatment options for a sore throat
- Outline the chemistry and mechanism of action of local anaesthetics
- Know when to refer a patient with a sore throat to another healthcare professional
- Question a patient to determine a differential diagnosis

Case study

Mrs JS is 34 years old and a mother of two small children. She is a regular visitor to your pharmacy for nappies and other healthcare products. On this particular day, she seems stressed and looks tired and pale. She asks for some throat lozenges because she has a sore throat.

❷ What questions would you need to ask Mrs JS?

Mrs JS says that she has had the sore throat for about 2 days. She has been sucking some 'soothers' but it's not getting any better. It is painful when she swallows and she is finding it difficult to eat.

❷ What is a sore throat? Explain the pathophysiology, signs and symptoms
❷ What treatment options are available to treat a sore throat?
❷ Describe the structure features of local anaesthetics used for sore throat and explain their mechanism of action

You sell Mrs JS some throat pastilles. She returns 2 days later. She has now lost her voice, which is causing her problems because she can't shout after her 2-year-old child. Her friend says that she should gargle with aspirin but she wasn't sure about this so thought she would ask for your advice.

- ❓ What advice would you give Mrs JS with regard to gargling with aspirin?
- ❓ What lifestyle advice can be recommended for patients with a sore throat?
- ❓ What criteria would lead you to refer someone with a sore throat to a GP?
- ❓ What other considerations are there relating to this case with regard to Mrs JS's children?

Case discussion

A sore throat is a very common minor ailment that pharmacists encounter, because only about 5% of patients with a sore throat will consult their doctor. Most sore throats with which a pharmacist is presented will be caused by a viral infection (approximately 90%) and therefore antibiotics would be inappropriate. Once a pharmacist has excluded any serious conditions, an OTC product is usually an appropriate recommendation.

— Questioning and differential diagnosis

A sore throat with no serious underlying cause will be self-limiting. However, to confirm this, the patient should be questioned to ensure that all the relevant information has been elicited. The following information is needed:

- The age of the patient
- How long she has had the sore throat
- The severity (this can be subjective so the pharmacist may want to prompt the patient based on what she considers severe)
- Any associated symptoms, e.g. cold, cough, elevated temperature; previous history and lifestyle
- Other medication and medical conditions.

If the patient is a woman of childbearing age, the pharmacist would also need to establish if she is pregnant or breastfeeding. Various acronyms can be used as an aid memoire for this questioning process, for example:

> WWHAM, ENCORE, ASMETHOD (see Case 5 in Section 3)

This may be helpful to ensure that relevant information is gathered to enable identification of symptoms that may indicate the possibility of a more serious condition requiring referral, or to recommend appropriate symptomatic treatment. In practice, often a combination or selected questions from these is used, depending on the patient's presentation.

— Pathophysiology

There are various possible causes of a 'sore throat' in a patient:

- Tonsillitis is inflammation due to infection of the tonsils
- Pharyngitis is inflammation of the oropharynx but not the tonsils
- In laryngitis, there are few visible signs of infection, but with soreness lower down the throat often associated with a hoarse voice
- An infection by the virus that causes croup in a young child may cause a cough or sore throat in an older child or adult
- Glandular fever.

— Signs and symptoms

There is a raw feeling at the back of the throat, discomfort on swallowing, occasional earache, redness and swelling of the throat, enlarged and tender lymph glands in the neck, and slight fever.

A sore throat is often the first part of a common cold. It tends to occur on the first day, and nasal discharge (rhinorrhoea) makes the diagnosis obvious the following day. If the sore throat is due to a viral infection, the symptoms are usually milder and often related to the common cold. It has been shown that it is very difficult to differentiate between a bacterial and a viral infection based on patient history and clinical findings.

— Treatment options

Many people do not seek professional advice for a sore throat, and most sore throats resolve within 1 week. Symptomatic treatment should be advised. Antipyretic analgesics, such as paracetamol and ibuprofen, are often helpful.

— Lozenges, pastilles and warm drinks

One of the most effective treatments for a sore throat is producing saliva to lubricate the throat and wash any infection away. For this reason, sucking any pastille, lozenge or boiled sweet (whether or not medicated) can help to relieve a sore throat. It is also helpful to drink plenty of fluids, and warm drinks may be especially soothing.

Lozenges are solid dosage forms that dissolve slowly in the mouth to lubricate and soothe irritated throat surfaces. They may contain drugs that have a local action in the throat, including local anaesthetics, antiseptics and antimicrobial agents. These were traditionally prepared from sugar and gums, but now are usually compressed tablets, prepared like conventional tablets, but without a disintegrant, which slowly release drug that dissolves in the saliva. Pastilles are a solid dosage form produced from a viscous liquid, usually a solution of starches, gums, gelatine, etc. that has been solidified. The liquid is poured into a lubricated mould and allowed to set and dry. Active components can be dissolved or suspended in the liquid, before pouring into the mould. Many pastilles contain demulcents (relieve irritation), e.g. glycerin or honey, which can safely be taken by most people to stop their throat from feeling dry. Honey should not be given to babies aged <12 months, while iodised lozenges should be avoided in pregnancy. People with diabetes should also be careful because many of these pastilles have a high sugar content. Sugar-free pastilles are available. Lozenges containing the NSAID flurbiprofen provide another option. Some pastilles also contain antiseptic agents, e.g. benzalkonium, dequalinium, cetylpyridinium and tyrothricin (a weak antibacterial drug). As most sore throats are caused by viral infections their value is questionable.

— Gargles and gargling

Salt water gargling can be a good way to relieve a sore throat. Gargles should not be swallowed, but spat out after completion of gargling. Salt water (a teaspoonful of salt in a glass of warm water) is a traditional therapy. For patients who can take aspirin, two or three 300 mg tablets of *soluble aspirin* can be dissolved in water and used as a gargle for 3–4 min. After gargling, the solution can be swallowed which may provide additional pain relief. There is, however, limited evidence to support the effectiveness of this or salt gargles.

Local anaesthetics for sore throat

Benzocaine and lidocaine are used in both lozenges and throat sprays. If there is difficulty swallowing due to a sore throat, these can be helpful and reduce pain. Children or elderly people should not use local anaesthetic lozenges or sprays because they may be more sensitive to their actions and therefore more likely to develop

adverse side effects. No one should use these products for more than 5 days.

benzocaine   lidocaine

— Chemical properties of local anaesthetics

Lidocaine displays the structural features typical of most local anaesthetics. It consists of a lipophilic group (a dimethylphenyl group) linked via an amide bond to a basic tertiary amino group. The tertiary amino group has a pK_a (for its conjugate acid) of around 7.8, so is approximately 70% ionised (protonated) at physiological pH. The amide nitrogen is not basic. Most other local anaesthetics have a similar structural arrangement: a lipophilic group linked via an amide (or ester) to a basic aliphatic amino group. Benzocaine is unusual in that it does not contain an aliphatic amino group; the aromatic amino group (attached to the lipophilic portion of the molecule) is only very weakly basic (pK_a = 2.8) due to overlapping of its lone pair of electrons with the delocalised aromatic system. Benzocaine is not charged at physiological pH and is poorly soluble in water.

The structural features of local anaesthetics are important to their ability to interact with their biological target, the neuronal voltage-gated sodium channel (VGSC). The protonated (charged) and deprotonated (uncharged) forms of lidocaine exist in equilibrium outside the cell at physiological pH. Only the uncharged form is sufficiently lipophilic to diffuse across the cell membrane into the intracellular environment (membranes are generally impermeable to charged molecules). Inflammation and local infection can reduce the pH of the extracellular environment, which can reduce the proportion of uncharged local anaesthetic available to diffuse across the membrane. This explains the often reduced effectiveness of local anaesthetics under these circumstances. Once inside the cell, some of the uncharged form becomes protonated again and is able to interact with its binding site within the open sodium channel (use-dependent block). Benzocaine is always uncharged at physiological pH and can therefore readily diffuse across the cell membrane to access the local anaesthetic binding site within the VGSC directly. It is possible that an additional VGSC binding site exists for uncharged local anaesthetics such as benzocaine.

— Antibiotics for sore throat

The vast majority of sore throats are self-limiting viral infections and, even when infection is bacterial, the value of antibiotics is small. Phenoxymethylpenicillin and macrolides, such as erythromycin and azithromycin, can be used. The Cochrane summary on the use of antibiotics in the treatment of sore throats (Spinks et al., 2006) advises that antibiotics confer relative benefits in the treatment of sore throat, but the absolute benefits are modest and at the cost of treating many with antibiotics who will derive no benefit. Antibiotics shorten the duration of symptoms, but by an average of only 1 day about half-way through the illness, and by about 16 hours overall. Phenoxymethylpenicillin is the drug of choice in bacterial infection because *Streptococcus* sp. is the suspected organism and it has no resistance to this drug. A 10-day course is required. Macrolides, such as erythromycin and azithromycin, can be used where there is allergy and a course need be for only 5 days. If the underlying diagnosis is glandular fever, which is most common in adolescents and young adults, amoxicillin and ampicillin should be avoided, because these lead to a rash, even in the absence of allergy to penicillin.

When to refer

Most sore throats are self-limiting and will resolve within 7–10 days. If the throat has not improved after a couple of weeks, the patient should see the GP. Hoarseness persisting for >3 weeks can (although relatively rare) be an indication of laryngeal cancer.

Dysphagia (difficult in swallowing) can be a sign of abscesses, glandular fever or infectious mononucleosis (glandular fever), which principally affects teenagers and young adults. Patients with glandular fever can be quite unwell, with very large and purulent tonsils, weakness and a long-lasting lethargy.

The presence of white spots or pus can be a sign of bacterial infection, warranting referral, as would the presence of white plaques, which could indicate an oral *Candida* (thrush) infection. This is most commonly seen in infants, very elderly people or immunocompromised patients.

A sore throat due to Coxsackievirus infection may be characterised by small blisters on the tonsils and roof of the mouth. The blisters erupt in a few days and are followed by a scab, which may be very painful. In streptococcal infection, the tonsils often swell and become coated and the throat is sore. The patient has an elevated temperature and foul-smelling breath, and may feel quite ill. In reality, it is not possible to tell on inspection if the infection is due to a virus or bacterium.

Complications of sore throat or upper respiratory tract infection include otitis media, usually confined to those aged <5 years, and sinusitis. A very rare complication can lead to severe swelling of the back of the throat (epiglottitis), which may restrict the airways and cause breathing difficulties. Failed medication, the presence of certain medications for which a sore throat is a criterion for referral, e.g. carbimazole, and recurrent bouts of infection would also prompt a referral.

— Lifestyle advice for patients with a sore throat

Smoking will aggravate a sore throat and it is important to keep teeth and gums clean to avoid secondary oral infections. Therefore, smoking cessation advice and good oral hygiene guidance would help recovery.

EXTENDED LEARNING

- Why is honey not considered safe to give to babies under one year old?

References and further reading

Blenkinsopp A, Paxton P, Blenkinsopp J (2009). *Symptoms in the Pharmacy: A guide to the management of common illness.* 6th edn. London: Wiley-Blackwell.

Edwards C, Stillman P (2006). *Minor Illness or Major Disease?*, 4th edn. London: Pharmaceutical Press.

Nathan A (2012). *Managing Symptoms in the Pharmacy*, 2nd edn. London: Pharmaceutical Press.

Rutter P (2013). *Community Pharmacy: Symptoms, diagnosis and treatment*, 3rd edn. London: Churchill Livingstone Elsevier.

Spinks A, Glasziou PP, Del Mar CB (2006). Antibiotics for sore throat. *Cochrane Database Syst Rev* 4:CD000023.

Case 5
Hay fever
LOUISE COGAN

LEARNING OUTCOMES

At the end of this case, you will be able to:

- Outline the pathophysiology, signs, symptoms and diagnosis of hay fever
- Discuss the various treatment options available to relieve the different symptoms
- Outline the chemistry of chlorphenamine and cetirizine, and relate this to the sedating effects of some antihistamines
- Counsel a patient on lifestyle changes that may help with their management of hay fever
- Know when to refer a patient to another healthcare professional

Case study

Jack is a 17-year-old A-level student who comes into your pharmacy looking for something to help with his hay fever. He has not had hay fever previously, but the pollen levels are currently high, and his cold-like symptoms have not gone, despite trying some Lemsip that he found at home. One of his friends has hay fever, and suggested that he should go to the pharmacy to see what they could offer him.

❷ Describe the signs and symptoms of hay fever, and discuss how they differ from those of a cold

You ask Jack a series of questions about his symptoms, and decide that he has hay fever. He's surprised, because he has never had hay fever before. He asks you what treatment would be most suitable for him.

❷ What questions should you ask a patient who is displaying possible hay fever symptoms?
❷ Is there a common age of onset of hay fever?
❷ How has the incidence of hay fever changed over recent decades?
❷ What oral treatment options are available to Jack? Are there any cautions or contraindications that you need to consider?
❷ Outline the structural features that give some antihistamines their sedating properties

Jack is given some oral antihistamine tablets to take, and is advised to return if his symptoms do not improve. Three weeks later he returns to your pharmacy, asking if there is something else he could try, because the tablets have helped a bit, but on certain days his nose is still blocked and his eyes are itchy.

❷ What further options are available to help Jack manage his symptoms? Discuss how the different dosage forms help to alleviate symptoms
❷ What lifestyle advice could be given to Jack to help minimise his symptoms?

Jack takes your advice, and buys some eyedrops to use alongside his tablets.

❷ When would you refer Jack to another healthcare professional? Why?

Case discussion

— Hay fever and its pathophysiology

Hay fever (or seasonal allergic rhinitis) occurs when a patient comes into contact with an allergen (most commonly pollen related). It affects about 10–30% of all adults. In susceptible individuals, the allergen activates IgE antibodies on the surface of mast cells in the nasal mucosa. This then causes mast cell degranulation and the release of chemical mediators, the main one being histamine. This response is known as the early phase allergic reaction, which gives rise to the classic symptoms of hay fever. Up to 12 hours after this initial reaction, the T-helper type 2 (TH2)-cell-mediated late-phase inflammatory reaction occurs, which causes mucosal swelling and prolonged nasal congestion. Allergic rhinitis is therefore a complex disorder that also involves distinct components of the immune system.

The main symptoms of hay fever include nasal itching, sneezing, runny nose, nasal congestion and red, itchy, watery eyes. The ocular symptoms of hay fever may impact significantly (sometimes more so than nasal) on the daily activities of sufferers and therefore impose an additional challenge to practitioners to achieve adequate and effective therapeutic relief. The symptoms are thought to arise from both direct allergen-triggered release of histamine from mast cell stimulation on the surface of the eye, and naso-ocular reflexes triggered by histamine release acting on inflamed sensory nerve endings in the nasal mucosa.

Cold symptoms are self-limiting and tend to last between 7 and 10 days, and are usually more common in winter. Hay fever symptoms last for as long as the individual is in contact with the pollen, and will occur on a seasonal basis, depending on to which pollens they are allergic.

- Tree pollen: March to May
- Grass pollen: May to August
- Fungal spores: September to October.

— Treatment options and choice of agent

Hay fever often first develops in school-age children and during the teenage years. Lifetime prevalence in the UK has been estimated to be up to 30%. In many cases, the condition improves or disappears after a number of years. There is some evidence that it is increasingly affecting more, and older, people. In patients with asthma, their symptoms can be triggered by hay fever.

There is a variety of OTC treatment options available to Jack. First-line treatment usually involves a once-daily antihistamine, such as loratadine. If nasal or eye symptoms persist, then the addition of a corticosteroid nasal spray and/or eyedrops can be recommended.

— Oral antihistamines: structural features and sedating properties

The use of oral antihistamines as first-line treatment for the allergic symptoms of hay fever is well established. These can be split into two groups: sedating and non-sedating antihistamines. The most common sedating antihistamine is chlorphenamine. As well as causing sedation as a side effect, chlorphenamine also has the disadvantage that it requires four to six times-a-day dosing. So-called second-generation, non-sedating antihistamines can still cause drowsiness, although this is very rare, and patients should always be counselled about this. OTC non-sedating antihistamines include cetirizine, loratadine and acrivastine, the last of which requires a dose to be taken every 8 hours, unlike the other two, which require once-daily dosing.

The structures of chlorphenamine and cetirizine are shown in the diagram. The tendency of an antihistamine to cause sedation is primarily a

chlorphenamine

cetirizine

consequence of polarity and the ability of the drug to diffuse across the blood–brain barrier (BBB) into the CNS. Chlorphenamine has much lower polarity than cetirizine. Cetirizine contains more electronegative atoms and has higher hydrogen-bonding potential. Cetirizine also contains three groups (two basic tertiary amino groups and one acidic carboxyl group) that may be charged at physiological pH. The presence of multiple charges on a molecule means that it is very unlikely to be able to diffuse across the lipophilic environment of the BBB cell membranes. Chlorphenamine contains a basic single tertiary amino group (as well as a weakly basic pyridine nitrogen that is very unlikely to be protonated at physiological pH), and the equilibrium proportion of uncharged drug at physiological pH will allow some distribution into the CNS through the BBB. Low-polarity, older antihistamines that penetrate the BBB can cause sedation as an unwanted side effect due to antagonism at central H_1-receptors.

Further treatment options and dosage forms

— Nasal preparations

Products of choice are the nasal corticosteroids beclometasone, fluticasone and triamcinolone. They work by reducing inflammation and easing nasal congestion, although they can take a couple of weeks to exert their full effect.

Drugs are primarily administered to the nasal cavity for the rapid treatment of local symptoms, as is the case in hay fever, without the side effects that may occur with oral dosage forms. Such drugs are administered using drops, sprays, ointments or creams. The traditional dosage form is the nasal drop. However, considerable dexterity is required to administer these appropriately and hence they are not convenient for patients to use. Moreover, drops require the inclusion of an antimicrobial preservative in their formulation, to prevent growth of contaminating microorganisms introduced into the container during use. Consequently, pressurised containers, without preservative and permitting accurate dosing, are becoming increasingly popular for nasal drug delivery.

— **Eye preparations**

The most commonly used eye preparation is sodium cromoglicate, which is a mast cell stabiliser. Sodium cromoglicate is formulated as a solution for administration to the eye in a conventional, sterile, eyedrop formulation containing an antimicrobial preservative and additional excipients to ensure that the product is isotonic with tears. The usual dose is one or two drops into the affected eye(s), four times a day. Other preparations are also available.

— **Lifestyle advice to help minimise symptoms**

Pollen levels are at their highest in the early morning, and between 4 pm and 7 pm, so when possible, sufferers should avoid going out during these times. Keeping windows in the house and car closed will reduce the amount of pollen coming in through them. Wearing sunglasses will help to protect the eyes from pollen exposure. Pollen may also stick to hair, so washing hair before going to bed will help to reduce symptoms during the night and first thing in the morning.

— **When to refer to another healthcare professional**

If a patient's symptoms are still not controlled despite taking an antihistamine and using both eyedrops and a nasal spray, then referral to a GP may be wise. There are many other products that can be considered on prescription.

If hay fever symptoms persist, then a patient may require immunotherapy, which is an extract of grass and tree pollen used to reduce symptoms. If so, the GP will need to refer the patient to a hospital specialist, for accurate diagnosis, assessment and treatment.

Each set of allergen extract usually contains vials for the administration of graded amounts of

allergen to patients undergoing hyposensitisation. Maintenance sets containing vials at the highest strength are also available. This can improve people's tolerance of the allergen and improve their quality of life, and has long-term results. However, immunotherapy may take months or even years to be effective.

Hypersensitivity reactions to immunotherapy can be life threatening: bronchospasm usually develops within 1 hour, and anaphylaxis within 30 minutes of injection. Patients therefore need to be monitored for an hour after injection.

— **Prescription-only and non-prescription medicines**

Some antihistamines are available over the counter in the UK, whereas others are supplied only with a prescription. The classification of medicines as prescription and non-prescription is common across the world. However, the actual products that are available without a prescription vary from country to country. Also, especially in low-income countries, regulation is limited and products that would be expected to be available only with a prescription can be readily purchased without. This has been controversial. Lack of access to medicines is a problem for people in many parts of the world, especially where health service infrastructure is not comprehensive. The ability to purchase from different providers, including pharmacists and other licensed sellers, enables continuity of supply for many people with long-term conditions.

EXTENDED LEARNING

- What nasal preparations are available for systemic drug delivery?
- What other local conditions are treated by nasal and ophthalmic preparations?

ADDITIONAL PRACTICE POINT

- How would you explain to a patient the correct administration procedures for nasal and ophthalmic products?

References and further reading

Baroody FM, Foster KA, Markaryan A, deTineo M, Naclerio RM (2008). Nasal ocular reflexes and eye symptoms in patients with allergic rhinitis. *Ann Allergy Asthma Immunol* **100**:194–9.

Bartra J, Mullol J, Montoro J et al. (2011). Effect of bilastine upon the ocular symptoms of allergic rhinoconjunctivitis. *J Invest Allergol Clin Immunol* **21**(Suppl 3):24–33.

Cassell HR, Katial RK (2009). Intranasal antihistamines for allergic rhinitis: examining the clinical impact. *Allergy Asthma Proc* **30**:349–57.

Joint Formulary Committee (2009). *BNF*. London: BMJ Group and RPS Publishing.

Martin BP, Lansley AB (2013). Nasal drug delivery. In: Aulton ME, Taylor KMG (eds), *Aulton's Pharmaceutics: The design and manufacture of medicines*, 4th edn. London: Elsevier, 657–74.

Rutter P (2009). *Community Pharmacy – Symptoms, diagnosis and treatment*, 2nd edn, London: Churchill Livingstone Elsevier.

Taylor-Clark T (2010). Histamine in allergic rhinitis. *Adv Exp Med Biol* **709**:33–41.

10
Skin cases

INTRODUCTION

This section contains seven cases centred on patients with conditions affecting the skin and nails, namely eczema, contact dermatitis, psoriasis, acne, fungal nail infections and head lice infestation.

Case 1
Atopic eczema ▶ 359

This case involves an adult patient with a history of eczema who has experienced a flare of the condition. First, the pathophysiology, signs, symptoms and diagnosis of eczema are outlined, before the potential triggers responsible for a flare of eczema are identified. Topical treatments are the mainstay of therapy and these are considered, including: emollients, corticosteroids, immunosuppressants, ichthammol, zinc oxide and potassium permanganate soaks. Special attention is given to the use of topical corticosteroids, including considerations of their potency, application (fingertip units) and adverse effects. Patients with more generalised eczema and recurrent flares may benefit from the use of antiseptics. The chemistry of the quaternary ammonium compound, benzalkonium chloride, used as an antiseptic and preservative is outlined. The case concludes with a consideration of the process of patch testing and its importance in determining adverse reactions to chemicals.

Case 2
Contact dermatitis ▶ 363

This case continues and extends some of the themes from the preceding case, describing a patient presenting with the symptoms of contact dermatitis, following occupational exposure to irritant(s) while working in a hairdressing salon. The three common forms of eczema (atopic eczema, allergic contact dermatitis, irritant contact dermatitis) are described and common allergens and sensitising agents, including those associated with hairdressing, are outlined. The barrier function of healthy skin and the changes associated with eczema are described. Emollients are frequently employed to soothe and hydrate the skin. Their use and formulation are described here. Most emollients contain an emulsifying agent, usually one of three types of surfactant (anionic, cationic, non-ionic). The classification and use of surfactants in pharmaceutical products are discussed.

Case 3
Management of an acute flare of psoriasis ▶ 366

This case outlines the pathophysiology, signs, symptoms and diagnosis of psoriasis, and the common triggers for a flare of the condition. There are a number of topical treatment options available for the management of an acute flare of mild-to-moderate psoriasis, including: emollients, topical steroids, vitamin D analogues and dithranol. These are considered together with the factors that influence the choice of treatment. Short contact therapy (with dithranol) in the management of psoriasis, together with the appropriate use, and possible adverse effects, of topical corticosteroids are considered in detail.

Case 4
Acne ▶ 369

This case outlines the pathophysiology, signs, symptoms and diagnosis of acne, and considers its common causes. The main aims of acne therapy and available treatments are described, with particular emphasis on the chemistry, properties and mode of action of benzoyl peroxide, which is widely used in topical formulations as an over-the-counter (OTC) medicine. The formulation and properties of topical semi-solid dosage forms – creams, ointments and gels – are outlined.

Although the large majority of treatments for acne are used topically, isotretinoin is used for the oral treatment of severe acne. There are a number of contraindications and risks associated with the use of isotretinoin and these, together with specific counselling points, are considered at the end of the case.

Case 5
Antibacterial treatment of acne in young people ▸ 372

This case continues the theme of acne with a focus on its antibacterial treatment and in the context of multiple pathologies. The properties of oral and topical antibacterial treatments commonly used for acne are described, and the chemical and physical properties of these treatments related to their indications and possible side effects. Treatments considered include: erythromycin/zinc acetate solution, azithromycin and doxycyline. The suitability of these treatments for patients taking other medicines for common conditions in adolescence, e.g. sexually transmitted infections, is considered. Unfortunately the organism primarily responsible for acne vulgaris (*Propionibacterium acnes*) has developed resistance to macrolide antibiotics. Some mechanisms of bacterial resistance to antibiotics are considered here. The risk factors for non-adherence to these treatments and ways to help young people get the best from their medicines are outlined.

Case 6
Fungal infection of the foot ▸ 376

This case involves a relatively healthy individual who has suffered with athlete's foot and has now developed a fungal infection of a toenail. The structure of the healthy nail is described and the differential diagnosis of fungal nail infections outlined. The various treatment options, both oral and topical, are considered. The structure, activity and side effects of the three oral antifungal drugs licensed for treating nail infections (onychomycosis), namely griseofulvin, itraconazole and terbinafine, are considered in detail. Topical drug delivery into the nail presents a major drug delivery challenge. The nature of the biological barrier, and the solution and lacquer formulation approaches, are considered.

Case 7
Treatment of head lice ▸ 380

This case outlines the pathophysiology, signs, symptoms and diagnosis of head lice infestation. The condition is commonly treated in the community using OTC products, and the various options for treating such an infestation are described. Insecticides have been the traditional treatment, and the chemical structures, properties and mechanisms of action of insecticides used to treat head lice are provided. Non-traditional pesticides such as dimeticone and 1,2-octanediol are considered, along with wet combing ('bug busting'), which is a first-line method for removing lice and their eggs. Misconceptions associated with head lice infestation, and the appropriate counselling of patients with respect to lifestyle changes that will help with their management of head lice, are described. The case concludes with a consideration of when patients should be referred to another healthcare professional.

Case 1
Atopic eczema
JAYMI MISTRY

LEARNING OUTCOMES

At the end of this case you will be able to:

- Outline the pathophysiology, signs, symptoms and diagnosis of eczema
- Identify potential triggers responsible for a flare of eczema
- Describe what topical products are available for the management of eczema
- Describe the use of topical corticosteroids, including potency, application (fingertip units) and adverse effects
- Describe the use and mode of action of emollients
- Outline the chemistry of benzalkonium chloride and its use in pharmaceutical products.
- Explain the process of patch testing and its importance in the determination of adverse reactions to chemicals

Case study

Miss FL is a 34-year-old patient with a history of eczema (her last flare occurred when she was 20 years old), asthma, hiatus hernia and hay fever. She is referred to the dermatology consultant after reporting a 3-month worsening of eczema affecting her eyelids, neck and trunk. She is diagnosed with an acute flare of eczema and is admitted to the dermatology day unit for intensive topical treatment.

❷ What is eczema and what are the common signs and symptoms?

Her drug history is shown in the box:

CASE NOTES

Drug history
- Omeprazole 20 mg once daily
- Terbutaline inhaler to be used when required for shortness of breath
- Loratadine 10 mg daily
- Bath emollient, which she uses each morning

❷ What are the main triggers for a flare of eczema?

❷ What treatment options are available for the management of eczema?

She is started on:

- *Emollient used as a soap substitute each morning*
- *Bath emollient*
- *Regular greasy emollient to be applied every 2 hours*
- *Clobetasone ointment to her face and trunk twice daily for 7 days.*

❷ What are emollients and how do they work?

After 1-week's treatment with emollients, there is no sign of improvement, and her skin appears to have become more red and inflamed. Through questioning, it is discovered that Miss FL's eczema initially began to flare after initiation of a bath emollient containing an antimicrobial agent (benzalkonium chloride). She undergoes patch testing to discover whether it is this compound causing the reaction.

❷ Chemically, what sort of compound is benzalkonium chloride?

❷ Why is it included in pharmaceutical products?

❷ What is patch testing?

The results of the patch testing return, which determine that the patient did develop a reaction to benzalkonium chloride. The doctors ask whether you can recommend an alternative emollient (to be used as a soap substitute and bath emollient) that does not contain this compound.

❷ What information sources will you use to inform your response?

Case discussion

— Eczema and its pathophysiology

Eczema can be divided into two types: exogenous or contact eczema (due to irritants, allergy or light sensitivity) and the endogenous type, such as atopic, seborrhoeic eczema. This case focuses on atopic eczema.

Atopic eczema is eczema that has an underlying genetic basis and tends to run in families. It normally presents in childhood and tends to resolve by adulthood. It results in the skin being unable to perform a core function (barrier function), which causes it to be easily irritated by external irritants and allergens, including microorganisms. Atopic eczema is a chronic inflammatory condition that causes the skin to become dry, red and scaly, and sometimes to weep. The main symptom of eczema is itchiness (which may also affect sleep). The itching can be so intense that patients may exhibit scratch marks and even bleed where they have scratched. Eczema can affect the whole body. However, it commonly affects the flexures (such as the crevices in the elbows, knees and neck).

— Possible triggers for a flare of eczema

Atopic eczema can be triggered by factors including:

- Irritants in the patient's environment (such as soap, detergent and excipients contained in topical products)
- Infection: *Staphylococcus aureus* is not part of the normal skin flora but can flourish wherever there is eczema, and the more heavy the colonisation the more active the eczema
- Stress.

Treatment options for the management of eczema

It should be noted that atopic eczema cannot be cured, only controlled and managed. Topical treatments are the mainstay of treatment and are used to reduce the inflammation, treat any associated infection and maintain the integrity of the barrier function of the skin.

— Emollients

There are various different emollients. The basic function of the emollient is to occlude and hydrate the skin and to help maintain the skin's barrier function (thus protecting the skin from external allergens and irritants). Emollients are available in a variety of consistencies – generally the greasier the emollient the better it occludes the skin, and therefore reduces water loss from the skin. Emollients should also be used as soap substitutes, because they remove dirt and organic material on the skin while also leaving a lipid layer (which forms an occlusive barrier). To achieve concordance, the patient should be encouraged to try out a range of emollients and bath oils before deciding which she prefers. Many emollients also contain antiseptics (benzalkonium chloride, triclosan, chlorhexidine) that may be suitable for use as a soap substitute.

— Corticosteroids

There are various corticosteroids differing in formulation and potency (Table 10.1). Corticosteroids reduce the inflammation associated with eczema (therefore helping to reduce the itchiness of the skin). There are seven points to consider for using topical corticosteroids:

1 It is important to be clear what condition is being treated and the cause, e.g. fungal infections that are very similar in appearance to eczema will change to strange forms if treated with steroids. In cases of contact eczema it is important to identify the cause, rather than reduce the inflammatory response by steroids.
2 Use only mild steroids on the face, e.g. 0.5–1% hydrocortisone, to prevent atrophy.
3 Use the lowest-potency corticosteroid to achieve symptom control. Some patients may need to start with a moderate-to-potent steroid to achieve symptom control; this would then be switched to a weaker potency steroid to suppress the symptoms.
4 Avoid using potent steroids in children.
5 Provide a suitable supply of steroid creams (this also applies to the supply of emollients).
6 Tell the patient how to apply and how much to apply, explaining the fingertip unit (1 FTU on each foot, 2.5 FTUs on face, 3 FTUs on the arm, 6 FTUs on the leg and 7 FTUs on the front and back of the trunk).
7 Tell the patients both the benefits and the risks of the treatment, including adverse effects (such as skin atrophy and stretch marks with prolonged use).

When choosing steroids, choose the lowest potency steroid that effectively controls the

▼ TABLE 10.1

Corticosteroid potency

Potency	Corticosteroid
Very potent	Clobetasol, diflucortolone valerate
Potent	Betamethasone valerate
Moderate	Clobetasone, fludroxycortide
Mild	Hydrocortisone (0.1–2.5%)

symptoms and ensure that the correct potency steroid is used for the area on the body to be treated (e.g. thinner areas of skin, such as found in the flexures and the face should be managed with mild-to-moderate potency steroids). Patients should be taught how to apply, and how much steroid to use – using the fingertip measure of steroids. One fingertip unit (measured from the tip of the adult index finger to the first crease) is sufficient to cover an area that is twice that of the flat adult palm. If multiple steroids are being used in different areas it is essential that the patient understands which corticosteroid is being used at which site. (It is important to mark on the label of the steroid very potent, potent, moderate or mild so that the patient can follow instructions effectively.)

Topical steroids have many side effects. A patient is more likely to experience more side effects with the more potent steroids, or if the application is on a large area. Rarely, the patient may experience side effects due to systemic absorption when large areas of the body are treated for prolonged periods.

Local adverse effects that may occur include:

* Spread or worsening of untreated skin infection
* Skin thinning (which may reduce, but not be fully reversible on cessation of therapy)
* Irreversible striae atropicae (stretch marks)
* Acne (or worsening of acne)
* Mild depigmentation (which may be reversible on cessation of therapy).

— **Antimicrobial/antibiotic creams**
Staphylococcus colonisation on the skin aggravates eczema. Creams containing antimicrobial agents (antibiotics) should be used only when the skin is infected and crusted (antifungal and antibacterial creams are available). They should be used when the skin is crusted and weepy. Topical antibiotics that are available include: chlortetracycline, sodium fusidate, gramicidin, neomycin, oxytetracycline and polymyxin B.

Note that tetracycline and clioquinol (an antiseptic) can discolour the skin and neomycin can be a skin sensitiser. Fucidin H and Fucibet are particularly good combinations of sodium fusidate with steroids for treating eczema aggravated by staphylococci.

— **Topical immunosuppressants**
Staphylococcus aureus produce exotoxins and these act as allergens that stimulate T lymphocytes

to produce large amounts of cytokines that are involved in the inflammatory process of eczema. Immunomodulators such as tacrolimus and pimecrolimus work by targeting calcineurin (a serine/threonine protein phosphatase controlled by intracellular calcium), and suppressing T-cell activation and proinflammatory cytokine production.

— **Oral antihistamines**
Many different oral antihistamines are available (sedating and non-sedating), which block the effects of locally released histamine from mast cells, thereby helping to relieve the itch associated with eczema. Sedating antihistamines such as hydroxyzine are especially helpful in patients whose sleep is affected due to itchiness.

— **Ichthammol**
This is available in combination with zinc, and also in a variety of preparations from pastes to bandages. It is a mildly antiseptic product that helps to reduce the itching and hyperkeratinisation associated with eczema.

— **Zinc oxide**
Available in combination with ichthammol, and also in a variety of preparations from pastes to bandages. It is an astringent, is soothing and plays a role in wound healing.

— **Potassium permanganate soaks**
Potassium permanganate is a mild antiseptic and also acts as an astringent. It is useful to dry up weeping/exudative areas. It is usually used as a 1 in 10 000 solution, prepared by dissolving a tablet (Permitabs) in water that can be used for soaking localised areas, or in the bath. Patients should be counselled that the solution will stain their clothes, skin and nails.

Patients with mild atopic eczema are less likely to benefit from antiseptics because these patients are usually colonised with Staphylococcus aureus, so the potential of any benefit is outweighed by the cause of irritation and contact allergy due to the antiseptic. However, patients with more generalised eczema with recurrent flares of the condition may benefit with the use of antiseptics.

— **Benzalkonium chloride**
Benzalkonium chloride is a cationic antimicrobial agent frequently used in pharmaceutical products as a preservative. It is a permanently charged quaternary ammonium compound with surface active properties. Benzalkonium chloride is in fact

a mixture of alkylbenzyldimethylammonium chlorides, with differing hydrocarbon chain lengths.

The general structure of the alkylbenzyldimethylammonium chlorides that make up benzalkonium chloride is shown in the diagram.

benzalkonium chloride

In addition to the two methyl groups and the benzyl group, the positively charged nitrogen atom is covalently bonded to an alkyl chain that contains an even number of carbon atoms, varying in length between 8 and 18 carbon atoms. The nitrogen atom's positive charge is permanent and therefore independent of pH. The charge arises from the presence of four covalent bonds, which comprise eight bonding electrons, four of which 'belong' to nitrogen. As nitrogen normally has five valence electrons, it is effectively one electron deficient in quaternary ammonium compounds.

Benzalkonium chloride is used as a skin antiseptic and is also frequently encountered as a preservative in ocular preparations, typically at a concentration of 0.01% w/v.

— Patch testing

Patch testing is the process in which dilute concentrations of substances thought to have caused eczema are incorporated into patches that are placed on to the skin. The patches are removed 48 hours later to observe for any reactions caused by the allergen.

Patch testing allows us to test a variety of materials that come into contact with the skin. Identification of offending substances allows the individual to avoid contact in the future.

When patch testing indicates a reaction to a component of a product, a suitable alternative will need to be supplied. Some information on the excipients used in topical products that are associated with sensitisation reactions is provided in the *British National Formulary* (*BNF*). The *BNF* also provides information on the components of topical formulations, and further information can be obtained from the products' summary of product characteristics (SmPC), available online.

— General management of patients with atopic eczema

Discuss the patient's condition and expectations of the treatment and explain realistically that the treatment only controls symptoms that may flare periodically:

- Give general advice to keep nails short (to avoid skin damage/bleeding through scratching) and try to wear cotton next to the skin; avoid wool
- Teach how to use emollients regularly and frequently after bathing
- Use a soap substitute such as aqueous cream or other similar products
- Teach the patients how to use topical steroids.

EXTENDED LEARNING

- Describe the anatomy and physiology of the skin and the implications for drug delivery to the skin (topical) and through the skin (transdermal)
- What is the immune response to skin damage?
- What systemic treatments are available for the management of severe eczema (including azathioprine, ciclosporin and alitretinoin), and how do they work?
- Describe the formulation of emulsions, creams and ointments.
- Why may more than one emollient be prescribed simultaneously?
- Miss FL's drug history shows that she is taking omeprazole and loratadine orally and using a terbutaline inhaler. What are the indications for each of these medications, and what is the mode of action of the drug substance in each case?

References and further reading

Joint Formulary Committee, British Medical Association and Royal Pharmaceutical Society (2013). *British National Formulary 65*. London: Pharmaceutical Press.

Moncrieff G, Cork M, Lawton S, Kokiet S, Daly C, Clark, C. (2013). Use of emollients in dry-skin conditions: consensus statement. *Clin Exp Dermatol* 38:231–8.

— Resources

British Association of Dermatologist: www.bad.org.uk
Electronic Medicines Compendium: www.medicines.org.uk

Case 2
Contact dermatitis
IMOGEN SAVAGE

LEARNING OUTCOMES

At the end of this case, you will be able to:

- Understand the three common forms of eczema: atopic eczema, allergic contact dermatitis, irritant contact dermatitis
- Outline the barrier function of the skin
- Outline the occupational exposure risks in hairdressers (and their clients)
- Identify possible irritants and/or allergens in topical emollient formulations
- Outline the use of emollients and how they are commonly formulated
- Differentiate between the different types of surfactants used in pharmaceutical products

Case study

Miss EF is a healthy 18-year-old young woman working full-time as a trainee in a busy hairdressing salon. At first, her main duties were to sweep and clean up after the stylists, but 2 weeks ago she graduated to more 'basin work', washing hair, and rinsing off perming and colouring products. She is supposed to wear gloves, but the stylists have priority and there aren't always enough to go round. However, she takes good care of her hands, washing them frequently during the day, and using an emollient afterwards. The salon supplies big tubs of emollient for all staff to use.

Miss EF is surprised when her hands suddenly start to feel dry, sore and itchy. Moisturising doesn't help much and within 48 hours both palms have become scaly and cracked and her fingertips are red, swollen, and very sore and itchy. The symptoms are particularly bad on her left hand, which she routinely uses to channel rinse water back from clients' foreheads into the basin. Her salon manager is horrified and says this is what happens when you don't use gloves. Unable to work, she is forced to visit her GP who tells her she is has contact dermatitis, a type of eczema. Given

her occupation, he suspects that hair dyes are to blame.

❓ What is 'contact dermatitis' and how is it different from atopic eczema?

The GP says the first thing is to heal the skin with a short course of a potent topical steroid plus intensive emollients. They must then do patch testing to identify exactly what she is allergic to, so she can avoid further contact. Miss EF is upset. Does this mean that she has to find a different job?

❓ Which hair products are the likely culprits?

❓ Comment on the use of topical steroid products. Which emollient products would you choose? How are emollients formulated?

Miss EF responds well to treatment. Subsequent patch testing at the hospital dermatology department confirms a strong allergy to p-phenylenediamine (PPD), a compound found in many types of dye. After advice from her NVQ training provider, she decides to switch to training as a beauty therapist to minimise the risk of further PPD contact.

Miss EF continues to take good care of her hands but runs out of her prescribed emollient. Her grandmother, who suffers from varicose eczema on her legs, offers her a tub of aqueous cream, saying the surgery always gives her too much on her repeat prescription. When Miss EF tries it, her hands sting and go red. Granny tells her she's imagining it; she's used aqueous cream for years and it is perfectly safe for eczema. It's a lot nicer than the emulsifying ointment they used to give her.

❓ Why are aqueous cream and emulsifying ointment prescribed? How should they be used?

❓ What ingredients might Miss EF react to?

Case discussion
— Differential diagnosis

The terms 'dermatitis' and 'eczema' actually mean the same thing: inflammation of the skin. Historically they have been used to distinguish inflammation with no obvious external cause (atopic eczema) from cases where the causal agent, either a specific allergen such as nickel (allergic contact dermatitis) or a general irritant such as detergent (irritant contact dermatitis), was known.

The current view is that these common conditions are all caused by the same thing: a defect in the barrier function of the skin. A nice analogy is to think of the outer layers of skin as a wall comprising bricks and mortar. The skin cells are the bricks; the mortar holding them together is a mix of lipids, water and keratin structures called desmosomes. If the mortar seal breaks down, water is lost, cracks appear and damaging chemicals or environmental agents can penetrate.

Epidermal skin cells are constantly regenerating and the outermost layer, the stratum corneum, is the end-product, consisting of dead keratinised cells (corneocytes) normally kept supple by sebum, plus a mix of amino acid products (natural moisturising factor) which help to retain water. Corneocytes last around 2 weeks before being shed. This is called desquamation, and it is triggered by action of stratum corneum chymotryptic enzyme (SCCE), which hydrolyses the desmosomes that hold cells together.

One theory is that people with atopic/allergic eczema have a change in the gene coding for SCCE, leading to increased desmosome breakdown. Opening up channels between cells enhances water loss and makes it easier for allergens to penetrate down to the basal layer, which contains blood vessels, nerves and antigen-presenting cells.

Clinically, the dry skin 'boils up' (the Greek origin of the word eczema), becoming inflamed, scaly and itchy, and it may blister or weep. Affected areas may then become cracked and prone to colonisation by bacteria, particularly *Staphylococcus epidermidis*, which can intensify and prolong the inflammatory response.

— **Occupational allergens and sensitising agents**
Eczema is very common; it is estimated that around 10% of the population has some form of eczema at any one time. Modern life brings most people into regular contact with irritants, such as soaps, detergents and solvents. These degrease the skin, and will cause irritant contact dermatitis in anyone if used often enough for a long time.

In addition, there are common contact allergens: metal (usually nickel) in jewellery and clothes' fastenings, rubber or latex in gloves, hair dyes and preservatives and fragrances in cosmetics and medicines. All these can cause a delayed-type IV T-cell-mediated response after exposure in a proportion of people. This type of allergic response requires prior exposure and is an exaggerated response of a normal immune reaction, in which the foreign antigen is presented to T-helper cells, which then release cytokines, resulting in macrophage build-up and activation of cytotoxic T cells. This produces localised inflammation and damage, usually some 24–48 hours after exposure.

Hairdressers are an example of an occupation with frequent exposure to skin irritants (shampoos, conditioners, cleaning products, etc.) plus PPD in hair dyes, ammonium persulfate in bleach and glyceryl monothioglycolate in perm solutions. Around half of all hairdressers have experienced a problem with their hands and junior staff have up to a 35% risk of developing occupational eczema (irritant and/or allergic) in their first 2 years of work.

— **Emollient products: choice and formulation**
Keeping the skin supple and avoiding contact with harsh soaps and irritants is key to eczema management. Emollients are designed to soothe, smooth and hydrate by depositing a fine film of oily ingredients (often paraffin based) on the skin. Diluted, they can also be used as wash products, to lift dirt from the skin in the same way as ordinary soap (although with less lather). A large range of proprietary washes, creams, lotions and bath products is available, but not all are prescribable on the NHS. Some dermatology clinics offer new patients a selection of products to try, because the most effective product is the one the patient prefers and so uses most.

The vast majority of emollients contain an emulsifying agent to allow the oily ingredients to mix with water, either on the skin or in the bath. Many will also contain a preservative. The emulsifying agent is likely to be one of three types of surfactant.

Anionic (dissociate to form negative ions) and cationic (positive ions) surfactants can be irritant to human skin, although cationic quaternary ammonium compounds, such as benzalkonium chloride, have useful bactericidal properties and can be used as preservatives and antiseptics. Amphoteric surfactants have varying charge, depending on the pH of the system. They are most often found in 'mild' shampoos and washes.

Non-ionic surfactants are a large group with low irritant potential, used in a wide range of formulations. Examples are sorbitan esters (Spans), polysorbates (Tweens) and fatty alcohol polyglycol ethers (cetomacrogol 1000).

Surfactants (also called surface active agents) are amphiphilic molecules, with hydrophilic (water-liking) and hydrophobic (water-hating) regions. This amphiphilic nature means that they tend to adsorb at the interfaces of solids, liquids and gases. This results in changes in the properties of that interface, e.g. changes in the surface tension of a liquid, resulting in adsorption at the air/liquid interface. In a mixture of oily and aqueous phases, as in an emulsion or cream, the adsorption of surfactant at the oil/water interface aids the dispersion of one phase in the other as droplets.

— **Aqueous cream and emulsifying ointment**
Emulsifying ointment and aqueous cream are two long-standing and widely prescribed generic British Pharmacopoeia emollient formulations. Emulsifying ointment contains white soft paraffin, liquid paraffin and emulsifying wax, which is a mix of cetostearyl alcohol (a non-ionic surfactant) and sodium laurylsulfate (SLS, an anionic surfactant also known as sodium dodecylsulfate, SDS). Aqueous cream is an oil-in-water emulsion produced by mixing emulsifying ointment with water and adding a preservative (phenoxyethanol).

Both can be prescribed as soap substitutes, either used directly on the skin before washing or added to water. Emulsifying ointment is much messier to use. The best way is to whisk up a small piece with hot water in a blender then add it to the bath.

Emulsifying ointment and aqueous cream are also classified in the *British National Formulary* (*BNF*) as 'leave on' emollient products. There is growing evidence that the high levels of SLS in these formulations can damage the skin barrier, in normal healthy skin, decreasing corneocyte size and increasing activity of the enzymes involved in desquamation.

A recent study in asymptomatic volunteers with a history of eczema found that twice-daily application of Aqueous Cream BP for 4 weeks increased transepidermal water loss and decreased stratum corneum integrity to 'damaged' levels found in volunteers with active eczema.

— **Use of topical steroids and prevention of recurrence**
For the management of symptoms of dermatitis, short-term use of a topical corticosteroid may be appropriate. To prevent any recurrence, strict avoidance of the causative agent must be advised. This may be wearing of protective gloves, or in some cases not engaging in activities that may cause problems.

EXTENDED LEARNING

- Describe the structural features of healthy and diseased skin
- Describe the structure, properties and pharmaceutical uses of surface active agents
- Outline the formulation, manufacture and properties of topical preparations
- What is the interrelationship of pH, pK_a and ionic charge?

References and further reading
Danby SG, Al-Enezi T, Sultan A, Chittock J, Kennedy K, Cork MJ (2011). The effect of aqueous cream BP on the skin barrier in volunteers with a previous history of atopic dermatitis. *Br J Dermatol* **165**:329–34

Eccleston GM (2013). Emulsions and creams. In: Aulton ME, Taylor, KMG (eds), *Aulton's Pharmaceutics: The design and manufacture of medicines*, 4th edn. London: Elsevier, 435–64.

Mohammed D, Matts PJ, Hadgraft J, Lane ME (2011). Influence of aqueous cream BP on corneocyte size, maturity, protease activity, protein content and transepidermal water loss. *Br J Dermatol* **164**:1304–10.

Nixon R, Roberts H, Frowen K, Sim K (2006). Knowledge of skin hazards and the use of gloves by Australian hairdressing students and practising hairdressers. *Contact Dermatitis* **54**:112–16.

Oranje AP, de Waard-van der Spek FB, Ordonez C, De Raeve L, Spierings M, van der Wouden JC (2010). Emollients for eczema. *Cochrane Database Syst Rev* **1**:CD008304.

Williams AC (2013). Topical and transdermal drug delivery. In: Aulton ME, Taylor, KMG (eds), *Aulton's Pharmaceutics: The design and manufacture of medicines*, 4th edn. London: Elsevier, 675–97.

Case 3
Management of an acute flare of psoriasis
JAYMI MISTRY

LEARNING OUTCOMES

At the end of this case, you will be able to:

- Outline the pathophysiology, signs, symptoms and diagnosis of psoriasis
- Understand common triggers for a flare of psoriasis
- Describe the topical treatment options available for the management of an acute flare of mild-to-moderate psoriasis, and understand the factors that would influence the choice of treatment
- Understand the use of short-contact therapy (with dithranol) in the management of psoriasis
- Outline the appropriate use, and possible adverse effects, of topical corticosteroids
- Describe the main counselling points for patients with psoriasis

Case study

Mrs PP is a 47-year-old white woman with a past medical history of chronic plaque psoriasis (diagnosed at the age of 6) and hay fever (seasonal). Her psoriasis has been stable for the last year, maintained on regular emollient twice daily. Mrs PP is divorced and lives with her two children (who are 21 and 24 years). She works full-time as a GP receptionist, but 4 weeks ago was made redundant; this has caused her much stress and anxiety. In the last 2 weeks, she has noticed the formation of widespread pink plaques on her body and limbs (arms and legs). The plaques are extremely itchy and she is having difficulty sleeping at night.

❷ What is psoriasis?
❷ What are the common signs and symptoms of psoriasis?
❷ What are the main triggers for an acute flare of psoriasis?

Mrs PP's last flare had been approximately a year ago. During that attack she was managed in the specialist dermatology clinic with regular

emollients, steroid ointments and short-contact dithranol treatment.

❷ What topical treatments are available for the management of psoriasis?
❷ What factors would influence the choice of treatment?

Mrs PP visits her dermatology consultant who admits her to the specialist dermatology unit for intensive topical treatment.

She is prescribed:

- *Regular 50% liquid paraffin and white soft paraffin emollient for application to the entire body four times daily*
- *A suitable emollient as a soap substitute once daily (when she showers)*
- *Dithranol for short-contact therapy application to all plaques in the morning*
- *Moderately potent corticosteroid ointment for application in the afternoon to all plaques*
- *A sedating antihistamine to be taken before bedtime*

❷ Explain the rationale for each topical product prescribed in the management of psoriasis
❷ What is short-contact dithranol therapy, how is it applied and how long is the normal course of treatment?

By the end of the treatment period Mrs PP's plaques are greatly reduced.

She is discharged on:

- *Regular 50% liquid paraffin and white soft paraffin emollient for application to the whole body four times daily*
- *A suitable emollient, as a soap substitute, once daily (when she showers)*
- *Moderately potent steroid to be used twice daily until reviewed by the consultant in clinic.*

❷ What should the patient be counselled about before discharge?

Case discussion

— Psoriasis and its pathophysiology

Psoriasis is a chronic condition characterised by the formation of bright red, elevated scaly plaques on the skin. It is a T-cell-mediated condition, thought to be autoimmune in origin.

The skin is a large, complex organ that fulfils many functions including: barrier function to protect the body from the external environment, a temperature regulator, an immune organ to detect infections, and a sensory organ to detect temperature, touch and vibration. If any of these functions fails, there can be serious consequences for the patient (e.g. if the skin is unable to perform its barrier function, patients are at risk of infection or excess fluid loss, which could contribute to the patient becoming dehydrated). The skin comprises three distinct layers: the epidermis, the dermis (vascular layer) and the subcutaneous layer (adipose tissue).

The epidermis is the thin, tough outermost layer responsible for providing the skin's barrier function. The epidermis is split into several layers: the lowermost layer being the basal layer and the outermost being the stratum corneum. Within the epidermis there is a constant transition of epidermal cells (keratinocytes) from the basal layer to the stratum corneum. The cornified (old) keratinocytes are shed from the stratum corneum and replaced by newer cells. This process helps to maintain the health and integrity of the skin surface. In healthy skin, this process takes approximately 28 days. In patients with psoriasis, the turnover of cells is much greater and is thought to occur in as little as 3–4 days, resulting in the formation of plaques.

— Common signs, symptoms and triggers of psoriasis

There are several different types of psoriasis – the most common being chronic plaque psoriasis which affects approximately 80% of all psoriasis patients. Psoriasis is characterised by red/pink lesions (also known as plaques) covered in silvery/white scales. Plaques vary according to size and type of psoriasis among individuals.

The plaques may be extremely itchy and inflamed, which may affect patients' ability to continue with their daily activities, or their ability to sleep. Sometimes, the plaques split, causing pain and distress.

The diagnosis of psoriasis should be based on full clinical assessments for symptoms and any clinical signs, as well as a complete history (including past medical history, drug history, social history and family history).

Common triggers of psoriasis include stress (or emotional upset), alcohol intake, sunlight, infection and medication (such as *β* blockers, lithium and NSAIDs).

— Treatment options for the management of psoriasis: choice and rationale

There are multiple factors affecting the choice of treatment for patients with psoriasis including:

- The type of psoriasis
- The size and distribution of plaques.

As topical treatments take several weeks to work, the choice of product should take into consideration therapeutic efficacy (including previous therapeutic effect) with cosmetic acceptability and local side-effect profile.

Emollients: used to moisturise the skin. They help to ease itching, reduce scaling and reduce dry, cracked skin. There are also studies to show how hydrated skin aids the penetration of other topical products.

Topical corticosteroids and vitamin D analogues: first-line therapy for most patients.

Corticosteroids: have anti-inflammatory, anti-proliferative and immunomodulatory properties, but they also have many local side effects.

Vitamin D: inhibits keratinocyte proliferation, normalises keratinisation and inhibits the accumulation of inflammatory cells in the skin, particularly neutrophils and T lymphocytes.

Tar preparations and dithranol: anti-mitotic medications that inhibit DNA synthesis and therefore reduce epidermal hyperproliferation.

Salicylic acid and urea: keratolytic agents that are used to reduce scales, but they also enhance the absorption of other topical agents used to treat psoriasis.

Sedating antihistamines such as hydroxyzine: may be useful to manage sleep affected by itching.

The severity of psoriasis is measured using a scoring system called the PASI (Psoriasis Area and Severity Index) score. The score considers the degree of severity, coverage, erythema, induration and scaling. A PASI will be carried out before starting treatment and regularly every couple of weeks during treatment to assess the efficacy of the treatment. Psoriasis is a very disfiguring disease and so an assessment of the patient's quality of life is also carried out using the Dermatology Life Quality Index (DLQI).

— Dithranol short-contact treatment

Dithranol (anthralin) is a synthetic hydroxyanthracenone compound derived from the bark of the South American araroba tree. On contact with the skin, dithranol oxidises and combines with proteins found in the stratum corneum where it exerts its anti-mitotic effect. It is this process that causes the characteristic yellowy-brown staining of the skin (as well as clothing, bedding and dressings). Dithranol can cause skin irritation and burning, as well as staining of the skin. To minimise this effect on the healthy perilesional areas, dithranol is usually prepared in a paste such as Lassar's paste, which also contains salicylic acid (a keratolytic) and zinc oxide (an astringent). Pharmaceutical pastes are high-viscosity, semi-solid formulations comprising a high concentration of drug (often >50%) dispersed as a solid in an ointment base. There is large variation in the concentrations of dithranol that can be tolerated from individual to individual.

In short-contact dithranol therapy, increasing concentrations of dithranol are applied (usually as Lassar's paste) over a period of time. Dithranol concentrations should not be increased more frequently than every 3–5 days. Most patients receiving dithranol treatment in an outpatient setting will start treatment on 1% dithranol, gradually increasing to 4% dithranol over the course of a couple of weeks. The overall treatment course is about 12–18 weeks depending on response.

— Counselling points

There is a fire hazard associated with paraffin-based skin products: paraffins (e.g. white and yellow soft paraffin, hard paraffin, liquid paraffin) are hydrocarbon compounds frequently used as ointment bases, being emollient and well retained on the skin. Other than undergoing combustion, paraffins are very stable and unreactive (the name paraffin is derived from the Latin *parum* + *affinitas* meaning 'little affinity'), which makes them good choices for topical pharmaceutical excipients.

Appropriate use of topical corticosteroids (fingertip dose unit):

1 fingertip unit (FTU) = 0.5 g.

In an adult, the typical corticosteroid requirements for the face and neck = 1.5 g (3 FTUs); trunk (front and back) = 7 g (14 FTUs); one arm = 1.5 g (3 FTUs); one hand = 0.5 g, one leg = 3 g and one foot = 1 g.

Adverse effects associated with the use of topical corticosteroids include:

- Skin atrophy and telangiectasia (reddening of skin due to dilatation of fine blood vessels near the skin surface)
- Bleaching of the skin
- Striae
- Masking of local infection
- Rebound of psoriasis on stopping therapy
- The transformation of stable psoriasis to pustular psoriasis
- Tachyphylaxis.

EXTENDED LEARNING

- Describe the main types of psoriasis and outline the differences between them
- Describe how scalp psoriasis is managed
- Describe the structure and function of the skin
- Differentiate between meiosis and mitosis

References and further reading

British Association of Dermatologists and Primary Care Dermatology Society (2009). *Recommendations for the initial management of psoriasis*. Available at: www.bad.org.uk (accessed 11 July 2013).

Joint Formulary Committee, British Medical Association and Royal Pharmaceutical Society (2013). *British National Formulary 6*. London: Pharmaceutical Press.

— Resources

Electronic Medicines Compendium: www.medicines.org.uk

Case 4
Acne
JAYMI MISTRY

LEARNING OUTCOMES

At the end of this case, you will be able to:

- Outline the pathophysiology, signs and symptoms, and diagnosis of acne
- Understand the common causes of acne
- Describe the main aims of acne treatment
- Outline the structure and properties of benzoyl peroxide
- Outline the formulation and properties of creams, ointments and gels
- Discuss alternative treatments for the management of acne
- Outline the use of isotretinoin for the oral treatment of severe acne, the contraindications for its use and specific counselling points

Case study

Collette is a 15-year-old girl (of average build and height) who started to develop acne when she first turned 13 years of age. Her acne was initially easily managed with daily use of soap and water. However, in recent months her acne has worsened in severity and as a result she has become embarrassed, anxious and upset about the appearance of her skin. She recently saw an advertisement on television for an anti-acne treatment that she is thinking about trying.

You are the pharmacist working in Collette's local community pharmacy. Collette comes to you one afternoon with her mother seeking advice about her acne. On examination of her skin, you notice that Collette has a large number of comedones covering her cheeks and T zone. Her skin is also red and inflamed.

- What is acne?
- What are the common signs and symptoms of acne?
- What are the main causes?
- What is T-zone acne?
- What are the main aims of acne treatment?

From further questioning, you discover that Collette has not previously used any products to manage her acne. She does not have any medical conditions and is not taking any medication. You decide to recommend the use of a benzoyl peroxide preparation.

- What is benzoyl peroxide and how does it work in the treatment of acne?
- Benzoyl peroxide is available as a pharmaceutical cream or gel. What are these dosage forms and why are they appropriate to treat this condition?
- What counselling would you give Colette?

Collette's mother mentions that a friend's daughter is taking a tablet called isotretinoin.

- What is isotretinoin and how does it work to manage acne?
- Do you think isotretinoin appropriate for this patient?

Case discussion

— Acne and its pathophysiology

Acne (acne vulgaris) is a common skin disorder that presents during puberty and usually resolves by the age of 20. It is normally found only on the face, neck and back. Acne targets teenagers in the most crucial years of life when social development and job searching are a high priority; therefore the scarring and the disfigurement associated with acne can lead to psychosocial problems and depression.

At puberty, there is an increase in androgen production, which is thought to have a stimulating effect in the production of sebum, and the proliferation of the keratinocytes lining the sebaceous follicle. This results in the production of a very sticky substance that blocks pores, forming an 'open comedone', also known as a 'whitehead'. Oxidation of the occlusion of a whitehead leads to the formation of a 'blackhead' or closed comedone. The pilosebaceous glands may also become colonised with *Propionibacterium acnes*, which may trigger the formation of inflammation and pus-filled spots. It should also be noted that certain medications can cause or exacerbate acne, including corticosteroids, isoniazid and androgens.

Acne initially presents as comedones but may progress to inflammatory lesions that are known as papules, and pustules that can further develop to nodules and cysts. Assessment of acne severity may be done with different tools including the Leeds Revised Acne Grading System, which consists of a series of pictures of patients that are graded with varying severity of acne. This method may be used in clinical investigations but in normal practice acne is graded as mild (comedone stage), moderate (few papules and pustules) and severe (many papules/pustules/some nodules or cysts.). The grade, together with a rough count and distribution, is usually documented in the patient's notes for assessing the effectiveness of the treatment.

The area of the face referred to as the T-zone that people often touch, includes the middle and sides of the forehead, down the middle and sides of the nose down to chin, where outbreaks of acne appear to be most frequent.

— **Treatment of acne**

The main aims of acne treatment are to reduce sebum formation, the bacterial population of the sebaceous glands, keratinisation of pores and inflammation. Acne cannot be cured, only managed. Treatment should always be started early to prevent permanent scarring.

— **Benzoyl peroxide: chemical structure, modes of action and formulation**

The structure of benzoyl peroxide is shown in the diagram. It consists of two benzoyl groups (C_6H_5CO-) joined via a peroxide group. This reactive functional group consists of a weak oxygen–oxygen single bond. Benzoyl peroxide has multiple mechanisms of action. It is sebostatic and has keratolytic activity (thus reducing sebum production and hyperkeratinisation). It also has antibacterial activity against *Propionibacterium acnes*, a Gram-positive anaerobic skin bacterium that is most commonly associated with acne breakouts.

benzoyl peroxide

Benzoyl peroxide is available as a gel, cream or wash. A pharmaceutical cream is a semi-solid formulation, comprising two phases, one dispersed in the other. Where the oily phase is dispersed in the aqueous phase, these are described as oil in water (O/W) creams. Water in oil (W/O) systems are less common systems. Formulations include emulsifiers (e.g. surfactants, polysaccharides) to provide structure to the cream and to maintain the integrity of the droplets. Creams spread easily and are well accepted by patients.

Pharmaceutical gels are also semi-solids. They are relatively transparent, and are usually water-based, though they can be alcohol-based. Gels contain gelling agents, which may be natural (e.g. alginate, tragacanth) or synthetic (e.g. cellulose derivatives, Carbopol).

Creams and gels contain a preservative to protect against microbial contamination of the product during use by the patient. Creams and gels are less viscous and occlusive than ointments, which are greasy, often anhydrous, semi-solid preparations, and hence creams or gels would be preferred to ointments in the treatment of acne.

Patients new to benzoyl peroxide should start treatment with the lower strength products and increase the concentration gradually.

— **Other treatments**

Azelaic acid: this has two main actions. It has antibacterial activity against *Propionibacterium acnes* and also reduces follicular hyperkeratosis.
Topical retinoids, similar to isotretinoin, work by inducing metabolic changes in keratinised epithelia. They help to increase proliferative activity of epidermal cells. Topical retinoids should, however, be avoided in severe acne covering large areas. The patient should be counselled to avoid contact with the eyes, mucous membranes, eczematous areas, or broken and sunburned skin. The patient should also avoid exposure to UV light. Common adverse effects may include dry or peeling skin.
Topical antibacterials (mainly clindamycin and erythromycin): have direct action against *Propionibacterium acnes*. Unfortunately there is a risk of antibacterial resistance of *Propionibacterium acnes* to this treatment.
Oral antibiotics such as tetracyclines: may be used which have antibacterial activity against *Propionibacterium acnes* and also an anti-inflammatory effect.

Oral contraceptives: include an anti-androgen (such as co-cyprindiol); they work by reducing sebum production.

Oral retinoids: isotretinoin is an oral retinoid that is effective in the management of severe acne, or acne that has caused scarring, or when other standard preparations for acne are ineffective.

— **Counselling points**

Patients should always be counselled that:

- They should not pick or squeeze their spots because this will aggravate their condition, and may lead to scarring.
- They may need to use a treatment for at least 2 months before they see any improvements.
- They may use an oil-free moisturiser if dryness of the skin is troublesome.

— **Use of isotretinoin for acne**

Isotretinoin is a synthetic retinoid (chemically related to vitamin A), which is licensed for the treatment of severe forms of acne (including those involved with scarring and acne resistant to adequate courses of other treatments). It acts by suppressing (by inhibiting proliferation of sebocyte cells) and reducing the size of the sebaceous glands. It is also thought to have anti-inflammatory activity.

Isotretinoin is contraindicated in patients with hepatic impairment, elevated blood lipid levels or raised vitamin A levels, or in those also receiving concomitant treatment with a tetracycline, and in women who are pregnant, breastfeeding or of child-bearing potential.

Isotretinoin should not be used in women unless they meet all of the conditions of the pregnancy prevention programme and acknowledge the risks involved with therapy:

- The patient must have severe acne that could not be treated with conventional topical or oral preparations.
- The patient understands the teratogenic risk.
- The patient understands the need for follow-up on a monthly basis.
- The patient understands the need to use regular contraception 1 month before starting treatment, during treatment and for 1 month after the cessation of treatment to prevent the risk of pregnancy. The patient must understand that she preferably will need to use two forms of contraception (one of which should be a barrier method).

- The patient must follow the advice even if she experiences amenorrhoea.
- The patient understands the risks of pregnancy and understands whom to contact should she become pregnant.
- The patient understands that she needs to have regular pregnancy tests (ideally every 4 weeks) during treatment and 5 weeks after the cessation of treatment.
- The patient should not give blood during treatment or for 1 month after cessation of treatment as there is a risk that the blood is given to a pregnant recipient (which may cause harm to the fetus).
- The patient understands that the supply of isotretinoin is only from the hospital pharmacy (where she is being seen) and she will receive only 1 month's supply at a time. The prescription will not be dispensed unless it is accompanied with a negative pregnancy test form that is dated similar to the date on the prescription.

The patient also needs to be counselled on other points relating to isotretinoin therapy, including:

- The risk of hepatic damage particularly if the patient is also on other hepatotoxic substances (this includes heavy alcohol consumption).
- The risk of reduced night vision: the patient needs to be warned not to operate machinery or drive at night should he or she have this side effect.
- The risk of myalgia particularly on exercise: the patient should be asked to reduce strenuous exercise.
- Patients need to ask a relative or close friend to observe them for changes in mood, because depression and suicidal thoughts are possible but rare.
- Patients should be told never to share their medication with others, particularly other women.
- Any isotretinoin capsules remaining after the course is complete need to be returned to a pharmacy.

EXTENDING LEARNING

- Outline the differences between acne and rosacea, and the differences in treating each condition

- Describe the formulation and manufacture of pharmaceutical semi-solids: creams, ointments, gels and pastes
- Outline the use of emulsifying agents in pharmaceutical systems
- Why should some pharmaceutical preparations include an antimicrobial preservative? What excipients are included as preservatives in medicines?
- How is the effectiveness of an antimicrobial preservative in a pharmaceutical product tested?

ADDITIONAL PRACTICE POINT

- Benzoyl peroxide-based creams have a powerful bleaching effect on contact with coloured fabrics, e.g. towels, bed linen, clothes, so patients should be warned against skin contact with such fabrics

during treatment. Also, some patients may react to initial treatment with severe irritation and reddening/dryness of the skin, so some care is needed when first applying, until a degree of skin tolerance is achieved

References and further reading

Eccleston GM (2013). Emulsions and creams. In: Aulton ME, Taylor, KMG (eds), *Aulton's Pharmaceutics: The design and manufacture of medicines*, 4th edn. London: Elsevier, 435–64.

Goodfield MJD, Cox NH, Bowser A et al. (2010). Advice on the safe introduction and continued use of isotretinoin in acne in the UK 2010. *Br J Dermatol* **162**:1172–9.

Williams AC (2003). *Transdermal and Topical Drug Delivery*. London: Pharmaceutical Press.

— Resources

British Association of Dermatologists: www.bad.org.uk
Electronic Medicines Compendium: www.medicines.org.uk

Case 5
Antibacterial treatment of acne in young people

NICOLA J GRAY, TIMOTHY J SNAPE AND GORDON BECKET

LEARNING OUTCOMES

At the end of this case, you will be able to:

- Describe the properties of some oral and topical antibacterial treatments commonly used for acne
- Relate the chemical and physical properties of these treatments to their indication and possible side effects
- Evaluate the suitability of these treatments for treating patients taking other medicines for common conditions in adolescence, e.g. STIs (sexually transmitted infections)
- Outline some mechanisms of bacterial resistance to antibiotics
- Evaluate the risk factors for non-adherence to these treatments during selection of the correct product for each young person

Case study

You are a community pharmacist who participates in a screening and patient group direction (PGD) treatment service for Chlamydia *sp. Miss MJ is a*

16-year-old student who has been notified through the screening service that her test for Chlamydia *sp. was positive.*

You conduct a private consultation with Miss MJ, and consult your patient medication record (PMR), and you are able to elicit the following information:

Miss MJ is 16 years of age (you have an existing PMR for her)

Miss MJ is currently having her period, and has had no sexual intercourse in the past month (she does not have a regular partner)

Miss MJ can identify two sexual partners in the past 6 months who could be notified and treated

Miss MJ has no known allergies to any antibiotics

Miss MJ has no abdominal pain or unusual/smelly discharge

Miss MJ has moderate acne and has been using Zineryt (erythromycin/zinc acetate solution) applied topically twice a day for the last 6 months (your PMR confirms this)

Miss MJ switched to Zineryt after a course of oral erythromycin as she found the GI side effects intolerable

Miss MJ is pleased with the results of her ongoing acne treatment, and there is little evidence of any spots or scarring (she is wearing very light make-up)

Miss MJ is very keen to look her best, and likes to use a sunbed at least once a month to help her skin and give her a constant light tan

You consult your PGD to determine which treatment is most appropriate for Miss MJ's chlamydia infection. Azithromycin (Zithromax), the first-line treatment, is closely related to erythromycin. You are concerned about using this macrolide antibiotic, in case Miss MJ gets pronounced GI side effects again.

- ❓ What are the common side effects of oral macrolide (e.g. erythromycin) antibiotics?
- ❓ Why do they occur?
- ❓ Discuss the issue of resistance with antibacterial therapy for acne
- ❓ What is the mechanism of action of Zineryt and how is it prepared in a pharmacy?
- ❓ Outline the non-antibacterial options for treating acne?

You decide that a 7-day course of doxycycline will be the most appropriate treatment for Miss MJ.

- ❓ How does the structure of doxycycline differ from that of the macrolide antibiotics?
- ❓ Why should sunlight be avoided when using doxycyline?
- ❓ How can the risk of non-adherence be minimised in young adults in general and in this case in particular?

Miss MJ knows that her friend who also recently had a chlamydia infection took a one-dose antibiotic, and wants to have it too. You explain the complication of the Zineryt treatment, and Miss MJ eventually agrees that she needs to treat this STI, and so she accepts the 7-day course of doxycycline. You provide spoken and written advice about how to take it, what to avoid while taking it, which side effects commonly occur with it, and what to do if side effects occur and make life difficult for her. You arrange for Miss MJ to come back and see you in a week's time, to discuss how she managed the treatment, and to talk about preventing future infection.

Case discussion

Propionibacterium acnes is the principal anaerobic organism implicated in the cause of acne vulgaris, a skin disease that most commonly affects young people during adolescence, and sometimes even into adulthood. The organisms feed on sebum in the skin, and the waste products formed by the bacteria give rise to redness and inflammation of skin pores, resulting in painful and unsightly pimples and papules, particularly on the face, chest, shoulders and back.

— Development of resistance to antibacterial therapy for acne

These bacteria have now become largely resistant to drugs such as erythromycin. The macrolide antibiotics inhibit bacterial growth by binding to the bacterial ribosome and interfering with protein synthesis, thus preventing the bacteria from replicating (they are bacteriostatic agents). Development of resistance to these antibiotics comes from modifications made to the rRNA of the ribosome by cellular enzymes, rendering the bacterial ribosome unable to bind the macrolide, yet still maintain the ability to synthesise bacterial proteins. Other potential methods of resistance to these compounds may involve mechanisms developed by the bacteria to efflux the medicine from the cell, or by chemically modifying the medicine's chemical structure through phase I or phase II metabolic reactions, rendering them inactive or more readily excreted. Both oral and topical antibacterial treatments have been linked with the formation of resistant *Propionibacterium acnes* strains.

The *BNF* suggests the following strategies for minimising the development of bacterial resistance to these preparations when using topical antibacterials for acne:

- When possible use non-antibiotic antimicrobials (such as benzoyl peroxide or azelaic acid)
- Avoid concomitant treatment with different oral and topical antibacterials
- If a particular antibacterial is effective, use it for repeat courses if needed (short intervening courses of benzoyl peroxide or azelaic acid may eliminate any resistant propionibacteria)
- Do not continue treatment for longer than necessary (however, treatment with a topical preparation should be continued for at least 6 months).

— Choice of treatment

The *BNF* (2012) states that:

For many patients with mild to moderate inflammatory acne, topical antibacterials may be no more effective than topical benzoyl peroxide or tretinoin. Topical antibacterials are probably best reserved for patients who wish to avoid oral antibacterials or who cannot tolerate them. Topical preparations of erythromycin and clindamycin are effective for inflammatory acne. Topical antibacterials can produce mild irritation of the skin, and on rare occasions cause sensitisation.

However, the *BNF* also states that, if topical treatments are ineffective, oral products may need to be used.

— Mechanism of action of Zineryt preparation in a pharmacy

Erythromycin and zinc acetate are used in combination in topical acne treatment. Erythromycin stops the replication of the *Propionibacterium* sp., and thus reduces the amount of allergens irritating the skin. Zinc preparations are traditionally associated with skin-healing properties. The zinc acetate in Zineryt combines with the erythromycin to form a chemical complex that is efficiently absorbed into the skin.

Topical treatments such as Zineryt need to be freshly prepared in the pharmacy and have a limited shelf-life. Erythromycin is acid sensitive and gives rise to decomposition products at low pH. It also contains a lactone (cyclic ester) which is potentially prone to hydrolysis. Although complexation of erythromycin to zinc salts, in the presence of suitable solvents and certain nitrogen-containing compounds, stabilises the drug and extends its shelf-life, it is known that ethanol is detrimental to the storage of zinc erythromycin unless the compositions are refrigerated or contain such nitrogen-containing stabilisers. Despite this, it is reconstituted in ethanol on dispensing. Erythromycin has a partition coefficient value (log *P*) of 3.06. It is insufficiently soluble in water to achieve the desired concentration and hence, in this product, ethanol is used as the solvent to produce the final concentration of erythromycin 40 mg/mL on reconstitution.

— Oral macrolides erythromycin and azithromycin: explaining common side effects, drug–drug interactions and dosing regimens

The *BNF* lists nausea, vomiting, abdominal discomfort and diarrhoea as common side effects with erythromycin; these are less common with azithromycin.

Motilin is a GI peptide hormone involved in regulating intestinal motility by acting on G-protein-coupled motilin receptors in the gut smooth muscle. Erythromycin, and its acid-catalysed degradation products, is a known motilin-receptor agonist, leading to some of the GI side effects observed. However, the lack of the carbonyl group (C=O) at C9 in azithromycin (see diagram on page 375), and its weakly basic tertiary amine prevents these antimicrobially inactive, yet powerful, motilin-receptor agonists from forming; thus it has reduced GI side effects.

Azithromycin also does not bind to the drug-metabolising cytochrome P450 (CYP) liver enzyme isoform CYP3A4, which reduces some of the drug–drug interactions observed with erythromycin. The enhanced acid stability and reduced metabolism of azithromycin, compared with erythromycin, also means that it has a longer half-life coupled with longer and greater tissue penetration. Reduced dosing frequency may thus improve adherence.

— The structure of doxycycline and macrolide antibiotics

As can be seen from their structures in the diagram (page 375), azithromycin and doxycycline differ greatly in their chemical structures and are members of entirely different classes of compounds. Aside from being highly functionalised with a few types of functional group (notably tertiary amino and secondary hydroxyl groups) in common, there is little similarity between them. Azithromycin contains a glycosylated, aliphatic, macrocyclic lactone, whereas doxycycline comprises a tetracyclic (four-ring) fused system, incorporating both aromatic and aliphatic rings. Interestingly, despite its different chemical structure and shape compared with the macrolides, doxycycline also binds to the bacterial ribosome, thus preventing protein synthesis and bacterial growth, but binding at a *different* site on the ribosome.

Azithromycin binds reversibly to the large 50-S subunit of the bacterial ribosome. On binding, azithromycin blocks the channel, preventing elongation of the polypeptide chain. Doxycycline binds to the smaller 30-S subunit of the bacterial ribosome and prevents the binding of the aminoacyl-tRNA to the acceptor site, which

erythromycin · azithromycin · doxycycline

subsequently prevents new amino acids from being delivered to the growing peptide chain.

— Avoiding sunlight when using doxycycline

The nature of its chemical structure means that doxycycline can easily absorb sunlight's UV radiation, and the resulting photoproducts may cause cellular toxicity. As a result, doxycycline causes sensitive skin and can therefore make you burn more easily when exposed to UV radiation. Studies into the mechanism of such phototoxicity suggest that the products caused on exposure to UV and the differing absorption spectra of the tetracycline antibiotics mean that they have different responses to radiation.

The precise mechanism of doxycycline photoallergy is not fully understood. The photosensitisation (phototoxicity or photoallergy) is usually caused by UVA radiation, which penetrates deeper into the skin. After UV irradiation and photon absorption, drug molecules in an excited energy state cause chemical reactions when they return to their energetic base level, resulting in the synthesis of photoproducts that generate an allergic reaction.

— Outline other options for treating acne

Benzoyl peroxide and azelaic acid are recommended for mild-to-moderate acne, and preparations containing these drugs are available without prescription. It is estimated that 30% of young people with acne need prescription medicines to control the condition satisfactorily. It might be useful for the pharmacist to give advice sensitively to young people who routinely buy over-the-counter medicines for acne.

Topical retinoids (tretinoin, isotretinoin and the related drug adapalene) are available to treat mild-to-moderate acne, and oral isotretinoin for severe acne. Stringent contraceptive practices must be employed by young women using these medicines because they have major teratogenic effects. (It should be noted, particularly in this case scenario, that concurrent use of oral doxycycline with oral retinoids can result in benign intercranial hypertension.)

See the relevant section of the *BNF* for a full description of the treatments available for acne vulgaris.

— Selecting the right medicine in this case

Important points to consider:

- Understand how the young person feels about his or her acne, and the effectiveness of the topical treatment
- Understand that any visible skin conditions are a source of overwhelming concern for young people, and may contribute to feelings of low mood or lack of self-confidence
- Emphasise the need for the 7-day course to clear the chlamydia infection
- Explain why it is not advisable to use a sunbed when taking doxycycline antibiotics, and how it could cause a sensitisation reaction that would be very visible.

— Creating a good pharmacy environment for helping young people to get the best from their medicines

Further points for consideration:

- All staff are welcoming to young people
- The pharmacy has leaflets that are relevant to, and aimed at, young people about services such as these
- The pharmacy staff have training in confidentiality and consent for young people, including an understanding of Gillick competence and Fraser guidance

- The pharmacist has time to listen, is non-judgemental, and encourages young people to come back and ask more questions about their medicines and health.

- What are the implications of increasing bacterial resistance to antibiotics? What roles can pharmacists play to optimise the use of antibiotics and reduce opportunities for antibiotic resistance to occur?

EXTENDED LEARNING

- What are the Gillick and Fraser guidelines for competency?
- What are the trends in STIs, pregnancy and long-term conditions (including acne) among young people?
- What are patient group directions?
- What is a partition coefficient? How is it determined and why is the partition coefficient a useful parameter to determine in pre-formulation studies?

References and further reading

Eady E.A, Cove JH, Holland KT, Cunliffe WJ (1989). Erythromycin resistant propionibacteria in antibiotic treated acne patients: association with therapeutic failure. *Br J Dermatol* **121**:51–7.

Kuznetsov AV, Weisenseel P, Flaig MJ, Ruzicka T, Prinz JC (2011). Photoallergic erythroderma due to doxycycline therapy of erythema chronicum migrans. *ActaDermato Venereol* **91**:734–6.

Department of Health (2011). *You're Welcome: quality criteria for young people-friendly health services.* London: Department of Health, Available at: www.dh.gov.uk.

— **Resources**

Association for Young People's Health: www. youngpeopleshealth.org.uk

YouthHealthTalk: www.youthhealthtalk.org.uk

Case 6
Fungal infection of the foot
IMOGEN SAVAGE

LEARNING OUTCOMES

At the end of this case, you will be able to:

- Understand the differential diagnosis of fungal nail infections
- Indicate ways in which the chemical structure and modes of action of antifungal agents influence their clinical use
- Outline the structure of the nail
- Appreciate the challenges of delivering drugs to and through the nail

Case study

Ms TM is a healthy 55 year-old woman who started taking simvastatin a year ago after dietary changes alone failed to reduce her elevated blood cholesterol levels. She has responded well to this drug, but the doctor hinted that she might need to start calcium channel blockers (CCBs) if her blood pressure (currently at the top of the normal range) goes up. Anxious to avoid any more regular medicines, Ms TM starts a range of exercise classes

at her local gym. This makes her feel good and after 6 months her weight and blood pressure have both dropped significantly. The only drawback is that wearing trainers tends to give her 'athlete's foot' which affects her toes and the soles of her feet.

One day, Ms TM notices that her right toenail has some creamy white areas with opaque streaks along one side of it. Over the next few months, the streaks start to spread under the top of the nail, which begins to look thicker with a roughened edge. Her toenails also seem to have lost their smoothness, and have fine vertical lines on them.

Ms TM starts to feel self-conscious about her feet and stops her swimming and yoga classes. She also begins to worry, because she has heard that nail changes can be a sign of heart disease. So she eventually makes a GP appointment.

- Which conditions can cause nail changes and what do they look like?

Ms TM's GP says that he is sure that this is just a common fungal nail infection called distal and lateral subungual onychomycosis. The keys to his diagnosis are the colour change in the nail, her history of fungal foot infection, which doesn't look to have cleared up, and the fact that just one nail is affected. If it were something else, he would expect to see symmetrical changes and evidence of skin disease or some other chronic condition.

Ms TM is relieved but says that she would like to get her nail back to normal. The GP sends nail scrapings off for mycology tests.

❓ Do we have to treat this condition with drugs? If so, what are the options?

The test results confirm Trichophyton rubrum infection. Ms TM and the GP discuss possible treatment options and agree that a topical nail varnish is best for her, but she will need to use it twice a week for at least 9 months. Ms TM is horrified at the length of time that this treatment will take.

❓ What reasons might the GP have for not prescribing oral antifungals in this case?
❓ What are the challenges in delivering therapeutic agents to the nail?
❓ Consider how would you explain the risks and benefits of treatment to Ms TM

Case discussion

— Conditions that cause changes to the nail and its appearance

The human nail is a plate of keratinised cells which protects the ends of the fingers and toes, and helps increase sensations of touch. Fingernails grow approximately 1 cm in 3 months; toenails grow three times slower than this.

A normal nail is clear, with the pink nail bed visible under the plate of keratin and a tight seal (the hyponychium) between nail and finger at the top. Most fungal nail infections (onychomycosis) are caused by dermatophytes with *Trichophyton rubrum* and *Trichophyton mentagrophytes* var. *interdigitale* being the most common. Yeasts such as *Candida* sp. are rarer causes, and more likely to infect nails on the hands.

The most common type of infection (distal and lateral subungual onychomycosis or DLSO) starts at the side edge of this junction, in the nail bed, then spreads to the nail itself, producing creamy opaque areas. There is nearly always evidence of coexisting fungal infection of the foot (tinea pedis). White crumbly patches on the nail itself may indicate the less common condition – superficial white onychomycosis. Infection starting at the

bottom of the nail is uncommon and would be a sign of intercurrent disease (an intervening disease during the course of another disease).

DLSO is most common in the big toe (often on the dominant side), because this nail has the largest surface area and is also most vulnerable to injury. As the infection progresses, the nail becomes misshapen and lumpy (subungual hyperkeratosis). The end of the nail lifts up, and the free edge erodes (distal onycholysis).

Changes to the shape and surface of nails can also be signs of skin disease (eczema, psoriasis), other autoimmune conditions or circulation problems, but changes are much more likely to be symmetrical and also to be visible on the hands. The same applies to nail colour changes from non-fungal causes, e.g. bacterial infection, liver disease and, rarely, chronic lung conditions. Iron deficiency can produce thin, curved, 'spoon-shaped' nails (koilonychia). 'Clubbing' of the fingertips, a well-known sign of heart disease and COPD (chronic obstructive pulmonary disease), will tend to curve the nails in the opposite direction.

Vertical 'wrinkling' on fingers and toenails is usually a normal part of ageing, when the nail may also thicken (onychogryphosis), although the appearance of pigmented streaks on just one nail would need investigation to rule out subungual melanoma. By contrast, any horizontal grooves or ridges (Beau's lines) or colour bands usually signal systemic disease or, possibly, exposure to toxins (e.g. after chemotherapy or from arsenic).

— Treatment options

A fungal nail infection is a relatively minor problem in a healthy person, but one that is unlikely to resolve on its own. Not treating this common condition therefore has public health implications. The psychological distress caused by ugly nails may mean people avoid certain activities, and progressive physical changes in the nail could lead to more serious foot problems in later life.

The aim of treatment is to eradicate the fungal organism from the nail plate and nail bed, but this can take several months. Surgical removal of the nail (avulsion) and subsequent topical treatment can work faster but requires surgery and carries the risk that the nail won't grow back normally.

Three systemic (oral) antifungal drugs – griseofulvin, itraconazole and terbinafine – are all licensed for onychomycosis. All need to be taken

terbinafine

griseofulvin

itraconazole

for at least 3 months and none is suitable for people actively planning a family, due to possible teratogenic effects on the fetus. The oldest drug, griseofulvin (derived from the mould *Penicillium griseofulvum*), is probably the safest, but also the least effective; it is not active topically. It gets incorporated into keratin and can then inhibit fungal cell division through tubulin binding and mitotic spindle function interference. Itraconazole is a synthetic triazole compound, with a broader antifungal spectrum, but both it and its major metabolite are potent inhibitors of the CYP3A4 drug-metabolising enzyme; therefore possible interactions with other medications need to be considered. Its use is also not advised in patients with heart disease or at increased risk of developing heart failure. It inhibits fungal ergosterol biosynthesis, thus interfering with normal membrane function and ultimately leading to fungal cell death. Long-term use also carries a risk of hepatotoxicity.

Terbinafine is a synthetic allylamine antifungal that is probably the most effective for dermatophyte infections, and possibly the safest in terms of clinically significant drug interactions, although it isn't suitable for everyone. However, its efficacy can be markedly reduced by potent enzyme inducers, and it may also interfere with other drugs metabolised via CYP2D6. Terbinafine also inhibits fungal ergosterol biosynthesis, but

through inhibition of the enzyme squalene epoxidase, involved in the synthesis of the fungal cell membrane. Due to the drug's very high lipophilicity, it distributes effectively into the nail bed and the nail itself, making it a good choice for nail-borne fungal infections. It can be taken orally or as a cream or powder for treating superficial skin infections.

In terms of tolerability: headache, GI disturbances and skin rashes are all listed as 'common' adverse effects for both itraconazole and terbinafine. Muscle (myalgia) and joint (arthralgia) pain are 'very common' with terbinafine.

The toenail cure rate with oral antifungals is said to be 70–80% (higher for fingernails), although there is little comparative evidence for the drugs used in the UK. Topical antifungal treatment is claimed to have a much lower and more variable success rate, but there have been very few studies on toenail infection. Only two topical antifungal nail formulations are currently available in the UK.

— The structure of the nail and topical drug delivery

Getting drugs into/across the nail (ungual or transungual drug delivery) poses a greater formulation challenge than drug delivery to the skin – itself a challenge! Nails comprise three structures: the outermost nail plate, the underlying nail bed and the nail matrix. The nail plate comprises approximately 25 layers of tightly bound, dead keratinised cells; it is up to 0.6 mm thick on the fingers and up to 1.3 mm thick on the toes. There are three main layers in the nail plate: the outer and inner ones are thin and made of softer skin-like cells, whereas the middle layer is arranged in harder hair-like filaments held together by sulfur-containing proteins. It contains a fair amount of water and is thought to behave like a hydrogel with the aqueous route playing the main role in drug penetration. The shape and curvature of the nail, and its permeability to water, vary greatly from person to person. The nail plate provides a formidable barrier to drug delivery. Hydrating the nail (or blocking normal outward diffusion of water) can increase permeability, as can filing the nail surface. Penetration enhancers can be included in formulations, such as solvents or compounds that break down keratin (e.g. urea and salicylic acid).

The two topical formulations currently licensed for fungal nail infections are Loceryl nail lacquer and Trosyl solution. Loceryl contains the morpholine antifungal amorolfine in an organic solution of an acrylic polymer. On loss of solvent, the polymer forms a film, which reduces transungual water loss and retains the drug on the nail plate, and from which drug diffuses to reach the nail bed. Trosyl solution contains the imidazole antifungal tioconazole and undecylenic acid (a natural fatty acid fungicide) in the organic solvent, ethyl acetate.

A fair amount of evidence exists for topical treatment of dermatophyte infections of the foot (topical terbinafine is probably the most effective choice). However, the evidence for drugs used to treat fungal nail infections in the UK is much weaker, and topical nail products have not yet been compared 'head to head' in a clinical trial.

EXTENDED LEARNING

- What is 'athlete's foot' and how do people self-treat it?
- What do the terms 'common' and 'very common' mean when considering manufacturer's information on drug side effects?
- What can Ms TM do to maximise the chances of successful treatment?
- What are the different classes and mechanisms of action of antifungal agents?
- Outline the role of cytochrome P450 in the metabolism of drugs and its role in drug interactions
- Describe the approaches to the formulation of therapeutic nail lacquers

References and further reading

Buxton OK, Mims-Jones R (2009). *ABC of Dermatology*, 5th edn. London; BMJ Books.

Crawford F, Hollis S (2007). Topical treatments for fungal infection of the skin and nails of the foot. *Cochrane Database Syst Rev* 3:CD001434.

Elkeeb R, AliKhan A, Elkeeb L, Hui X, Maibach HI (2010). Transungual drug delivery: current status. *Int J Pharmaceutics* 384:1–8.

Murdan S (2002). Drug delivery to the nail following topical application. *Int J Pharmaceutics* 236:1–26.

Murthy SN, Maibach H, eds (2012). *Topical Nail Products and Ungual Drug Delivery*. Boca Raton, FL: CRC Press.

Case 7
Treatment of head lice
LOUISE COGAN

Case study

Mrs B brings her 4-year-old daughter, Chloe, into your pharmacy. She tells you that a letter has gone round Chloe's pre-school, telling parents that some children have got head lice, and she is worried that Chloe may have nits. She wants you to help.

- What is the difference between head lice and nits?
- What symptoms may indicate that a head lice infestation is present?
- How would a diagnosis of head lice be confirmed?

After looking at Chloe's hair and asking questions about her symptoms, you are able to confirm that Chloe does indeed have head lice. Mrs B is horrified, because she washes Chloe's hair every night, and can't understand how she has got them.

- What are the common myths/beliefs about head lice infestation?
- Discuss how head lice are transmitted. What steps can Mrs B take to reduce transmission of head lice to other members of the family?

You discuss treatment options with Mrs B. You check if Chloe takes any other medication or has any medical conditions. You recommend an appropriate treatment for head lice eradication.

- What treatment options are available over the counter?
- How do the drugs differ in their mode of action?
- Are there any cautions or contraindications that you need to consider?
- What benefits do the different dosage forms offer?

Mrs B thanks you for your advice, but is still not happy that Chloe has got head lice, and is worried that the product won't work. She also isn't entirely happy with the thought of Chloe using chemicals on her hair. Furthermore, she is concerned that she will have to keep Chloe off pre-school until the head lice have gone.

- What lifestyle and counselling advice can you give Mrs B to ensure that she uses the product most effectively?
- Are there any 'natural' products available that have been shown to be effective?

Case discussion

— Head lice infestation

Head lice are wingless parasitic insects (*Pediculus humanus capitis*) that can be transmitted only via head-to-head contact and, despite some long-held beliefs, they cannot jump or fly between heads. They are more prevalent in children of primary school age, and girls tend to be affected more than boys because they often play closer together. Lice can infest regardless of the length of hair or its cleanliness, or standards of personal hygiene. Lice are unlikely to be transmitted by sharing hair combs, hair brushes, towels or clothes because they cannot survive more than 12 hours away from a host.

The female louse lays eggs at the base of the hair shaft at night. These eggs attach to the scalp hair, and hatch about a week later. An adult louse can live for up to a month feeding on blood from the host. Unlike the body louse (*Pediculus humanus humanus*), the head louse is not known to carry any infectious diseases, so is not considered a health-risk as such. They do not burrow into the skin. Once the eggs have hatched, the empty egg case remains attached to the hair, and it is these empty egg cases that are referred to as 'nits'.

— Signs and symptoms of infestation

One of the first signs of head lice infestation is an itchy scalp, but is not necessarily experienced by all those who have head lice. Itching is the result of an allergic reaction to the saliva of the lice that is injected into the scalp during feeding. Other signs that head lice may be present include white eggs stuck to hair roots or small bite marks on the scalp and/or the back of the neck.

— Diagnosis

A firm diagnosis can be made only once live lice have been seen. This can be done by wet combing, which aims to remove the lice and eggs from the person's head and hair.

Treatment options

— Wet combing

Wet combing with a fine-tooth comb and conditioner can be used as a first-line method for removal of lice and eggs. To wet comb, hair must be washed and plenty of conditioner applied to make it slippery. The wet and conditioned hair is sectioned from the scalp and a fine-tooth comb (designed for the purpose) is slowly dragged from the hair root to the end. A systematic approach, combing out a small amount with each stroke, is essential for successful eradication. After each stroke, the comb is wiped on a tissue to check for the presence of lice or eggs. The process should take approximately 30 min. Wet combing should be continued for 2 weeks, repeated after 5, 9 and 13 days, until no lice are found on three consecutive sessions (to match the lifecycle of lice: eggs hatch after 7 days).

Products available over-the-counter

There are several treatment options available, which can be categorised as traditional insecticides, non-traditional insecticides and wet combing ('bug busting').

— Insecticides: structure and properties

The main insecticides available OTC include malathion and permethrin.

Permethrin is a synthetic pyrethroid derivative based on the structure of the pyrethrins, natural product insecticides extracted from chrysanthemum flowers. Permethrin is a neurotoxin that binds to, and prolongs the opening time of, nerve membrane sodium channels, thereby interfering with insect nerve conduction (hyperexcitability). The drug is only of low toxicity to most mammals because it is rapidly metabolised if absorbed into the systemic circulation. Permethrin is suitable for children aged >6 months, and for children and people who have asthma. It is applied to towel-dried hair after washing, left in place for 10 minutes, and then rinsed off. The hair is then wet combed. Side effects include itching and stinging sensations.

permethrin

Malathion is an organophosphate acetylcholinesterase inhibitor. In insects, malathion is bioactivated to a toxic phosphorothioate (in which the P=S group is replaced by P=O) metabolite called malaoxon. Selective toxicity in insects is possible because malathion is poorly absorbed transdermally in humans and any drug that reaches the systemic circulation is rapidly hydrolysed by plasma esterases to form rapidly excreted metabolites. This hydrolysis does not occur in insects. Malathion is also suitable for children aged >6 months and people with asthma. It is applied to dry hair and left for 12 hours to dry naturally, then rinsed off as normal. The hair is then wet combed. Side effects include skin irritation. Hair driers should not be used to speed up the drying process because the chemical is inactivated by heat.

malathion

Treatment with pesticides should be recommended only if live lice are found. Two treatments of pesticides should be conducted 7 days apart.

— **Non-traditional insecticides**

The main non-traditional pesticide is dimeticone, which is suitable for children aged >6 months and those with asthma or eczema.

Dimeticone is a polydimethylsiloxane $(CH_3)_3SiO[SiO(CH_3)_2]_nSi(CH_3)_3$. Silicone-based products immediately immobilise lice and their lethality has been related to disrupting the organism's ability to manage its water balance. Dimeticone is applied to the hair, left in place for 8 hours and then rinsed off. Dimeticone has a good safety profile but it can cause an itchy, flaky scalp.

Other similarly acting non-traditional pesticides include cyclomethicone (decamethylcyclopentasiloxane) and isopropyl myristate $(CH_3(CH_2)_{12}CO_2CH(CH_3)_2)$, which are suitable for children aged >2 years and for those with asthma or eczema. It is applied to dry hair and left for 10 min. Then the hair is combed through using a fine-tooth comb and washed out with a non-conditioning shampoo.

A newer, non-traditional pesticide also available is Activdiol (1,2-octanediol). It is a non-oily formula that is applied to the hair and left to dry. It can be left on the hair during the day or overnight with no need for combing, and is then rinsed out when convenient. According to the manufacturer, the compound works by stripping away the louse's waxy cuticle, causing it to dehydrate. This has the same mechanism of action as seen with other lipophilic derivatives containing long alkyl chains (such as isopropyl myristate, above).

A common alternative treatment that is sometimes used for head lice is tea tree oil. However, there is no scientific evidence (including from recent studies) that it is effective.

— **Product selection**

When recommending treatment, pharmacists must consider an appropriate formulation: lotions are preferred for head lice because of the long contact time advised. Lotions are low-to-medium viscosity topical formulations, which may be solutions, suspensions or emulsions. Cream rinses and shampoos are water based and tend not to be as effective as lotions because they are diluted by water in use. Therefore, the concentration of pesticide is lower and they have a short contact time. Alcohol-based products are not recommended for broken skin, or for people with eczema or asthma. Pregnant women are advised only to use dimeticone or wet combing.

— **When to refer patients to another healthcare professional**

Head lice infestation is a minor condition but, if left untreated, it can cause severe itching and scratching, sometimes resulting in a secondary bacterial infection, such as impetigo.

As diagnosis can only be confirmed once live lice have been seen, and an itching scalp could indicate other conditions such as dandruff or seborrhoeic dermatitis, then these should also be considered as possible causes of the itching.

EXTENDED LEARNING

- What is impetigo and how is it treated?
- Should children with head lice be kept away from school until the head lice have all gone?
- What do we mean by the term 'viscosity'? How is viscosity measured, and why may it be an important property of pharmaceutical liquids and semisolids?

References and further reading

Barnett E, Palma KG, Clayton B, Ballard T (2012). Effectiveness of isopropyl myristate/cyclomethicone D5 solution of removing cuticular hydrocarbons from human head lice (*Pediculus humanus capitis*). *BMC Dermatol* **12**:15.

Joint Formulary Committee, British Medical Association and Royal Pharmaceutical Society (2013). *British National Formulary 65*. London: Pharmaceutical Press.

Mistry R (2011). Heads up on head lice – how parents can keep their children's head clear. *Pharmaceut J* **286**:198.

Rutter P (2009). *Community Pharmacy – Symptom, diagnosis and treatment*, 2nd edn. London: Churchill Livingstone Elsevier.

Special cases

INTRODUCTION

This section comprises six individual and diverse cases. The cases focus on paediatric pharmacokinetics, falls in elderly people, benign prostatic hyperplasia (BPH), pain management in palliative care, human papillomavirus (HPV) immunisation and the use of black cohosh for menopausal symptoms.

Case 1
Paediatric pharmacokinetics in a newborn preterm infant ▶ 385

This case features a 26-week gestational male neonate, weighing 750 g. The important physiological changes that occur after birth and how they may affect treatment choices are described. The different pharmacokinetics of neonates and children are identified and the ways in which medicine use is influenced by these parameters are explored. The nutritional requirements of neonates, including parenteral nutrition, are outlined. An 'apnoeic attack' is defined and its treatment with methylxanthines described. The case concludes by highlighting the differences that may present in neonates, children and adults when managing some symptoms and conditions.

Case 2
Falls and care of elderly people ▶ 389

This case considers an elderly woman who is admitted to hospital due to shortness of breath and chest pain, and a history of multiple falls in the past year. The common risk factors that contribute to falls are reviewed, particularly focusing on examples of medication. The mechanism of action of anticoagulants, the types of condition where anticoagulant therapy may be

advocated and the probable side effects are outlined. Treatment of osteoporosis is presented. The case concludes with a description of good prescribing practice in older people.

Case 3
Treating a patient with benign prostatic hyperplasia ▶ 396

This case concerns a male patient who has symptoms associated with BPH, and who the pharmacist believes would be a good candidate to try over-the-counter (OTC) tamsulosin. The signs and symptoms of BPH are outlined and the treatment options (e.g. α-blockers and the 5α-reductase inhibitors) described. The chemistry and mechanism of action of tamsulosin and finasteride are detailed. The circumstances when BPH can be managed 'over the counter' are explained.

Case 4
Pain management using strong opiates in palliative care ▶ 399

This case considers a woman with advanced metastatic breast cancer whose pain is no longer controlled on her current medication. The core questions for assessment of pain in palliative care are outlined. The principles of titrating oral opiate doses and converting between different routes and preparations are described. The principles with regard to opiates and addiction in palliative care are explored. The use of anticipatory medicines at the end of life, including drug choices and appropriate doses are examined.

Case 5
Human papillomavirus and cervical cancer ▶ 404

This case focuses on a parent seeking advice from the pharmacist about the need for her 12-year-old daughter to receive the HPV immunisation at school. The different types of human papillomavirus (HPV), their mode of transmutation and the resultant infections are described. The link between HPV immunisation and cervical cancer is outlined. The HPV immunisation programme in the UK, including the targeted age group and consent, available vaccines, their possible side effects and the national implementation are summarised. Finally, the rationale for cervical screening and its place after implementation of the national HPV programme is explained.

Case 6
Black cohosh for menopausal symptoms ▶ 406

This focuses on a woman who asks the pharmacist for information about the safety and any possible risks to her health from taking a product containing the herb black cohosh to alleviate her menopausal symptoms. The regulation of herbal medicines is explained. The issues involved in the controversy over the safety of the common herbal medicine black cohosh are described. The place of systematic reviews as a source of research evidence is discussed. Ways in which 'traditional' medicines and 'western' approaches may coexist are also discussed.

Case 1
Paediatric pharmacokinetics in a newborn preterm infant
STEPHEN TOMLIN

LEARNING OUTCOMES

At the end of this case you will be able to:

- Outline important physiological changes after birth and how they may affect treatment choices
- Identify ways in which use of medicines is influenced by the different pharmacokinetics of neonates and children
- Outline the nutritional requirements of neonates, including parenteral nutrition
- Outline what is meant by an apnoeic attack and describe its treatment with methylxanthines
- Explain how metabolic pathways of some analgesics differ in neonates and the implications for their use

Case study

— Day 1

Baby ST is a 26-week gestational male neonate who is born on the labour ward (weight = 750 g). The baby was born by emergency caesarean section after the mother had a hypertensive crisis. Baby ST is tachypnoeic (rapid breathing) and cyanotic (bluish skin due to inadequate blood oxygenation), and needs to be mechanically ventilated. Respiratory distress syndrome (RDS) is diagnosed.

- Describe how preterm this baby is and the likely initial problems from being born prematurely
- What would you expect to see on the drug chart in the first hour of life? (Give reasons and discuss dosing)

Baby ST is stabilised and sent to the NICU (neonatal intensive care unit). Later on that day, an intravenous long line is introduced and total parenteral nutrition (TPN) commenced.

- Why would TPN be started so quickly?
- Describe the main requirements of TPN compared with an adult and the fluid volumes that would be required for its delivery

— Days 2 and 3

Mechanical ventilation and TPN continue.

— Day 4

Baby ST is gradually being weaned off the ventilator and it is decided to start therapy to prevent apnoeic attacks. The plasma bilirubin levels are now high at >200 μmol/L indicating neonatal jaundice. Unfortunately, the TPN has had a small extravasation (fluid leakage around the infusion site) and the area around the line looks inflamed and painful. It is decided that pain control and topical steroids may be useful.

- What is an apnoeic attack and what medicine can be used to prevent it?
- Describe, based on pharmacokinetic and dynamic properties, why this is a unique medicine for babies
- What is the significance and probable reasons for the raised bilirubin and how might it be treated?
- Explain why extravasation in newborns is a common problem and discuss the issues associated with the choice of topical treatment and possible pain control

Case discussion

There are some significant differences for neonates, children and adults that can have profound consequences with respect to drug handling. These variations, in both pharmacokinetics and pharmacodynamics, are most acute in infancy and especially in neonates and preterm babies. Once a child is aged >3 years, there are fewer significant kinetic and dynamic differences between children and adults.

It is fairly easy to understand the main problems of prematurity if you consider that the baby is still supposed to be inside the mother. Importantly, the lungs and gastrointestinal (GI) tract are not employed *in utero* and after early delivery they are not ready to function adequately. The most important issue at birth is the ability to breathe, but with lung (pulmonary) surfactant only being produced by a baby from about 30 weeks' gestational age, a preterm baby (especially <30 weeks' gestation) will struggle to maintain lung function.

— **What would you expect to see on the drug chart in the first hour of life?**

There are three types of medicine that you would expect to see just post-birth on a drug chart for a baby of this age:

- Pulmonary surfactant
- Antibiotics
- Vitamin K.

The need for surfactant to be delivered into the lungs as soon after birth as possible is critical to support breathing. It is a simple replacement of fluid (pulmonary surfactant) that the baby is not yet making for him- or herself at this stage. Pulmonary surfactant comprises phospholipids, particularly dipalmitoyl phosphatidylcholine, and other minor components, including proteins and cholesterol. It modulates surface tension at the alveolar air/tissue interface, allowing inflation of the wet surface of the airways. Replacement surfactant is provided by an endotracheal tube.

Antibiotics are given to most preterm babies immediately after birth and continued for 48 h to prevent infection. These provide cover for streptococci and Gram-negative bacteria (*Escherichia coli*). The dosing of these medicines illustrates some important differences in drug handling by neonates.

i.v. benzylpenicillin 50 mg/kg twice daily
i.v. gentamicin 5 mg/kg 36-hourly

The doses per kilogram differ from those for adults for a number of reasons. At birth, the neonate has a relatively poor immunity to infection and so the chances of developing severe bacteraemia are high. Also, at birth, approximately 85% of the neonate's body mass is water (compared with approximately 60% for adults). Thus, for drugs distributed in body water, a larger dose per kilogram will be required to achieve a similar concentration.

As renal function is relatively undeveloped, many of these drugs will be less rapidly cleared, therefore dosing is less frequent. However, renal function does increase quickly after birth and, by the age of 1 month, a four times daily dose of penicillin may be administered.

The gentamicin dose may appear low compared with what is usual for adults and older children (commonly 6–8 mg/kg). This lower dose is to avoid toxicity from accumulation.

The antibiotics are given intravenously because of the need to cover severe infection quickly, but also because the GI tract is not absorbing well at this age. In addition, in the first few months of life the gastric contents are of comparatively low acidity (higher pH). This can affect the absorption of orally administered drugs. For acidic drugs such as the penicillins, the higher pH will mean that a greater proportion of the drug is in the deprotonated, ionised form – both in the stomach and at the site of absorption, the small intestine. The absorption of weak acids and bases is highly influenced by the pH at the site of absorption and the lipid solubility of the unionised drug. Diffusion through the lipid membrane is generally limited to small, unionised (and so low polarity) drugs. The pH of the gastric contents can also influence the stability of an orally administered drug. Many penicillins demonstrate poor chemical stability at low pH and, in adults, are best administered before food or on an empty stomach, when the gastric pH is higher

The proportion of an acidic or basic drug that is ionised or unionised at a particular pH can be calculated using the Henderson–Hasselbalch equation, given knowledge of the pK_a value(s) of the acidic or basic functional group(s). Despite being predominantly ionised at a particular pH, many drugs are still effectively absorbed after oral administration. The small proportion of unionised drug present gets absorbed and the acid dissociation equilibrium adjusts itself so that more unionised drug is produced (the ratio of unionised and ionised drug concentrations remains constant). This continuous mechanism, referred to as the pH partition hypothesis, can result in the absorption of substantial amounts of the drug from the GI tract.

Vitamin K is given to all babies at birth (including those born at term) to prevent haemorrhagic disease of the newborn. An interesting point is that it is administered to premature babies as an intramuscular (i.m.) injection. Intramuscular injection is generally avoided in young children because their muscle mass is low and thus it is very painful, and also in the sick newborn infant the muscles are poorly perfused and inactive. Thus, it is a poor route of administration for most drugs. However, the one dose of vitamin K distributes out of the muscle very slowly over the next few weeks making it ideal in this instance, because cover is required for this period of time.

— TPN for the preterm infant

Before delivery, a foetus is receiving constant nutrition from the mother; a preterm neonate will not have built up sufficient of its own energy stores to meet his or her requirements. At birth, this maternal source of nutrients will abruptly come to an end, and blood glucose levels can fall to a critical level very quickly. Although administration of intravenous glucose may provide an energy source, within a couple of days there will be a deterioration in the condition of the neonate as the nitrogen pool and essential fatty acids (used in most enzyme processes) are depleted. It is essential therefore to start full nutrition in the first day or two of life. However, because of undeveloped renal and hepatic function at this time, the nutrition has to be closely matched to actual requirements, as neither deficiencies nor over-supply will be tolerated well by the premature infant.

Parenteral nutrition (PN) involves the infusion of nutrient fluids via a peripherally inserted long line into a large vein. This has obvious risks and is considered only when enteral nutrition (nutrient fluids by nasogastric tube) is not possible. When the nutrient fluid comprises amino acids, glucose, electrolytes, trace elements, essential vitamins and a concentrated energy source (e.g. a lipid emulsion) then it is termed 'total parenteral nutrition'. Pharmacists are directly responsible for the preparation and formulation of these fluids (under strict aseptic conditions) in addition to providing comprehensive medical information for physicians.

To support life and promote rapid growth, the carbohydrate and nitrogen supply for a neonate has to be substantial. Whereas an adult may require about 40 kcal/kg per day, a preterm infant will require about 100 kcal/kg per day. Thus an intravenous glucose infusion of at least 10% as a normal fluid may be indicated. The volumes of PN, on a per kilogram basis, are also relatively large. For the first 4 days of life the newborn infant will need 60, 90, 120 and 150 mL/kg per day, respectively. This low start and fast increase in fluid requirement is partly explained by the rapid rise in renal function after birth. The neonate then remains on 150 mL/kg per day for the first month or so of life. If an adult of 70 kg

were to receive this level of fluid they would be receiving 10 L a day instead of the required 2–3 L. At the age of 1 year, a baby would require about a litre (approximately half of an adult requirement).

— Apnoea and its management

An apnoeic attack is defined as a cessation of breathing for at least 15 seconds. The easiest explanation of neonatal apnoea is that the preterm neonate just 'forgets' to breathe; the neonate should still be *in utero* and therefore not required to breathe for him- or herself. However, the fact that the apnoeic episodes generally resolve with maturation suggests that it may relate to inadequate myelination of brain-stem axons involved in the breathing reflex. A mild central respiratory stimulant (e.g. in the form a methylxanthine, such as theophylline or caffeine) may be expected to be effective therapy in this case. Caffeine is preferred to theophylline in treating apnoea and its consequences in neonates, because it is less toxic (having a wider therapeutic range) and has a longer half-life in the newborn, enabling once daily dosing. The half-life decreases over the first month of life as the liver matures rapidly; twice daily dosing may be required by a 4–6 week old if apnoea is still a problem.

— Pharmacokinetic and pharmacodynamic properties of theophylline in neonates

Interestingly, theophylline is largely converted to caffeine by the liver in premature newborns, but, due to immaturity of the newborn liver CYP cytochrome system, the relative rates of conversion may be unpredictable. The exact mechanism by which the methylxanthines stabilise neonatal respiration is not entirely understood, but may well involve antagonistic effects exerted on central adenosine A_1 (and particularly A_{2A}-type) receptors present on central γ-aminobutyric acid (GABA)-ergic inhibitory interneurons involved in the medullary respiratory circuit. This case also indicates how extrapolation of drug pharmacokinetic parameters from adults to neonates could be potentially dangerous, increasing the risk of toxic side effects. It is therefore important to be aware that very young children may, or may not, metabolise drugs in the same way as older children and adults.

— Raised bilirubin in neonates and its management

It is not uncommon for a baby at term to have a raised bilirubin level (and therefore appear jaundiced) in the first few days after birth. This becomes more significant the more preterm the baby is at birth. At birth, fetal haemoglobin is destroyed and replaced by the baby's own red blood cells. This destruction leads to high levels of bilirubin, which the very immature liver cannot deal with. Protein binding is also significantly reduced in neonates, leading to a lot of free bilirubin. A further complication can arise in that, as the blood–brain barrier is not fully formed, bilirubin may cross this barrier and cause a potentially fatal disease called kernicterus.

Phototherapy exposure to narrow-spectrum blue fluorescent tube light (wavelength 460–490 nm) or more recently, from equivalent light-emitting diode (LED) devices, may be used to help detoxify the bilirubin and convert it to a more water-soluble form excreted in the bile, allowing blood levels to decrease more quickly. This photoexposure is not as effective in adults with jaundice, because the skin is thicker.

— Extravasation in neonates: topical treatment and pain control

Similar to the skin, the blood vessels of newborns are very thin and fragile. Thus, they are prone to extravasation (blood/fluid leakage into surrounding tissues). Inflammation of the skin (whether due to extravasation or nappy rash) may benefit from the application of a steroid cream. But, although this may be helpful for a short-term problem, prolonged use can be dangerous; absorption through the very thin neonatal skin is high. A 1-week course of regular use of a medium strength corticosteroid cream has led to development of cushingoid symptoms in a neonate. Any topical application of steroids should therefore be minimal and with caution.

— Pain management in neonates: drug handling and analgesics

Pain control in neonates is still relatively poorly understood and therefore difficult to put into practice. Some common analgesics demonstrate important variation in kinetics and metabolism. Paracetamol is the most commonly used analgesic in children, but for many years was not given to neonates.

Paracetamol metabolism in the liver includes glucuronidation. Glucuronidation is the last hepatic pathway to develop in the neonate. This process is very poor in a week-old preterm baby, but is reasonably well developed in a 1-month old

term baby. However, paracetamol is now used in all neonates and babies. This is because it has been found that a neonate will sulfonate the paracetamol instead. In each case, metabolism produces a much more polar metabolite (glucuronide or sulfate), which is more readily eliminated in the urine. This further illustrates the difficulties in predicting drug handling and effects in the newborn. Paracetamol is available as an oral suspension for pain relief in children, and also as suppositories for rectal administration.

paracetamol

Morphine is also commonly used for pain control for children. This has two main glucuronide metabolites (morphine-3-glucuronide [M3G] and morphine-6-glucuronide [M6G]), one of which (M6G) is associated with higher levels of respiratory depression. As neonates (unlike older children) produce more of this metabolite, they are more prone to respiratory depression. The impact can be enhanced by the fact that the drug will also more readily pass through the immature blood–brain barrier.

EXTENDED LEARNING

- Understand the Henderson–Hasselbalch equations and pH partition theory of drug absorption

- How are parenteral nutrition fluids formulated, prepared and administered?
- How are suppositories formulated and manufactured? What advantages does the rectal route offer over alternative routes of drug administration?

References and further reading

Fluhr JW, Pfistere S, Gloor M (2000). Direct comparison of skin physiology in children and adults with bioengineering methods. *Pediatr Dermatol* 17:436–9.

Henderson-Smart DJ, De Paoli AG (2010). Methylxanthine treatment for apnoea in preterm infants. *Cochrane Database Syst Rev* 12:CD000140.

Heinmann G (1980). Enteral absorption and bioavailability in children in relation to age. *Eur J Clin Pharmacol* 18:43–50.

Mathew OP (2011). Apnea of prematurity: pathogenesis and management strategies. *J Perinatol* 31:302–10.

Mohammadizadeh M, Eliadarani FK, Badiei Z (2012). Is the light-emitting diode a better light source than fluorescent tube for phototherapy of neonatal jaundice in preterm infants? *Adv Biomed Res* 1:51.

Morselli PL, Franco-Morselli R, Bossi L (1980). Clinical pharmacokinetics in newborns and infants, age related differences and therapeutic implications. *Clin Pharmacokinet* 5:485–527.

Ritschel WA, Kearns GL (1999). Paediatric pharmacokinetics. In: *Handbook of Basic Phamacokinetics*, 5th edn. Washington DC: American Pharmaceutical Association, 304–21.

Weiss CF, Glazko AJ, Weston JK (1960). Chloramphenicol in the newborn infant: a physiological explanation of its toxicity when given in excessive doses. *N Engl J Med* 262:787–94.

West DP, Worobec S, Solomon LM (1981). Pharmacology and toxicology if infant skin. *J Invest Dermatol* 76:147–50.

Case 2
Falls and care of elderly people

ANA ARMSTRONG

LEARNING OUTCOMES

At the end of this case, you will be able to:

- Describe the common risk factors that can contribute to a fall
- Give examples of medications that can contribute to falls
- Outline the mechanism of action of anticoagulants, the types of condition in which anticoagulant therapy may be advocated and the probable side effects
- Give examples of the types of medications that may be used to treat osteoporosis
- Describe good prescribing practice in older people

Case study

Mrs JB is a frail 83-year-old white woman. She has been experiencing increased shortness of breath and chest pain for the past week. She lives alone and is independent in her daily activities. She is admitted to your medicine for the elderly ward for further investigation.

CASE NOTES

Presenting complaint
- Shortness of breath and chest pain

Past medical history
- Multiple falls in the last year, hypertension, atrial fibrillation, stroke, diabetes, glaucoma

Drug history
- Digoxin 250 micrograms daily
- Bendroflumethiazide 2.5 mg daily
- Ramipril 7.5 mg daily
- Atenolol 50 mg daily
- Simvastatin 40 mg at night
- Aspirin 75 mg daily
- Dipyridamole MR 200 mg twice a day
- Lansoprazole 30 mg daily
- NovoMix 30 (biphasic insulin) 30 units in the morning and 10 units in the evening
- Temazepam 10 mg at night as required
- Levobunolol 0.5% eyedrops 1 drop into both eyes twice a day
- Latanoprost eyedrops 1 drop into both eyes at night

> **On examination**
> - Blood pressure: 98/76 mmHg
> - Pulse: 54 beats/min
> - Apyrexial

Diagnosis
- *Bilateral pulmonary embolism*
- *Recent falls*
- *Hypotension and bradycardia, possibly secondary to medication*

After some consideration, the junior doctor has decided to start Mrs JB on warfarin for her pulmonary embolism. The junior doctor also decides to refer Mrs JB to the local falls service.

- ❓ Outline the types of condition where warfarin anticoagulant therapy may be advocated
- ❓ Outline the mechanism of warfarin's anticoagulant effects
- ❓ Draw the structure of warfarin and explain the importance of acidity and stereochemistry to its clinical use
- ❓ What is the mechanism of interaction of warfarin with aspirin?
- ❓ What is the link between warfarin plasma binding and gastric bleeding risk?
- ❓ Outline the main counselling points for warfarin
- ❓ What factors might have contributed to Mrs JB's falls?
- ❓ Of the medication that Mrs JB is taking, list the ones that could have contributed to her falls. Explain how these medications could increase Mrs JB's risk of falls
- ❓ On attending the falls clinic, what medication might you expect Mrs JB to be started on to protect her bones?

The junior doctor is worried about Mrs JB's hypotension and bradycardia, and suspects that some of her medication might be responsible. He asks you to review all of Mrs JB's medication, with a view to improving her blood pressure and pulse rate, and optimising her prescription.

- ❓ Outline the questions that you would consider when reviewing a prescription for an elderly person

Mrs JB is now medically fit to be discharged back home, but, when you counsel her on her discharge medication, she confesses to you that she gets easily muddled with all her medication and has been struggling to take her medicines as prescribed.

- ❓ What is adherence? How can adherence be improved in elderly people?

Case discussion

— Falls in elderly people

Every year more than 400 000 older people in England will attend accident and emergency departments (A&Es) after a fall. Falls are a major cause of disability and the leading cause of mortality due to injury in people aged >75 in the UK. Many falls do not cause a serious injury. However, the consequences for an individual can be wide reaching, and can include:

- Loss of mobility leading to social isolation and depression
- Increase in dependency and disability
- Psychological problems, e.g. fear of falling and loss of confidence in being able to move about safely.

Standard 6 of the National Service Framework for Older People aims to reduce the number of falls that result in serious injury and to ensure effective treatment and rehabilitation for those who have fallen.

It is widely accepted that there is rarely a single specific cause for an elderly patient to fall, with, more often than not, more than one contributory factor. It is for this reason that the National Institute for Health and Care Excellence (NICE, 2013) published the clinical guideline *Falls: Assessment and prevention of falls in older people*. This advocates the use of a multifactorial falls risk assessment and multifactorial interventions as part of a specialist falls service.

NICE recommends that the multifactorial assessment may include the following:

- Identification of falls' history
- Assessment of gait, balance and mobility, and muscle weakness
- Assessment of osteoporosis risk
- Assessment of the older person's perceived functional ability and fear of falling
- Assessment of visual impairment
- Assessment of cognitive impairment and neurological examination
- Assessment of urinary incontinence
- Assessment of home hazards

- Cardiovascular examination and medication review.

NICE also states that, if a multifactorial intervention programme is to be successful, it should include the following components:

- Strength and balance training
- Home hazard assessment and intervention
- Vision assessment and referral
- Medication review with modification/ withdrawal.

— Medications that can contribute to a fall

Although NICE advocates a medication review when a patient has a fall, the only class of medication that has been shown to increase the risk of falling as such is psychotropic medication (i.e. any drug capable of affecting the central nervous system or CNS). Any older person taking psychotropic medication should be reviewed, by a specialist if necessary, with a view to discontinuing the medication if possible. Alcohol can also contribute to falls, and should not be overlooked in elderly people as a potential cause.

Other medication can contribute to falls, so the aim of a medication review is to reduce the risk of falls by eliminating any medication-related causes. Table 11.1 summarises common medications that may be implicated in falls. It is worth noting that the list is not exhaustive, and all medications should be reviewed for their potential to cause falls.

— Conditions in which warfarin therapy may be advocated

Warfarin is a synthetic dicoumarol derivative that is widely used in medicine to inhibit blood clotting, and therefore to reduce the incidence of serious thromboembolic events in patients with coronary heart disease, atrial fibrillation, deep vein thrombosis or for those undergoing major heart surgery, e.g. fitting of artificial replacement valves.

— Outline the mechanism of warfarin's anticoagulant effects

Warfarin decreases blood coagulation by inhibiting the enzyme *vitamin K epoxide reductase*, responsible for recycling oxidised vitamin K_1 to its reduced hydroquinone form (vitamin KH_2), effectively depleting active vitamin K_1, and therefore interfering with the carboxylation and function of the blood coagulation proteins, e.g. prothrombin and factor VII. A major concern with the use of warfarin (a drug that binds strongly to plasma proteins, see below) is its possible interaction with several other commonly prescribed medications, herbal medicines or even certain food products rich in vitamin K_1 (green vegetables such as spinach and broccoli), thereby altering its effectiveness. As a result of potential interactions, leading to an enhanced effect of warfarin, patients should avoid cranberry juice and grapefruit juice. It is also dangerous to binge drink or get drunk while taking warfarin, because this increases the effect of warfarin and consequently the risk of bleeding.

— Warfarin structure, acidity and stereochemistry: implications for clinical use

Warfarin is a weakly acidic molecule because of the hydroxyl (-OH) group, which has a pK_a of 5.1. At a pH <5.1, the hydroxyl group remains protonated, but when the pH is >5.1, the proton dissociates leaving a negative charge on the oxygen atom. As a consequence of this acidity, warfarin can be formulated as the more polar sodium salt, which aids dissolution from tablets and is sufficiently water soluble for formulation as an injection. After oral administration, a significant proportion of a dose of warfarin is in the uncharged (protonated) form at the pH found in the small intestine. This uncharged form is of much lower polarity and is efficiently absorbed from the GI tract. Once absorbed, >99% of a dose of warfarin is in the charged (deprotonated) form.

warfarin

Warfarin is chiral and is manufactured and administered as a racemic mixture of *R*-warfarin and *S*-warfarin. The *S*-enantiomer is largely responsible for the anticoagulant activity. The two enantiomers of warfarin are also metabolised differently because their different shapes result in different abilities to interact with the active sites of drug-metabolising enzymes. The biologically active *S*-warfarin is metabolised primarily by CYP2C9 (cytochrome P450 2C9 isoenzyme), resulting in clinically significant drug–drug interactions with other drugs that can induce or inhibit this isoform.

Common medication that may be implicated in falls

Medication groups	Class and examples
Antiarrhythmics Used to control how the heart beats and help keep its rhythm	Digoxin, amiodarone, flecainide Dizziness and drowsiness are signs of possible digoxin toxicity Flecainide has many drug interactions and can also cause dizziness
Antibiotics Used to treat bacterial infections	Gentamicin, tobramycin, isoniazid Gentamicin and tobramycin may cause vestibular damage if dosed incorrectly. Dose should be determined by renal function and levels should be monitored Isoniazid can cause neuropathy
Antidepressants Used to lift mood (some also for neuropathic pain and to assist sleeping)	**Tricyclic antidepressants (TCAs):** amitriptyline, dosulepin, imipramine and clomipramine **Others:** trazodone, venlafaxine, maprotiline, mirtazepine and MAOIs May cause confusion, drowsiness, blurred vision, constipation, urinary retention and low blood pressure TCAs can also cause cardiac dysrhythmias
Anti-diabetic drugs Used to control blood sugar levels	Glibenclamide, gliclazide, glipizide, tolbutamide, acarbose, metformin and insulins Dizziness can occur due to low blood sugar, but usually avoidable with appropriate dose
Antiepileptics (anticonvulsants) Prevent seizures in people with epilepsy and some are also used for neuropathic pain, mood disorders and migraine	Carbamazepine, clonazepam, gabapentin, lamotrigine, phenobarbital, phenytoin, sodium valproate, topiramate, vigabatrin Phenytoin side effects such as dizziness, blurred vision, etc., may be signs of drug-related toxicity Dizziness, drowsiness and blurred vision are dose-related side effects of carbamazepine, especially on initiation
Antihistamines Used in hay fever, itching and to control nausea, vomiting and vertigo	Those most likely to cause drowsiness include: chlorphenamine, diphenhydramine, promethazin, cyclizine **Others:** loratadine, desloratadine, cetirizine, acrivastine, cinnarizine Hypotension with cinnarizine is dose related
Antihypertensives Various classes of drug used to treat hypertension, angina, heart failure, oedema, heart abnormalities, or after a heart attack	**ACE inhibitors and ARBs:** captopril, enalapril, lisinopril, ramipril, perindopril, quinapril, fosinopril, trandolapril, losartan, valsartan, irbesartan, candesartan, eprosartan, telmisartan Greater risk of hypotension if recently started and if also taking a diuretic, particularly furosemide **α-Blockers:** doxazosin, indoramin, prazosin, terazosin Doses used for treating prostate problems are less likely to cause hypotension and dizziness than those required to treat hypertension **β-Blockers:** atenolol, bisoprolol, metoprolol, nebivolol, acebutolol, oxprenolol, propranolol, carvedilol, sotalol Dizziness may be due to postural hypotension **Calcium channel blockers:** diltiazem, verapamil, amlodipine, felodipine, lacidipine, nifedipine Dizziness, hypotension and other cardiac effects possible **Diuretics:** bendroflumethiazide, chlortalidone, indapamide, metolazone, furosemide, bumetanide, amiloride, triamterene, spironolactone Can cause dehydration, dizziness, confusion and postural hypotension Intravenous furosemide, if administered too quickly, may cause vestibular damage **Centrally acting antihypertensives:** clonidine, methyldopa, moxonidine Can cause sedation, dizziness, bradycardia and postural hypotension
Anti-muscarinic drugs (anticholinergics) Used to treat incontinence, Parkinson's disease and to control effects some antipsychotics have on movement	Oxybutynin, tolterodine, orphenadrine, procyclidine, trihexylphenidyl Oxybutynin may cause acute confusion in elderly people, especially those with pre-existing cognitive impairment All can cause drowsiness, dizziness, blurred vision, restlessness, hallucinations and confusion

Medication groups	Class and examples
Antipsychotics including atypicals Used to treat schizophrenia, manic depression and other conditions such as aggression associated with dementia	**'Typicals'**: chlorpromazine, haloperidol, trifluperazine, prochlorperazine, flupentixol, zuclopentixol **'Atypicals'**: amisulpiride, clozapine, olanzapine, risperidone, sertindole, quetiapine, zotepine 'Typicals' are frequently implicated in drug-induced parkinsonism, i.e. extrapyramidal symptoms Also: drowsiness, dizziness, low BP and arrhythmias
Benzodiazepines and hypnotics Sleeping tablets	**Benzodiazepines**: nitrazepam, diazepam, temazepam, lorazepam, chlordiazepoxide **Others**: clomethiazole, chloral betaine, zolpidem, zopiclone May cause hangover effects the next day Also: balance disturbance, memory loss and restlessness
Dopaminergic drugs Used to treat Parkinson's disease	Amantadine, bromocriptine, levodopa, lysuride, pergolide, selegiline, apomorphine Sudden excessive daytime sleepiness can occur Also: dizziness and hypotension
Eyedrops and ointments	Most eye preparations can cause visual disturbances, as can an untreated eye condition Also consider if the eyedrops may cause other side effects typical of their class of medication if they are absorbed systemically after topical administration
Nitrates Used to ease and prevent angina	Glyceryl trinitrate, isosorbide mononitrate and dinitrate Dizziness may be due to postural hypotension
Opiate analgesics Used to relieve moderate-to-severe pain	Morphine, buprenorphine, codeine, tramadol, co-codamol (especially 30/500), co-dydramol, dihydrocodeine Confusion is common with tramadol Drowsiness and sedation are common upon starting treatment or dose titration
Quinine Used to treat malaria and leg cramps	Can cause visual disturbances, confusion and hypoglycaemia, although these are most common when using higher doses for the treatment of malaria or when given intravenously
Respiratory medication Used to treat asthma and COPD	Theophylline and salbutamol Can cause arrhythmias especially at higher doses
Ulcer healing medication Used to treat or prevent GI ulcers and reflux	**H_2-histamine receptor antagonists and proton pump inhibitors** Can cause dizziness

ACE, angiotensin-converting enzyme; ARB, angiotensin-receptor blockers; COPD, chronic obstructive pulmonary disease; MAOIs, monoamine oxidase inhibitors.

— Mechanism of interaction of warfarin with aspirin: plasma binding and gastric bleeding risk

Partly as a consequence of its negative charge at physiological pH, warfarin is very highly (>95%) bound to plasma proteins. The free, unbound drug is responsible for the anticoagulant activity. Other highly plasma protein-bound drugs (such as aspirin) have the potential to compete for plasma protein-binding sites and displace warfarin. This can increase the concentration of unbound warfarin in the plasma and therefore lead to toxicity and bleeding. The propensity of aspirin to cause gastric bleeding in addition to its own anti-platelet activity exacerbates the dangers associated with this interaction.

— Main counselling points for warfarin

The pharmacokinetic properties of warfarin, narrow therapeutic range and potential interactions discussed above can lead to serious adverse effects. Thus, counselling of patients is very important. On starting warfarin therapy, patients will be provided with an 'anticoagulant record book' that they should carry at all times. They will be asked to attend for regular blood tests. The main adverse effect is haemorrhage, which may be apparent from unusual bruising, bleeding or blackened stools. Dietary advice as discussed above should also be given. Tablets come in different strengths and colours and understanding of, and adherence to, the correct regimen is also important to achieve optimal outcomes.

— **On attending the falls clinic, what medication might you expect Mrs JB to be started on to protect her bones?**

Older people with osteoporosis are at a higher risk of sustaining a fracture if they fall. People at risk of developing osteoporosis include those with a low body mass index (BMI = mass (kg)/[height (metres)]^2), those who have taken prolonged courses of corticosteroids, women who have had a hysterectomy or a premature menopause (thus lacking in oestrogens), people who have previously sustained a fragility fracture, people with a family history of osteoporosis, people with another disease state that may increase their risk, and people who smoke a lot or have chronic alcohol problems.

Older people at risk of developing osteoporosis should be encouraged to get sufficient dietary calcium and vitamin D, to undertake regular weight-bearing exercise and to stop smoking. If patients are unable to meet their dietary calcium requirements, then they may benefit from calcium and vitamin D supplements.

There are several different classes of medication licensed for the prevention and treatment of osteoporosis. The exact licensing details should be checked in the summary of product characteristics, but the most commonly prescribed class of drugs is the bisphosphonates (e.g. pamidronate, alendronate, risedronate) and other drugs that affect bone metabolism. Other options available, if a patient is unable to take a bisphosphonate, include hormone replacement therapy, strontium ranelate, raloxifene (an oral selective oestrogen receptor modulator [SERM]), calcitonin, parathyroid hormone (PTH) or the recombinant PTH analogue teriparatide. (Note that, although PTH released naturally in the body from the parathyroid glands generally acts to *increase* bone resorption, when it is injected therapeutically in small intermittent amounts it can apparently *stimulate* new bone formation over resorption, and therefore can be used effectively in osteoporosis treatment.) Denosumab is a monoclonal antibody that is given by 6-monthly subcutaneous injections. It may be an option for those who are unable to comply with instructions for alendronate and either risedronate or etidronate.

— **Reviewing a prescription for an elderly person**
One of the most common interventions a doctor can make is to prescribe medication for a patient.

Elderly patients, who normally have more medical conditions, will typically be prescribed more medications. Polypharmacy, usually defined as four or more regular medications, is common.

There are seven broad rules to prescribing that should always be considered when reviewing a prescription:

— **1. Is it indicated?**

- If a patient describes a new symptom, consider whether that symptom could be a side effect from an existing medication that could be changed, e.g. constipation caused by opioid analgesia.
- Ensure that the patient receives optimal treatment for all his or her conditions. Elderly patients should not be denied beneficial treatment on the basis of their age, polypharmacy or potential side effects, without a reasonable trial period.
- Remember that many clinical trials exclude elderly patients, so there may not be much reliable evidence. If an elderly patient is biologically fit and well, and understands the rationale for the medication, then preventive medication is usually appropriate. However, if a patient has a limited life span for other reasons, e.g. extreme frailty or terminal cancer, then preventive medication is not usually warranted.

— **2. Are there any contraindications?**

- Think about drug–disease contraindications, and whether they are absolute contraindications. An elderly patient with mild renal impairment may still be able to take ACE inhibitors if they are monitored appropriately.

— **3. Are there any likely interactions?**

- Think about drug–drug interactions. Do there need to be any dose adjustments or changes to timing as a result of an interaction? Could an interaction be causing a new symptom or treatment failure?

— **4. What is the best medication?**

- Think about which class of medication will work best for a particular patient. Take into account those medications that may have a more acceptable side-effect profile, or those that have the potential for dual action.

— **5. What should the starting dose be?**

- In elderly patients the general rule is to 'start low and go slow'. Medications can normally be started at lower doses than normal, and titrated upwards if well tolerated. However, it is important to make sure that doses used are therapeutic.

- An elderly patient will also have some degree of renal impairment. For those medications that require dose adjustments in renal impairment it is worth checking renal function using either the Cockcroft–Gault formula or the estimated glomerular filtration rate (eGFR). A creatinine blood test result that falls within the upper levels of normal in an elderly patient should always be treated with suspicion.

— 6. **How will the impact be assessed?**

- For each medication the patient is taking, think about how to monitor for efficacy, toxicity and side effects.

— 7. **What is the timeframe?**

- Some medication is intended for long-term use, e.g. antihypertensives. Some medication is intended for short-term use only, e.g. antibiotics. However, sometimes medication is continued unintentionally when there is no longer a clinical indication, e.g. analgesics or laxatives.
- If a medication that is no longer required has been identified, care should be taken when discontinuing it, to avoid rebound problems.

— **Adherence**

Adherence may be broadly defined as the extent to which a patient is able to follow his or her given medical advice and take the medication as prescribed. Patients can be non-compliant with their medication for many reasons, and it is not a problem that is specific to elderly people. However, it often becomes more apparent in elderly people because they are prescribed more medication.

Non-adherence can be grouped into intentional (deliberate deviation from prescribed regimen by the patient) or non-intentional adherence (where the patient, if able to, would have taken medicines as prescribed). Intentional non-adherence is when the patient chooses not to take the medication as prescribed. Common reasons for this might include the patient having unacceptable side effects or lack of knowledge, or the medication not fitting well into the patient's lifestyle. The best way to reduce intentional non-adherence is to discuss the issue with the patient to identify and address

any concerns that they have. If a patient has unacceptable side effects then there may be a suitable therapeutic alternative to which he or she could be switched. A common example of deliberate non-adherence in elderly people is a patient refusing to take furosemide on shopping days because of a fear of not finding a toilet. A compromise could be reached whereby the patient takes the furosemide slightly later on those days, once he or she gets back home.

Non-intentional non-adherence is when patients either want to take their medication and something prevents them, or they are unaware that they are taking their medication incorrectly. Counselling a patient on how they should be taking their medication correctly is very important. However, in non-intentional non-adherence the patient may require further help. The best way to address non-intentional non-adherence is to make the patient's life simpler with regard to the medication. Simplifying medication regimens by the use of combination products or modified-release preparations, to minimise the 'pill burden' and the frequency of administration, may help. If these simple measures are insufficient, the patient would probably benefit from a more in-depth assessment to find out what specific help may be required. Other things that may help adherence are setting up a home delivery system with a local pharmacy, large print labels, non-child-proof bottle tops, a medication record card or a multi-compartment compliance aid.

It is worth remembering that each patient is different and what works for one patient will not necessarily suit the next. If, however, all the above measures fail, the patient may need additional help from carers.

EXTENDED LEARNING

- What is a creatinine clearance rate? How is it determined and what is its significance?
- How would you expect renal impairment to affect drug pharmacokinetics?
- What do you understand by the terms 'prothrombin time' (PT) and 'international normalised ratio' (INR)? How are they determined and interpreted?
- New oral anticoagulants are increasingly prescribed as alternatives to warfarin. What

are these agents and why might they be preferred?

- In relation to patient adherence, what do you understand by the terms 'compliance', 'adherence' and 'concordance'?

ADDITIONAL PRACTICE POINT

- What types of compliance aid are available and how are they used?

References and further reading

Bloch F, Thibaud M, Dugué B, Brèque C, Rigaud AS, Kemoun G (2011). Psychotropic drugs and falls in the elderly people: updated literature review and meta-analysis. *J Aging Health* **23**:329–46.

Department of Health (2001) *National Service Framework for the Older Person*. London: Department of Health. Available at: www.gov.uk/government/publications/quality-standards-for-care-services-for-older-people (accessed 27 June 2013).

Kannus P, Sievänen H, Palvanen M, Järvinen T, Parkkari J (2005) Prevention of falls and consequent injuries in elderly people. *Lancet* **366**:1885–93.

National Institute for Health and Care Excellence (2013). *Falls: Assessment and prevention of falls in older people*. NICE Clinical Guidance CG161. London: NICE. Available at: www.nice.org.uk/CG161 (accessed 27 June 2013).

National Institute for Health and Clinical Excellence (2010). *Osteoporotic Fractures – Denosumab*. NICE Technology Appraisal Guideline 204. London: NICE. Available at: http://guidance.nice.org.uk/TA204 (accessed: 7 April 2014).

National Patient Safety Agency (2007). *Slips, Trips and Falls*. Available at: www.nrls.npsa.nhs.uk (accessed 27 June 2013).

Nutescu EA, Shapiro NL, Ibrahim S, West P (2006). Warfarin and its interactions with foods, herbs and other dietary supplements. *Expert Opin Drug Safety* **5**:433–51.

Case 3
Treating a patient with benign prostatic hyperplasia

ADAM TODD AND ANDY HUSBAND

LEARNING OUTCOMES

At the end of this case, you will be able to:

- Outline the signs and symptoms of benign prostatic hyperplasia (BPH)
- Describe the treatment options associated with BPH
- Describe the chemistry and mechanism of action of tamsulosin and finasteride
- Examine the circumstances when BPH can be managed 'over the counter'

Case study

Mr TT is a 58-year-old man who has just come into your pharmacy; he looks rather anxious and explains that he would like some advice 'in private'. You take him into the consultation room where he whispers that he is having problems with his 'waterworks'. He explains that, when he goes to the toilet, he finds it difficult to start urinating; there is no pain, but it happens all of the time, especially during the night when he has to get up at least three times to empty his bladder.

You think that Mr TT has symptoms associated with BPH and decide he would be a good candidate to try OTC tamsulosin.

- What is BPH?
- What are the signs and symptoms of BPH?
- How is it diagnosed?
- What information is required before a supply of OTC tamsulosin can be made?
- When should tamsulosin not be supplied OTC?

Mr TT returns to the pharmacy 2 weeks' later. He explains that his symptoms have significantly improved and would like a further supply of tamsulosin.

- What is the mechanism of action of tamsulosin?
- What is the guidance for using tamsulosin to manage symptoms associated with BPH?

Six months later, you get a prescription for Mr TT; his GP has prescribed him finasteride 5 mg once daily to take in combination with tamsulosin.

- What is the mechanism of action of finasteride?
- What is the rationale for using it in combination with tamsulosin?

- Are there any other pharmaceutical interventions that can be used to manage Mr TT's symptoms?
- What lifestyle advice could be offered to a patient with BPH?

Case discussion

— BPH and its pathophysiology

BPH (benign prostatic hyperplasia) is a term used to describe a prostate measuring larger than normal (a 'normal' prostate is around 4 cm in diameter and weighs around 20 g). The prostate is a doughnut-shaped organ that encircles the urethra; thus, an increase in size affects bladder outflow. The pathophysiology of BPH is complex and not fully understood, although there are a number of factors that are thought to be associated with the development, these include:

- **Age:** as men get older, the size of the prostate gland increases; half of men aged >60 years have BPH symptoms
- **Tissue remodelling:** in BPH tissue, the balance of cellular proliferation and apoptosis shifts in favour of proliferation – possibly due to increased expression of transforming growth factor β_1 (TGF-β_1) and Bcl-2 (an apoptosis regulator protein)
- **Hormonal:** increased dihydrotestosterone (DHT) levels have been reported in BPH tissue
- **Metabolic effects:** men with metabolic syndrome have a faster growing BPH compared with men without metabolic syndrome; elevated blood pressure, high insulin and low high-density lipoprotein (HDL)-cholesterol levels may also be risk factors for BPH
- **Inflammation:** chronic inflammation has been identified in BPH and higher levels have been associated with larger prostates.

— Signs, symptoms and diagnosis of BPH

Some patients with BPH may be asymptomatic, whereas in other cases lower urinary tract symptoms (LUTSs) may be present (although there is a lack of convincing evidence to relate prostate size to the severity of LUTSs). Broadly speaking, clinical symptoms of BPH are caused by problems with either storing or passing urine and include:

Storage symptoms (storing urine):

- Increased urinary frequency (the patient may report the need to pass small volumes of urine several times each night)
- Urgency (a compelling need to pass urine that cannot be deferred):

Voiding symptoms (passing urine):

- Hesitancy (patient can often have difficulty initiating micturition)
- Poor urinary flow (and an associated increase in time taken to urinate)
- Incomplete bladder emptying (the sensation of still having urine in the bladder)
- Dribbling.

BPH can lead to the development of urinary retention. This can be acute, which can be painful and is considered a medical emergency, or chronic, which, although not immediately life threatening, can lead to renal impairment.

From the case outlined above, Mr TT described that he was up several times a night to pass urine (i.e. increased urinary frequency) and he finds it difficult to start urinating (i.e. hesitancy). He is therefore showing both voiding and storage symptoms, which can be associated with BPH.

To quantify how much these symptoms are affecting the patient, a screening tool, consisting of eight questions, known as the International Prostate Symptom Score (IPSS), can be used. Patients are asked to rate their urinary symptoms on a scale of 1–5 and to rate their quality of life on a scale of 1–6. The results are then quantified to give an overall score. Scores between 0 and 7 indicate mild symptoms, between 8 and 19 moderate symptoms, whereas between 30 and 35 is considered to be indicative of severe symptoms.

— Treatment options

Patients with a low IPSS (<7) can often be managed with lifestyle advice and watchful waiting, e.g. patients can be advised to reduce their fluid intake before bedtime and, if possible, reduce the consumption of caffeine-containing products. Pharmacists should also be aware of any medication that could exacerbate the LUTSs (e.g. the timing of administration for diuretics) and advise accordingly.

For patients with more troublesome symptoms, pharmaceutical intervention can be offered with the aim of reducing smooth muscle tone in the bladder or reducing the size of the prostate. *α-Adrenoreceptor blockers:* the first class of agent that can be used is the α-adrenoreceptor blockers; they antagonise α_{1A}-receptors in the bladder neck (and prostate) and α_{1D}-receptors present mainly in

tamsulosin

finasteride

the bladder detrusor smooth muscle, causing relaxation, thus improving urinary flow. Less selective, older-generation α-blockers (e.g. terazosin and doxazosin) antagonise α_1-adrenoceptors throughout various body systems (including α_1-adrenoceptors within the cardiovascular system), causing cardiovascular side effects, whereas the newer agents (e.g. tamsulosin) have a relatively higher affinity for α_{1A} and α_{1D}-subtype adrenoreceptors in the bladder, versus α_{1B}-subtype receptors present in peripheral blood vessels, and are therefore associated with fewer cardiovascular side effects (such as postural hypotension). Apparently, this selectivity difference of tamulosin may be due to a slower dissociation of the antagonist molecule from α_{1A}-receptors compared with α_{1B}-receptors. However, although the α-blockers improve urinary flow (typically by 2–3 mL/s) and other LUTSs, they do not reduce the size of the prostate or the rate of prostate growth and, ultimately, the need for surgical intervention.

5α-Reductase inhibitors: the next class of agent that can be used is the 5α-reductase inhibitors (5ARIs); they inhibit the enzyme 5α-reductase, which prevents the normal formation of dihydrotestosterone (DHT) from testosterone. DHT is around three times more potent than testosterone and is a driving force for prostate growth. In contrast to α-blockers, 5ARIs improve LUTSs, but also reduce prostate size (around 20–30% reduction in prostate volume has been

observed), making them very useful agents for the management of BPH.

5ARIs are indicated for men with LUTSs, substantially enlarged prostate glands (typically >30 g) and in patients with a high risk of disease progression (e.g. older men). There are two 5ARIs licensed for the treatment of BPH: finasteride and dutasteride.

In view of the varying mechanism of action of α-blockers and the 5ARIs, the combined use of these agents is pharmacologically favourable. Indeed, an α-blocker will provide immediate relief of symptoms, whereas, longer term, the 5ARI will reduce the size of the prostate (and the subsequent need for surgical intervention). Positive results have been reported with the combined use of dutasteride and tamsulosin; similarly, dutasteride and tamsulosin used together have been reported to be more effective at slowing clinical progression of BPH compared with using each agent alone. Both tamsulosin and finasteride (and dutasteride) should be used with caution in patients with hepatic impairment. Similar to many low polarity drugs, they undergo extensive metabolism in the liver, which is the primary means by which they are cleared from the systemic circulation.

— Managing BPH OTC in a community pharmacy

In the UK, tamsulosin is now licensed for OTC sale in community pharmacies for the treatment of symptoms of BPH. It can be sold to men, aged 45–75 years, who have experienced LUTSs (such as urinary hesitancy or increased urinary frequency) for >3 months. A 2-week initial supply can be made to patients: if there is an improvement in symptoms after this time, a further 4-week supply can be made. After 6 weeks, patients should be advised to see their GP for assessment of their symptoms and confirmation that continued use of tamsulosin is appropriate. Patients should be offered advice, such as to limit the intake of caffeine, and be alerted to the possibility of first-dose postural hypotension and ejaculation dysfunction, when initially taking tamsulosin.

EXTENDED LEARNING

- Discuss the structure and function of the prostate

- How might BPH be distinguished from prostate cancer?
- What is the evidence base for using saw palmetto in the treatment of BPH?

ADDITIONAL PRACTICE POINT

- What are the red flag warning symptoms requiring urgent referral?

References and further reading

Husband AK, Todd A (2012). Benign prostatic hyperplasia: Clinical features and diagnosis. *Clin Pharmacist* 4:42–6.

Husband AK, Todd A (2012). Benign prostatic hyperplasia: Management. *Clin Pharmacist* 4:47–50.

National Institute for Health and Clinical Excellence (2010). *Lower Urinary Tract Symptoms: The management of lower urinary tract symptoms in men.* Clinical Guideline 97. London: NICE. Available at: www.nice.org.uk/Guidance/CG97 (accessed 22 July 2014).

Roehrborn CG, Schwinn DA (2004). Alpha1-adrenergic receptors and their inhibitors in lower urinary tract symptoms and benign prostatic hyperplasia. *J Urol* 171:1029–35.

Sato S, Hatanaka T, Yuyama H et al. (2012). Tamsulosin potently and selectively antagonizes human recombinant α(1A/1D)-adrenoceptors: slow dissociation from the α(1A)-adrenoceptor may account for selectivity for α(1A)-adrenoceptor over α(1B)-adrenoceptor subtype. *Biol Pharm Bull* 35:72–7.

Urological Sciences Research Foundation. *International Prostate Symptom Score (IPSS).* Available at: www.usrf.org/questionnaires/AUA_SymptomScore.html (accessed 16 August 2012).

Yamada S, Ito Y (2011). α(1)-Adrenoceptors in the urinary tract. *Handbook Exp Pharmacol* 202:283–306.

Yoshimura K, Kadoyama K, Sakaeda T et al. (2013). A survey of the FAERS database concerning the adverse event profiles of α1-adrenoreceptor blockers for lower urinary tract symptoms. *Int J Med Sci* 10:864–9.

Case 4
Pain management using strong opiates in palliative care

LOUISE SEAGER AND JO BARTLETT

LEARNING OUTCOMES

At the end of this case, you will be able to:

- Outline the core questions for assessment of pain in palliative care
- Outline the principles of titrating oral opiate doses and converting between different routes and preparations
- Describe the principles surrounding opiates and addiction in palliative care
- Describe the use of anticipatory medicines at the end of life, including drug choices and appropriate doses

Case study

Mrs WL is a 56-year-old woman with advanced metastatic breast cancer. She has been pain controlled on morphine sulfate MR 40 mg twice daily, paracetamol 1 g four times a day and 10 mg morphine sulfate liquid 10 mg/5 mL as required for the past few months. She is unable to take NSAIDs due to a previous history of a GI bleed.

Lately, she has noticed that her pain is no longer controlled on her current medication.

- What questions would you need to ask in order to assess her pain appropriately?
- Why is morphine usually formulated and administered as the sulfate salt?
- How is the maintenance and breakthrough pain dose of morphine usually calculated?

Mrs WL describes the pain as a generalised constant dull ache that is relieved partially when she takes her morphine liquid. She states that she is taking 10 mg (5 mL) which helps a little, but she is scared to take it any more often than 4-hourly because she is concerned that she will become addicted. She is currently taking 4 × 5 mL (10 mg) doses per day.

- How would you address the issue of addiction in this case?
- How would you adjust her regular and breakthrough analgesia?

Over the next few months Mrs WL deteriorates and she is now struggling to swallow her oral medication, namely morphine sulfate MR capsules 90 mg twice a day plus 15 mL (30 mg) morphine sulfate oral liquid 10 mg/5 mL, when needed, approximately two doses over 24 hours. The district nurses would like to set up a continuous subcutaneous infusion (CSCI) via a syringe driver device and deliver her medication this way. You are asked by the district nurses for your advice.

- ❓ What dose of morphine will they need to use via CSCI over 24 hours?
- ❓ What dose of subcutaneous morphine would they need for breakthrough pain?

The district nurses would also like anticipatory (just in case) subcutaneous medication, for use as required, available in the house for nausea, agitation and excessive respiratory secretions.

- ❓ What drug and dose would you recommend for each symptom, and why?

Case discussion

— Core questions for assessment of pain in palliative care

Pain is a symptom with many different definitions, reflecting its subjective nature. These definitions have a common theme, which is that pain not only has a physical component but also important emotional, spiritual, functional and psychosocial contexts.

The starting point of pain management is its comprehensive assessment. The aim is to determine the nature of the pain and where possible the cause of the pain, which in turn will influence the best course of action. As pain is multifactorial the assessment should encompass the factors in Table 11.2.

Patients may have more than one type of pain, so the assessment process should be repeated for each type of pain.

There may be other factors contributing to the pain:

- Anxiety or depression
- Fear or a feeling of 'unfinished business' in life
- Family or social issues
- Other physical symptoms such as coughing and vomiting.

Non-verbal indicators of pain, such as body language, e.g. frequently adjusting position, and facial expressions, e.g. grimacing, are a useful part of the assessment process.

Accurate assessment of pain and the patient's goals for treatment are essential when choosing a treatment plan. The success or failure of a

▼ TABLE 11.2
Factors for pain assessment

Location	Where is the pain? Does it radiate to other area(s)? Is there more than one site?
Intensity	How bad is the pain?
Constant/ Intermittent	Is it there all the time? Does it come and go and if so how long does it last?
Exacerbating factors	What makes it worse?
Relieving factors	What makes it better?
Time line	When did the pain start?
Effect	What effect does it have on function, i.e. sleep, mobility and wellbeing?
Other factors	Are there any changes in sensation or loss of power associated with the pain?
Analgesic history	What medication has been tried or is currently being used? How effective was/is it? What doses were used and how was it tolerated?

Adapted from Laverty (2009) and Cox (2010).

treatment plan needs to be monitored, e.g. by scoring the severity of pain on a numerical rating scale:

If 0 = no pain and 10 = worst possible pain, how would you rate your pain?

It is important to regularly reassess pain, because it can change in response to other treatments, such as radiotherapy or as a consequence of disease progression or infection.

— Principles of titrating oral opiate doses and converting between different routes and preparations

There are different types of strong opioid analgesic available in a wide range of formulations. It is important to be aware of what drugs and formulations are available and when and how to convert between them.

All strong opioids are agonists at the G-protein-coupled μ-opioid receptor, but they also act at other opioid receptors, of which there are four in total (historically, μ, δ, κ, σ, although nowadays the σ receptor is not generally regarded as a true opiate receptor, but is still considered to be involved physiologically in pain processing, by acting as a 'molecular chaperone' to modulate opiate-mediated anti-nociception [Zamanillo et al., 2013]; the fourth member of the opiate receptor family is now referred to as the N-receptor or nociception-orphanin FQ receptor [Cox, 2013]). Different affinities for these receptors possibly explain patients' different tolerability and efficacy.

The most commonly prescribed strong opioid in palliative care is morphine. However, other opioids are used when morphine cannot be tolerated, renal function is impaired or the transdermal route is preferred.

Morphine is usually formulated and administered as the sulfate salt. The nitrogen atom in morphine is a basic centre and will accept a proton to become positively charged when the pH is below around 8 (the pK_a value of the conjugate acid of morphine). When treated with a dilute solution of sulfuric acid, morphine sulfate is produced, in which there are two positively charged protonated morphine cations for each sulfate anion. The sulfate salt of morphine is around 300 times more water soluble than morphine free base, due to considerably increased polarity in the ionic form. This makes the salt ideal for formulation in an aqueous vehicle for preparation of an oral solution. Dissolution of morphine sulfate from an immediate-release solid oral dosage form (tablet) is also more rapid.

morphine sulfate

Some of the currently listed opiate analgesics in the *BNF* (apart from morphine) are: alfentanil, buprenorphine, codeine, diamorphine (heroin), dihydrocodeine, dipipanone, fentanyl, hydromorphone, meptazinol, oxycodone, pentazocine, pethidine, tapentadol and tramadol.

The starting dose of an oral opioid depends on the analgesia that the patient has had previously and its effectiveness. The patient's age, severity of pain, weight and renal function may also influence the dose prescribed. It is common practice to start on immediate-release morphine (2.5–10 mg) as needed in response to pain; however, the dose prescribed should be guided by individual circumstances. Immediate-release morphine is available in tablet or liquid form; onset of action is usually within 20–30 min and lasts for approximately 4 hours. There is no maximum dose and patients should take it when pain occurs; in some cases this can be as frequently as every hour. Patients are encouraged to document doses taken, time taken and its effect.

— **Calculation of maintenance and breakthrough pain doses of morphine**

If patients are regularly requiring immediate-release morphine they should be converted to a slow-release morphine preparation. The most commonly prescribed slow-release morphine is the twice-daily preparation, with an onset of action of 2 hours and duration of action of 12 hours. There are once-daily slow-release morphine preparations available, but these are not commonly prescribed.

CONVERTING IMMEDIATE-RELEASE MORPHINE TO A SLOW-RELEASE PREPARATION

Calculate the total daily dose (TDD) of morphine – the total amount of morphine taken in milligrams over 24 hours.

Dose of 12-hourly slow release morphine the patient should be prescribed is the TDD divided by 2, e.g. morphine immediate release 10 mg prescribed as required. The patient takes the following:

06.00 h 10 mg

09.30 h 10 mg

12.30 h 10 mg

16.00 h 10 mg

18.45 h 10 mg

22.00 h 10 mg

TDD = 60 mg

Dose of 12-hourly slow-release morphine = 60/2 = 30 mg twice daily.

A breakthrough dose of immediate-release morphine should always be prescribed; this is calculated as one-sixth of the TDD.

Using the example above the as required immediate release morphine dose would be: 60/6 = 10 mg immediate-release morphine

These principles of calculating doses of opioids are the same regardless of the type of opioid prescribed.

Modified release of a drug administered via the oral route involves manipulating the release rate until the dosage form reaches the required site within the GI tract. This may be to target specific anatomical sites, avoid degradation of drug in the stomach, prevent irritation of the stomach by a drug or, as in this case, extend the release of the drug, prolonging the presence of drug at therapeutic levels in the bloodstream. The dosage form can be a single entity (monolithic), e.g. a tablet, or can be prepared from multiple units, for instance granules or pellets (often produced by extrusion spheronisation) filled into hard gelatin capsules. Modified-release drug can be achieved using a matrix approach, with drug dispersed in a polymer matrix, or with a system whereby the dosage unit, e.g. a tablet, is coated with a rate-limiting membrane that controls the drug release rate.

Different strong opioids have varying receptor affinities and bioavailabilities and their relative potency to morphine is different. If changing to a different opioid, then the dose needs to be calculated carefully; this is done using its morphine equivalence. Conversion charts and ratios are widely available and can be a very useful aid to clinical practice; however, when converting to an equivalent dose, always remember dose equivalents/ratios are approximate.

When changing the route of administration, the opioid dose must be recalculated. This is because, when a drug is administered via a different route, its bioavailability can vary. Again conversion charts and ratios are widely available to aid the conversion process.

— **Principles surrounding opiates and addiction in palliative care**

Several barriers to successful treatment of pain have been identified, one of which is fear of addiction (psychological dependence) to opioids. In palliative care patients, addiction is rare; however, opioids should still be used with caution in patients with a current or past history of drug misuse. It may still be appropriate to use opioids in this patient group but the preparation and dose should be chosen with care.

Opioid analgesics are a class of medicines that are produced from substances controlled under the international drug control conventions. It is recognised that in many, principally poorer, countries people who could benefit from these drugs do not have access to them. The WHO has estimated that over 5 billion (of total 7 billion world population) people live in countries with little or no access. These include patients with end-stage HIV/AIDS, terminal cancer, sickle cell disease, injuries from accidents or violence, and also in labour pain, recovering from surgery. In fact, the richest 20% of the world's population account for >90% of global consumption. Why is this? Morphine is cheap and it can be easily stored and administered. The reasons for the lack of access are largely attributed to lack of awareness among health professionals as well as patients of the effectiveness of these drugs. Patients and health professionals may be deterred by the stigma of using a drug perceived as addictive, fear of addiction itself or the regulation about controlled drugs that is often not correctly interpreted.

As chemotherapy for cancers is often not available, opioids have an important role in ensuring people with terminal illness do not suffer unnecessary pain. However, in both rich and poor countries, a common barrier to starting opiates in palliative care is the idea that they may signify the end of life. It is important to address these fears with both the patient and, where appropriate, their carers.

— **Use of anticipatory medicines at end of life, including drug choices and appropriate doses**

Dysphagia usually occurs towards the end of life and swallowing tablets can become a problem. Subcutaneous administration of medication is the preferred route at end of life because it is:

- Less invasive than intravenous administration
- Less painful and more predictable than intramuscular administration
- Quicker than transdermal administration to titrate drug doses.

Although it can be difficult to predict how and when a patient's condition will deteriorate, there are common symptoms that can worsen in the last days of life, such as pain, nausea, agitation and excessive bronchial secretions. Anticipatory prescribing of medicines ensures that, should these symptoms develop, treatments are available for administration without delay wherever the patient is being cared for.

Nausea and vomiting: the choice of antiemetic depends on the underlying cause and suitability for administration via the subcutaneous route. Commonly prescribed antiemetics include:

- Cyclizine 50 mg when required, up to three times a day
- Haloperidol 1.5–5 mg when required, up to three times a day
- Levomepromazine 6.25–12.5 mg when required, up to three times a day
- Metoclopramide 10–20 mg when required, up to four times a day.

Agitation: there can be reversible causes of agitation that should be addressed before starting drug treatment; these include urinary retention, pain, etc. If agitation is still present, or no clear cause can be identified, it may be appropriate to prescribe medication. Commonly prescribed anxiolytics are:

- Midazolam 2.5–5 mg 4- to 6-hourly when required
- Haloperidol 1.5–5 mg 4- to 6-hourly when required
- Levomepromazine 6.25–12.5 mg 6- to 8-hourly when required.

The frequency of administration should be judged by the patient's response: some patients may need higher doses.

Excessive bronchial secretions: in the last days of life, progressive muscle weakness can prevent patients from coughing or swallowing effectively. An inability to clear secretions in the upper respiratory tract causes noisy or bubbly breathing. Commonly prescribed drugs are:

- Hyoscine butylbromide 20–40 mg 4- to 6-hourly as required
- Hyoscine hydrobromide 400 micrograms 4- to 6-hourly as required

If any of these medications is being used repeatedly, it should be administered by continuous subcutaneous infusion. This is achieved using a syringe driver, which is a small portable infusion device that administers medication at a set rate over a 24-hour period. More than one medication can be prescribed to be mixed in the syringe, but drug compatibility should be checked. Reference sources are available, e.g. the Syringe Driver Survey Database.

EXTENDED LEARNING

- What are the causes of nausea and vomiting in palliative care and what informs the choice of antiemetic?
- Discuss the use of opioids delivered via the transdermal route in palliative care
- Discuss opioid choice in renal failure
- Outline the formulation and manufacture of modified-release oral and non-oral dosage forms
- How are transdermal patches formulated and manufactured?

References and further reading

Bartlett J, Seager L (2012). Palliative care: principles and pharmacy roles *Clin Pharmacist* 4:317–21.

Bartlett J, Seager L (2012). Palliative care: end of life medicines management. *Clin Pharmacist* 4:322–4.

Cox F (2010). Basic principles of pain management: assessment and intervention. *Nursing Stand* 25(1):36–9.

Cox BM (2013). Recent developments in the study of opioid receptors. *Mol Pharmacol* 83:723–8.

Ellershaw J, Sutcliffe J, Saunders C (1995). Dehydration and the dying patient. *J Pain Symptom Manag* 10:192–7.

Greenstreet W (2001). The concept of total pain: a focused patient care study. *BJN* 10:1248–55.

Higgs R (1999). The diagnosis of dying. *J R Coll Physicians* 33:110–12.

International Association for the Study of Pain (2012). Pain terms: a current list with definitions and notes on usage. *Pain* S3:215–21.

Laverty D (2009). The assessment and management of patients with chronic pain. *Cancer Nursing Pract* 8(10):17–20.

Law PY, Reggio PH, Loh HH (2013). Opioid receptors: toward separation of analgesic from undesirable effects. *Trends Biochem Sci* 38:275–28.

McCaffery M, Beebe A (1994). *Pain: A clinical manual for nursing practice*. London: Mosby.

McConnell EL, Basit AW (2013). Modified-release oral drug delivery. In: Aulton ME, Taylor KMG (eds), *Aulton's Pharmaceutics: The design and manufacture of medicines*, 4th edn. London: Elsevier, 550–65.

Mika J (2008). The opioid systems and role of glial cells in the effects of opioids. *Advances in Palliative Care Med* 7: 185–96.

National Institute for Health and Clinical Excellence (2012). *Opioids in Palliative Care: Safe and effective prescribing of strong opioids for pain in palliative care of adults*. NICE Clinical Guideline CG140. London: NICE. Available at: http://guidance.nice.org.uk/CG140 (accessed 3 October 2013).

Scottish Intercollegiate Guidelines Network (SIGN) (2008). *Control of Pain in Adults with Cancer: A national clinical guideline*, Number 106. Edinburgh: SIGN. Available at: www.sign.ac.uk/pdf/SIGN106.pdf. (accessed 03 October 2013).

Taylor J (2010). Vets get more pain training than doctors and nurses. *The Times Raconteur Media*. Available at: http://bit.ly/RS3izm (accessed 18 April 2013).

Twycross R, Wilcock A, eds (2011). *Palliative Care Formulary*, 4th edn. Nottingham: Palliativedrugs.com Ltd. Available at: www.palliativedrugs.com (accessed 18 May 2013).

Zamanillo D, Romero L, Merlos M, Velam JM (2013). Sigma 1 receptor: A new therapeutic target for pain. *Eur J Pharmacol* 716(1–3):78–93.

Case 5
Human papillomavirus and cervical cancer

ZOE ASLANPOUR

LEARNING OUTCOMES

At the end of this case, you will be able to:

- Outline the link between HPV immunisation and cervical cancer
- Describe the HPV immunisation programme, including the targeted age group and consent, available vaccines, their possible side effects and the national implementation
- Outline the principles and processes in the production of an effective vaccine
- Outline the rationale for cervical screening and its place after implementation of the national HPV programme

Case study

Mrs H has been a regular customer at your pharmacy for the last 12 years, and you have known her daughter, NH, since she was born. Mrs H comes in with a letter from NH's school which explains that the school nurse will be immunising year 8 students (aged 12–13 years) with HPV vaccine the following week and seeking parental consent. Mrs H comments that NH is not sexually active and asks whether the immunisation is necessary at this time. She asks you if you know about the HPV immunisation programme and what it entails.

❓ How would you respond to Mrs H's request?

Eight months later, Mrs H comes to your pharmacy again and you ask her about NH and her immunisation. She tells you that NH has had 2 doses of Gardasil vaccine already and is due for a third one the following day. However, NH is unwell with flu and is running a high temperature. Mrs H

asks your advice as to whether NH should give the final dose a miss.

❓ What is your advice to Mrs H?

Next time Mrs H visits your pharmacy she tells you that she has received a letter from her GP asking her to go for cervical screening. She comments that at least NH won't need to go for cervical screening now that she has been immunised.

❓ How would you respond to Mrs H's comment?

Case discussion

— Different types of HPV

There are more than 100 different types of HPV, with around 40 types affecting the genital area. Infection with some high-risk types of HPV can cause abnormal tissue growth as well as other cell changes that can lead to cervical cancer.

Infection with other types of HPV may cause:

- Genital warts: small growths or skin changes on or around the genital or anal area; these are the most common viral STI in the UK
- Skin warts and verrucas
- Vaginal cancer or vulval cancer (although these types of cancer are rare)
- Anal cancer or cancer of the penis
- Some cancers of the head and neck
- Laryngeal papillomas (warts on the larynx or vocal folds).

Combined with cervical screening, HPV immunisation is an important step towards preventing cervical cancer. It is estimated that about 400 lives could be saved in the UK every year as a result of immunising girls before they are infected with HPV.

— Being immunised

The HPV vaccine is part of the national immunisation programme and is given to secondary school girls aged 12 and 13 years. Special precautions may need to be taken if the person being immunised has certain health conditions, or has ever had a severe allergic reaction.

— Before vaccination
If the child is 12–13 years old, the parent(s) will usually receive information about the immunisation schedule and a consent form before the immunisation takes place.

— The vaccine
Gardasil vaccine is a suspension of HPV, of four types (quadrivalent), prepared by recombinant technology and administered by intramuscular injection.

The vaccine, rather than containing deactivated viral particles, consists of the L1 major capsid (protein shell) proteins from four separate strains of HPV (types 6, 11, 16 and 18), which together are associated with around 70% of cases of cervical cancer (see below) and around 90% of cases of genital warts and recurrent respiratory papillomatosis. The four individual HPV L1 capsid proteins (one from each strain) are produced commercially from the fermentation of genetically-engineered *Saccharomyces cerevisiae* yeasts. For each HPV strain, the gene encoding for the L1 capsid protein has been cloned and then integrated into the yeast cells. The recombinant yeast cells (which can be frozen and stored for future use) are then cultured and produce the desired L1 capsid proteins in large quantities. The capsid proteins are isolated from the culture by homogenising and lysing the cells, followed by extraction and purification. Each of the four HPV L1 capsid proteins is separately produced in this way and incorporated into the vaccine. The proteins corresponding to each strain self-assemble to give virus-like particles that resemble the real virions for each HPV strain, but which lack any viral DNA so are unable to cause infection. The virus-like particles are, however, antigenic and bring about an immune response in the vaccine recipient. Antibodies to all four strains found in the vaccine are produced, which can prevent subsequent infection on exposure to live HPV (of the types on which the vaccine is based).

The vaccine formulation also contains aluminium hydroxyphosphate sulfate. Aluminium salts are often used in vaccines, as so called vaccine adjuvants, which enhance the immune response and lead to increased production of antibodies.

— The immunisation schedule
The HPV vaccine is given as an injection into the muscle of the upper arm or thigh (upper leg). The immunisation consists of three doses and all three injections are needed to ensure full protection against the virus. Girls given the HPV vaccine as part of the national immunisation programme are given the Gardasil vaccine.

The schedule for Gardasil is as follows:

- The first dose is given
- The second dose is given at least once month after the first dose
- A third and final dose is given at least 3 months after the second dose.

All three doses should be given within a 12-month period. In some circumstances it may be possible for the immunisation schedule to be more flexible.

— Who should not be immunised?
As with any medicine or vaccine, the HPV vaccine should not be used if you have had:

- A confirmed anaphylactic reaction (severe allergic reaction) to any of its ingredients
- A confirmed anaphylactic reaction to a previous dose of the vaccine.

If you are due to have the vaccine and have a severe illness with a high temperature (fever), the immunisation should be delayed. This is because symptoms of the illness may be confused with side effects from the vaccine, and this could result in the wrong diagnosis being made. However, there is no reason to delay immunisation for a mild illness, such as the common cold, that does not cause a fever or systemic upset (symptoms affecting the entire body).

— The need for continuation of cervical screening
The most common high-risk types of HPV (HPV-16 and HPV-18) are responsible for about 70% of cervical cancer cases. If the immune system does not deal with a high-risk HPV infection, it can lead to cell changes (dyskaryosis) and abnormal growth of pre-cancerous cells in the cervix. This is also known as cervical intraepithelial neoplasia (CIN). CIN is not cancer but, if left untreated, it can develop into cancer in some women. This can take up to 10 years. This is why regular cervical screening continues to play an important role in

detecting potentially cancerous cell changes in the cervix. The HPV vaccine does not treat an existing case of cervical cancer.

EXTENDED LEARNING

- Identify the most recent local and national recommendations about immunisation programmes
- Gardasil vaccine product information carries a black triangle symbol. What does this mean?
- What is recombinant technology? Describe some of its applications in pharmacy and medicine

- What other vaccines based on recombinantly produced, virus-like particles or virus surface antigens are listed in the *BNF*? What are the immunisation schedules (in adults) for these vaccines?
- What are the differences of primary, secondary and tertiary prevention strategies?
- What other vaccine adjuvants are available?

References and further reading

Haedicke J, Iftner T (2013). Human papillomaviruses and cancer. *Radiother Oncol* 108:397–402.
Patel PR, Berenson AB (2013). Sources of HPV vaccine hesitancy in parents. *Hum Vaccin Immunother.* **9**:2649–53.

Case 6
Black cohosh for menopausal symptoms

ELIZABETH M WILLIAMSON

LEARNING OUTCOMES

At the end of this case, you will be able to

- Understand how herbal medicines are regulated to protect the patient and explain traditional herbal registration (THR) as an indicator of quality and safety
- Describe the issues involved in the controversy over the safety of the common herbal medicine black cohosh
- Identify the place of systematic reviews as a source of research evidence
- Comment on how 'traditional' medicines and 'western' approaches may exist side by side

Case study

Mrs EE is a 52-year-old woman who has been taking a product containing the herb black cohosh to alleviate her menopausal symptoms for several years, and finds it helpful. She has now been admitted to hospital (for an unrelated matter) and, as the medical admissions pharmacist taking her drug history, you are aware of warnings issued by the MHRA (Medicines and Healthcare products Regulatory Agency) that products containing this herb have been taken off the market and that it

may cause liver damage. Mrs EE wishes to continue to take the product and asks you to look into its safety and any possible risks to her health, to put her mind at rest. She takes no other regular medication and has no family history of breast cancer or liver disorders.

- Is there any evidence for the use of black cohosh to treat menopausal symptoms?
- Is there any reason to believe that black cohosh can cause liver damage?

Ms EE tells you that she always takes a particular branded product, which you discover has a THR.

- What does that mean?
- Is it the same as a food supplement?
- Is the reported toxicity related to the quality of the product?
- How is quality assured for herbal products?
- Would you recommend that Mrs EE continues to take this product?

Case discussion

— Is there any evidence for the use of black cohosh to treat menopausal symptoms?
Black cohosh (derived from the North American flowering plant *Actea racemosa* – see below) is a popular and commonly used traditional herbal

remedy for relief of menopausal symptoms. There have been a number of trials to examine the effectiveness and safety of black cohosh for menopausal symptoms and a systematic review by the Cochrane Collaboration (a highly regarded research organisation). This particular review included 16 studies involving a total of over 2000 women; however, because of the uncertain quality of many studies, the authors were unable to conclude that there was sufficient clinical evidence for the product to receive a full marketing authorisation.

The aim of a systematic review is to draw together research papers on a subject of interest, to answer a specific research question. The authors take a planned approach to identify relevant studies in the literature and 'synthesise' the findings of these studies into a body of evidence. This provides a summary of the evidence on a topic in terms of the range of issues or outcomes that have been investigated and an assessment of the quality of this evidence. Thus, a key part of the process is 'critical appraisal', which involves assessment of the strengths and weaknesses of previous studies, and taking these into account when reporting the likely reliability of the findings of the review. Sometimes additional analysis of the findings of the previous studies is undertaken, e.g. bringing together data from previous quantitative studies can provide a larger pool of data to which further analytical procedures can be applied. This is referred to as meta-analysis.

As a systematic review brings together findings of all high-quality and relevant previous studies in a scientific way, they are considered a robust source of evidence in healthcare and medicines use. However, although providing a valuable overview on the extent and quality of evidence on a research question, as they apply strict eligibility criteria, they may be narrow in scope and limited in terms of their generalisability.

The MHRA, as the UK's medicines' regulator is responsible for ensuring that medicines prescribed and supplied in the UK meet stated standards relating to their quality, safety and efficacy. Medicines that meet these standards are granted a marketing authorisation (formerly known as a product licence). Thus, products containing the herb black cohosh are usually sold as either food supplements or as registered herbal medicines under THR.

— **Is there any reason to believe that black cohosh can cause liver damage?**

The use of black cohosh has been associated with reports of liver toxicity. The MHRA has issued several press releases following cases of liver failure suspected to have been caused by the herb. Since 2006, the MHRA has asked all manufacturers of black cohosh products to ensure that an appropriate warning about possible liver problems is included on the label.

However, it has also been suggested that these rare cases of liver toxicity may actually be due to contamination with a related herb. Black cohosh is the common name of *Actaea racemosa* L. (synonym *Cimicifuga racemosa* (L.) Nutt.), and is specified as such in the European, British and United States Pharmacopoeias. A particular brand of capsules was recalled after some batches were found to contain an undeclared plant species: the product was labelled 'black cohosh', but tests carried out showed that it also contained other *Actaea/Cimicifuga* species (probably *Actaea foetida*), and it was suggested that this particular 'black cohosh' extract may also be present in other unlicensed medicines. *Actaea foetida* is not used in western herbal medicine and its properties and safety have not been evaluated. It is therefore not suitable for inclusion in THR and should not be present in any products licensed under the THMPD (traditional herbal medicinal product directive). However, whether contamination with this species is responsible for the liver toxicity reports is not known.

— **Herbal product registration as an indicator of quality**

Under the THMPD, for a THR to be granted, the manufacturer has to show that the product is of good quality and safe, but there is no requirement to prove efficacy. (This is replaced by the need to demonstrate that the herb, in the form used in the product, e.g. the dried aqueous extract, has been used without problems in the European Union for at least 30 years [or 15 years within the EU and 15 years outside].) The aim is to protect the patient from poor quality, adulterated or fraudulent medicines, although not suggesting that THR products are of proven efficacy.

The MHRA always recommends that registered herbal products be used. These can be recognised by the THR registration number or logo on their packaging.

THR products have been assessed and quality checked to ensure that they are acceptably safe to use and are accompanied by a Patient Information Leaflet (PIL) which contains appropriate information on how to use the product, possible side effects, contraindications, etc. Unlicensed products do not have the THR logo or registration number, do not require a PIL, and are unlikely to have been assessed for quality.

— Food supplement legislation

Many herbs are also sold as food supplements, which do not have to comply with the same stringent requirements as medicines, although they are regulated by the EU Food Supplements Directive 2002/46. They are not allowed to make medicinal claims and do not have to contain a patient information leaflet. This means that the patient may not receive suitable information about drug interactions, side effects or contraindications

— Ensuring the quality of herbal products

Unlicensed products are of unknown and highly variable quality. A product marketed as a 'food supplement' was recently removed from the market because it contained black cohosh 1000 mg, which equates to 50 times the dose approved for traditional herbal medicinal products used to relieve menopausal symptoms. It is not known what risks are associated with such a high level of black cohosh.

Many popular herbal medicines, and most of those used in THR products, are the subject of British or European Pharmacopoeia monographs, and compliance with these is considered a suitable measure of quality. The usual way of analysing herbal materials is both botanically (morphology and microscopy) and chemically, using TLC (thin-layer chromatography) and HPLC (high-performance liquid chromatography). In the case of *Actaea* spp., HPTLC (high-performance thin-layer chromatography) has been shown to be a suitable way of detecting adulteration.

Chromatographic methods of separation and analysis depend on the relative abilities of components in a mixture to partition between an immobilised stationary phase and a mobile phase, which constantly moves through/over the stationary phase. Components that partition strongly into the stationary phase spend little time in the mobile phase and so are eluted slowly; compounds that partition weakly into the stationary phase spend more time in the mobile

phase and are eluted quickly. Chromatography therefore allows separation of the components of a mixture according to their physicochemical properties. With the notable exception of GC (gas chromatography, which separates components largely on the basis of molecular mass), most chromatographic methods separate components on the basis of their polarities.

TLC most commonly uses polar silica gel (coated in a thin layer on an aluminium or glass plate) as the stationary phase and a mixture of low-polarity organic solvents (ethyl acetate, chloroform) as the mobile phase. Low-polarity components migrate further than high-polarity ones. HPTLC is a more efficient, automated process. HPLC generally uses a lipophilic ('reverse phase') stationary phase, packed into a steel column, and a mixture of water and a miscible organic solvent (methanol, acetonitrile) as the mobile phase. High-polarity components elute more quickly than low-polarity ones. Chromatographic separation of complex herbal extracts allows examination of the relative amounts (and identities, when coupled with mass spectrometry) of components in the mixture and comparison with known standards. Such analysis permits both qualitative and quantitative characterisation for quality control.

— Advising Mrs EE on the use of this product

Mrs EE has been taking the product for several years without evidence of harm and strongly believes that it is helping her symptoms. You discover that the product she is taking does indeed have THR status so you can be reasonably assured of its quality. As she wishes to continue, and as there are no medical reasons (previous side effects, known liver disorders, drug interactions or contraindications) to suggest otherwise (despite the rather weak clinical trial evidence to support it), there is no pressing reason why Mrs EE should not do so. However, if any adverse effects arise, she should be encouraged to report them via the Yellow Card scheme.

The Yellow Card scheme is operated by the MHRA and the Commission on Human Medicines (CHM), the UK government's independent scientific advisory committee on medicines, as a means of collecting information on suspected side effects of marketed medicines, vaccines, herbal and complementary medicines. Yellow Card reports have traditionally been made using yellow forms, included in the *BNF*, but they are now more usually submitted online: https://yellowcard.mhra.gov.uk

— Black cohosh and 'traditional' remedies

The herb black cohosh was traditionally used by Native Americans. Its wider use today illustrates how different approaches to healthcare (often referred to as pluralism in healthcare) can exist side by side and that the interface is dynamic. In most countries, 'western' (allopathic, biomedicine) dominates provision in the formal healthcare sector. An exception is China, where, traditional Chinese medicine is practised alongside 'western' medicine at every level of the healthcare system. Other significant examples of alternative approaches include Ayurvedic medicine in India, indigenous healers, e.g. in Africa, and herbalists in many parts of the world. So-called 'traditional' care is often evolving and changing in response to new knowledge and patients' needs. Although, there is some scepticism, it can be a valuable complement to a biomedical approach, e.g. alternative providers may offer more 'holistic' approaches to supporting patients with health needs in their daily lives. Furthermore, there are many examples where therapies used routinely by local herbalists have led to the identification of effective remedies that have then become available more widely.

Although these alternative approaches are commonly associated with traditional societies and settings in particular parts of the globe, in our increasingly multicultural communities throughout the world, there is evidence of pluralism. People seeking care in all communities may make an assessment of the type of practitioner who may best assist them. There is evidence of patients with long-term illness seeking advice from allopathic and alternative therapists concurrently.

EXTENDED LEARNING

- What are the most common symptoms of menopause? How are they usually treated with conventional medicines and what are the risks involved?
- What are the routes to market for herbal products, and what are their implications?
- How are the manufacture and marketing of conventional medicines regulated?

- What are the methods of quality assurance and analysis for herbal products?
- Consider patient choice, ethics, and dilemmas of regulating and recommending unproven medicines

ADDITIONAL PRACTICE POINT

- What are the quality criteria for patient information leaflets (according to the MHRA)?

References and further reading

Royal Pharmaceutical Society of Great Britain (2013). *Herbal Medicines*, 4th edn. London: Pharmaceutical Press.

Leach MJ, Moore V (2012). Black cohosh (*Cimicifuga* spp.) for menopausal symptoms. *Cochrane Database Syst Rev* **9**: CD007244.

Teschke R, Frenzel C, Glass X, Schulze J, Eickhoff A (2013). Herbal hepatotoxicity: a critical review. *Br J Clin Pharmacol* **75**:630–6.

Teschke R, Schwarzenboeck A, Schmidt-Taenzer W, Wolff A, Hennermann KH (2011). Herb induced liver injury presumably caused by black cohosh: a survey of initially purported cases and herbal quality specifications. *Ann Hepatol* **10**:249–59.

— Useful documents from the MHRA website

Black cohosh risk of liver problems: www.mhra.gov.uk/home/groups/comms-po/documents/websiteresources/con2024119.pdf

Press release (Oct 2012): Liver failure case highlights need to use Black Cohosh remedies carefully: www.mhra.gov.uk/NewsCentre/Pressreleases/CON199545

Press release: MHRA action on safety concerns over black cohosh and liver injury www.mhra.gov.uk/NewsCentre/Pressreleases/CON2024116

Public assessment reports of liver toxicity: www.mhra.gov.uk/home/groups/es-herbal/documents/websiteresources/con2024279.pdf

Example THR documents for registration of a black cohosh product: www.mhra.gov.uk/home/groups/par/documents/websiteresources/con126267.pdf

Recall of black cohosh capsules due to contamination: www.mhra.gov.uk/Safetyinformation/Generalsafetyinformationandadvice/Herbalmedicines/Herbalsafetyupdates/Allherbalsafetyupdates/CON207203

Analytical issues (pp 15–20): www.ga-online.org/files/Graz/WS-4_Klier.pdf

HPTLC analysis of herbal drugs including black cohosh (pp 28–35) www.qia.go.kr/downloadwebQiaCom.do?id=20407

Black cohosh product withdrawn from the market due to dose issues: www.mhra.gov.uk/NewsCentre/Pressreleases/CON137768

The THR scheme: www.mhra.gov.uk/Safetyinformation/Generalsafetyinformationandadvice/Herbalmedicines/TheTHRscheme/Index.htm

Food supplement legislation: www.dh.gov.uk/prod_consum_dh/groups/dh_digitalassets/@dh/@en/documents/digitalasset/dh_132124.pdf

Index